ONE HEALTH CASE STUDIES

Addressing Complex Problems
in a Changing World

ONE HEALTH CASE STUDIES

Addressing Complex Problems in a Changing World

Edited by

Susan C. Cork

David C. Hall

Karen A. Liljebjelke

First published 2016

Published by
5M Publishing Ltd,
Benchmark House,
8 Smithy Wood Drive,
Sheffield, S35 1QN, UK
Tel: +44 (0) 1234 81 81 80
www.5mpublishing.com

A Catalogue record for this book is available from the British Library

ISBN 978-1-910455-55-5

Book layout by
Keystroke, Neville Lodge, Tettenhall, Wolverhampton

Printed by
Replika Press Pvt. Ltd, India

Photos by contributors unless otherwise credited in the text

Table of contents

Contributors

Japatee Akeeagok, Iviq Hunters and Trappers Organization, Grise Fiord, Nunavut, Canada

William Anyan, Noguchi Memorial Institute for Medical Research, University of Ghana, Accra, Ghana, WAnyan@noguchi.ug.edu.gh

Edi Basuno, socioeconomics researcher, Indonesian Centre for Agricultural Socio Economic and Policy Studies (ICASEPS), Bogor, West Java, Indonesia

Stephanie Behrens, Department of Environment & Natural Resources, Government of the Northwest Territories (NWT), Canada

Jackie Benschop, Infectious Disease Research Centre, Hopkirk Research Institute, IVABS, New Zealand, 4442

Kathryn Berger, Department of Veterinary Medicine, University of Cambridge, UK

Sandra Black, Department of Ecosystem & Public Health, Faculty of Veterinary Medicine, University of Calgary, Canada; Calgary Zoo Animal Health Centre, Calgary, Canada

Bonnie Buntain, Professor Emerita, University of Calgary, Canada and fellow of the University of Wales, Aberystwyth, Wales

Theresa Burns, Centre for Coastal Health, Nanaimo, British Columbia, Canada

Anja M. Carlsson, Department of Ecosystem and Public Health, Faculty of Veterinary Medicine, University of Calgary, Canada

Aurelie Castinel, Cawthron Institute, Nelson, New Zealand

Sylvia Checkley, Department of Ecosystem & Public Health, Faculty of Veterinary Medicine, University of Calgary, Canada

Julie M. Collins-Emerson, Infectious Disease Research Centre, Hopkirk Research Institute, IVABS (Institute for Veterinary, Animal and Biomedical Science), New Zealand

Susan C. Cork, Department of Ecosystem and Public Health, Faculty of Veterinary Medicine, University of Calgary, Canada

Lisa Crump, Swiss Tropical and Public Health Institute, Basel, Switzerland; University of Basel, Switzerland

Luis A. Cruz-Martinez, Ross University School of Veterinary Medicine, Basseterre, St Kits

Ishwari P. Dhakal, Dean, Faculty of Animal Science, Veterinary Sciences and Fisheries, Agricultural and Forestry University (AFU), Rampur, Chitwan, Nepal

Brent Dixon, Bureau of Microbial Hazards, Food Directorate, Health Canada, Ottawa, Ontario, Canada

Jambay Dorjee, National Centre for Animal Health, Department of Livestock, Ministry of Agriculture & Forests, Thimphu, Bhutan

Tshering Dorji, Department of Public Health, Ministry of Health, Thimphu, Bhutan

Padraig Duignan, Department of Ecosystem & Public Health, Faculty of Veterinary Medicine, University of Calgary, Canada

Kinzang Dukpa, National Centre for Animal Health, Department of Livestock, Ministry of Agriculture & Forests, Thimphu, Bhutan

Stanley G. Fenwick, Department of Infectious Disease and Global Health, Cummings School of Veterinary Medicine, Tufts University, North Grafton, MA; Emeritus Professor, Murdoch University, Perth, Australia, S.Fenwick@murdoch.edu.au

Sabine Gilch, Department of Ecosystem and Public Health, Faculty of Veterinary Medicine, University of Calgary

Tessa R. Grasswitz, Plant Extension Services, University of New Mexico, USA

Ratna B. Gurung, National Centre for Animal Health, Department of Livestock, Ministry of Agriculture & Forests, Thimphu, Bhutan

Ernesto Guzman-Novoa, Honey Bee Research Centre, University of Guelph, Ontario, Canada

David C. Hall, Department of Ecosystem and Public Health, Faculty of Veterinary Medicine, University of Calgary, Calgary, Alberta, Canada, dchall@ucalgary.ca

Patrick Hanington, School of Public Health, University of Alberta, Edmonton, Canada, pch1@ualberta.ca

Jennifer Hatfield, University of Calgary, Faculty of Veterinary Medicine, Department of Ecosystem and Public Health; Cumming School of Medicine, Department of Community Health Sciences

Grant Hopkins, Cawthron Institute, Nelson, New Zealand

Ron Jackson, EpiCentre, Institute of Veterinary, Animal and Biomedical Sciences, Massey University, Palmerston North, New Zealand

Richard Jakob-Hoff, Manager, Conservation Science and Research, Auckland Zoo, Auckland, New Zealand

Peter Jolly, International Development Group, Institute of Veterinary, Animal and Biomedical Sciences, Massey University

Gretchen E. Kaufman, Veterinary Initiative for Endangered Wildlife, Pullman, Washington, USA

Susan J. Kutz, Department of Ecosystem and Public Health, Faculty of Veterinary Medicine, University of Calgary, Canada; Canadian Wildlife Health Cooperative, Alberta node, Calgary, Canada

Quynh Ba Le, Dept. Ecosystem and Public Health, Faculty of Veterinary Medicine, Calgary, Alberta, Canada

Stefano Liccioli, Department of Ecosystem and Public Health, Faculty of Veterinary Medicine, University of Calgary, Canada; Parks Canada, Alberta, Canada

Karen A. Liljebjelke, Department of Ecosystem & Public Health, Faculty of Veterinary Medicine, University of Calgary, Canada

Mahamat Bechir, Centre de Support en Santé Internationale, N'Djaména, Chad

Alessandro Massolo, Department of Ecosystem and Public Health, Faculty of Veterinary Medicine, University of Calgary, Canada; O'Brien Institute for Public Health, Cumming School of Medicine, University of Calgary, Canada

Joanna McKenzie, International Development Group, Institute of Veterinary, Animal and Biomedical Sciences, Massey University

Susan K. Mikota, Elephant Care International, 166 Limo View Lane, Hohenwald, TN 38462 USA

Stephanie Montesanti, Department of Community Health Sciences, Cumming School of Medicine, University of Calgary

Ngandolo Bongo Nare, Institut de Recherche en Elevage pour le Développement, N'Djaména, Chad

Michelle North, University of Calgary, Faculty of Veterinary Medicine, Calgary, Alberta, Canada

Karin Orsel, University of Calgary, Faculty of Veterinary Medicine, Department of Production Animal Health; Cumming School of Medicine, Department of Community Health Sciences

Richard Popko, Department of Environment & Natural Resources, Government of the Northwest Territories (NWT), Canada

Anak Agung Gde Putra, epidemiologist, Disease Investigation Center, Denpasar, Bali, Indonesia

Stephen Raverty, Ministry of Agriculture, Abbotsford, British Columbia, Canada

Thomas G. Rawdon, Investigation & Diagnostic Centre, Ministry for Primary Industries, Wallaceville, New Zealand

Carl S. Ribble, Professor, Department of Ecosystem and Public Health Faculty of Veterinary Medicine, University of Calgary Alberta, Canada

Judit E.G. Smits, Department of Ecosystem & Public Health, Faculty of Veterinary Medicine, University of Calgary, Canada

Wlodek L. Stanislawek, Investigation & Diagnostic Centre, Ministry for Primary Industries, Wallaceville, New Zealand

Craig Stephen, Canadian Wildlife Health Cooperative and Western College of Veterinary Medicine, University of Saskatchewan, Canada

Naresh Subedi, National Trust for Nature Conservation, Lalitpur, Nepal

Tenzin Tenzin, National Centre for Animal Health, Department of Livestock, Ministry of Agriculture & Forests, Thimphu, Bhutan

Nirmal K. Thapa, National Centre for Animal Health, Department of Livestock, Ministry of Agriculture & Forests, Thimphu, Bhutan

Wilfreda (Billie) E. Thurston, Department of Ecosystem and Public Health, Faculty of Veterinary Medicine, University of Calgary; Department of Community Health Sciences, Faculty of Medicine University of Calgary

Lorraine Toews, University of Calgary, Health Sciences Library and Faculty of Veterinary Medicine, Calgary, Alberta, Canada

Frank van der Meer, University of Calgary, Faculty of Veterinary Medicine, Department of Ecosystem and Public Health; Cumming School of Medicine, Department of Community Health Sciences

Alasdair M. Veitch, Department of Environment & Natural Resources, Government of the Northwest Territories (NWT), Canada

Karma Wangdi, Department of Public Health, Ministry of Health, Thimphu, Bhutan

Trisha Westers, Department of Population Medicine, Ontario Veterinary College, University of Guelph, Canada

Keri L. Williams, Department of Community Health Sciences, Faculty of Medicine University of Calgary, Canada

Iwan Willyanto, veterinary health consultant, Surabaya, Indonesia

Jessica Wu, Department of Health, Government of Nunavut, Iqaliut, Nunavut, Canada

John Woodford, Veterinary Consultant, Le Coderc, La Rochebeaucourt et Argentine, France

Jakob Zinsstag, Swiss Tropical and Public Health Institute, Basel, Switzerland; University of Basel, Basel, Switzerland

Acknowledgements

The origins of our idea to explain and teach One Health through case studies was derived from discussions based on the experiences of colleagues from the veterinary faculties from the Universities of Calgary, Saskatchewan, Guelph, Montreal and Prince Edward Island. For more than 20 years, veterinary students in their final year at these universities have joined from across Canada to engage in experiential One Health learning during a two week ecohealth rotation delivered by one of the veterinary faculties across Canada. We would like to thank our colleagues within Canada as well as those across the globe who have inspired us to bring together the case studies outlined in this book. In addition, we would like to thank Brenda Moore and Lori Starkey, both based at the University of Calgary, Faculty of Veterinary Medicine for administrative and editorial support.

Dedication

We would like to dedicate this book to Dr Bruce Hunter of the Ontario Veterinary College, University of Guelph. Dr Hunter was a widely respected wildlife and poultry veterinarian, as well as being one of the foundational ecohealth course developers and teachers. He proposed assembling One Health case scenarios in a textbook format complete with case scenarios, data, photographs, and other materials. Bruce unfortunately died before the book could be well developed. We hope that this textbook is a fitting tribute to his passion for the use of case studies in teaching and learning more about One Health.

Preface

More than 1,000 years ago, Greek philosophers wrote about health as a function of climate and water supply. Similar accounts of identifying a link between the environment and human, animal and plant health are recorded in the oral and written histories of many cultures. Over the past two centuries there have been profound advances in our level of understanding of how the 'health' of our environment and our interactions with it influence health outcomes in human populations as well as in the health of our animals and plants. Emergence of disease in animals (including humans) and plants can frequently be traced to interactions between the biophysical and socioeconomic components of the world in which we live. How well we manage the complexity of those interactions can have a great deal to do with the probability and degree of success in safeguarding the health and well-being of human, animal and plant populations.

In this book, we present a number of case studies from around the world describing various approaches to addressing health management problems. All of these studies illustrate the value of working across health disciplines while also drawing on other areas of expertise. We venture from the African plains to the oceans of New Zealand, to rural Afghanistan and Nepal, the Canadian Prairies and the Arctic. We consider the case of the disappearing salmon in British Columbia, the impact of climate change on Arctic ecosystems, coordinated responses to

wildlife conservation and plant protection, dealing with declining bee populations, emerging concerns regarding antimicrobial resistance and the importance of ensuring that the food and water supply is safe. We have grouped the chapters into four themes reflecting the nature of the case studies: systems and disease; environmental complexity; agricultural sustainability (and resources); and concepts and knowledge transfer. These four principal themes capture the key characteristics of the One Health and ecohealth approach while providing a coherent/logical method for grouping the case studies presented. At the same time, we recognize that there are several cross-cutting topics that arise in several of the cases outlined in the book: biosecurity; climate change; community engagement; education; human development; knowledge translation and communication; policy formulation and support; and public health.

While the concept of One Health is not new, the term is often misunderstood or used in a manner that is too narrow, and several authors have used it as an alternative to the term 'One Medicine'. The issue of terminology can pose challenges for researchers and means of overcoming this, especially when undertaking a review of the literature, are outlined in the Appendix. In this book we use the term 'One Health' to encompass an interdisciplinary and multifaceted approach to addressing complex problems that impact human, animal and environmental health. The term 'ecohealth' has also been used in some chapters in order to take into consideration the broader ecosystem and social dynamics that impact human, animal and environmental health. It is easy to become overwhelmed by the wide range of terms used when promoting the value of taking a broad interdisciplinary (or holistic) approach. In this book, we would like readers to focus instead on the case studies presented in each chapter, whereby our chapter contributors aim to illustrate what is meant, in practical terms, by applying the 'One Health' approach.

Foreword: the challenge of One Health

Biomedical sciences increasingly examine more and more elementary processes of living beings through focusing and reducing to ever smaller entities. This is fundamental to an exponentially growing, uninterrupted increase of knowledge in the biomedical sciences over the past decades. However, this reductionist approach comes with a cost of losing the big picture and encountering problems that require a broader perspective and an integrative view on the public's health. There is a frontier where more detailed knowledge no longer leads implicitly to better health because its broader context is ignored. This boundary is crossed when diseases in humans occur because public health and veterinary authorities do not talk with each other or when international organizations concentrate solely on provision of human health ignoring that continuous reinfection of humans can only be prevented by an intervention in the animal reservoir, to state only two examples.

When compared to the ongoing reductionist biomedical research, integrative approaches are often considered to be below the cusp of knowledge and can be difficult to fund. Consequently, interdisciplinary projects need a stringent theoretical foundation based on rigorous methods demonstrating that they yield more and better results than can be achieved through one field alone. The concept of One Health seeks to demonstrate better health for humans and animals from closer cooperation of human and veterinary medicine. In the first place, this necessitates an understanding of how humans and animals relate and which are the critical interfaces. But understanding how humans and animals relate is well established and not enough to fulfil the aspirations of One Health. An integrated One Health study of human and animal health must show a synergistic benefit or added value of human and animal health, financial savings or improved ecosystem services that could not be achieved if the study concentrated only on human or animal health. To prove such added value is not simple and requires novel study designs that combine biomedical, mathematical, economic and social science methods. It cannot be overlooked that One Health, concentrating on human and animal health only, is limited by the inability to relate directly to ecosystem aspects of health. One Health is thus clearly embedded into the broader conceptual thinking of ecosystem approaches to health and health in social-ecological systems.

Unfortunately, the term 'One Health' is currently often misused as a fashionable term in cases where it only points to how humans and animals are related. Ignoring the theoretical stringency and inherent difficulty to demonstrate synergistic effects of integrated human and animal health research, the true meaning of One Health as an important concept for future health development is diluted, and its reputation is diminished. We urgently need more robust examples of quantitative and qualitative additional benefits from human and veterinary medicine working better together in support of the One Health postulate. This book provides an important contribution along this pathway, and I wish the authors success and a broad readership.

Jakob Zinsstag
Basel, Switzerland
6 February 2016

INTRODUCTION

chapter 1

Introduction to One Health Concepts

David C. Hall and Susan C. Cork

Abstract

One Health developed from very early concepts of health as a function of the features of the environment around us. It developed with encouragement of interdisciplinary engagement, and currently includes systems thinking and informed input to policy formulation. Much of recent One Health development has been guided by 'ecohealth' principles, although disagreement regarding terminology has sometimes complicated development of the One Health concept. This text defines One Health as a transdisciplinary approach to the sustainable management of complex health problems arising from the interaction of animals, humans and their environment. Case studies are presented under four principal characterizing themes: concepts and knowledge transfer; systems and disease; environmental complexity; and agricultural sustainability.

1.1 Introduction

In 425 BCE, Aristotle wrote about health as a function of climate and water supply in *Airs, Waters, Places* (Chadwick and Mann, 1978). Since that time there has been profound development in the details of our understanding that the condition of the world around us and our interactions with it influences health outcomes. If there have been great leaps forward in the health sciences, then surely among them we can include recognizing the need for clean water, the development of vaccines and awareness of zoonoses. Nevertheless, as important as advances in the biological sciences have been and will continue to be in controlling emerging infectious diseases, recent global health concerns including avian influenza and Ebola virus remind us of the need for greater consideration of the social science aspects of disease control as well as the need to work in interdisciplinary teams that include community members.

This book collects a number of case studies describing various aspects of health management problems, all of which illustrate the value of working across health disciplines while also drawing on other areas of expertise. For many of our colleagues who embrace this interdisciplinary[1] approach, the term 'One Health' has been applied. For others, 'ecohealth' is a more appropriate term. For this reason we set out in this chapter a brief history of One Health/ecohealth concepts and our definitions of terminology.

1.2 A brief history of the One Health philosophy

The term 'One Health' is often misunderstood. Several authors have used it as an alternative to the term 'One Medicine' to imply a more sustainable ecological approach to solving complex problems that impact human, animal and environmental health. The term 'ecohealth' has also been used to take into consideration the broader ecosystem and social dynamics that impact human, animal and environmental health. It is easy to get confused by the plethora of terms used when promoting the value of taking a broad interdisciplinary (or holistic) approach, so in this book we would like readers to focus on the case studies presented in each chapter whereby the authors hope to illustrate what is meant, in practical terms, by applying the 'One Health' approach.

The American veterinarian Calvin Schwabe has been widely credited with coining the phrase 'One Medicine' (Kaplan and Scott, 2011) and he makes reference to the writings of several innovative thinkers such as Virchow, Osler and others (see Schwabe, 1984, 1991). Subsequent use of this term has tended to reflect a focus on linkages between human and animal health with limited attention given to the broader environmental aspects of One Health. However, there are earlier references to taking a 'One Medicine' approach (Cass, 1973; Cardiff et al., 2008) and some of these do make reference to the importance of environmental health, especially if we consider more philosophical sources such as the writings of Plato. As early as 200 BCE, surviving texts indicate that the Egyptian and Greek healers of that period gained much

of their knowledge from treating both humans and animals and making observations about patterns of disease linked to environmental factors. Similar references are found in ancient Chinese and Indian literature, although the provenance of these is often unclear due to uncertainties around dates and the unknown accuracy of translation.

The issue of terminology continues to pose challenges for translators and researchers to this day. For example, many parts of the world in which rural people retain a strong cultural connection to the land (for example, Bhutan, Nepal, Peru) practise what we might consider a One Health approach when dealing with human, animal and plant health, and yet they do not use that term and would not immediately identify with it. Similarly, looking to the field of economics, writings of early philosophers in India (e.g., Chanakya) and Greece (e.g., Xenophon) recognized that a healthy local economy relied on healthy interactions between communities and their leaders who came from different walks of life, including life on the land and in the city. Illness was a result of disruption of those actions and intercommunity relationships. This idea has survived and been extended in economics for centuries, through the writings of Adam Smith – in which he recognized that the welfare of communities relies on cooperation between members of different communities – to the recent writings of Eleanor Ostrom, who recognized that unsustainable levels of resource exploitation due to poor management (particularly those that lack an interdisciplinary approach) are doomed to becoming weakened to the point of ill health and possibly collapse. The message from agriculture and economics for the past several centuries seems to be that we do better as individuals when we directly concern ourselves with doing better as a community, which of course includes the absence of disease.

On the international scene, the trigger for formally adopting the One Health approach in recent years was, in part, a result of the 1997 outbreak of highly pathogenic avian influenza (HPAI) in Asia. Due to fears that this virus (H5N1) would mutate into a virus capable of spreading from poultry to humans, and subsequently mutating to cause a human influenza pandemic, the human and animal health authorities recognized the need to work together (FAO, 2008). This followed a series of other dramatic zoonotic disease outbreaks including the West Nile virus outbreak starting in New York in 1999 and, more recently, the severe acute respiratory syndrome (SARS) outbreak in 2003. These events, and the associated media coverage and public interest, led to unprecedented political support and a call for much closer international collaboration for disease surveillance and control. As a consequence, several major global agencies with an interest in human and animal health, in particular the World Health Organization (WHO), the Food and Agriculture Organization of the United Nations (FAO) and the World Organisation for Animal Health (OIE), UNICEF and the World Bank developed a framework for reducing the risks of infectious diseases at the human–animal–ecosystems interface (FAO et al., 2010).

Reference was made earlier in this chapter to the term 'ecohealth', which has been used separately from 'One Health'. The origins of the term 'ecohealth' lie with an approach to ecosystems health research driven largely by the International Development Research Centre (IDRC) in Ottawa, Canada (Forget and Lebel, 2001; Lebel, 2003.) As outlined by Charron (2012), in addressing global health problems and human development, the ecohealth approach advocates attention to ecosystems as well as social and economic inequities. The ecosystem approach is guided by six principles that can be seen as guide posts to the implementation of ecohealth research (rather than a checklist assuring success), informing process and expected outcomes. These six principles are well explained by Charron (2012) and are:

incorporating a systems approach to thinking; embracing transdisciplinarity; assuring stakeholder participation in the process; identifying environmentally sound and socially sustainable solutions; taking into account addressing social and economic inequities; and applying a 'knowledge-to-action' approach (as opposed to knowledge translation), which influences policy change, increasing support for solutions.

There has been strong support in project and peer-reviewed literature for the use of either or both terms by different practitioners. Advocates of both approaches are finding common ground and overlap while maintaining their differences (Zinsstag et al., 2011, 2012; Zinsstag, 2012), allowing for a strengthened approach to managing health outcomes.

1.3   Characterizing One Health

It would be incorrect to conclude that a One Health approach must by definition include particular characteristics (e.g., veterinarians and physicians working together to prevent zoonotic disease transmission). Yet this has been a common misunderstanding. Hall and Coghlan (2011, 2012) examined more than 45 case studies, project reports, articles and discussion papers that used the phrases 'One Health' or 'ecohealth' in their project titles or descriptions and found that they all addressed prevention of spread of zoonotic disease. Most of the projects were led by either veterinarians or physicians working together, and rarely addressed the role of wildlife or environmental factors, the importance of regional networks, and funding sustainability. However, all the case studies did address several characteristics we believe are more important to a One Health approach – transdisciplinarity, complexity and a strong sense of community-level participation in the project.

With the collection of case studies presented in this book we are not advocating that a One

Health approach be based on a particular collection of conditions. The recent tendency to label any health response that includes more than one health discipline a One Health approach is misleading. For example, an emergency room physician treating a car accident victim requiring physiotherapy follow-up and pain management counselling might struggle to consider this a One Health approach, even though one could argue case follow-up is complex and the social fabric of the community is damaged due to loss of income suffered by the accident victim.

The point is that overzealous application of the term 'One Health' to any situation in which more than one health discipline is involved risks diluting one of the key messages of One Health. That is, transdisciplinarity requires us to move out of our individual silos of knowledge and bridge gaps in developing solutions to health problems by working in teams with other experts and community members with whom we traditionally would not normally work.

1.4   Presentation of case studies in this book

With this book we offer a number of case studies that characterize the approach and benefits of a One Health philosophy. We have grouped cases into one of four themes reflecting the nature of the case studies: systems and disease; environmental complexity; agricultural sustainability and concepts and knowledge transfer. These four principal themes seem to us to capture nearly completely the characteristics of One Health and ecohealth approaches described above while providing a convenient method for grouping the cases. At the same time, we recognize that there are a number of cross-cutting concepts that arise in several cases: biosecurity, climate change, community engagement, education, human development, knowledge translation and communication,

policy formulation and support, and public health.

Systems and disease

Awareness and examination of the complexity of systems is an important part of disease ecology and integral to a One Health approach in managing disease. Case studies in this section cover a diverse range of One Health applications including control of emerging infectious disease policy development during a response to a rabies epidemic in Bali, Indonesia, and an example of a local approach to a global health problem (leptospirosis in New Zealand). An appreciation for the complexity of systems and investigation into the impact on humans within their environment is apparent in all the cases presented in this section. This anthropocentric view is not entirely without concern for the care of the local and global environment in which we live; many of the cases highlight a need for better understanding of the importance of managing the environment in order to mitigate undesirable health outcomes to humans. Nevertheless, the focus is on human health as well as animal health within a system.

Environmental complexity

In contrast to the 'systems and disease' theme, the cases clustered under the 'environmental complexity' theme view humans as stewards of the environment we share with animals and other systems. Without due sustainable care and attention to this stewardship role we are bound to generate imbalances in the general equilibrium of a system which can take generations to correct.[2] Uncontrollable outbreaks of disease in this context can be considered a clinical sign of a system that is in disequilibrium.

Agricultural sustainability

Lebel (2003) has referred to agroecosystems as being coherent geographical and functional entities where agricultural production takes place. Farms, rural communities, and catchment basins can be considered agroecosystems; these agroecosystems and others are considered in various cases under the theme 'agricultural sustainability'. There is no question that progress in mono-cropping of both plants and animals (improved hybrid vigour, more efficient irrigation methods) has resulted in tremendous gains in production efficiency. However, when undesirable outcomes include loss of essential insect life, newly emerging prion diseases or threatened extinction of a species, one has to ask is there not a better way to manage our natural resources? This does not suggest we should abandon mono-cropping and feed the global human and domesticated animal population with close-to-home small-scale farms or rooftop garden plots (admirably sustainable small-scale methods but insufficient to feed eight billion people). Rather, the suggestion is we look more closely at how we manage our natural resources in larger-scale intensive farming and other agroecosystems where short-term gains can result in long-term undesirable outcomes leading to negative impact on the health of humans, animals, and the environment in which they live.

Concepts and knowledge transfer

The concept of One Health can be interpreted to mean different things to different people based on his or her role in a health management problem, perceived impact on daily life, or effect on the ecozone/ecological community. Chapters and cases under this theme cover the basic concepts of One Health and summarize case studies where knowledge exchange and transdisciplinarity play key roles in the One Health scenario.

These cases also help to introduce a recurring theme in this text that has been referred to by many One Health authors: the inextricable links between humans, animals and their environment that are reflected in the health of the individual.

It is important to note that there are many clearly One Health problems requiring transdisciplinary approaches that do not immediately bring to mind cooperation between primarily health science personnel. Some such problems are identified in this text. A current example is the devastation caused to pine forests in western North America by the mountain pine beetle.[3] This small creature, insignificant in size and voice, non-threatening as an intermediate host or vector, is slowly destroying enormous swaths of pine forest that serve as home to hundreds of other forest species. When pine beetle populations are small, they prefer stressed, mature or over-mature (>80 years) pine but as beetle populations grow, any pine including healthy trees can be killed. In this example, the devastation to forests upsets ecosystem dynamics and also threatens the economic future of regions that rely on forestry and tourism. These industries are key to the sustainability of many small communities in North America and unless pine beetles are brought back into balance, many small communities, as well as the health of the surrounding ecosystem, will continue to decline.

1.5 Conclusions

The intended outcome of a One Health approach is essentially engagement of key stakeholders in better risk management of health outcomes. From early philosophers such as Xenophon who advocated transdisciplinarity as a way of improving community welfare to Carl Schwabe and other recent leaders of One Health who reminded us to be aware of the interactions of humans and animals with their environment, there is a common message: we do better as individuals and as a community when we concern ourselves with the health of others and interactions of ourselves and other species with the environment around us. Essential competencies, actors and institutions are less clearly defined and do change with context. However, what *is* clear and what we illustrate from the case studies presented in this text is that we can do a better job of preventing, controlling and recovering from unwanted health outcomes when we consider and include the ideas, knowledge and experience of disciplines that are traditionally outside our own.

Our focus on survival as humans revolves around a healthy food supply and healthy animals around us, which in turn demands a healthy environment. As populations grow and peri-urban areas become more integrated into our cities, we are under increasing pressure to manage our resources efficiently. An implicit expectation of controlled growth is freedom from disease risks, but the outcome we hope for is not always the consequence we generate. By neglecting to engage in a One Health approach to risk management of health outcomes, we jeopardize the health of our communities and the health of others, as we have seen during recent epidemics of emerging infectious disease including highly pathogenic avian influenza and the Ebola virus.

This text is not founded on a Malthusian belief that a 'doom-and-gloom' outcome for our world is inevitable. We document many examples of positive changes occurring in health education, adoption of transdisciplinary approaches to solving complex health problems, recognition of the central role of communities in sustainable solutions and acknowledgement of the need for policy formulation to facilitate sustainability of those solutions. Many more examples are shared in annual reports of health development agencies, presented at transdisciplinary conferences, discussed during community meetings and pre-sented in textbooks authored by our colleagues. We encourage wide sharing of these case studies for all students and practitioners of transdisciplinary approaches to management of health outcomes.

Recommended recent texts

For those readers who would like to extend their knowledge of the One Health and ecohealth literature beyond our collection of case studies, apart from references cited in chapters in this book, we can recommend three excellent texts all published in the last five years. *One Health: The Theory and Practice of Integrated Health Approaches* (2015, CABI, edited by Zinsstag et al.) provides a compendium of One Health research from the past decade by leaders in the field. *Ecohealth Research In Practice: Innovative Applications of an Ecosystem Approach to Health* (2012, Springer, edited by Charron and freely available online at IDRC) presents a collection of summaries from foundational ecohealth research projects, highlighting both achievements and shortfalls. Finally, although it references neither One Health nor ecohealth in the title, those readers particularly interested in the application of a One Health approach to conservation will find *New Directions in Conservation Medicine: Applied Cases of Ecological Health* (2012, Oxford, edited by Aguirre et al.) contains superb examples of the practical value of a One Health approach applied to health management problems of the biosphere.

Key words

Complexity: if the emergent behaviour of a system cannot be understood by merely understanding the component parts then the system is considered complex; complex systems can change state unexpectedly.

Ecohealth: a transdisciplinary, participatory approach to sustainable management of health problems that includes consideration for complexity, gender and social equity, and policy support for solutions.

Interdisciplinarity: working together with disciplines outside one's own in order to expand both the understanding of and identification of solutions to complex problems.

Knowledge translation: the synthesis, dissemination, exchange, and application of knowledge.

One Health: a transdisciplinary approach to sustainable management of complex health problems arising from the interaction of animals, humans, and their environment.

Transdisciplinarity: working together with disciplines outside one's own in order to expand the understanding of complex problems and identify solutions that would not be apparent otherwise.

Endnotes

1 More correctly, a transdisciplinary approach, a term we define later in this chapter.
2 While outbreaks of several zoonotic diseases have been made worse by mismanagement of our interaction with the environment in which we live (avian influenza for example), better examples of long-term imbalances exist in the annals of wildlife conservation. For example, excessive hunting of the plains bison associated with western migration and expansion of the US and Canada led to near extinction of the plains bison gene pool. It has taken more than three human generations to begin to recover much of that lost genetic diversity.
3 The mountain pine beetle (*Dendroctonus ponderosae Hopkins*), a member of the bark beetle family, is a small bark beetle about 4.0–7.5mm in length. Its consumption of pine has affected particularly lodgepole, jack, ponderosa, whitebark, limber and Scots pine species.

References

Cardiff, R.D., Ward, J.M. and Barthold, S.W. (2008). 'One Medicine – one pathology': are veterinary and human pathology prepared? *Laboratory Investigation*, 88, 18–26.

Cass, J. (1973). One Medicine – human and veterinary. *Perspectives in Biology & Medicine*, 16(3), 418–426.

Chadwick, J. and Mann, W. (1978). Airs, waters, places. In G.E.R. Lloyd (ed.), *Hippocratic Writings*. Harmondsworth: Penguin, pp. 148–169.

Charron, D. (2012). Ecohealth: origins and approach. In D. Charron (ed.), *Ecohealth Research In Practice: Innovative Applications of an Ecosystem Approach to Health*. New York: Springer, pp. 1–30.

FAO (2008). *In Collaboration with the OIE/WHO/ UNICEF/World Bank and UN System-Influenza Coordination, Contributing to One World, One Health: A Strategic Framework for Reducing the Risks of Infectious Diseases at the Human–Animal–Ecosystems Interface*. Consultation document at the international ministerial conference on avian and pandemic influenza at Sharm El-Sheikh, Egypt.

FAO, OIE and WHO (2010). *The FAO-OIE-WHO Collaboration: Sharing Responsibilities and Coordinating Global Activities to Address Health Risks at the Animal– Human–Ecosystems Interfaces. A Tripartite Concept Note*. Geneva: FAO.

Forget, G. and Lebel, K. (2001). An ecosystem approach to human health. *International Journal of Occupational and Environmental Health*, 7(2), S1–S38.

Hall, D.C. and Coghlan, B. (2011). *Implementation of the One Health Approach in Asia and Europe: How To Set Up A Common Basis For Action and Exchange of Experience*. Brussels: European External Action Service.

Hall, D.C. and Coghlan, B. (2012). *Common Themes and Missed Opportunities of One Health and Ecohealth Case Studies*. Presentation at the International Society For Veterinary Epidemiology and Economics conference, 20–25 August, Maastricht, Netherlands.

Kaplan, B. and Scott, C. (2011). *One Health History Question: Who Coined the Term 'One Medicine'?* www.vetmed.ucdavis.edu/onehealth/local-assets/pdfs/ schwabe_coins_onemedicine#schwabe_coins_one-medicine.pdf.

Lebel, J. (2003). *Health: An Ecosystem Approach*. Ottawa: International Development Research Centre, www.idrc.ca/EN/Resources/Publications/openebooks/012-8/index.html.

Schwabe, C.W. (1984). *Veterinary Medicine and Human Health*, 3rd edn. Baltimore: Williams and Wilkins.

Schwabe, C.W. (1991). History of the scientific relationships of veterinary public health. *Scientific & Technical Review of the Office International des Epizooties*, 10, 933–949.

Zinsstag, J. (2012). Convergence of Ecohealth and One Health. *EcoHealth*. 9:371-373.

Zinsstag, J., Schelling, E., Waltner-Toews, D. and Tanner, M. (2011). From 'One Medicine' to 'One Health' and systemic approaches to health and well-being. *Preventive Veterinary Medicine*, 101, 148–156.

Zinsstag, J., Mackenzie, J.S., Jeggo, M., Heymann, D.L., Patz, J.A. and Daszak, P. (2012). Mainstreaming One Health. *EcoHealth*, 9, 107–110.

SYSTEMS AND DISEASE

chapter 2

One Health approaches to rabies control in Bali, Indonesia

David C. Hall, Anak Agung Gde Putra, Iwan Willyanto and Edi Basuno

Abstract

In 2008, Bali, Indonesia saw its first case of rabies. Initially the response was to cull unconfined dogs with limited vaccination, a response that did not control the epidemic. Following engagement with villagers, epidemiologists, ecologists and NGOs, and with assistance from the FAO and international researchers, a One Health approach was adopted focusing on understanding the complexity of dog ecology in Bali, community engagement and improved communication. The current approach follows a capture, vaccination, collar and release plan for unconfined dogs. Domesticated dogs are vaccinated and sterilization encouraged. At least half of all dogs on Bali are thought to have been vaccinated, and cases of human rabies have declined since 2010, although the epidemic continues.

2.1 Introduction

Rabies is one of the first reported diseases in written history. As early as 2200 BCE, writings from Mesopotamia link dog bites with illness in humans exhibiting rage-like symptoms (Adamson, 1977; Theodorides, 1974; Pritchard, 1955). In the eighth century BCE, Homer wrote in *The Iliad* of '*menin*' to describe the rage of Achilles and '*lyssa*' in reference to Achilles' rage, from which we derive the words meningitis[1] and lyssavirus.[2] By the sixth century BCE, rabies was in China and thought to have expanded into Asia. More than four millennia after the first writings on canine rabies and despite development of a vaccine by Pasteur and Roux in 1885, rabies is still a major disease burden for many parts of the world, causing not just death but also economic stress on health systems where post-exposure prophylaxis (PEP) treatment and vector control campaigns are mobilized. This chapter explores an epidemic of rabies in Bali, Indonesia, and examines elements of a One Health approach used in the epidemic and the impact of that approach.

The island of Bali is known for its beautiful beaches, Hindu culture and temples, and terraced rice fields amid integrated agricultural communities. Prior to late 2008, unlike most of Indonesia, there was no record of rabies in

Bali. However, in November 2008 the death two months earlier of 46-year-old Putu Linda was diagnosed as being a result of rabies, probably brought to the island several months before that on a fishing boat from neighbouring Flores (Putra, 1998; Putra and Gunata, 2009).

The response to controlling the rabies epidemic in Bali presents a compelling case study for supporting a One Health approach to health management. All six of the classic pillars of ecohealth are present, briefly identified here. Understanding the complexity of the epidemiology of the rabies epidemic has required learning about canine ecology on the island as well as the social and cultural importance of the dog in Bali society. Consideration of various alternative strategies to control the spread of the disease has taught that community participation is essential, particularly for sustainability of control. Social inequity plays a role where members of lower-income communities are less likely to have attained higher levels of formal education allowing clearer understanding of the etiology of rabies and the importance of rapid post-exposure treatment to dog bites. Finally, learning from past efforts can inform local and national rabies policy, particularly with respect to how to engage with communities in order to foster sustainable approaches to control.

This chapter will briefly explain the history of the rabies epidemic in Bali, the approaches to control used thus far, and recommendations for furthering a One Health sustainable approach to managing control and local elimination of rabies in Bali and neighbouring islands in Indonesia.

2.2 Rabies in Bali – an outline of the epidemic

Until 2008, Bali was known as one of the very few Indonesian provinces that had never seen a case of rabies, in part due to the fact it is an island but also due to strict quarantine measures for dogs brought onto the island. Although the latter control measure was generally respected by fishermen who travelled with their dogs as companions between the islands in the area, the index case of canine rabies was most likely in a dog brought to Bali by a fisherman probably from neighbouring Flores Island, where rabies was known to exist. This is supported by phylogenetic analysis of the rabies strain in Bali (Mahardika et al., 2014), which is a descendent of the Kalimantan 00-18 strain, correspondingly an ancestor of the Flores and Sulawesi strains. By November 2008, two villagers had died of clinical signs consistent with rabies, and on 30 November, the governor of Bali declared rabies present on the island.

With full awareness of the importance of a rapid response to the introduction of this fatal zoonotic disease, in December 2008 the provincial government of Bali began a two-pronged approach to rabies control: (1) culling of unconfined dogs in the rabies confirmed regencies of Denpasar and Badung with the use of strychnine bait and blow-dart methods; and (2) vaccination of dogs at selected locations with a locally produced vaccine that required a booster three months after first vaccination. From a survey of dog owners in Badung Peninsula (Putra et al., 2011), it was estimated that up to 40 per cent of all known dogs in Badung and Denpasar were vaccinated by March 2009; of those, slightly more than half received a booster vaccination by June 2009, suggesting effective protection of about one quarter of the owned dog population.

The low coverage of vaccination combined with other factors to suggest this approach would not be successful. For example, dog density is about one in eight in Denpasar, and most dogs are communally owned, fed and free-roaming (Morters et al., 2014), meaning human/dog encounters resulting in bites from unvaccinated dogs would not be uncommon. By September 2010, rabies was confirmed present in 221 or one-third of all villages in Bali. It was

Table 2.1 Timeline of rabies in Bali, Indonesia

Jan–May 2008	Rabies probably arrives via a dog from a neighbouring island (e.g., Flores Island); settles in Ungasan Village, Bukit Peninsula, Bali.
Jul 2008	Dog from Flores, normally placid, bites owner (Mr TA) and is claimed to have bitten a friend in August; this is thought to be the first human infection with rabies in Bali.
6 Sep 2008	Female child (Miss L) bitten in Ungasan village.
9 Sep 2008	Male adult (Mr MA, aged 32) bitten.
16 Sep 2008	Male adult (Mr KW, aged 28) bitten in Ungasan village.
17 Sep 2008	Miss L dies (thought to be first human death of rabies in Bali).
Sep 2008	Ms Putu Linda (aged 46) dies of rabies, diagnosed on post-mortem examination.
19 Oct 2008	Muhammad Oktav Rhamana Putra (male, aged 3) in Ungasan Village bitten by stray dog; PEP denied at Sanglah Hospital, Denpasar, Bali due to presumed absence of rabies on Bali.
14 Nov 2008	Mr MA dies.
21 Nov 2008	Muhammad Oktav dies after exhibiting clinical signs consistent with rabies.
23 Nov 2008	Mr KW dies.
24 Nov 2008	Regent of Badung requests rabies vaccines be sent to Bali.
26 Nov 2008	Human bitten in Kedonganan by a dog that later dies and is diagnosed positive for rabies using fluorescent antibody technique.
30 Nov 2008	Indonesian Department of Agriculture declares rabies present on Bali.
Dec 2008	Provincial government of Bali launches canine cull and vaccination campaigns.
16 Jan 2009	Mr TA dies (six months post-infection).
Apr 2013	130 people reported dead from rabies; PEP administered to more than 130,000 people following dog bites.
July 2015	Rabies deaths in humans has started to rise again; one in 2013 to 12 by July 2015.

accepted that the rapid response had failed to control the rabies epidemic.

Involvement of NGOs and outside agencies

By 2010, a number of charitable organizations as well as outside government aid agencies had begun to participate in the efforts to reduce rabies in Bali. These included the Bali Animal Welfare Association (BAWA), the World Society for the Protection of Animals (WSPA, now called World Animal Protection), the Australian government (AusAID), the United States government (USAID), the International Development Research Centre of Canada (IDRC) and the Food and Agriculture Organization of the United Nations (FAO). BAWA and AusAID led the charge in late 2010 to use vaccination (as well as sterilization) rather than culling as the sole tactic in the rabies containment and elimination strategy for Bali. This was through a Memorandum of Understanding developed in agreement with the governor of Bali and most regencies of Bali, indicating an early willingness of key stakeholders to discuss and agree on approaches for control, particularly when it included funding support for costly vaccines.

The strategy developed in late 2010 included several components that can be seen as incorporating a One Health approach. These included a transdisciplinary approach to a vaccination strategy (dog ecology was recognized as important, as well as understanding the epidemiology of the disease and a communication plan) intending to vaccinate 70 per cent of the dogs in Bali; a community education component, recognizing the importance of collaboration and community participation; and addressing equity by offering free vaccination for those who could not afford to pay to vaccinate their dogs. As many as 239,000 of the more than 500,000 dogs in Bali were thought to have been vaccinated under this first stage of vaccination. A second stage was due to vaccinate 235,000 dogs, and a third round would cover 250,000 additional vaccinations. By the time of the second stage, responsibility for second implementation of the vaccination programme and subsequent phases had been assumed by the governments of Bali and Indonesia with strong technical cooperation assistance from FAO. Although a red collar programme existed, it was not possible to collar most free-roaming dogs (the majority of dogs in Bali) and thus it was not clear how many dogs were being revaccinated.

An additional element critical to surveillance for rabies was the integrated bite case management (IBCM) system, generated through cooperation between animal and human health authorities and designed to improve both surveillance for rabies cases and medical response to human exposure. Bali is also home to a large number of chick hatcheries, and the ICBM system benefitted from Indonesia's and Bali's need for effective One Health surveillance experience with highly pathogenic avian influenza (HPAI), which resulted in several outbreaks in Bali as well as human illness and death. The experience with HPAI outbreaks led to development and collaboration of a veterinary Participatory Disease Surveillance and Response (PDSR) programme and a human health District Surveillance Office (DSO) programme; it was around the experi-

ence and success of these HPAI surveillance and response programmes that the ICBM system was developed. An important part of the ICBM system has been a coordinated SMS messaging protocol used to communicate events and alert system members to possible rabies-linked events, accelerating response time and in order to ensure both animal and human health officials are aware of possible need for medical or other intervention.

Although the strategy was admirable in its efforts to bring together government, local and international agencies, and community members, the full logistics of the strategy were slow to roll out, delaying a second stage until May 2011. This difficulty in logistics (in hindsight, 'operationalizing' the One Health approach) may have been a costly opening in the vaccination coverage that began to roll out in 2010. From that point forward, the government of Bali with directive from the government of Indonesia and continuing input from FAO took charge of the rabies control campaign. Different stakeholders have varying views on reasons for this, but the summary conclusion seems to be concern on the part of the government that rabies cases were not decreasing rapidly enough under a vaccination-only campaign, and it has since resorted to occasional sweeps of culling free-roaming dogs.

In hindsight, there was considerable progress towards a 70 per cent coverage in several regencies by 2012 – including Denpasar, Badung, Gianyar and Bangli – which saw more than 235,000 dogs vaccinated in each of the two vaccination campaigns (Putra et al., 2013). However, it is impossible to say how many dogs were repeat vaccinates, how many escaped vaccination altogether and how many were simply inaccessible, leaving the claim of 70 per cent total coverage on the island unclear. Further challenges in the 2010 and 2011 campaigns were cold chain management, varying access to and supply of vaccine, funding liquidity and data reporting and management.

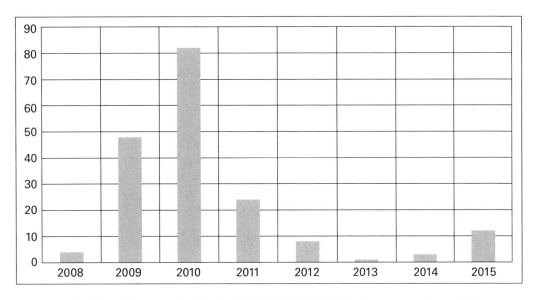

Figure 2.1 Confirmed human rabies deaths in Bali, 2008–2015 (2015 data are up to June 2015)

At time of writing, rabies remains in the dog population in Bali. By July 2015 there were 12 more human deaths from canine rabies and there continue to be human/dog confrontations with dog bites numbering around 150 a year (see Figure 2.1). As a result, the official target for freedom from rabies in Bali has been pushed out to 2016. The government of Bali continues to recognize vaccination and sterilization as valid options for rabies control but also actively and vigorously pursues culling of free-roaming dogs (Erviani, 2014), noting that in their opinion, control results from vaccination alone have been slow and not completely satisfactory.

2.3 Dogs in Bali

The dog plays an important cultural role in Balinese society, adding further complexity to the mix of dog ecology and stakeholder interaction that continues to be a part of the investigation of rabies epidemiology in Bali. The fact that most Balinese dogs are free-roaming further confounds the issue. Both the cultural

role and free-roaming as an issue for disease control are described here.

The dog has long been a part of community life in Bali, functioning as a guard dog for house and garden, a companion in hunting and fishing, and a pet (Putra et al., 2011). Most Balinese are Hindu; in Hindu culture, the dog is referred to as the guardian of Heaven and Hell. Caring for dogs is thus considered a conduit to Heaven, as well as a way to avert calamity (Lodrick, 2009). As well, certain colours of dogs are used in cultural ceremonies by the Balinese, who also believe dogs may cure certain diseases and prevent misfortune. Clearly, killing off all the dogs would not be a culturally respectful nor reasonable approach to rabies control.

Dog ecology

Dog ecology has been studied and reported as part of understanding, designing and interpreting the sero-epidemiology of rabies in Bali by Putra and colleagues in several Balinese publications (Putra and Gunata, 2009; Putra et al.,

2009, 2011). It was also noted as an important part of a transdisciplinary, ecohealth-based approach to policy formulation to address rabies in Bali (Willyanto et al., 2012). These studies have identified several important findings with respect to free-roaming indigenous (*kampung*) dog ecology including:

- There are close to half a million free-roaming dogs in Bali and about 10,000 'high bred' dogs (i.e., not free-roaming and kept as house pets).
- The free-roaming dog-to-human ratio is about 1:8.
- The largest age group of free-roaming dogs captured, vaccinated and released are less than one year of age.
- The majority of free-roaming dogs observed are three years of age or younger.
- Dog density is highest around urban areas at 256/km^2, with density in peri-urban at 184/km^2 and rural village areas at 129/km^2.
- Puppies are least likely to be born during the wet season (December to May).
- Free-roaming dogs tend to congregate near sites associated with people and food including temples, garbage drops, markets and beaches.
- Among *kampung* dog-keepers (e.g., fishermen, guard dog needs), there is a preference for an intact male dog.

In a rabies control and elimination campaign, knowledge of dog ecology can be highly valuable to increasing efficacy. From the work conducted in Bali, we know a well-planned strategy would target truly free-roaming dogs (such as catch, vaccinate, tag and release tactics) as well as contained dogs, although the former are far more difficult to handle and vaccinate. A strategy should also consider that free-roaming dogs tend to stay close to human habitation, very young dogs will require a second booster in a matter of months, and vaccination programmes would be

best to target two seasons: first, the pre-breeding season in the first two months of the year and, second, in October and November with the appearance of new-born puppies.

From the above data and estimates from Putra et al. (2011, 2013), it seems the coverage rate of free-roaming dogs in the first two waves of vaccination was closer to 10 per cent, which was far from the minimum of 70 per cent required to stop maintenance of the disease in the dog population. As well as the challenges noted above, understanding of dog ecology in Bali as well as the role of communities and cooperative coordination with government was crucial to mounting a successful catch-and-release vaccination campaign.

2.4 Community/participatory approach

The response to the Bali rabies epidemic has demonstrated the need for a participatory approach to solving a complex problem, involving numerous stakeholders including several levels of government, health professionals including veterinarians and physicians, epidemiologists and ecologists, communications and logistics experts and, of course, members of the local community. The village community plays a particularly important role in Bali in part because of the free-roaming nature of the dogs, making it difficult for outsiders to identify locally cared-for dogs that are fed and considered part of the community.

Communication is a vital element of a successful participatory approach to rabies control as much for human post-exposure treatment as prevention and control of rabies in dogs. Of 104 cases of human rabies investigated from 2008 to 2010 (Susilawathi et al., 2012), 92 per cent had history of a dog bite but fewer than 6 per cent had their wounds treated and received PEP vaccine (none received PEP immunoglobulins).

The authors concluded this was primarily due to lack of awareness of rabies risk, understanding of rabies in dogs or the need for urgent post-bite care, and limited awareness or availability of PEP treatment. Because Bali had been free of rabies up to 2008, there was a general lack of awareness or concern for either rabies following a dog bite or for control of rabies in communities. Thus communication and educational programmes would be essential to raising public awareness and assisting in identifying rabies cases in dogs, helping human bite victims seek urgent medical care, and implementing a surveillance and rapid response mechanism.

Effective collaboration with community partners can take several years to foster and maintain, but in a transdisciplinary participatory approach, community members are as vital a stakeholder as governments and scientists. Components of effective collaborations with communities in Bali vary depending on the regency and community, but there are several commonalities:

• Communities are a part of the government-led PDSR/DSO and ICBM programmes.
• Multilevel age-appropriate training and education programmes in recognizing the threat of rabies and management of free-roaming dogs in the community.
• Heightened awareness of how to respond to dog bites.
• Improved participation in mass rabies vaccination of dogs including post-vaccination marking with a long-lasting collar to prevent culling of vaccinated dogs.
• Training and signposted identification of community members who act as village rabies awareness wardens; children are taught to seek help from these respected community members in the event of dog threats or attacks.
• Community environmental management to reduce the risk of rabies including garbage management.

• Improved animal welfare of free-roaming dogs including veterinary care and awareness of sterilization as a healthy option to prolong the life and welfare of all dogs.

It is worth noting the importance of a community-based One Health approach in rabies control has been appreciated in other countries in Asia, notably Bhutan. The dog-neutering programme in Bhutan ensures that feral dogs are also vaccinated against rabies during concurrent public awareness campaigns and vaccination of pet dogs. The neuter and vaccination programme is well described in Tenzin et al. (2012a, 2012b), and engages veterinary professionals, para-professionals and community members. The awareness programme engages professionals from human and animal health and includes the development of new inter-sectoral government guidelines for the prevention of rabies in humans. The ongoing collaborations (at all levels of government service) and the joint disease investigations conducted by field staff from the Department of Public Health and Department of Livestock in Bhutan demonstrate a genuine commitment to the One Health approach.

2.5 Impact on tourism

More than 40 per cent of tourism income in Indonesia comes from Bali (*Bali Daily*, 25 January 2013), generating more than US$5.4 billion in 2012, up from US$4 billion in 2011. The economic impact on tourism in Bali attributable to fear of rabies has not been calculated. However, despite travel warnings for Bali because of rabies that have been issued by the governments of Australia, UK and the US, arrivals to Bali have increased significantly every year since the first case was reported (Figure 2.2) and show no sign of decreasing. The absence of evidence of a slowdown in tourism is made more surprising given that Indonesia is the second highest

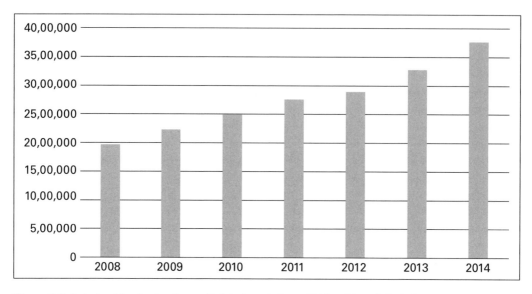

Figure 2.2 Arrivals of foreign tourists to Bali, Indonesia from 2008 to 2014. Calculations by Hall using data from Bali provincial government.

reported country after Thailand for travellers who were bitten by animals and received rabies PEP (Gautret et al., 2015). Despite these data being made available to travellers online and via health personnel, there seems to be a general lack of awareness among travellers of the risks, as well as a lack of pre-travel advice issued by health professionals. Furthermore, most travellers neither seek nor receive pre-exposure rabies vaccination (Gautret et al., 2015), and of those who are bitten, less than a third seem to seek any medical care at all (Piyaphanee et al., 2012). Our conclusion is that rabies has had no appreciable impact on tourism in Bali, but that travellers and health professionals may not be well aware of either the epidemic or pre-travel prevention options.

Policy development

Prior to the rabies epidemic in Bali, no policies existed for dog control, dog-bite surveillance or canine rabies vaccination. Today there are multiple informal policies in place to address these matters, including the guidelines for engagement and support of the PDSR, DSO and ICBM programmes described above. A formal rabies control and elimination policy recognized by provincial and federal governments and formulated with the cooperation of all stakeholders, whether it be a set of standard operating procedures or a provincial decree, has not been developed in Bali. Current vaccination policy is guided by two main elements: first, technical cooperation agreements that are developed between the governments of Bali and Indonesia and partners including FAO, international donors and NGOs; and, second, community-led initiatives that operate as part of wider programmes.

Well-developed One Health policies are needed for broad zoonotic control and elimination programmes to guide science-based decision-making and allocation of resources in a coordinated manner with understanding of longer-term needs such as the role of surveillance, while being cognisant of shorter-term demands including controlling free-roaming biting dogs and having urgent access to PEP treatment. But just as is the case for HPAI in Southeast Asia (Cork et al., 2015), policy to support rabies control in Bali faces a challenge: how to formulate strict and enforceable standards while minimizing disruption of property rights. The benefits of a One Health approach to this policy formulation problem include the opportunities for dialogue and agreement among stakeholders by taking a participatory approach, recognition of the complexity of a health problem allowing changing standards and methods, and adopting a transdisciplinary approach that reduces marginalization of important stakeholders while bringing together critical expertise.

Among the policy challenges Bali faces in rabies control and elimination are two important barriers that have yet to be overcome: a reliance on foreign aid for programme inputs including vaccines, and clear distinction between community, provincial and central government policy intent and results. Of Indonesia's total revenue from tourism, at least 40 per cent is generated by Bali (Bali provincial government, 2015), amounting to several billion US dollars per annum. This is clearly worth protecting, but so too does it seem extraordinary that a fraction of these funds are not used to completely cover the costs of maintaining vaccine and PEP supplies. The second barrier is harder to overcome, in part due to the devolution of Indonesian governance structure and responsibility, but here One Health offers part of a means to solution through participatory approaches to problem-solving, and recognition of the importance of addressing social inequities in zoonotic disease control.

2.6 The Rabies vaccination/culling debate

For many infectious diseases for which (1) consequences of human infection are devastating to health or economics or both, (2) there exists an identified non-human animal reservoir or vector, and (3) an effective animal vaccine exists, passionate longstanding debates have arisen regarding elimination of the animal reservoir/vector versus vaccination. Two examples are the debate over elimination versus vaccination for brucellosis of bison in Canada's vast Wood Buffalo National Park (Nishi et al., 2006) and elimination of tuberculosis maintained by badgers in farming areas of the UK (Enticott et al., 2012). The polemic of rabies control through vaccination versus culling has generated considerable heated debate in Bali and shows little sign of resolving. This section serves to identify elements of the debate but not to take sides in order to highlight the need for objective assessment of options as well as point out vulnerabilities of both approaches.

This chapter has pointed out that there has been progress, albeit slow, in controlling rabies in Bali, predominantly through transdisciplinary approaches involving investigation in ecology, community engagement, communications and control of virus movement through primarily vaccination and, to a lesser extent, culling. For a rabies vaccination programme to be successful in Bali (i.e., eliminate the virus) several elements are required including: sufficient coverage of all dogs in Bali (greater than 70 per cent); no gaps in vaccination coverage either in time or geographic location; effective delivery of long-term single-dose vaccine, available whenever needed; and a well-coordinated delivery system that includes participation of communities and local government.

Townsend and colleagues (2013) have demonstrated the importance of several of these factors and the need for effective surveillance to detect rabies positive cases. Under poor surveillance conditions, which reflect the reality of low income and low technical capacity situations, the authors also show that vaccination is more effective at controlling rabies than is culling. They also demonstrate that high rates of vaccination coverage are critical to achieving high control or elimination of rabies in Bali, and even the slightest breaks in coverage jeopardize success.

An analysis of the economic efficiency of vaccination versus culling including the option of PEP for humans is yet to be rigorously developed for Bali. Despite limited support and under challenging logistic conditions, Zinsstag and colleagues have shown that rabies control using vaccination and PEP can be achieved cost-effectively in parts of Africa (Zinsstag et al., 2009, 2015). Their analysis noted the need for vigilant prolonged efforts and that the results are highly context-dependent.

From a practical viewpoint, the Bali provincial government has demonstrated little patience with epidemiologic simulations that argue in support of expensive and logistically demanding high vaccination coverage when canine cases and human deaths continue, and Governor Made Pangku Pastika has been very vocal about his support for culling (*Jakarta Post*, 2014). At the same time, to encourage home containment of dogs and vaccination, the Bali provincial government is enforcing a rabies prevention bylaw enacted in 2009 that stipulates dog owners must keep their dogs at home and have them vaccinated regularly or face a maximum of six months in prison or a fine of Rp 50 million (US$4,100).

Both strategic sides of the control and elimination argument have weaknesses. It is clearly incorrect to jump to a conclusion that either method will never work to control rabies;[3] under perfect conditions either method would contain and eliminate rabies. A more sensible analysis, recognizing that perfect conditions are next to impossible, would clearly state programme objectives (control versus elimination under an achievable time horizon), assess the limitations of each method, examine the resources available and realistic constraints to utilization, and develop a corresponding strategy that engages all stakeholders in a transdisciplinary, participatory approach. At time of writing, this debate shows no sign of resolving, much like the situation with brucellosis in bison in Canada and tuberculosis in badgers in the UK.

2.7 Rabies as a One Health problem

Rabies is most burdensome for both humans and dogs in countries in Africa and Asia in which resources for tackling public health problems, mostly human and financial capital, are highly constrained. As a result, high-profile diseases including malaria and influenza get first priority, leaving rabies on the WHO list of neglected tropical diseases (Holmes, 2015). It is the lowest income and less well-educated communities that one finds highest rates death from rabies, identifying the social inequity of rabies prevention.

For these reasons, successful control and elimination of rabies requires a well-coordinated, sustainably funded, and carefully planned approach that includes participation of all stakeholders as well as integration of health disciplines, appropriately targeted communication programmes, and supporting policies for sustainable implementation. Add to this the necessity of understanding dog ecology and the complexity of the disease, and it is clear addressing rabies requires a One Health approach. The WHO has noted that key among the limiting factors in a successful programme are access and affordability of dog vaccination and PEP biologicals (Holmes, 2015) as well as rapid response to seek treatment following a dog bite. All three of these factors are most constrained in low-income communities.

It is also unfortunate that human health and animal health disciplines are not always working together to tackle rabies. In Bali, this has not been the case, where primary healthcare providers have trained and developed rabies PEP planning in consult with communities and animal health workers who are most likely to be the first persons aware of a person being bitten by a dog. However, shared communication systems and data obstacles remain, despite willingness to exchange knowledge of dog bites and persons or communities at risk. This reduces the efficiency of surveillance and of planned prevention and response efforts, particularly with respect to which communities should be targeted.

Similarly, a key outcome of shared knowledge and improved cooperation between animal and human health professionals is awareness of risk of exposure following a dog bite. If health professionals are sharing knowledge of risk and of vaccination status of dogs in communities, the overuse of PEP treatment can be avoided, avoiding mistakes of overuse and prolonged unnecessary concern for rabies such as occurred in Bhutan (Léchenne et al., 2015; Tenzin et al., 2011).

2.8 Conclusions

Dogs have shared our environment for millennia, as has the rabies virus. The response to rabies in Bali has gone through several stages of culling, vaccination and combinations thereof under various manifestations of institution-led response and stakeholder engagement. In 2015, there still is no clear unwavering policy established in terms of mechanism of prevention and response, although there has been considerable progress in surveillance, understanding of dog ecology, cooperation between animal and human health authorities and participation of all key stakeholders in controlling rabies. Strong differences of opinion continue to influence rapid response to new rabies cases, but at least it is clear that in 2014, cases of dog bites, dog rabies, and human deaths in Bali were markedly reduced from what they were in 2009 and 2010.

A number of factors led to the One Health response that developed in fighting the rabies epidemic in Bali. The initial culling strategy resulted in a backlash of bad press, both domestic and international, which was unexpected in

part because the local government did not place substantial weight on the somewhat unconventional bond between the community and the free-roaming dogs. Once that had been realized and the role of NGOs accepted, the strategy included mass vaccination, but there still were missing pieces of the transdisciplinary approach. Key among these was better understanding of dog ecology and ways and means to engage with community partners. At the same time, it was clear that solving the rabies problem would require a partnership between human and animal health personnel, as had worked for HPAI.

A recognition of the need to address social equity as well as communication became evident early in the campaign as programmes accommodated low-income village residents who needed access to vaccines and PEP treatment as well as improved understanding at the village level of how to prevent and respond to dog bites. Technology and transdisciplinary approaches were modified and adopted to complement these programmes and to support and encourage community participation.

As the campaign to rid Bali of rabies approaches its fifth wave of dog vaccination in 2015, Bali has learned that an integrated, transdisciplinary, participatory approach to zoonotic disease control and elimination is preferable to and more likely to be successful than a centrally coordinated effort. This has been an evolving One Health strategy that has come about through necessity as well as reflection on successes and constraints. There are opportunities to learn from the One Health approach developed in Bali to address rabies and other zoonotic diseases elsewhere, including many of the WHO neglected tropical diseases found in many lower-income countries.

Endnotes

1 Meningitis is inflammation of the lining of the brain, one of the clinical consequences of rabies.

2 *Lyssa* translates not only as rage but is also the name for the Greek goddess of anger. Lyssaviruses are closely related to the rabies virus and are classified in the same family, the *Rhabdoviridae*.

3 Rabies was eliminated from the UK in the early twentieth century through culling combined with licensing and muzzling of dogs. In contrast, a declaration in 2007 by the CDC of the elimination of rabies from dogs in the US noted that the primary reason for this success was vaccination of pets, both in the past and ongoing.

References

Adamson, P.B. (1977). The spread of rabies into Europe and the probable origin of this disease in antiquity. *The Journal of the Royal Asiatic Society of Great Britain and Ireland*, 2(2), 140–144.

Bali Provincial Government (2015). President Joko Widodo recognizes tourism as leading sector, www.balitourismboard.org/news.html.

Cork, S.C., Geale, D.W. and Hall, D.C. (2015). One Health in policy development: an integrated approach to translating science into policy. In J. Zinsstag, E. Schelling, D. Waltner-Toews, M. Whittaker and M. Tanner (eds.), *One Health: The Theory and Practice of Integrated Health Approaches*. Oxfordshire: CABI.

Enticott, G., Maye, D., Ilbery, B., Fisher, R. and Kirwan, J. (2012). Farmers' confidence in vaccinating badgers against bovine tuberculosis. *Veterinary Record*, 170(8), 204.

Erviani, N.K. (2014). Stray dogs must be culled, Bali governor says. *The Jakarta Post*, 27 June.

Gautret, P., Harvey, K., Pandey, P., Lim, P.L., Leder, K., Piyaphanee, W., Shaw, M., McDonald, S.C., Schwartz, E., Esposito, D.H. and Parola, P. (2015). Animal-associated exposure to rabies virus among travelers, 1997–2012. *Emerging Infectious Diseases*, 21(4), 569–577.

Holmes, P. (2015). *Investing to Overcome the Global Impact of Neglected Tropical Diseases: Third WHO Report on Neglected Diseases 2015*. Geneva: World Health Organization.

Léchenne, M., Miranda, M.E. and Zinsstag, J. (2015). Integrated rabies control. In J. Zinsstag, E. Schelling, D. Waltner-Toews, M. Whittaker and M. Tanner (eds.), *One Health: The Theory and Practice of Integrated Health Approaches*. Oxfordshire: CABI.

Lodrick, D.O. (2009). The sacred and the profane: the dog in South Asian culture. *Man In India*, 89, 497–523.

Mahardika, G.N.K, Dibia, N., Budayanti, N.S., Susilawathi, N.M., Subrata, K., Darwinata, A.E., Wignall, F.S., Richt, J.A., Valdivia-Granda, W.A. and Sudewi, A.A. (2014). Phylogenetic analysis and victim contact tracing of rabies virus from humans and dogs in Bali, Indonesia. *Epidemiology and Infection*, 142, 1146–1154.

Morters, M.K., Bharadwajb, S., Whay, H.R., Cleaveland, S., Damriyasae, I.M. and Wood, J.L.N. (2014). Participatory methods for the assessment of the ownership status of free-roaming dogs in Bali, Indonesia, for disease control and animal welfare. *Preventive Veterinary Medicine*, 116, 203–208.

Nishi, J.S., Shury, T. and Elkin, B.T. (2006). Wildlife reservoirs for bovine tuberculosis (*Mycobacterium bovis*) in Canada: strategies for management and research. *Veterinary Microbiology*, 112, 325–338.

Piyaphanee, W., Kittitrakul, C., Lawpoolsri, S., Gautret, P., Kashino, W., Tangkanakul, W., Charoenpong, P., Ponam, T., Sibunruang, S., Phumratanaprapin, W. and Tantawichien, T. (2012). Risk of potentially rabid animal exposure among foreign travelers in Southeast Asia. *PLS Neglected Tropical Disease*, 6, e1852.

Pritchard, J.B. (ed.) (1955). *Ancient Near Eastern Texts Relating to the Old Testament*. Princeton: Princeton University Press.

Putra, A.A.G. (1998). *Monitoring Rabies di Pulau Flores*. Report BPPH VI Denpasar, October 1998.

Putra, A.A.G. and Gunata, I.K. (2009). Epidemiologi rabies: Suatu kajian terhadap wabah rabies di Bali. *Workshop Kesehatan Hewan Regional VI*, June.

Putra, A.A.G, Dartini, N.L., Faizah, Soegiarto and Scott-Orr, H. (2009). Surveilans seroepidemiologi rabies di Bali. *Buletin Veteriner Balai Besar Veteriner Denpasar*, 21(75), 52–61.

Putra, A.A.G., Gunata, I.K., and Asrama, I.G. (2011). Dog demography in Badung district, the Province of Bali and their significance to rabies control. *Buletin Veteriner Balai Besar Veteriner Denpasar*, 23, 14–24.

Putra, A.A.G., Hampson, K., Girardi, J., Hiby, E., Knobel, D., Mardiana, I.W., Townsend, S. and Scott-Orr, H. (2013). Response to a rabies epidemic, Bali, Indonesia, 2008–2011. *Emerging Infectious Diseases*, 19(4), 648–651.

Susilawathi, N.M., Darwinata, A.E., Dwija, I.B.N.P., Budayanti, N.S., Wirasandhi, G.A.K., Subrata, K., Susilarini, N.K., Sudewi, R.A.A., Wignall, F.S. and Mahardika, G.N.K. (2012). Epidemiological and clinical features of human rabies cases in Bali 2008–2010. *BMC Infectious Diseases*, 12, 81.

Tenzin, Dhand, N.K. and Ward, M.P. (2011). Human rabies post exposure prophylaxis in Bhutan, 2005–2008: trends and risk factors. *Vaccine*, 29, 4094–4101.

Tenzin, Dukpak, Tshering, Y. and Thapa, L. (2012a). Status of notifiable animal diseases in Bhutan, 2011–2012, www.ncah.gov.bt/reports.php?page=2.

Tenzin., Ward, M.P. and Dhand, N.K (2012b). *Epidemiology of Rabies in Bhutan: Geographic Information System Based Analysis. The Reality of Rabies; Setting the Scene*. Compendium of the OIE Global Conference on Rabies Control

Theodorides, J. (1974). *Proceedings of the International Congress of the History of Medicine in 1972*. Brussels: Societas Belgia Historiae Medicinae.

Townsend, S.E., Sumantra, I.P., Pudjiatmoko, Bagus G.N., Brum, E. et al. (2013). Designing Programs for Eliminating Canine Rabies from Islands: Bali, Indonesia as a Case Study. *PLOS Neglected Tropical Diseases*, 7(8), e2372.

Willyanto, I., Putra, A.A.G., Basuno, E. and Hall, D.C. (2012). *Optimizing Rabies Control Program in Bali: An Ecohealth Approach*. BECA policy brief. Building Ecosystem Capacity in Asia project, IDRC and AusAID.

Zinsstag, J., Durr, S., Penny, M.A., Mindekem, R., Roth, F., Menendez Gonzalez, S., Naissengar, S. and Hattendorf, J. (2009). Transmission dynamics and economics of rabies control in dogs and humans in an African city. Proceedings of the National Academy of Science, 106(35), 14996–15001.

Zinsstag, J., Choudury, A., Roth, F. and Shaw, A. (2015). One Health economics. In J. Zinsstag, E. Schelling, D. Waltner-Toews, M. Whittaker and M. Tanner (eds.), *One Health: The Theory and Practice of Integrated Health Approaches*, Oxfordshire: CABI.

chapter 3

Integrating a One Health approach to avian influenza control in New Zealand

Wlodek L. Stanislawek, Thomas G. Rawdon and Susan C. Cork

Abstract

With the unprecedented spread of avian influenza (subtype H5N1) across Asia in 2004, and the potential for a new influenza pandemic in humans, New Zealand enhanced its wild bird and poultry surveillance activities. The government also put together an interdisciplinary team to update its pandemic preparedness plan. Pandemic planning requires coordinated global actions as well as actions at the national level. Good governance, public education and stakeholder engagement is essential. In this chapter we outline the complex biology of avian influenza and illustrate the importance of interagency cooperation when developing disease preparedness and response plans.

3.1 Introduction

The emergence of a number of new strains of avian influenza (AI) in recent years (To et al., 2014) as well as other zoonotic viruses, such as H1N1 influenza virus from pigs and severe acute respiratory syndrome (SARS), Nipah and Hendra viruses from bats (Ksiazek et al., 2003, Field et al., 2007) triggered organizations working in the human and animal health fields to seriously examine disease transmission risks between animals and humans. Due to the frequent movement of animals and humans within and between countries, viruses not currently endemic continue to pose a potential risk to countries such as New Zealand. Significant disease outbreaks caused by any infectious disease can be economically, socially, medically and environmentally costly. Given the complex ecology of potentially zoonotic diseases such as avian influenza, developing effective plans for disease prevention and control demands an effective interdisciplinary and interagency solution. The 'One Health' approach engages a wide range of experts to deal with the varied challenges required to prevent and control zoonotic diseases such as avian influenza. This collaborative approach has also been adopted by policymakers in New Zealand in response to a recognized need for more effective and sustainable measures to address emerging diseases (Barrett et al., 2011).

In 2004, the New Zealand government established the interagency National Centre for Biosecurity and Infectious Disease (NCBID). This reflected a recognition of the value of the implementing the One World, One Health concept.[1] The aim was to facilitate enhanced collaboration between organizations such as the Investigation and Diagnostic Centre[2] (Ministry for Primary Industries, MPI, previously known as the Ministry of Agriculture & Forestry), Environmental Science and Research (ESR), AgResearch and AsureQuality to more efficiently coordinate the management of zoonotic diseases in particular (Hope, 2009). ESR provides core diagnostic and surveillance support for the Ministry of Health[3] whereas AgResearch[4] and AsureQuality[5] are semi-commercial enterprises that provide technical support to the Ministry of Primary Industries and Industry stakeholders.

A key motivator for developing enhanced collaborations between these government agencies is the fact that approximately 75 per cent of emerging infectious diseases in the human population have originated from domestic and wild animals (Jones et al., 2008; WHO, 2008).

3.2 The National Centre for Biosecurity and Infectious Diseases

In 2008, the World Health Organization (WHO) published a document on behalf of the World Organisation for Animal Health (OIE), the Food and Agriculture Organization of the United Nations (FAO) and WHO, suggesting the need for a reliable mechanism for sharing information and surveillance data to ensure a coordinated international response and risk reduction process in order to improve the management and prevention of zoonotic diseases (WHO et al., 2008). At a country and local level, New

Zealand has demonstrated a strong commitment to enhance collaborations between agencies responsible for human and animal health in order to prevent and manage emerging zoonotic diseases. An important step was the establishment of a group of co-located organizations responsible for diagnostic and epidemiological work in both the animal and human health fields. Establishing supporting infrastructure and expertise on a single site has fostered cross-collaboration, resulting in a coordinated team approach to problem-solving. A decade later, the establishment of NCBID has provided an excellent example of proximity, breaking the barriers created by years of separated disciplines and narrow thinking.

The international concerns about the risk of human infection with influenza type A (H1N1) in 2009 demonstrated the value to the human health sector of engaging the diagnostic and epidemiological expertise of the animal health sector in New Zealand. MPI's epidemiologists and disease response personnel worked effectively alongside staff in the Ministry of Health and ESR to assess potential risks from pigs. At the same time, the Animal Health Laboratory scientists worked side-by-side with ESR laboratory staff to examine samples collected as part of disease surveillance activities. Effective sharing of ideas and technical resources was possible because of the establishment of NCBID. This interagency collaboration has built resilience by cross-skilling, which is crucial to ensure sustainable scientific and technical capability and capacity given the small population pool and remoteness of New Zealand. Interagency partnerships between human and animal scientists and technical staff at NCBID and other institutions has also facilitated ongoing collaborations for the development of assays and field testing of a mobile PCR system developed by Lincoln University, testing mobile sequence analysis technology (O'Keefe, 2009; Hope, 2009).

Veterinary Public Health (VPH) was defined by the WHO consultation on 'Future Trends in Veterinary Public Health' held in Teramo, Italy in 1999 as 'the sum of all contributions to the physical, mental and social well-being of humans through an understanding and application of veterinary science' (www.who.int/zoonoses/vph/en).

3.3 Influenza viruses and their genomic characteristics

Avian influenza viruses are commonly found in wild waterfowl and frequently cause no clinical signs in these birds. However, the ecology of avian influenza viruses is complex and changes in viral genetic structure can result in increased virulence and enhanced risk of transmission from their natural reservoirs to other species. Although humans exposed to avian influenza viruses can become infected, in most cases this does not result in clinical disease unless the viral strains have become adapted to humans or the viral load is high enough to overcome natural levels of specific and non-specific immunity.

Influenza viruses are members of the *Orthomyxoviridae* family. These are enveloped viruses that contain a segmented single-stranded RNA genome. There are three genera of influenza virus: influenza type A, influenza type B and influenza type C. Influenza types A and C infect multiple species, while influenza type B almost exclusively infects humans. Only viruses of the influenza A genus are known to infect birds. Influenza A viruses (Plate 1) are typically classified into different subtypes based on the antigenic properties and genetic sequences of their surface haemagglutinin (HA) and neuraminidase (NA) glycoproteins. HA subtypes H1-16 and NA subtypes N1-9 are found in a wide range of avian species, whereas subtypes H17-18 and N10-11 are found in bats (To et al., 2014).

The two external glycoproteins are particularly important as the HA glycoprotein is responsible for virus attachment to the target cell, and the NA glycoprotein is needed for virion maturation and release (Hampson, 2002).

Wild birds have been found to be infected with all known subtypes of Influenza A viruses (Kawaoka et al., 1988; Alexander, 2000; Olsen et al., 2006). Water birds, including anseriformes (e.g., ducks, geese and swans, etc.) and charadriiformes (e.g., gulls, terns, knots, plovers etc.), are recognized as the primary natural reservoirs of influenza A viruses (Webster et al., 1992; Olsen et al., 2006; Hurt et al., 2006; Krauss and Webster, 2010). Passerine birds (e.g., sparrows, crows etc.) may also serve as reservoirs for avian influenza viruses but the low prevalence of infection in these birds suggests that they are primarily spillover hosts from avian influenza (AI) virus-infected poultry or water birds (Vandergrift et al., 2010). The importance of AI viruses in wild birds was not fully appreciated until the connection between viruses in these birds, outbreaks in poultry and the potential for the development of human pandemic strains was realized. Influenza virus transmission in wild and domestic animals and humans is intimately connected. Evidence suggests that viral transmission – particularly in domestic poultry with subsequent spillover to other domestic animals – may cause human pandemics.

For influenza A viruses to become highly pathogenic, the haemagglutinin glycoprotein that is produced as a precursor (HA0) requires post-translational cleavage by host proteases. The HA0 precursor proteins of low pathogenic strains of avian influenza (LPAI) have a single basic amino acid (arginine) at the HA0 cleavage site but highly pathogenic strains (HPAI) contain a series of basic amino acids at the cleavage sites of the HA0, which allows the virus to replicate widely in many tissues throughout the infected host resulting in severe disease and death (Rott, 1992; Stieneke-Grober et al., 1992;

Walker et al., 1992). Therefore, sequences of multiple basic amino acids at the cleavage site of HA0, along with other virulence characteristics, can determine pathogenic properties of the virus. In most cases, only AIV subtypes H5, H7 and (more recently) H10 have been shown to cause serious disease outbreaks in susceptible poultry. However, H9 and other subtypes have also caused disease in cases where there are concurrent infections in poultry flocks i.e. bacteria, mycoplasma, viruses etc. (Capua and Alexander, 2009).

Low pathogenic avian influenza subtypes H5 and H7 viruses are generally regarded as potential precursors of HPAI strains and their detection in a commercial poultry flock results in the implementation of disease control measures. At least two key mechanisms may contribute to the development of highly pathogenic strains: antigenic drift and antigenic shift.

Antigenic drift is a process of gradual accumulation of mutations (or insertion) primarily of HA and NA surface antigens. Mutations in other genes (PB2, PB1, PA and NS) also play an important role in virus pathogenicity (Hampson, 2002; Krauss and Webster, 2010; Neverov et al., 2014). The segmented genome of influenza virus (Plate 1) can also exchange segments if different strains co-infect the same host, which can lead to a new gene constellation and new virus. This process is called reassortment or antigenic shift. Most known major influenza epidemics in humans were the result of virus mutations caused by such reassortment events. This was the case for the 1957 (H2N2) and the 1968 (H3N2) pandemics, as well as for the swine flu in 2009 (H1N1) (Lindstrom et al., 2004; Bastien et al., 2010).

An important factor in the development of virulence is tissue tropism, i.e., the ability of the virus to attach to the host cell (Baigent and McCauley, 2003). Influenza A viruses attach to host cells by binding of the haemagglutinin (HA) protein to sialosaccharides on the host cell surface. The HAs of influenza A viruses

from different host species typically have different binding preferences. Sialic acid (SA) is linked to different carbohydrates either by α-2,3 (SAα-2,3Gal) or α-2,6 (SAα-2,6Gal) glycosidic bond. The HAs of human influenza A bind preferably to SAα-2,6Gal whereas avian influenza HAs favor SAα-2,3Gal. The latter are prominent in avian species (Rogers and Paulson, 1983; Suzuki, 2005; Connor et al., 1994).

Therefore, the type and distribution of SA is considered to be an important factor in the susceptibility of different host species to influenza A viruses and is believed to be one of the major factors preventing strains of AI crossing the species barrier (Suzuki et al., 2000).

Since all genes in the virus are linked to each other, any mutations in one gene, or any changes in gene constellations in the virus, will lead to the creation of a new virus subtype or different genotypes within a virus; for example, at least nine different genotypes of avian influenza H5N1 have been identified (Li et al., 2004).

3.4 Avian influenza in New Zealand

The first published report on avian influenza viruses (AIV) in New Zealand birds was a result of work conducted between 1975 and 1978 by researchers from the Medical Council of New Zealand Virus Research Unit. This group recognized the importance of influenza surveillance in wild birds in order to obtain information on the ecology of influenza A viruses and the influenza status of New Zealand's waterfowl. Samples were collected from 286 birds (terns, gulls, shearwaters and mallard ducks) in Dunedin (Otago area, South Island) New Zealand. A number of AI viruses were isolated in this study but only from mallard ducks (*Anas platyrhynchos,* introduced to New Zealand by European and North American settlers from as early as 1860s). Isolates characterized included subtypes H1N3, H4N6 and H11N3 (Austin and Hinshaw, 1984). Such studies provide important baseline data, which can be used to identify AI viruses currently in the country and to help predict the arrival or development of new strains in the future.

Two further surveys of wild birds were conducted by the Ministry of Agriculture and Forestry (MAF; now Ministry for Primary Industries, MPI) in 1989 (Stanislawek, 1992; Stanislawek et al., 2002). These studies focused primarily on mallard ducks (*Anas platyrhynchos*) and the first H5N2 AI low pathogenic influenza (LPAI) virus was isolated in 1997 (Temuka, South Island of New Zealand) in addition to H4N6 and H6N4 subtypes. In all these studies, cloacal swabs were collected from ducks in various locations in the North Island and South Island of New Zealand.

Since 2004, MAF/BNZ has also carried out surveillance for AI on selected species of migratory birds (i.e., shorebirds crossing the Asia-Pacific flyway) and also resident birds (predominantly mallard ducks) in response to the spread of strains of highly pathogenic avian influenza (HPAI) H5N1 around the world and with the potential for introduction of new avian influenza viruses to New Zealand. (Stanislawek et al., 2013).To date, more than 10,000 birds have been sampled from both islands of New Zealand (Plate 2a and b). Samples were collected from red knot (*Calidris canutus*), bar-tailed godwits (*Limosa lapponica*) and turnstones (*Arenaria interpres*) as the representatives of migratory birds and from mallard ducks (*Anas platyrhynchos*), paradise shelducks (*Tadorna variegate*), grey teal (*Anas gracilis*), black-billed gulls (*Chroicocephalus bulleri*), black backed gulls (*Larus dominicanus*), little blue penguins (*Eudyptula minor*), yellow-eyed penguins (*Megadyptes antipodes*), sooty shearwaters (*Puffinus griseus*) and wrybils (*Anarhynchus frontalis*) as representatives of resident birds of New Zealand.

New Zealand is not on the common migration pathway for key species of waterfowl, although vagrant waterfowl from Australia are occasionally encountered (Williams et al., 2004). Non-migratory waterfowl, predominantly mallard ducks, are sampled in the summer months throughout New Zealand, with a particular focus on coastal areas where they may have had contact with migratory shorebirds, or where large numbers of juvenile ducks congregate (Plate 2a). The absence of waterfowl migration substantially limits the potential of introduction of avian influenza viruses into New Zealand. Thus far, all New Zealand AIV isolates have been obtained from wild mallard ducks including subtypes: H1, H2, H3, H4, H5, H6, H7, H9, H10, H11 and H12. All nine neuraminidase types associated with these viruses were detected (Stanislawek, unpublished data). All the H5 and H7 isolates were pathotyped and confirmed to be LPAI based on the HA cleavage site assessment (Stanislawek et al., 2007; Langstaff et al., 2009).

Initiatives that build on the One Health concept and MPI's commitment to stakeholder consultation and engagement included New Zealand's commercial poultry surveillance programme (2008–2009) (Rawdon et al., 2010). These are important activities with regard to the government mandate to protect the 'public good' because AIV are potentially zoonotic diseases and disease prevention and control is a joint responsibility that requires both government and stakeholder support. In addition, New Zealand is a member of the international community and the OIE, the latter requires regular disease surveillance for diseases such as AI that are relevant to trade.

The AI surveillance programme carried out in commercial poultry flocks in New Zealand required extensive consultation with the poultry industry. This was in order to determine appropriate trigger-points for disease reporting and intervention and was important because of the potential financial and market access repercussions of any detection of AIV in commercial poultry. It was also important to agree on a comprehensive communications plan for the public in order to reduce fear and unjustified concerns over food safety. The latter was especially important due to growing international concerns over the pandemic potential of H5N1 avian influenza strains and the wide, and often reactive, coverage by the national and international media.

The poultry industry in New Zealand is considered small in comparison to many other developed countries. Approximately 16 million meat chickens (broilers) are present at any one time on about 170 farms across the country. Around 3.3 million layer hens are also present on around 150 commercial farms (with more than 100 birds per farm). Every year, there are also approximately 1.5 million ducks and turkeys in commercial flocks. Although most poultry production is for the New Zealand market, there is also a growing export market of hatching eggs, live one-day-old chickens and meat product to neighbouring countries (Kerry Mulqueen, pers. comm., 2015).

Active surveillance of all the key sectors making up New Zealand's commercial poultry industry (for egg and meat production), including broiler, caged/barn layer, free range layer, pullet rearer and turkey broilers, was carried out using an epidemiologically robust cross-sectional design. An extensive serological survey found no evidence of antibodies to H5 or H7 AIV (i.e., OIE reportable subtypes) in commercial chickens or turkeys, indicating that there was no active infection with these subtypes. This provided evidence of good compliance with biosecurity practices in the poultry industry. However, the survey did identify evidence of historic exposure to LPAI subtypes on a single free-range layer farm (Rawdon et al., 2010). The latter identifies a potential risk pathway posed by free-range operations. This is not unexpected and is most likely a result of contact with wild birds and sources of environmental contamination.

In addition to formal surveillance activities, NCBID staff also developed a collaborative research project to examine birds in backyard poultry farms adjacent to wetlands with waterfowl. This surveillance initiative included sampling of humans on the selected farms. During the study, interdisciplinary partners had to examine key research questions from a range of new perspectives and to deal with a wide range of stakeholders from both the public health and livestock sectors. The study was complicated due to the range of approvals required and the ethical compliance processes that had to be navigated on both the human and animal side as well as the need for confidentiality. Due to the potential concerns over finding AIV-positive birds and also the need to educate the public about disease risk, the Ministry of Health and MPI developed common risk communication plans. The studied farms were monitored for a year and staff gathered information on biosecurity practices, assessed risk pathways and looked for seasonal risk patterns. Research findings confirmed exposure of backyard flocks to LPAI viruses and the differential exposure-risk levels between chicken and duck flocks on these farms (Zheng et al., 2010). As well as encouraging the development of strong working relationships across the human and animal health sectors, findings from the research also identified key disease risk pathways such as direct contact with wild birds or use of drinking water contaminated with AIVs for both humans and poultry. With this in mind, an enhanced passive surveillance programme has been put in place to monitor bird disease and mortality events, for all bird populations in New Zealand, reported via MPI's exotic disease reporting hotline.

The MPI hotline is a freephone number that allows immediate contact 24/7 with MPI telephone operators dedicated to directing calls to on-call specialists including veterinarians, horticulturalists and marine biologists covering New Zealand's primary sectors. Bird events are sent to an on-call veterinarian who triages cases following a standardized approach, and follows up with appropriate sampling and testing in order to rule in or rule out suspected cases of AI and other exotic diseases (McFadden et al., 2007; Rawdon et al., 2007b).

3.5 Avian influenza in humans

Avian influenza viruses have been reported to cause disease in humans as early as 1959. However, infection with avian influenza in humans was not really taken seriously as a global public health concern until 1997 when new strains of the H5N1 virus surfaced, causing 33 per cent human mortality in Hong Kong. Historically, the avian influenza subtypes involved in human infection, in addition to H5N1, were H6N1, H7N2, H7N3, H7N7, H7N9, H9N2, H10N7 and H10N8 (To et al., 2014). However, as demonstrated by the emergence of the H7N9 zoonotic strain in China in 2013, pandemic emergence remains a concern in the region and globally, and a new strain with the potential to infect humans could arise at any time. Given the complex biology of AI, and the difficulties in implementing effective biosecurity and effective disease control policy across developing countries, it is likely that surveillance for new and emerging AIV in animals (especially in pigs and poultry) and humans will need to continue. ESR's National Influenza Centre in Wellington, New Zealand conducts seasonal human influenza A and B diagnosis and also the capability to detect (using specific RT/PCRs and virus isolation) H5N1 and H7N9 viruses. The recent emergence of H10N8 AIV in China prompted ESR to develop appropriate PCR based assays to detect this virus if needed.

No human infections with avian influenza viruses have been detected in New Zealand to date (Sue Huang, pers. comm., 2014).

3.6 Pathways of introduction for AI viruses to New Zealand

The location of New Zealand as an island in the Pacific Ocean provides a high degree of natural biosecurity. However, a number of possibilities have been identified for the entrance of new AIV in to New Zealand, these are (1) migratory birds and vagrants; (2) contaminated export products or equipment; (3) people travelling; and (4) smuggling illegal live birds or products. New Zealand lies at the south-eastern extremity of the East Asian-Australasian Flyway, which was (and still is) of particular relevance for the introduction of novel AIV in the region, especially given the spread of H5N1 across Asia from 2004. The isolation of AIV from migratory shorebirds in Australia (Hurt et al., 2006) highlights the potential risk of introducing novel strains into New Zealand, but this presents a low risk pathway for New Zealand (Langstaff et al., 2009).

During the global spread of H5N1, wild bird surveillance activities were enhanced. However, because of New Zealand's geographical isolation, relatively few Arctic-breeding migratory shorebirds actually reach the country. In total, about 200,000 birds representing 47 species arrive, but the vast majority of these comprise only three species: bar-tailed godwits, red knots and ruddy turnstones (Williams et al., 2006). Godwits are believed to fly directly to New Zealand, knots have stopovers in East Asia and turnstones have a number of stops in the Pacific before they reach New Zealand (Williams et al, 2006) (Plate 3). For these birds to introduce AIV to New Zealand, they would have to be infected before or during migration. On arrival, they could then shed the virus while cohabiting with endemic shorebirds, gulls, waterfowl and other species, and thereby introduce infection. However, surveillance carried out between 2004 and 2010 indicates that migratory birds pose a very low risk for the introduction of AI into New Zealand, as no AIV has been isolated from migratory birds over the seven years of surveillance. Since 2011, New Zealand has focused on resident waterfowl mallard ducks (Stanislawek et al., 2013). Sample collection from wild birds is a very specialized procedure that requires the expertise of organizations involved in studies of bird ecology, i.e., Department of Conservation (DOC), Fish and Game Councils and ornithological societies in New Zealand. These organizations work together with MPI to share expertise and learn what can be expected in the event of sampling in an outbreak situation. Wild birds, particularly waterfowl such as mallard ducks, grey ducks, paradise ducks, geese and swans are the natural reservoir for AIV, and these water birds also are more likely to mingle with backyard poultry.

The increasing importation of products/ equipment and the movement of people (potentially infected with influenza viruses or bringing infected products, such as contaminated feathers and poultry products) dramatically increases the possibility of the introduction of influenza A viruses into New Zealand (Pharo, 2003). The human entry pathway is of particular relevance to pig herds given their susceptibility to human influenza viruses. The intensive management systems employed on pig farms also makes disease spread more likely if a new virus was introduced. Pigs are regarded as a 'mixing vessel' for influenza viruses because any co-infection of humans with human and avian influenza viruses may lead to the creation of new viruses with human pandemic potential (i.e., due to antigenic drift). Despite very rigid biosecurity procedures at airports and ports around New Zealand, the above are the most likely routes of introduction of novel influenza viruses into the country. It also remains difficult to implement rigorous screening of human passengers for disease, although this has been attempted in the face of disease outbreaks such as SARS.

3.7 A governance framework for Avian Influenza response planning and delivery

The need to increase interdisciplinary cooperation between the key scientific and professional groups, such as human and animal researchers, conservationists, commercial poultry operators and relevant government ministries, in the management of AI is well-recognized internationally. Due to the complex ecology and zoonotic potential of AIV, avian influenza requires a One Health approach. Policies developed for the prevention and control of AIV also have to consider the potential disease risks to wild birds, this is especially important in New Zealand, which is home to many unique flightless birds (e.g., the kiwi (*Apteryx* spp.), takahe (*Porphyrio hochstetteri*) and kakapo (*Strigops habroptilus*) and some of the world's most endangered species, including the black stilt (*Himantopus novaezelandiae*), Campbell island teal (*Anas nesiotis*) and orange-fronted parakeet (*Eupsittula canicularis*).

The Ministry of Primary Industries (MPI) looks after policy related to the forest, agricultural and fisheries sectors. MPI has expertise in risk assessment and in animal and plant health. The mandate of MPI also includes responsibility for fisheries, wildlife and food safety. For avian influenza response planning, MPI engaged a two-tiered One Health team, comprising a multisectoral and multidisciplinary Technical Advisory Group (TAG), complemented by a similarly diverse Stakeholder Advisory Group (SAG). The approach separates the technical/ scientific aspects of disease prevention and response planning, from the consideration of the socioeconomic aspects that relate to the government responsibility to consider 'public good'. The approach cements interdisciplinary relationships and helps avoids duplication and conflict of interest. The approach also helps ensure coordination and effective communication, under the complex setting presented by AI. Government leadership of a response to AIV would be MPI in the case of an outbreak in poultry, but this lead would be handed over to the Ministry of Health in the case of an outbreak of AIV in humans. In either case, both ministries and other agencies such as the police, social services and emergency management would need to work closely with municipalities and the relevant stakeholders to deliver a timely well-coordinated response. There is no magic formula for the success of a One Health approach. Success requires strong governance, agreed goals, clear communication and a common, unambiguous language. Importantly, these integral components have to be delivered within a framework of cooperation and partnership.

3.8 Development of a response policy for avian influenza

The basis for all biosecurity investigation and response in New Zealand is the Biosecurity Act 1993. Under the Act, the chief technical officer is responsible for the overall management, coordination and leadership during an initial investigation and a response to an incursion of an exotic animal disease. A generic policy governing an MPI response to risk organisms such as AI sets out MPI's framework for response to organisms that could harm people, the environment, and/or the economy (Ministry of Agriculture and Forestry, 2008). The MPI's *Technical Response Policies for AIV of Regulatory Concern* builds on this generic framework and principles and provides an overview of approved policies following interdepartmental, TAG, SAG and industry consultation (Ministry of

---

Technical decision-making and operational elements

The TAG is comprised of experts with scientific competencies such as virologists, epidemiologists, biologists, ornithologists and veterinarians who review the context of the situation and the associated risks. The TAG reviews and recommends appropriate technical response management option(s) to the chief technical officer (CTO). Along similar lines, the SAG is tasked with reviewing response management option(s) developed in consultation with the TAG in light of primary production/commerce, environment, social (including human health) and cultural values. TAG and SAG members are paid by MPI and sign a conflict of interest document for confidentiality and scientific impartiality throughout the advisory and review process.

The SAG is comprised of individuals with relevant skills and experience particular to AIV and its potential impacts, including policy advisers from the MoH and DOC and industry advisers from the Poultry Industry Association of New Zealand (PIANZ), Egg Producers Federation of New Zealand (EPFNZ), Ostrich and Emu Standards Council (OESC), Australasian Regional Association of Zoological Parks and Aquaria (ARAZPA), Game Preserves and the MPI Maori Strategic Unit with knowledge of Tikanga Maori (Maori customs). Tikanga Maori includes as a core value 'Kaitiakitanga', a term meaning guardianship, protection and preservation of *Taonga*. *Taonga* refers to all natural resources such as forests, rivers and lakes, plants and animals. Inclusion of Maori cultural input is critical when agreeing and implementing disease management approaches in New Zealand, given the potential affects any interventions may have on land, vegetation and protected animals.

Agriculture and Forestry, 2006). Both the TAG and SAG were instrumental in the embedding and adoption of the Technical Response Policies.

Due to the complex disease ecology of avian influenza and the range of susceptible species (including humans), the policy sets out a matrix of response actions. As indicated earlier, a 'whole-of-government' response would be adopted for AIV strains affecting animals that could affect humans, such as H5N1 (Ministry of Agriculture and Forestry, 2011). In the event of this scenario, each agency has defined roles and has identified key documents and legislation that could be relevant while controlling a pandemic (Howell, 2006, Rooney, 2008). On the other hand, a response to non-zoonotic strains would be led by MPI and managed within the MPI's Memorandum of Understanding (MOU) on biosecurity activities between MPI and DOC, Ministry of Fisheries (now amalgamated with MPI) and the MOH (October 2006), and operational guidelines developed between DOC and MPI (December 2008).

3.9 A foundation for poultry sector response preparedness

Due to the zoonotic implications, especially to poultry farmers and workers on both commercial and backyard farms, and because of the possibility of widespread disruption and economic impacts in the commercial poultry sectors, a number of broad collaborative projects have been developed. These projects aim to fill gaps in knowledge around poultry farm locations, bird types and numbers, and importantly the various husbandry, biosecurity and human health protection practices in place. Factors that could influence the potential disease transmission or exposure risk for farmers and farm workers, the farm's poultry and other poultry farms connected by industry networks, were also assessed.

Initiatives included:

- an ongoing census of all commercial poultry farms, with locations and bird types and numbers recorded online in Agribase – this ensured that farm locations and population demographics were immediately available in the event of an incursion (Sanson and Scott, 2003; Lockhart et al, 2010a);
- surveys of biosecurity practices, animal husbandry and human protective measures on commercial and backyard farms – important in understanding appropriate intervention points and modifiable behaviours to mitigate risk to other farms and humans from potential AIV transmission pathways (Geale et al., 2006, p. 778; Lockhart et al., 2010a, 2010b; Rawdon et al., 2007a, 2007b, 2008, 2012a, 2012b; Zheng et al., 2010);
- studies of movement patterns of poultry and other conveyors in and between the commercial and backyard sectors – findings were incorporated into network analyses to understand which farms would be important contributors to disease spread, and how risk varied by season and across the country (Lockhart et al., 2010b; Rawdon and Stevenson, 2011);
- development of a disease spread simulation model covering both the commercial and backyard sectors, that incorporated many of the population demographic and movement pattern parameters elucidated through the various other studies – outputs were important to understand likely spread scenarios and the contingency arrangements and resource requirements for a response to AIV (Rawdon and O'Leary, 2010; Stevenson et al., 2013).

The approach was designed to prepare New Zealand should exotic or emerging strains of AIV be detected, although the outputs would play an important role and prepare a strong foundation for resilience to any disease threat. Many of these preparedness initiatives had their foundation in a cross-sector partnership approach across the human and animal health sectors. Learnings from poultry sector preparedness work in turn have had preparedness benefits for diseases in other livestock sectors.

3.10 Conclusion

The government response to avian influenza provides a good example of effectively applying the One Health approach in New Zealand. The preparedness activities and collaborative studies undertaken by human and animal health organizations have provided a solid foundation for working together on other zoonotic diseases. This chapter demonstrates the value of a collaborative and coordinated approach with many valuable opportunities for joint surveillance and response preparedness. The 2009 response to influenza A (H1N1) demonstrated the value to the human health sector of diagnostic and epidemiological expertise in the animal sector, with MPI's epidemiologists and response personnel working with the Ministry of Health and ESR, and laboratory scientists and technical staff working with ESR staff. This was possible because of the proximity of staff at NCBID and the key relationships in place that fostered effective communication. This collaborative approach also allowed the sharing of resources and has built resilience due to enhanced information-sharing and cross-skilling. The latter is crucial in order to ensure sustainability of scientific and technical capability and capacity given the small population pool and remoteness of New Zealand.

Endnotes

1 www.oie.int/for-the-media/editorials/detail/article/one-world-one-health.

2 www.biosecurity.govt.nz/pests/animals/ahl.
3 www.esr.cri.nz/capabilities/Pages/NCBID.aspx.
4 www.agresearch.co.nz.
5 www.asurequality.com.

References

Alexander, D. (2000). A review of avian influenza in different bird species. *Veterinary Microbiology*, 74, 3–13.

Austin, F.J. and Hinshaw, V.S. (1984). The isolation of influenza A viruses and paramyxoviruses from feral ducks in New Zealand. *Australian Journal of Experimental Biology Medical Science*, 62(3), 355–360.

Baigent, S.J. and McCauley, J.W. (2003). Influenza type A in humans, mammals and birds: determinants of virus virulence, host-range and interspecies transmission. *Bioessays*, 25, 657–671.

Barrett, M.A., Bouley, T.A., Stoertz, A.H. and Stoertz, R.W. (2011). Integrating a One Health approach in education to address global health and sustainability challenges. *Frontiers in Ecology and the Environment*, 9(4), 239–245.

Bastien, N., Nick, A., Antonishyn, N.A., Brandt, K., Wong, C.E., Chokani, K., Vegh, N., Horsman, G.B., Tyler, S., Graham, M.R., Plummer, F.A., Levett, P.N. and Li, Y. (2010). Human infection with a triple-reassortant swine influenza A (H1N1) virus containing the hemagglutininand neuraminidase genes of seasonal influenza virus. *The Journal of Infectious Diseases*, 201, 1178–1182.

Capua, I. and Alexander, D.J. (2009). Ecology, epidemiology and human health implications of avian influenza virus infection. In I. Capua and D.J. Alexander (eds.), *Avian Influenza and Newcastle Disease: A Field and Laboratory Manual*, pp. 1–18.

Connor, R.J., Kawaoka, Y., Webster, R.G. and Paulson, J.C. (1994). Receptor specificity in human, avian, and equine H2 and H3 influenza virus isolates. *Virology*, 205, 17–23.

Field, H.E., Mackenzie, J.S. and Daszak, P. (2007). Henipaviruses: emerging paramyxoviruses associated with fruit bats. *Current Topics in Microbiology and Immunology*, 315, 133–159.

Geale, D.W., Gerber, N.D., Marks, D.A., Tana, T.A., Rawdon, T.G. and Murray, A. (2006). *Biosecurity Risk Profile: A Foundation for Poultry Sector Exotic Disease Contingency Planning*. Proceedings of the 11th Symposium of the International Society for Veterinary Epidemiology and Economics, Cairns, Australia.

Hampson, A.W. (2002). Influenza virus antigens and 'antigenic drift'. In C.W. Potter (ed.), *Influenza: Perspectives in Medical Virology*, 7th edn. Amsterdam: Elsevier, pp. 49–85.

Hope, V. (2009). One World, One Health: where to from here? *Vetscript*, 22(9), 1–3.

Howell, M. (2006). *Proceedings of the 14th FAVA Congress and the Food Safety and Biosecurity, and Epidemiology and Animal Health Management Branches of the NZVA*. FCE Publication No. 253, January.

Hurt, A.C., Hansbro, P.M., Selleck, P., Olsen, B., Minton, C., Hampson, A.W. and Barr, I.G. (2006). Isolation of avian influenza viruses from two different trans-hemispheric migratory shorebird species in Australia. *Archives of Virology*, 151, 2301–2309.

Jones, K.E., Patel, N.G., Levy, M.A., Storygard, A., Balk, D., Gittleman, J.L. and Daszak, P. (2008). Global trends in emerging infectious diseases. *Nature*, 451, 990–993.

Kawaoka, J., Chambers, T.M., Sladen, W.L. and Webster, R.G.(1988). Is the gene pool of influenza viruses in shorebirds and gulls different from that in wild ducks? *Virology*, 163, 247–250.

Krauss, S. and Webster, R.G. (2010). Avian influenza virus surveillance and wild birds: past and present. *Avian Diseases*, 54(S1), 394–398.

Ksiazek, T.G., Erdman, D., Goldsmith, C.S., Zaki, S.R., Peret, T., Emery, S. et al. (2003). A novel coronavirus associated with severe acute respiratory syndrome. *New England Journal of Medicine*, 348(20), 1953–1966.

Langstaff, I.G., McKenzie, J.S., Stanislawek, W.L., Reed, C.E.M., Poland, R. and Cork, S.C. (2009). Surveillance for highly pathogenic avian influenza in migratory shorebirds at the terminus of the East Asian-Australasian Flyway. *New Zealand Veterinary Journal*, 57, 160–165.

Li, K.S., Guan, Y., Wang, J., Smith G.J.D., Xu, K.M., Duan, L., Rahardjo, A.P., Puthavathana, P., Buranathai, C., Nguyen, T.D., Esteopangestie, A.T.S., Chaisingh, A., Auewarakul, P., Long, H.T., Hanh, N.T.H., Webby, R.J., Poon, L.L.M., Chen, H., Shortridge, K.F., Yuen, K.Y., Webster, R.G., Peiris, J.S.M. (2004): Genesis of a highly pathogenic and potentially pandemic H5N1 influenza virus in eastern Asia. *Nature* 430, 209-213.

Lindstrom, S.E., Cox, N.J. and Klimov, A. (2004). Genetic analysis of human H2N2 and early H3N2 influenza viruses,1957–1972: evidence for genetic divergence and multiple reassortment events. *Virology*, 328, 101–119.

Lockhart, C.Y., Stevenson, M.A. and Rawdon, T.G. (2010a). A cross-sectional study of ownership of backyard poultry in two areas of Palmerton North, New Zealand. *New Zealand Veterinary Journal*, 58(3), 155–159.

Lockhart, C.Y., Stevenson, M.A., Rawdon, T.G., Gerber, N. and French, N.P. (2010b). Patterns of contact within the New Zealand poultry industry. *Preventative Veterinary Medicine*, 95, 258–266.

McFadden, A., Rawdon, T., Bingham, P. and Loth, L. (2007). Public reports of avian mortality. Part 2: spatial and temporal trends. *Surveillance*, 34(3), 14–17.

Ministry of Agriculture and Forestry (2006). *Technical Response Policies for Avian Influenza Viruses of Regulatory Concern (Version 2.4)*, www.biosecurity.govt.nz/files/pests/avian-influenza/response-policies.pdf.

Ministry of Agriculture and Forestry (2008) *MAF's Response to Risk Organisms*, www.biosecurity.govt.nz/files/biosec/policy-laws/response-policy-risk-organisms.pdf.

Ministry of Agriculture and Forestry (2011). *Whole-of-Government Biosecurity Response Guide*, August 2011 http://brkb.biosecurity.govt.nz/Portals/1/BRKB/Reference/whole-of-govt-bs-response-guide.pdf.

Neverov, A.D., Lezhnina, K.V., Kondrashov, A.S. and Bazykin, G.A. (2014). Intrasubtype reassortments cause adaptive amino acid replacements in H3N2 influenza genes. *PLOS Genetics*, 10(1), e1004037.

O'Keefe, J. (2009), H1N1 emergency response work at NCBID – Wallaceville. *Biosecurity*, 93, 20, www.biosecurity.govt.nz/files/biosec/pubs-media/pubs/biosecurity-magazine/issue-93/biosecurity-93.pdf.

Olsen, B., Munster, V.J., Wallensten, A., Waldenstrom, J., Osterhaus, A.D.M.E. and Fouchier, R.A.M. (2006). Global patterns of influenza A virus in wild birds. *Science*, 312, 384–388.

Pharo, H. (2003). The impact of new epidemiological information on a risk analysis for the introduction of avian influenza viruses in imported poultry meat. *Avian Diseases*, 47, 988–995.

Rawdon, T.G. and O'Leary, B. (2010). *Infectious Disease Modelling of New Zealand's Poultry Industry using InterSpread Plus*. Australian College of Veterinary Scientists – Epidemiology Chapter. Gold Coast, Queensland, Australia, 1–4 July.

Rawdon, T.G. and Stevenson, M.A. (2011). *Disease Spread Risk Associated with Backyard Poultry Movements in New Zealand*. Australian College of Veterinary Scientists – Epidemiology Chapter. Gold Coast, Queensland, Australia, 30 June–2 July.

Rawdon, T., Thornton, R., McKenzie, J. and Gerber, N. (2007a). Biosecurity risk pathways in New

Zealand's commercial poultry industry. *Surveillance*, 34(3), 4–9.

Rawdon, T., McFadden, A., Stanislawek, W.L. and Bingham, P. (2007b). Public reports of avian mortality. Part 1: Risk profiling and investigation. *Surveillance*, 34(3), 10–13.

Rawdon, T., Tana, T., Frazer, J., Thornton, R. and Chrystal, N. (2008). Biosecurity risk pathways in the commercial poultry industry: free-range layers, pullet-rearers and turkey broilers. *Surveillance*, 35(4), 4–9.

Rawdon, T., Zheng, T., Adlam, B., Williman, J. and Huang, S. (2012a). Disease risk pathways associated with backyard poultry-keeping in New Zealand. Part 1: animal health implications. *Surveillance*, 38(2), 12–19.

Rawdon, T., Zheng, T., Stanislawek, W., Adlam, B., Williman, J. and Huang, S. (2012b). Disease risk pathways associated with backyard poultry keeping in New Zealand. Part 2: human health implications. *Surveillance*, 39(1), 7–11.

Rawdon TG, Tana T, Thornton RN, McKenzie JS, Stanislawek WL, Kittelberger R, Geale D, Stevenson MA, Gerber N, Cork SC (2010) *Surveillance for avian influenza subtypes H5 and H7 in chickens and turkeys farmed commercially in New Zealand.* New Zealand Veterinary Journal, 58(6)

Rogers, G.N. and Paulson, J.C. (1983). Receptor determinants of human and animal influenza virus isolates: differences in receptor specificity of the H3 hemagglutinin based on species of origin. *Virology*, 127, 361–373.

Rooney, J. (2008). Avian and pandemic influenza preparedness activities: 2007. *Biosecurity Magazine*, 82(15).

Rott, R. (1992). The pathogenic determinant of influenza virus. *Veterinary Microbiology*, 33(1–4), 303–310.

Sanson, R.L. and Scott, D.J. (2003). Agribase and its potential for use in NZ traceability and verification. In *Proceedings of the 3rd Pan Commonwealth Veterinary Conference: Plenary Sessions and Proceedings of the Industry and Food Safety & Biosecurity Branches of the NZVA*. FCE Publication No. 231, pp 69–74.

Stanislawek, W.L. (1992). Survey of wild ducks for evidence of avian influenza virus, 1988–90. *Surveillance*, 19(1), 21–22.

Stanislawek, W.L., Wilks, C.R., Meers, J., Horner, G.W., Alexander, D.J., Manvell, R.J., Kattenbelt, J.A. and Gould, A.R. (2002). Avian paramyxoviruses and influenza viruses isolated from mallard ducks (*Anas patyrhynchos*) in New Zealand. *Archives of Virology*, 147(7), 1287–1302.

Stanislawek, W.L., Cork, S.C., Rawdon, T., Thornton, R.N. and Melville, D.S. (2007). Surveillance for avian influenza in wild birds in New Zealand. In *Conference Proceedings: Option for the Control of Influenza VI*, Toronto, Canada, pp. 358–360.

Stanislawek, W.L., Frazer, J., Rawdon, T., McFadden, A. and Lee, E. (2011). Avian influenza surveillance programme. *Surveillance*, 38(3), 19–21.

Stanislawek, W.L., McFadden, A. and Tana, T. (2013). Avian influenza surveillance programme. *Surveillance*, 40(3), 19–22.

Stevenson, M.A., Sanson, R.L., Stern, M.W., O'Leary, B.D., Sujau, M., Moles-Benfell, N. and Morris, R.S. (2013). InterSpread Plus: a spatial and stochastic simulation model of disease in animal populations. *Preventive Veterinary Medicine*, 109, 10–24.

Stieneke-Grober, A., Vey, M., Angliker, H., Shaw, E., Thomas, G., Roberts, G., Klenk, H.D. and Garten, W. (1992). Influenza virus hemagglutinin with multibasic cleavage site is activated by furin, a subtilisin-like endoprotease. *EMBO Journal*, 11(7), 2407–2414.

Suzuki, Y. (2005). Sialobiology of influenza: molecular mechanism of host range variation of influenza viruses. *Biological and Pharmaceutical Bulletin*, 28, 399–408.

Suzuki, Y., Ito, T., Suzuki, T., Holland, R.E., Chambers, T.M., Kiso, M., Ishida, H. and Kawaoka, Y. (2000). Sialic acid species as a determinant of the host range of influenza A viruses. *Journal of Virology*, 74, 11825–11831.

To, K.W.K., Tsang, A.K.L., Chan, J.F.W., Cheng, V.C.C., Chen, H. and Yuen, K.Y.Y. (2014). Emergence in China of human disease due to avian influenza A (H10N8) –cause for concern? *Journal of Infection*, 68, 205–215.

Vandergrift, K.J., Sokolow, S.H., Daszak, P. and Kilpatrick, A.M. (2010). Ecology of avian influenza viruses in a changing world. *Annals of the New York Academy of Sciences*, 1195, 113–128.

Walker, J.A., Sakaguchi, T., Matsuda, Y., Yoshida, T. and Kawaoka, Y. (1992). Location and character of the cellular enzyme that cleaves the hemagglutinin of a virulent avian influenza virus. *Virology*, 190(1), 278–287.

Webster, R.G., Bean, W.J., Gorman, O.T., Chambers, T.M. and Kawaoka, Y. (1992). Evolution and ecology of influenza viruses. *Microbiology Review*, 56, 152–179.

Williams, M., Gummer, H., Powlesland, R., Robertson H., and Taylor, G. (2006). *Migrations and Movements of Birds to New Zealand and Surrounding Seas.* Science and

Technical Publishing, Department of Conservation, PO Box 10–420, Wellington, New Zealand.

WHO (2008). *The Global Burden of Disease: 2004 Update*. Geneva: World Health Association Press.

WHO, FAO and OIE (2008). *Zoonotic Diseases: A Guide to Establishing Collaboration Between Animal and Human Health Sectors at the Country Level*, www.oie.int/doc/ged/D12060.PDF.

Zheng, T., Adlam, B., Rawdon, T.G., Stanislawek, W.L., Cork, S.C., Hope, V., Buddle, B.M., Grimwood, K., Baker, M.G., O'Keefe, J.S. and Huang, Q.S. (2010). A cross-sectional survey of influenza A infection, and management practices in small rural backyard poultry flocks in two regions of New Zealand. *New Zealand Veterinary Journal*, 58(2), 74–80.

chapter 4

Applying a One Health, multi-scale approach to understanding and preventing zoonotic parasite transmission in urban ecosystems: *Echinococcus multilocularis* and Alveolar echinococcosis in North America

Alessandro Massolo and Stefano Liccioli

Abstract

Echinococcus multilocularis is an emerging zoonotic parasite of the family Taenidae, and it is the causative agent of alveolar echinococcosis (AE) in humans, a disease with a case mortality rate of up to 90 per cent when untreated. The natural cycle of the disease involves wild canids as definitive hosts and rodents that serve as intermediate hosts. Infection of humans occurs by accidental ingestion of parasite eggs through contaminated food or close interactions with infected domestic dogs. In this chapter we describe the complex transmission dynamics of *E. multilocularis* at the interface of wildlife, domestic animals, humans and the environment, focusing on the emerging situation in a North American urban setting. We describe key ecological and socioeconomic factors that affect parasite distribution and the subsequent risk for humans at different geographical (*local*, *regional* and *global*) and temporal (*seasonal* and *pluriannual*) scales. We also present various parasite control and risk management options based on a hazard analysis and critical control point (HACCP) approach.

4.1 Introduction

Echinococcus multilocularis is a parasitic cestode of the family Taenidae, and it is the causative agent of alveolar echinococcosis (AE) in humans, a disease with a case mortality rate of up to 90 per cent when untreated (Craig et al., 1996).

Infection of humans occurs by accidental ingestion of parasite eggs through contaminated food or close interactions with infected domestic dogs (Salb et al., 2008; Vaniscotte et al., 2011; Massolo et al., 2014). According to a 2014 report of the World Health Organization (WHO) and the UN's Food and Agriculture Organization (FAO), *E. multilocularis* represents the third most significant food-borne parasite worldwide (FAO and WHO, 2014). Alveolar echinococcosis is estimated to affect more than 18,000 people each year on a global scale, with more than 90 per cent of these cases recorded in China (Torgerson et al., 2010), but with increasing rates in Europe since the 1990s (Davidson et al., 2012; Deplazes et al., 2015). Effectiveness of medical treatment for AE has improved in recent decades, and the reduction of life expectancy due to AE in 2005 (2–4 years) is significantly improved from what was observed in the 1970s (reduction of 18–20 years) (Torgerson et al., 2008). However, AE is still a severe disease that requires long-term (often lifelong) and highly expensive medical treatment (McManus et al., 2003; Vuitton et al., 2011). This is aggravated by (1) the high incidence of the disease in areas of the world where public healthcare is limited (e.g., China) and many infected people might not have access to proper diagnosis (Torgerson et al., 2010; Hegglin and Deplazes, 2013); (2) the pathogen cannot be eradicated, and that control is costly and temporary (Hegglin and Deplazes, 2008, 2013); and (3) the long latency (5–15 years) in human patients, which further complicates epidemiological studies (Craig et al., 1996).

In North America, besides the cases documented in the historic AE hotspot of St Lawrence Island (Alaska) (Rausch and Schiller, 1954, 1956; Fay and Rausch, 1964; Rausch et al., 1990a, 1990b), only two other cases of AE were reported as being locally acquired, until the most recent finding in Edmonton, Alberta, Canada (Massolo et al., 2014). Even though *E. multilocularis* is quite widely distributed in North America and its prevalence can be fairly high in wild hosts, it is unclear why only few human cases have been discovered until now (Massolo et al., 2014; Jenkins et al., 2015).

Echinococcus multilocularis relies on a complex transmission cycle involving domestic or wild canids as definitive hosts and small rodents and few lagomorph species as intermediate hosts

(Figure 4.1). The cycle is primarily sylvatic (i.e., maintained by wild host species), but in some circumstances (e.g., China) domestic dogs can play a relevant role in spreading and transmitting the parasite (Moss et al., 2013).

The transmission ecology of *E. multilocularis* is determined by the predator–prey interactions between definitive and intermediate hosts that occur at various geographical and temporal scales. These complex interactions between host(s), the parasite and the environment affect the degree of environmental contamination and the subsequent disease risk for people (Giraudoux et al., 2003, 2007). From the very first cases of AE diagnosed in Germany in 1855 (Vuitton et al., 2011) to the most recent discovery of numerous human cases in a hyper-endemic area in rural China (Craig et al., 1992, 2000), it has become evident that the degree of human exposure also depends on a number of socioeconomic factors (e.g., hygiene, dog management, type of vegetable cultivations; McManus et al., 2003; Torgerson et al., 2010). This can be particularly relevant in population dense urban settings (Liccioli et al., 2015a), where the proximity of the parasite to people and pets may further increase the risk of zoonotic transmission.

For these reasons, tackling *E. multilocularis* represents a challenge well-suited for a multidisciplinary, collaborative and coordinated approach. In the following study we illustrate the value of applying the One Health framework to protect the health of animals, humans and the environment.

This chapter aims to describe the complex system that characterizes the transmission dynamics of *E. multilocularis* at the interface of wildlife, domestic animals and humans, focusing on the emerging situation in North American urban settings. We will examine the key ecological and socioeconomic factors that affect parasite distribution and risk for public health at different geographical scales (local, regional and global) and various parasite control and risk management options will be explored.

In addition we present a framework, based on a hazard analysis and critical control point (HACCP) approach at multiple temporal and spatial scales, to help develop risk mitigation options to prevent the potential emergence (or re-emergence) of this parasite in urban settings in North America.

4.2 Disease ecology

The lifecycle of Echinococcus multilocularis

Echinococcus multilocularis is a dixenous (i.e., requiring two hosts to complete its development) cestode that is typically maintained in a sylvatic lifecycle (Figure 4.1) involving wild and domestic canids (i.e., foxes *Vulpes* spp., coyote *Canis latrans* and wolf *Canis lupus*; domestic and sylvatic dogs) as definitive hosts, and small mammals (mainly rodents and pikas) as intermediate hosts (Eckert and Deplazes, 2004).

In the definitive host, adults of *E. multilocularis* develop in the small intestine. Eggs of the parasite are shed through the faeces into the environment, where they can be accidentally ingested by an intermediate host. After the eggs hatch in the intestine, the larval stage migrates to the target organs and develop in to the cystic stage (i.e. metacestode). In intermediate hosts, the multiplication of metacestodes causes a multivesicular and infiltrating structure that grows rapidly and brings the development of the infectious stages (protoscolices) in 2–4 months (Eckert and Deplazes, 2004). At advanced stages of infection, the larval mass may extend through a metastatic process from the liver (the main target organ) to other organs of the abdominal cavity (e.g., spleen, pancreas, gastrointestinal tract) and reproductive organs as the structure grows (McManus et al., 2003). The parasite completes its cycle when infectious intermediate hosts are ingested by the competent definitive host, i.e., canids. Humans typically act as dead-end (i.e., accidental) hosts,

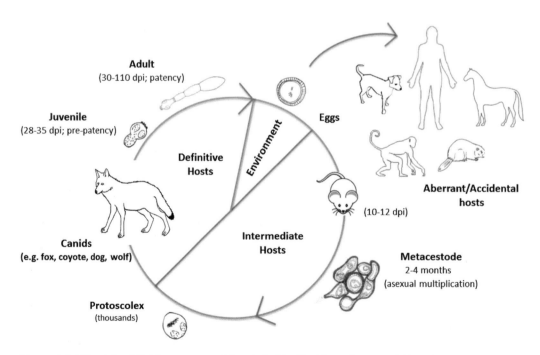

Figure 4.1 Life cycle of *Echinococcus multilocularis*. Modified from Gesy et al. (2013).

who acquire infection by ingesting parasite eggs through contaminated food (e.g., berries and vegetables), soil, or through direct contact with faecal material from infected dogs (McManus et al., 2003).

4.3 The ecology of *Echinococcus multilocularis* in North America

Given the broad latitudinal distribution of the parasite across North America (Gesy et al., 2013), wild hosts of *E. multilocularis* are very diverse depending primarily on the local predator–prey communities. In the Northern Tundra Zone (NTZ) of Alaska and Northern Canada, the parasite is historically maintained in a cycle involving the arctic fox *Vulpes lagopus* and its prey species, such as the northern vole *Microtus oeconomus*, the brown lemming *Lemmus sibiricus* and the northern red-backed vole *Myodes rutilus* (Massolo et al., 2014). After the 1960s, parasitological surveys have progressively delineated a second area of distribution – the Northern Central Region (NCR) – which today includes up to 13 states in the USA (North Dakota, South Dakota, Iowa, Minnesota, Montana, Wyoming, Nebraska, Illinois, Wisconsin, Indiana, Ohio, Missouri and Michigan), the prairie provinces of Canada (Alberta, Saskatchewan and Manitoba) and most recently, British Columbia (see Massolo et al., 2014, for a review).

The parasite exists globally in 18 different strains or genotypes (Nakao et al., 2009; Massolo et al., 2014), two of which are considered characteristic of North America (N1, Tundra zone and Alaska; N2, Central region; Nakao et al., 2009). However, while two Asian mitochondrial haplotypes have been reported in St Lawrence Island, Alaska (Nakao et al., 2009), recent research has provided evidence of European haplotypes in wild hosts in Canada (British Columbia, Alberta and Saskatchewan; Jenkins et al., 2012; Gesy et al., 2014; Massolo et al., 2014). This finding

has potential consequences for public health (Jenkins et al., 2012; Massolo et al., 2014), given that genetic differences among strains are hypothesized to be associated with variability in development and pathogenicity of larval stages (Bartel et al., 1992).

In the ecosystems of the central region of North America, coyotes and red foxes are the main definitive hosts, while the deer mouse (*Peromyscus maniculatus*) and meadow vole (*Microtus pennsylvanicus*) are considered to be the most important intermediate hosts (Eckert and Deplazes, 2004), although other species may become locally relevant depending on habitat characteristics as is the case for the southern red-backed vole (*Myodes gapperi*) (Liccioli et al., 2013).

Scientific evidence is still needed to ascertain whether the range of the parasite in North America is actually expanding, or whether it has instead passed undetected in previous studies (Davidson et al., 2012). However, coyotes have dramatically expanded their range in North America (40 per cent expansion in the past 50 years; Laliberte and Ripple, 2004), and have become increasingly common in urban areas (Baker and Timm, 1998). Today, aside from human–wildlife conflict issues (e.g., coyotes are considered by some as nuisance animals due to predation on pets, and to safety and health issues; Gehrt et al., 2009, 2010). Their presence inside urban settings has become a potential concern with regard to their role in the circulation of *E. multilocularis*, especially in recreational areas highly utilized by people and their dogs (Catalano et al., 2012; Liccioli et al., 2014). Indeed, the growth of urban red fox populations in the 1990s have been linked to the increase of AE incidence observed in endemic areas of Europe such as Lithuania (Bružinskaitė et al., 2007) and Switzerland (Schweiger et al., 2007).

Several ecological factors influence the presence and transmission dynamics of *E. multilocularis* in urban settings. Infection in definitive and intermediate hosts varies spatially within a region, with areas of low parasite occurrence interspersed with pockets characterized by high parasite prevalence (Liccioli et al., 2014). Preliminary results suggest that local variations in the proportion of competent intermediate host species in the prey assemblage are significant in the development of foci of hyper-endemicity (Liccioli et al., 2014), thus further stressing the importance of considering the entire range of available prey species (Giraudoux et al., 2003; Liccioli et al., 2015a; Baudrot et al., 2016), as opposed to approaches focused on the abundance of intermediate host population alone (Saitoh and Takahashi, 1998; Raoul et al., 2010). Habitat characteristics determining the local distribution and relative abundance of small mammal species influence the epidemiology of the parasite. Furthermore, infection rates of small mammal intermediate hosts are reported to fluctuate temporally, in accordance with their population dynamics and seasonal variations of climatic conditions. Specifically, highest prevalence is documented during fall and winter (Liccioli et al., 2014), when the age structure of intermediate host populations is highly skewed towards adult classes (which had longer exposure to parasite eggs; Burlet et al., 2011) and the survival of parasite eggs in the environment is longer (Veit et al., 1995). Other factors possibly influence the epidemiology of the parasite on a number of levels. At the individual level, host susceptibility may further increase the heterogeneity of parasite infection. At a landscape scale, the configuration and connectivity of natural patches within urban settings are likely to influence parasite transmission (Liccioli et al., 2015a). Indeed, gradients in urban densities (e.g., high-density versus low-density residential areas) may affect habitat permeability to hosts (and parasite) movements within urban green areas (e.g., Adkins and Stott, 1998), and between city settings and surrounding habitats (Beier and Noss, 1998). Similarly, urban landscape composition may affect the diversity of the host community, with important

consequences on the dynamics and resilience of parasite transmission (Giraudoux et al., 2007).

Although recent work has significantly advanced our knowledge of *E. multilocularis* in North America (Catalano et al., 2012; Liccioli et al., 2012, 2013, 2014, 2015b; Gesy et al., 2013, 2014; Klein and Massolo, 2015; Massolo et al., 2014), further research is needed to fully understand the ecology of this parasite in urban settings. In particular, future research efforts should focus on (1) the role of rural areas in the maintenance of the urban lifecycle of the parasite; (2) predator response to variations in small mammal assemblages; (3) differences in intermediate and definitive host susceptibility to parasite infection; and (4) the role of definitive host community composition and intra species competition.

4.4 Socioeconomic determinants of disease transmission

Although *E. multilocularis* is typically maintained in a sylvatic lifecycle, the risk of zoonotic transmission can be highly dependent on social and economic factors (Rausch et al., 1990b; Craig et al., 1996; Vuitton et al., 2003). This likely explains why the highest incidence of AE is observed in the rural communities of the Tibetan plateau (China Autonomous Region), where financial resources are limited (per capita annual income < US$500; Budke et al., 2005b) and education and hygiene are poor (Craig et al., 1992). In these settings, domestic dogs can play an important role in the parasite lifecycle and are often the primary source of infection of humans (Craig et al., 2000; Budke et al., 2005a) due to their close contact with owners. Analogous socioeconomic conditions were found in the historically infected area of St Lawrence Island (Alaska), where the incidence of AE in humans during 1950–1990 was among the highest ever recorded in the world, ranging from seven to

98 cases/100,000 inhabitants (Nakao et al., 2009; Rausch and Schiller, 1956; Rausch et al., 1990a, 1990b; Schantz et al. 1995). However, the situation is generally much different in the rest of North America, where only three locally acquired cases of AE have been described, with the latest occurrence documented in 2013 in an immunosuppressed patient in Alberta (Massolo et al., 2014). Although human cases seem to be generally very rare, lack of data and possible misdiagnosis (Somily et al., 2005; Massolo et al., 2014) severely limit the current knowledge about the impact of AE in North America (Massolo et al., 2014).

At present, there is no reliable information available to assess the risk of human infection occurring through direct contact with domestic dogs exposed to the parasite within urban areas. Indeed, the only published study that evaluated the role of dogs in the circulation of *E. multilocularis* refers to a control programme conducted in St Lawrence Island (Rausch et al., 1990b). However, preliminary results available for the metropolitan area of Calgary, Canada, suggest that in urban parks – and hyper-endemic areas in particular – the infection risk in dogs is not negligible (Massolo et al., 2014).

4.5 Parasite control and management of risk

As the parasite's natural reservoir is mainly represented by wildlife species, AE is considered a not-eradicable disease (Ito et al., 2003), for which disease prevention is the most effective solution (Hegglin and Deplazes, 2013). Frequent anthelmintic treatment of dogs – to be achieved through increased awareness of public and veterinary practitioners – certainly represents one of the management strategies to be implemented at the individual and community level (Hegglin and Deplazes, 2013; Takahashi et al., 2013; Massolo et al., 2014). Locally, anthelmintic treatment of wild reservoir species (i.e., foxes) has achieved interesting results in Japan (Takahashi et al., 2013) and Europe (Hegglin and Deplazes, 2008, 2013), although only in the short term unless regular treatment is maintained. Nonetheless, treatment of wild definitive hosts is still considered one of the few actions that could be undertaken to reduce the prevalence and hence the subsequent risk of zoonotic transmission (König et al., 2008).

At a regional scale, landscape changes (e.g., deforestation) can have dramatic effects on wildlife population dynamics, host densities and parasite prevalence, and thus ultimately can influence parasite transmission dynamics. Although empirical data are available for high endemic areas of China and Europe (Giraudoux et al., 2003, 2007; Vuitton et al., 2003), such information has not been obtained yet for North America.

At a global scale, humans have a very important role in shaping the distribution of *E. multilocularis*. The presence in North America of genetic variants closely related to European strains (Gesy et al., 2013) could suggest that pet travel has had an influence on the globalization of the parasite (Davidson et al., 2012). If this is the case, further introduction of new strains of the parasite is possible unless preventive measures and regulation (i.e., mandatory anthelmintic treatment of dogs imported from outside North America) will be established (Massolo et al., 2014).

4.6 Conceptual model of a One Health, multi-scale approach

The framework presented below is based on the hazard analysis and critical control points (HACCP) approach. HACCP (www.fda.gov/Food/GuidanceRegulation/HACCP/default.htm), is based on a series of steps: (1) hazard analysis; (2) critical control points (CCPs); (3)

critical limits; (4) monitoring procedures; (5) corrective actions; (6) verification procedures; and (7) record-keeping and documentation procedures. Although more typically used in food safety quality control (FAO 1997; www.fao.org/docrep/005/y1579e/y1579e03.htm), we have applied a modified HACCP to parasitic transmission excluding some of the typical steps in HACCP (6 and 7).

Ecological mechanisms and processes are spatially and temporally distributed. In this chapter we propose a multi-scale and temporally explicit approach for identifying hazards and critical control points to mitigate the risk of *E. multilocularis* transmission using the Calgary urban setting as a model.

We identify three key spatial scales (Figure 4.2):

1. *Local* (i.e., city, or district-wide). At this scale, different city parks may be characterized by different parasite prevalence in sylvatic hosts, thus affecting the risk for dogs to get infected during their off-leash activities and,

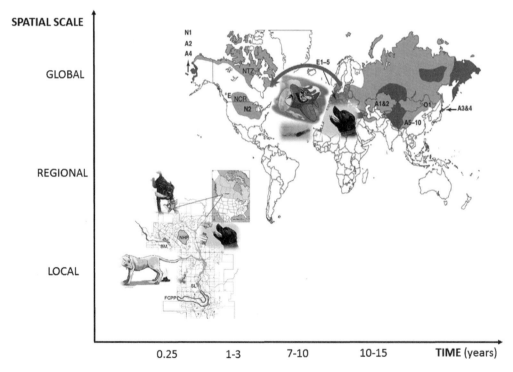

Figure 4.2 Spatial and temporal scales of corrective actions and monitoring of the critical control points for the management of *Echinococcus multilocularis* infection risk. Modified from Catalano et al. (2012) and Torgerson et al. (2010). Illustrations by James Butler; http://jamb-art.blogspot.co.uk. At a local scale, interventions in city parks to reduce the prevalence in definitive hosts (baiting of wild canids and deworming of domestic dogs using an effective anthelmintic) are to be conducted on seasonal or annual basis. At regional scale, deworming of dogs and monitoring of human cases are the actions to be implemented in one to three years, whereas at global scale, policy of deworming dogs that travel from areas of endemism (grey and dark grey areas) of different strains should be developed and implemented in a medium-long timescale (10–15 years) to avoid the spread of the different strains across the globe.

consequently, for people to be exposed through their dogs.

2. *Regional* (i.e., provincial or regional). At this scale the parasite is distributed within the population or metapopulations of definitive hosts, and the processes of diffusion or invasion of allochthonous (i.e., originating in a different place) parasite strains may occur.

3. *Global* (i.e., continental and intercontinental). At this scale are the socioeconomic processes (e.g., wild and domestic canid mobility for trade or personal purposes) that facilitates invasions of allochthonous strains (or species) across or among continent/s.

We also identified critical time windows.

1. At *local* scale, most of the transmission among sylvatic hosts likely occurs in the *winter* (transmission from rodents to coyotes and potentially to dogs) and late *summer* (transmission from coyotes to rodents) seasons.

2. At *regional* and *global* scales, there is no specific time at which the processes seem to occur, but monitoring should be carried out over *several years* to monitor the potential emergence of new human cases.

HACCP analysis: Calgary as a case study

Local scale

HAZARD IDENTIFICATION
At this scale the main hazard is the presence of infectious intermediate hosts that is directly related to their relative abundance (relative to the overall small mammal assemblage that coyotes and dogs can prey upon) and affects the risk for coyotes and dogs to get infected.

CRITICAL CONTROL POINTS (CCPs)
Parasite prevalence in definitive and intermediate hosts are typically correlated. As prevalence

in definitive hosts is much (10–100 times) higher than in intermediate hosts, the former should be used as critical control point.

CRITICAL LIMITS
• Winter/spring prevalence in coyotes (definitive host) in parks should be <40±5 per cent (i.e., significantly below average regional prevalence).
• Winter/spring prevalence in dogs (definitive hosts) should be ≤0.5 per cent (0/300 examined dogs).

MONITORING PROCEDURES
Routine faecal collection of coyotes and dogs should be conducted in parks that are mostly used by owners to walk their dogs off-leash and that are used by resident coyotes during the winter and spring seasons. Faeces should be then submitted to screening for presence of *Taeniidae* eggs and positive cases submitted to further molecular analysis for species confirmation.

CORRECTIVE ACTIONS
At this scale, the interventions should be focused primarily on the main reservoir species (coyote), and on dogs that may act as a vector for the parasite into houses.

1. Deworming campaign:

   a. Implement deworming of wild host canids with anthelmintic baits in the parks where prevalence in coyotes or dogs is above the critical limits.
   b. Promote contemporary deworming of dogs at risk (walked off-leash and chasing mice) through information campaigns to dog-owners and veterinarians.

2. Enforcing dog management rules:

   a. Be in control of dogs even when off-leash and impede them from predating/eating mice, as rodents affected by *E. multilocularis* are very likely to be preyed upon or found dead.

b. 'Pick up after your dog' to reduce spread of *E. multilocularis* eggs from dogs.

TEMPORAL SCALE

Anthelmintic baiting should be implemented just before and during winter, when most of the transmission to definitive hosts is known to occur in this ecosystem.

Monitoring of the status of infections in wild hosts should be: (1) implemented and carried out on a yearly basis during a single season (late winter–early spring) to optimize the likelihood to detect the peaks of infections in definitive hosts; (2) carried out consecutively for three years after the control campaign, and (3) if successful, carried out on a 3–4 years basis (corresponding to a likely turnover of the resident population of urban coyotes).

KEY AGENCIES AND STAKEHOLDERS INVOLVED

Monitoring and corrective actions should be implemented by a local government agency (e.g., municipality) in collaboration with animal and bylaws services and Fish and Wildlife. The engagement of animal health professionals (i.e., Veterinarian Association) is key to promoting and implementing deworming and education campaigns.

Regional scale

At regional scale the priority is to keep the number of human cases of alveolar echinococcosis locally acquired (i.e., not caused by infections acquired abroad) to zero. Implementation of personal hygiene for at risk categories, in particular immuno-depressed patients, is key.

HAZARD IDENTIFICATION

Hazards that should be monitored include the ingestion of contaminated food (i.e., berries or vegetables) and the presence of the European strain, which is known to be highly pathogenic for humans.

CRITICAL LIMITS

• The incidence of human cases of alveolar echinococcosis locally acquired should be equal to zero.

MONITORING PROCEDURES

Human patients that show undiagnosed hepatic lesions or anomalies should be tested for AE through immunohisto-chemistry testing and liver biopsies (histological and molecular diagnostic tools). Monitoring immune-depressed patients is priority as they can be considered as sentinels of AE outbreaks in new geographical regions (Chauchet et al., 2014). Collaboration with the healthcare services is critical in this phase.

CORRECTIVE ACTIONS

• General public education campaigns on foodborne transmission and deworming of dogs for at-risk owner categories.

• Inform dog owners of the risk of travelling with dogs in highly endemic areas (e.g., Central Europe, Asia) and promote deworming of dogs exposed to such strains.

TEMPORAL SCALE

Initially, continuous actions and monitoring should be implemented for a minimum of ten years, and follow-ups should be planned on a five-year basis.

KEY AGENCIES AND STAKEHOLDERS INVOLVED

State or provincial government/s should be engaged to promote education and information campaigns. The healthcare system/s should be engaged to prospectively monitor new cases and retrospectively investigate possible misdiagnosed cases. Importantly, information sessions with health professionals (e.g., surgeons, diagnostic professionals, infectious disease specialists) should be promoted.

At this level, veterinary associations can play an important role in educating customers on proper deworming practices. As with the healthcare system, information sessions should be promoted to inform the animal health professionals of the new information available on the parasite.

Global scale

Invasion of allochthonous and potentially more pathogenic strains of *E. multilocularis* from Europe and Asia through dog movements (e.g., rescued dogs and owned dogs) is likely happening or to happen (see Figure 4.2), as no policy is in place to impose deworming of dogs before travel (see Canada Food Inspection agency, www.inspection.gc.ca).

Regulating the translocation of potential hosts (e.g., dogs and foxes) is key for preventing the risk of introducing these new strains or new host species within new ecosystems and animal communities.

HAZARD
Introduction of allochthonous strains (or allochthonous species) of *E. multilocularis* that may have a higher level of virulence for humans.

CRITICAL LIMITS
No imported/travelling canids should be positive for *E. multilocularis*.

CORRECTIVE ACTIONS
Implement a policy for deworming of canids when from areas with different strains of *E. multilocularis*.

MONITORING PROCEDURES
Imported canids should be randomly tested for *E. multilocularis* at their arrival to make sure the prevalence is below the critical threshold.

TEMPORAL SCALE
Continuous actions and monitoring should be implemented for a minimum of ten years, and follow-ups should be planned on a five-year basis. Implementation of new policies on mandatory of anthelmintic treatment on canids translocated from Asian or European endemic areas may take longer and so a longer timeline might be expected.

KEY AGENCIES AND STAKEHOLDERS INVOLVED
National and international agencies should be engaged (e.g., Canadian Food Inspection Agency, European committee), along with government and non-government agencies that assess the health risk and develop import health standards for dogs coming from endemic countries such as China and Europe.

4.7 Conclusions and recommendations

Recent research on the epidemiology of AE and the ecology of *E. multilocularis* worldwide has emphasized the value of undertaking surveillance studies aimed at detecting areas of higher risk for zoonotic transmission. From a management standpoint, field studies based on the collection and analysis of faecal samples collected from wild and domestic carnivores are invaluable, as they provide information on local environmental contamination (Deplazes et al., 2004). Sites with hyper-endemicity in wild hosts represent areas where intervention strategies could be attempted or prioritized.

Although very difficult to prevent, the risk of exposure to *E. multilocularis* can be reduced with simple interventions and by involving different government/regulatory agencies and stakeholders. Mostly, education on food hygiene and deworming of dogs are the two key interventions that should be implemented at local and regional scales. At a more local scale, the critical intervention is reducing the level of infection in wild canids and domestic dogs. To achieve this, intervention should focus on deworming campaigns of local wild and domestic host populations, as well as preventing dogs from at risk behaviours (i.e., chasing and predating upon mice). Field data identified fall and winter as the seasons during which infection of definitive hosts is more likely to occur, so baiting programmes should ideally take place just before and during winter.

At a larger scale, the effects of translocations of domestic and wild hosts should be regulated and mandatory anthelmintic treatments implemented between areas where different strains are endemic. Current policies on the import and export of domestic dogs should be reassessed to include treating (with proper follow-up) for *E. multilocularis*.

At present, we believe that it is a priority to understand what the current incidence of human AE in North America is, and we recommend that regional authorities collaborate with research groups to conduct retrospective studies to assess the cases that have been misdiagnosed or simply not diagnosed (Somily et al., 2005; Massolo et al., 2014). Similarly, it is a priority to provide adequate information to animal and human health professionals to help prevent infections in dogs, and support early detection of human infections of alveolar echinococcosis.

Through this case study we wanted to illustrate the importance of taking a One Health, multi-scale approach to identify and mitigate disease risks to humans associated with an emerging zoonotic parasite (*Echinococcus multilocularis*). Identifying critical control points at different spatial and temporal scales to prevent disease transmission is a key component of an effective disease prevention and control programme. To implement such an approach, we need to engage a multidisciplinary team made of animal and human public health professionals, experts in ecology, parasitology, veterinary medicine, human medicine, as well as managers in charge of policy development and implementation at local, regional and global scales.

References

Adkins, C.A. and Stott, P. (1998). Home ranges, movements and habitat associations of red foxes *Vulpes vulpes* in suburban Toronto, Ontario, Canada. *Journal of Zoology*, 244(3), 335–346.

Baker, R.O. and Timm, R.M. (1998). Management of conflicts between urban coyotes and humans in Southern California. *Proceedings of the Vertebrate Pest Conference*, 18, 299–312.

Bartel, M.H., Seesee, F.M. and Worley, D.E. (1992). Comparison of Montana and Alaska isolates of *Echinococcus multilocularis* in gerbils with observations on the cyst growth, hook characteristics, and host response. *Journal of Parasitology*, 78(3), 529–532.

Baudrot, V., Perasso, A., Fritsch, C., Raoul, F (2016) Competence of hosts and complex foraging behavior are two cornerstones in the dynamics of tropically transmitted parasites. *Journal of Theoretical Biology*. 397, 158–168.

Beier, P. and Noss, R.F. (1998). Do habitat corridors provide connectivity? *Conservation Biology*, 12(6), 1241–1252.

Bružinskaitė, R., Marcinkutė, A., Strupas, K., Sokolovas, V., Deplazes, P., Mathis, A., Eddi, C. and Šarkūnas, M. (2007). Alveolar echinococcosis, Lithuania. *Emerging Infectious Diseases*, 13(10), 1618–1619.

Budke, C.M., Campos-Ponce, M., Qian, W. and Torgerson, P.R. (2005a). A canine purgation study and risk factor analysis for echinococcosis in a high endemic region of the Tibetan plateau. *Veterinary Parasitology*, 127(1), 43–49.

Budke, C.M., Jiamin, Q., Qian, W. and Torgerson,P.R. (2005b). Economic effects of echinococcosis in a disease-endemic region of the Tibetan Plateau. *The American Journal of Tropical Medicine and Hygiene*, 73(1), 2–10.

Burlet, P., Deplazes, P. and Hegglin, D. (2011). Age, season and spatio-temporal factors affecting the prevalence of *Echinococcus multilocularis* and *Taenia taeniaeformis* in *Arvicola terrestris*. *Parasites & Vectors*, 4, 6.

Catalano, S., Lejeune, M., Liccioli, S., Verocai, G.G., Gesy, K.M., Jenkins, E.J., Kutz, S.J., Fuentealba, C.,

Duignan, P.J. and Massolo, A. (2012). *Echinococcus multilocularis* in urban coyotes, Alberta, Canada. *Emerging Infectious Diseases*, 18(10), 1625–1628.

Chauchet, A., Grenouillet, F., Knapp, J., Richou, C., Delabrousse, E., Dentan, C., Millon, L., Di Martino, V., Contreras, R., Deconinck, E., Blagosklonov, O., Vuitton, D.A. and Bresson-Hadni, S. (2014). Increased incidence and characteristics of alveolar echinococcosis in patients with immunosuppression-associated conditions. *Clinical Infectious Diseases*, 59(8),1095–1104.

Craig, P.S., Deshan, L., MacPherson, C.N., Dazhong, S., Reynolds, D., Barnish, G., Gottstein, B. and Zhirong, W. (1992). A large focus of alveolar echinococcosis in central China. *Lancet*, 340(8823), 826–831.

Craig, P.S., Rogan, M.T. and Allan, J.C. (1996). Detection, screening and community epidemiology of taeniid cestode zoonoses: cystic echinococcosis, alveolar echinococcosis and neurocysticercosis. *Advances in Parasitology*, 38, 169–250.

Craig, P.S., Giraudoux, P., Shi, D., Bartholomot, B., Barnish, G., Delattre, P., Quere, J.P., Harraga, S., Bao, G., Wang, Y., Lu, F., Ito, A. and Vuitton, D.A. (2000). An epidemiological and ecological study of human alveolar echinococcosis transmission in south Gansu, China. *Acta Tropica*, 77(2), 167–177.

Davidson, R.K., Romig, T., Jenkins, E., Tryland, M. and Robertson, L.J. (2012). The impact of globalisation on the distribution of *Echinococcus multilocularis*. *Trends in Parasitology*, 28(6), 239–247.

Deplazes, P., Hagglin, D., Gloor, S. and Romig, T. (2004). Wilderness in the city: the urbanization of *Echinococcus multilocularis*. *Trends in Parasitology*, 20(2), 77–84.

Deplazes, P., Gottstein, B. and Junghanss, T. (2015). Alveolar and cystic echinococcosis in Europe: old burdens and new challenges. *Veterinary Parasitology*, 213(3–4), 73–75.

Eckert, J. and Deplazes, P. (2004). Biological, epidemiological, and clinical aspects of Echinococcosis, a zoonosis of increasing concern. *Clinical Microbiology Reviews*, 17(1), 107–135.

FAO (1997). *Hazard Analysis and Critical Control Point (HACCP) System and Guidelines for its Application: The Codex Alimentarius Commission and the FAO/WHO Food Standards*. Rome: FAO, Corporate Document Repository.

FAO and WHO (2014). *Multicriteria-Based Ranking for Risk Management of Food-Borne Parasites*. Rome: FAO.

Fay, F.H. and Rausch, R.L. (1964). The seasonal cycle of abundance of *Echinococcus multilocularis* in naturally infected Arctic foxes. In *Proceedings of the First International Congress of Parasitology*. London: Pergamon Press, pp. 465–476.

Gehrt, S.D., Anchor, C. and White, L.A. (2009). Home range and landscape use of coyotes in a metropolitan landscape: conflict or coexistence? *Journal of Mammalogy*, 90(5), 1045–1057.

Gehrt, S.D., Riley, S.P.D. and Cypher, B.L. (2010). *Urban Carnivores: Ecology, Conflict, and Conservation*. Baltimore: Johns Hopkins University Press.

Gesy, K., Hill, J.E., Schwantje, H., Liccioli, S. and Jenkins, E.J. (2013). Establishment of a European-type strain of *Echinococcus multilocularis* in Canadian wildlife. *Parasitology*, 140(9), 1133–1137.

Gesy, K.M., Schurer, J.M., Massolo, A., Liccioli, S., Elkin, B.T., Alisauskas, R. and Jenkins, E.J. (2014). Unexpected diversity of the cestode *Echinococcus multilocularis* in wildlife in Canada. *International Journal for Parasitology: Parasites and Wildlife*, 3(2), 81–87.

Giraudoux, P., Craig, P.S., Delattre, P., Bao, G., Bartholomot, B., Harraga, S., Quere, J.P., Raoul, F., Wang, Y., Shi, D. and Vuitton, D.A. (2003). Interactions between landscape changes and host communities can regulate *Echinococcus multilocularis* transmission. *Parasitology*, 127, S121–S131.

Giraudoux, P., Pleydell, D., Raoul, F., Vaniscotte, A., Ito, A. and Craig, P.S. (2007). *Echinococcus multilocularis*: why are multidisciplinary and multiscale approaches essential in infectious disease ecology? *Tropical Medicine and Health*, 35(4), 293–299.

Hegglin, D. and Deplazes, P. (2008). Control strategy for *Echinococcus multilocularis*. *Emerging Infectious Diseases*, 14(10), 1626–1628.

Hegglin, D. and Deplazes, P. (2013). Control of *Echinococcus multilocularis*: strategies, feasibility and cost-benefit analyses. *International Journal for Parasitology*, 43(5), 327–337.

Ito, A., Romig, T. and Takahashi, K. (2003). Perspective on control options for *Echinococcus multilocularis* with particular reference to Japan. *Parasitology*, 127, S159–S172.

Jenkins, E.J., Peregrine, A.S., Hill, J.E., Somers, C., Gesy, K., Barnes, B., Gottstein, B. and Polley, L. (2012). Detection of European strain of *Echinococcus multilocularis* in North America. *Emerging Infectious Diseases*, 18(6), 1010–1012.

Jenkins, E.J., Simon, A., Bachand, N. and Stephen, C. (2015). Wildlife parasites in a One Health world. *Trends in Parasitology*, 31(5), 174–180.

Klein, C. and Massolo, A. (2015). Demonstration that a case of human alveolar echinococcosis in

Minnesota in 1977 was caused by the N2 strain. *American Journal of Tropical Medicine and Hygene*, 92(3), 477–478.

König, A., Romig, T., Janko, C., Hildenbrand, R., Holzhofer, E., Kotulski, Y., Ludt, C., Merli, M., Eggenhofer, S., Thoma, D., Vilsmeier, J. and Zannantonio, D. (2008). Integrated-baiting concept against *Echinococcus multilocularis* in foxes is successful in southern Bavaria, Germany. *European Journal of Wildlife Research*, 54(3), 439–447.

Laliberte, A.S. and Ripple, W.J. (2004). Range contractions of North American carnivores and ungulates. *BioScience*, 54(2), 123–138.

Liccioli, S., Catalano, S., Kutz, S.J., Lejeune, M., Verocai, G.G., Duignan, P.J., Fuentealba, C., Hart, M., Ruckstuhl, K.E. and Massolo, A. (2012). Gastrointestinal parasites of coyotes (*Canis latrans*) in the metropolitan area of Calgary, Alberta, Canada. *Canadian Journal of Zoology – Revue Canadienne De Zoologie*, 90(8), 1023–1030.

Liccioli, S., Duignan, P.J., Lejeune, M., Deunk, J., Majid, S. and Massolo, A. (2013). A new intermediate host for *Echinococcus multilocularis*: the southern red-backed vole (*Myodes gapperi*) in urban landscape in Calgary, Canada. *Parasitology International*, 62(4), 355–357.

Liccioli, S., Kutz, S.J., Ruckstuhl, K.E. and Massolo, A. (2014). Spatial heterogeneity and temporal variations in *Echinococcus multilocularis* infections in wild hosts in a North American urban setting. *International Journal for Parasitology*, 44(7), 457–465.

Liccioli, S., Giraudoux P., Deplazes, P. and Massolo, A. (2015a). Wilderness in the 'city' revisited: different urbes shape transmission of Echinococcus multilocularis by altering predator and prey communities. *Trends in Parasitology*, 31(7), 297–305.

Liccioli, S., Rogers, S., Greco, C., Kutz, S.J., Chan, F., Ruckstuhl, K.E. and Massolo, A. (2015b). Assessing individual patterns of *Echinococcus multilocularis* infection in urban coyotes: non-invasive genetic sampling as epidemiological tool. *Journal of Applied Ecology*, 52(2), 434–442.

Massolo, A., Liccioli, S., Budke, C.M. and Klein, C. (2014). *Echinococcus multilocularis* in North America: the great unknown. *Parasite*, 21(73), 23.

McManus, D.P., Zhang, W., Li, J. and Bartley, P.B. (2003). Echinococcosis. *Lancet*, 362, 1295–1304.

Moss, J.E., Chen, X., Li, T., Qiu, J., Wang, Q., Giraudoux, P., Ito, A., Torgerson, P.R. and Craig, P.S. (2013). Reinfection studies of canine echinococcosis and role of dogs in transmission of *Echinococcus*

multilocularis in Tibetan communities, Sichuan, China. *Parasitology*, 140(S13), 1685–1692.

Nakao, M., Xiao, N., Okamoto, M., Yanagida, T., Sako, Y. and Ito, A. (2009). Geographic pattern of genetic variation in the fox tapeworm *Echinococcus multilocularis*. *Parasitology International*, 58(4), 384–389.

Raoul, F., Deplazes, P., Rieffel, D., Lambert, J.-C. and Giraudoux, P. (2010). Predator dietary response to prey density variation and consequences for cestode transmission. *Oecologia (Berlin)*, 164(1), 129–139.

Rausch, R. and Schiller, E.L. (1954). Studies on the helminth fauna of Alaska. XXIV. *Echinococcus sibiricensis* n. sp., from St. Lawrence Island. *Journal of Parasitology*, 40(6), 659–662.

Rausch, R. and Schiller, E.L. (1956). Studies on the helminth fauna of Alaska. XXV. The ecology and public health significance of *Echinococcus sibiricensis* Rausch & Schiller, 1954, on St. Lawrence Island. *Parasitology*, 46(3–4), 395–419.

Rausch, R.L., Fay, F.H. and Williamson, F.S. (1990a). The ecology of *Echinococcus multilocularis* (Cestoda: Taeniidae) on St. Lawrence Island, Alaska, USA. II. Helminth populations in the definitive host. *Annales de Parasitologie Humaine et Comparee*, 65(3), 131–140.

Rausch, R.L., Wilson, J.F. and Schantz, P.M. (1990b). A programme to reduce the risk of infection by *Echinococcus multilocularis*: the use of praziquantel to control the cestode in a village in the hyperendemic region of Alaska. *Annals of Tropical Medicine and Parasitology*, 84(3), 239–250.

Saitoh, T. and Takahashi, K. (1998). The role of vole populations in prevalence of the parasite (*Echinococcus multilocularis*) in foxes. *Researches on Population Ecology*, 40(1), 97–105.

Salb, A.L., Barkema, H.W., Elkin, B.T., Thompson, R.C., Whiteside, D.P., Black, S.R., Dubey, J.P. and Kutz, S.J. (2008). Dogs as sources and sentinels of parasites in humans and wildlife, northern Canada. *Emerging Infectious Diseases*, 14(1), 60–63.

Schantz, P.M., Chai, J., Craig, P.S., Eckert, J., Jenkins, D.J., MacPherson, C.N.L. and Thakur, A. (1995). Epidemiology and Control of Hydatid Disease. In R.C.A. Thompson and A.J. Lymbery (eds.), *Echinococcus and Hydatid Disease*. Oxford: CAB International, pp. 233–331.

Schweiger, A., Ammann, R.W., Candinas, D., Clavien, P.-A., Eckert, J., Gottstein, B., Halkic, N., Muellhaupt, B., Prinz, B.M., Reichen, J., Tarr, P.E., Torgerson, P.R. and Deplazes, P. (2007). Human alveolar echinococcosis after fox population increase, Switzerland. *Emerging Infectious Diseases*, 13(6), 878–882.

Somily, A., Robinson, J.L., Miedzinski, L.J., Bhargava, R. and Marrie, T.J. (2005). Echinococcal disease in Alberta, Canada: more than a calcified opacity. *BMC Infectious Diseases*, 5(34), 1–7.

Takahashi, K., Uraguchi, K., Hatakeyama, H., Giraudoux, P. and Romig, T. (2013). Efficacy of anthelmintic baiting of foxes against *Echinococcus multilocularis* in northern Japan. *Veterinary Parasitology*, 198(1–2), 122–126.

Torgerson, P.R., Schweiger, A., Deplazes, P., Pohar, M., Reichen, J., Ammann, R.W., Tarr, P.E., Halkik, N. and Müllhaupt, B. (2008). Alveolar echinococcosis: from a deadly disease to a well-controlled infection. Relative survival and economic analysis in Switzerland over the last 35 years. *Journal of Hepatology*, 49(1), 72–77.

Torgerson, P.R., Keller, K., Magnotta, M. and Ragland, N. (2010). The global burden of alveolar echinococcosis. *PLOS Neglected Tropical Diseases*, 4(6), e722.

Vaniscotte, A., Raoul, F., Poulle, M.L., Romig, T.,

Dinkel, A., Takahashi, K., Guislain, M.H., Moss, J., Tiaoying, L., Wang, Q., Qiu, J., Craig, P.S. and Giraudoux, P. (2011). Role of dog behaviour and environmental fecal contamination in transmission of *Echinococcus multilocularis* in Tibetan communities. *Parasitology*, 138(10), 1316–1329.

Veit, P., Bilger, B., Schad, V., Schaefer, J., Frank, W. and Lucius, R. (1995). Influence of environmental factors on the infectivity of *Echinococcus multilocularis* eggs. *Parasitology*, 110(1), 79–86.

Vuitton, D.A., Zhou, H., Bresson-Hadni, S., Wang, Q., Piarroux, M., Raoul, F. and Giraudoux, P. (2003). Epidemiology of alveolar echinococcosis with particular reference to China and Europe. *Parasitology*, 127, S87–S107.

Vuitton, D.A., Wang, Q., Zhou, H.-X., Raoul, F. and Knapp, J. (2011). A historical view of alveolar echinococcosis, 160 years after the discovery of the first case in humans. Part 1: what have we learnt on the distribution of the disease and on its parasitic agent? *Chinese Medical Journal*, 124(18), 2943–2953.

chapter 5

Mycobacterium tuberculosis in elephants in Asia: taking a One Health approach

Susan K. Mikota, Gretchen E. Kaufman,
Naresh Subedi and Ishwari P. Dhakal

Abstract

Tuberculosis is the leading cause of human death from a single infectious agent and has been designated a global public health crisis by the World Health Organization (WHO). The disease is endemic in many parts of South and Southeast Asia. There are a number of Mycobacteria known to cause tuberculosis in humans and animals, several are zoonotic, but *M. tuberculosis* is considered to be an obligate human pathogen with no known animal reservoirs. Animals that have close interactions with humans are known to have become infected with human strains. Tuberculosis in elephants is most often a result of infection with *M. tuberculosis* and has most often been reported in captive Asian elephants (*Elephas maximus*). Due to the complex ecology of the disease and the challenges of dealing with a 'reverse zoonosis' in a country where the disease is endemic in humans, it has been important to take a One Health approach to disease prevention and control. In this chapter we present a case study from Nepal.

5.1 Introduction

Tuberculosis (TB) is universally recognized as one of the most important and challenging diseases affecting the world today. It impacts both humans and animals and is found on every continent. Because of its ubiquitous nature, attempts to control or eradicate TB must utilize One Health principles to be most effective. In this chapter we will describe the case of tuberculosis shared by elephants and humans in the country of Nepal, a country in the heart of Asia.

Tuberculosis (TB) is caused by bacteria in the genus Mycobacterium, which includes more than 100 species. Seven species comprise the major disease-causing mycobacteria and these are grouped together in the Mycobacterium tuberculosis complex (MTBC). Of the seven species, *M. tuberculosis* (the human form) and *M. bovis* (the bovine form) are of most concern for humans and animals.

5.2 Tuberculosis (TB) in humans

TB has been designated a global crisis by the World Health Organization (WHO) and is the leading cause of death from a single infectious agent. In 2013 there were an estimated nine million new TB cases and 1.5 million deaths worldwide (WHO, 2014). Of the nine million people who developed TB, 56 per cent were in the Southeast Asia and Western Pacific regions. TB in humans is a chronic, insidious disease spread by respiratory droplets dispersed during common behaviours such as coughing and sneezing. Symptoms include fever, chills, weight loss, chest pain, night sweats and coughing blood. Of the two billion people estimated to be infected worldwide, approximately 10 per cent will develop active disease; in most cases the body's immune system is able to sequester the infection and prevent it from spreading.

In humans, a positive finding on a tuberculin skin test (TST) or acid-fast stain (AFS) is typically followed by a chest radiograph and a sputum culture to confirm a diagnosis. Mycobacteria are in a group of microorganisms (including nocardia, rhodococcus and some protozoa) that are highlighted when stained by acid-fast techniques such as Ziehl-Neelsen. This technique is not specific for mycobacteria and a positive stain could indicate the presence of any of these organisms. Isolation of the organism is the 'gold standard' to diagnose TB and facilitates drug sensitivity testing and correct antibiotic selection. However, in much of the developing world where the TB burden is high and laboratory capacity may be lacking, the AFS is the major test used. If the AFS test is positive, treatment is initiated according to standard protocols. Some of the tests used to diagnose TB are listed in Table 5.1

5.3 Tuberculosis (TB) in animals

While *M. tuberculosis* is an obligate human pathogen with no known animal reservoirs (Comas et al., 2013), various related strains of TB affect a wide range of mammalian species. *M. bovis* (bovine tuberculosis or bTB) is more common in non-human mammalian species than *M. tuberculosis*; domestic cattle are the natural reservoir. Bovine TB also affects humans and significant efforts have been put in place in most developed countries to eliminate bTB from domestic cattle. Recent spillover of *M. bovis* from cattle into wildlife has become a serious problem and is threatening conventional bTB control methods and sanitary policies. Affected species include badgers (*Meles meles*) in the UK, white-tailed deer (*Odocoileus virginianus*) in the US, brushtail possums (*Trichosurus vulpecula*) in New Zealand, Cape buffalo (*Syncerus caffer*) in South Africa, and wild boar (*Sus scrofa*) in Spain (Fitzgerald and Kaneene, 2013).

In contrast, TB in elephants is most often a result of infection with *M. tuberculosis*, the human strain, and has most often been reported in captive Asian elephants (*Elephas maximus*). One case has been reported in a wild African elephant that had previous human contact (Obanda et al., 2013) and one case has been reported in a wild Asian elephant (Perera et al., 2015). In elephants, signs of TB are often absent until the disease is quite advanced. Elephants have never been truly domesticated and, like other wild animals, tend to mask signs of disease as a

Table 5.1 Diagnostic tests for TB

Direct tests*	Indirect tests**
Culture	Tuberculin skin test
Acid-fast stain	ELISA
Nucleic acid amplification tests (PCR)	Serology
	Gamma-interferon assays

* Direct tests detect the TB organism
** Indirect tests detect antigens or antibodies or measure cellular reactivity against TB antigens

survival strategy against predators. Weight loss is the most common sign observed in elephants; dyspnoea (difficulty breathing) may also occur in advanced cases. In some cases, elephants died of other primary causes although TB was also detected during post-mortem examination.

The diagnosis of TB in elephants is complicated by their large body size, which precludes performing chest radiographs. In addition, the TST commonly used in people and in cattle is not an accurate test for many non-cattle species, including elephants (Mikota et al., 2001; Gavier-Widen et al., 2002; Lewerin et al., 2005; Moller et al., 2005). A trunk-wash procedure (comparable to obtaining a sputum sample from humans) has evolved as the preferred method to collect respiratory samples from elephants for culture (Isaza and Ketz, 1999; Abraham and Davis, 2008), however, the sensitivity is low and negative trunk-wash culture results are not uncommon in infected elephants (false negative). In an outbreak among elephants in a Swedish zoo, only seven of 189 trunk-wash samples collected over time were culture positive from five elephants with confirmed TB at necropsy (Moller et al., 2005); similar findings were reported in a study conducted in Thailand (Angkawanish et al., 2010). Intermittent shedding, contamination, overgrowth by other bacteria and difficulties with obtaining a sample from the lower respiratory tract through the long trunk may account for some of the discrepancies.

Commercial serological tests that detect antibodies against the TB organism have been developed for a variety of domestic and wild species. These assays vary in accuracy but have demonstrated surprising sensitivity and specificity in elephants (Greenwald et al., 2009; Lyashchenko et al., 2012).

5.4 Tuberculosis (TB) is a zoonotic One Health disease

Various strains of mycobacteria have a preferred reservoir host, but are shared across the mammalian species. Recent molecular studies have shown that TB has been co-evolving with humans for tens of thousands of years and that animal-adapted TB strains diverged from human strains before the Neolithic Demographic Transition, the period when humans transitioned from a hunter-gatherer dominated to an agricultural lifestyle (Comas et al., 2013; Anon., 2008; Wirth et al., 2008).

The zoonotic transmission of TB (usually *M. bovis*) is well-documented and occurs through ingestion of infected material or direct contact with an infected animal. Transmission of *M. tuberculosis* and *M. bovis* from humans to dogs (Erwin, 2004), cattle (Ocepek et al., 2005) and wild animals (Michel et al., 2003; Fritsche et al., 2004) has also been documented.

Evidence suggests that *M. tuberculosis* may also move back into humans from an infected animal (e.g., human to elephant and back to human). Staff TST conversions are common following the diagnosis of TB in an elephant in a zoo or private facility, although most are not reported in the scientific literature. In one case, the same strain of TB was found in an elephant handler and three elephants at a private facility but the direction of transmission (elephant-to-human or human-to-elephant) could not be determined (Michalak et al., 1998). More definitive support for elephant-to-human transmission was demonstrated by an epidemiologic investigation of a TB outbreak at the Elephant Sanctuary in Tennessee in which nine staff members had skin-test conversions (Murphree et al., 2011). Although the exact mode of transmission is unknown, in this case it was thought to be due to aerosolization from high-pressure cleaning. Human skin-test conversions have also been reported in other outbreaks involving elephants and chimpanzees (*Pan troglodytes*) (Stephens et al., 2013), a rhinoceros (*Diceros bicornis*) and three Rocky Mountain goats (*Oreamnos americanus*) (Oh et al., 2002).

5.5 Why tuberculosis (TB) matters for the conservation of elephants in Asia

Asian elephants (*Elephas maximus*) are an endangered species. They have been listed on Appendix I of the Convention on Trade in Endangered Species of Wild Fauna and Flora (CITES) since 1975. Accurate data on the number of wild Asian elephants is lacking; the most recent figures estimate that ~43,000 elephants remain in the 13 range countries (Fernando and Pastorini, 2011). The vast majority of wild elephants are found in India and Sri Lanka; five countries have less than 200 elephants (see Table 5.2). Figures on the numbers of Asian elephants in captivity are also lacking.

Asia has one of the highest rates of human TB in the world (WHO, 2014). Currently, the burden of TB in wild and captive elephants in Asia is unknown. The case study in Nepal described below illustrates the challenges of managing TB in captive elephants and mitigating the potential impact on the conservation of this endangered species.

Table 5.2 Asian elephant range countries

Bangladesh*	Malaysia
Bhutan*	Myanmar
Cambodia	Nepal*
China*	Sri Lanka
India	Thailand
Indonesia	Vietnam*
Laos	

* countries with less than 200 wild elephants

5.6 Nepal Case Study

Nepal has a population of approximately 30 million people; 45 per cent are infected with TB and 5,000–7,000 people die from the disease every year (National Tuberculosis Center, 2014). The National Tuberculosis Center and the Nepal Anti-tuberculosis Association (NATA) are the two main TB agencies.

Of the 400 laboratories in Nepal capable of diagnosing TB using AFS, only three perform cultures and only two have the capability to perform drug susceptibility testing. The latter is critical in managing drug-resistant infections. In 1996, Nepal instituted a Directly Observed Therapy Short Course (DOTS) programme in which healthcare workers observe patients taking their medications to ensure compliance with treatment (see Plate 4). Multidrug resistance is a significant problem with estimates of 2.9 per cent in new cases and 11.7 per cent in recurrent cases (Poudel et al., 2013).

Nepalese people live in close proximity to domestic animals. Most of the meat consumed in Nepal is from buffalo and goat; cows are sacred among the largely Hindu population and are neither consumed nor euthanized if found to be bTB reactors. However, milk consumption is common and pasteurization of milk, which would prevent transmission of TB, is not universally practised. In one study, 24 per cent of TB-positive Nepalese commonly consumed raw milk (Pandey et al., 2012).

Thus far, in the cases where culture has been performed, the causative agent of TB in elephants in Nepal has been *M. tuberculosis*, however, elephants are at risk for infection with *M. bovis* due to intermingling with domestic cattle and buffalo.

History of the Nepal elephant healthcare and TB surveillance programme

Tuberculosis was first diagnosed in captive elephants in Nepal in 2002 (Gairhe, 2002). Between 2002 and 2009, a total of seven captive elephants died due to TB; several were valuable government patrol elephants in their prime (Pradhan, et al., 2011). Captive elephants in Nepal are used to patrol the national parks and other protected areas and for conservation, research and tourist activities, which brings them into close proximity to wild elephants, rhinoceros and other TB-susceptible species. Wildlife officials in Nepal were concerned that TB could spread from captive elephants and threaten these wild populations.

In 2006, a comprehensive elephant TB screening programme was conducted in the Chitwan district by a team of US and Nepalese veterinarians, technicians, veterinary students and wildlife officials. A battery of tests – including culture and several commercial and experimental serological assays – were used to screen 120 elephants. Based on the results, elephants were assigned to one of four risk groups (high, moderate, low and undetermined) and management recommendations for each group were made to government authorities (Mikota et al., 2015).

The following year, Elephant Care International (ECI), and the Institute of Agriculture and Animal Science established a fellowship for a graduate veterinarian to continue monitoring the elephant population for TB. A workshop was held with key stakeholders during which the 2006 results were reviewed and a TB Action Plan was drafted. World Wildlife Fund (WWF) Nepal and ECI were awarded funding from the United States Fish and Wildlife Service (USFWS) Asian Elephant Conservation Fund in 2008 to continue the TB work. Efforts were directed toward constructing a segregation stable, conducting

TB testing of all mahouts (elephant caretakers), continuing surveillance of elephants and initiating treatment. A field office and small laboratory was established at the National Trust for Nature Conservation (NTNC), a local NGO, to provide a home for the elephant TB programme.

Building on the TB Action Plan drafted at the 2007 workshop, partners continued to develop a comprehensive written plan to manage TB in Nepal elephants with input from the Department of National Parks and Wildlife Conservation (DNPWC), WWF-Nepal, NTNC, international wildlife veterinary consultants and representatives from the human medical community in Nepal. In 2011, as part of Nepal's Elephant Action Plan, the Nepal Elephant Tuberculosis Control and Management Action Plan (2011–2015) (NETCMAP) was approved by the government of Nepal, Ministry of Forests and Soil Conservation, Department of National Parks and Wildlife Conservation (DNPWC, 2011). The Plan outlines methods to diagnose, treat and manage TB in elephants in Nepal.

The overarching goals of the Plan are to eliminate TB in captive elephants and any staff that work closely with them, to prevent transmission to the wild and to safeguard tourism, an important source of revenue for Nepal. The strategy to achieve these goals includes instituting and enforcing a sustainable testing, segregation and treatment programme for captive elephants and their handlers, and preventing TB-suspect or infected elephants from entering Nepal. The day-to-day activities of the Plan are managed by a veterinarian who is employed by NTNC with financial and technical support from international agencies.

NETCMAP and the programme that supports it is managed by DNPWC in collaboration with NTNC, WWF-Nepal, the Buffer Zone Management Committee (BZMC) and Hotel Association Nepal (HAN), Chitwan Chapter. The complete Plan is available online (see supplementary materials).

Testing methods and sampling strategy

The cultures that were performed on trunk-wash samples collected in 2006 from elephants in Nepal were non-diagnostic due to contamination, storage and transportation issues and did not yield any MTBC isolations from either the National TB Center in Nepal or the National Veterinary Services Laboratories in Ames, Iowa, USA (Mikota et al., 2015). Because of the known limitations of culture as a primary diagnostic technique, a decision was made by the One Health team to prioritize serological results in developing the management group algorithm. Improving culture and PCR methods remained a goal and the NETCMAP includes instructions for the collection of respiratory samples for culture and research.

The ElephantTB Stat-Pak test was licensed in the US as a screening test for elephants, in 2006; the DPP VetTB® test was not licensed until 2012. However, at the time that the NETCMAP was written, the DPP had been used as a research tool in Nepal for several years and positive results had correlated with confirmation of infection by culture in several elephants that had died. The DPP was therefore incorporated into the testing algorithm (see Plate 5).

Overview of management groups

Four management groups were established.

- *Group 1 TB-free* includes elephants that were non-reactive on the ElephantTB Stat-Pak test. These elephants were screened every other year with no segregation or work restrictions.
- *Group 2 TB-suspect* includes elephants reactive on the ElephantTB Stat-Pak assay and non-reactive on the DPP VetTB® test. There are two options for elephants in this group: (1) initiate prophylactic treatment; or (2) repeat the DPP test in six months. If the DPP is reactive at this time, the elephant changes to Group 3. If the DPP remained non-reactive, the elephant is tested annually with the DPP.
- *Group 3 TB-infected* includes elephants that are reactive on both the ElephantTB Stat-Pak and DPP VetTB® tests and/or from whom MTBC organisms have been identified using culture or molecular techniques. The NETCMAP describes protocols for segregation, treatment and post-treatment monitoring (see Plate 6).
- *Group 4 Untested* includes calves not yet trained for blood collection and elephants that have recently entered Nepal.

The complete testing algorithm can be viewed in the NETCMAP in the supplementary materials.

Management recommendations

The NETCMAP document describes specific activities including programme management, testing, preventing the entry of infected elephants into Nepal, criteria for participation in elephant events, segregation, treatment, grazing practices, dung disposal, post-mortem examination, human screening and education. Some of these topics are discussed in more detail below.

Testing

The NETCMAP outlined the following guidelines for testing:

- All captive elephants in Nepal will be TB tested every one to two years.
- Any elephants purchased or hired from outside of Nepal will be tested within 30 days prior to arrival.
- Procuring elephants from outside of Nepal is discouraged.

- The TB Plan veterinarian will have the authority to test (or retest) new elephants upon arrival in Nepal.
- All elephants participating in events such as elephant races or polo must have a current non-reactive test or have completed treatment.

All the captive elephants in Nepal have a TB programme number and are entered into a database that tracks changes in ownership. Most elephants are microchipped, so follow-up has not been a problem in Nepal. This may not be the case in other countries where elephants frequently change owners and are given new names.

Segregation

Segregation was designated to be an important management tool and segregation of infected elephants from wild elephants and other species (especially rhinoceros) was a stated priority. Segregation rather than treatment was considered to be an acceptable alternative for aged elephants.

Treatment

The detailed treatment regimens described in the NETCMAP are based on the protocols established in the Guidelines for the Control of Tuberculosis in Elephants developed in the US (Anon, 2010; also see supplementary material). TB drug dosages, methods for direct oral or rectal administration, monitoring during treatment and management of potential side-effects are described in detail (see Plate 7).

Minimizing tuberculosis transmission between humans and elephants

A strategy for minimizing the risk of disease transmission between humans and elephants was implemented as an 'integrated TB management programme'. This includes conducting further research and surveillance to better understand the ecology of TB across the environment and instituting measures to reduce the risk of transmission. All elephant handlers and any other staff working in close proximity to elephants are to be tested annually; new employees are to be tested before starting work. Workers testing positive must complete four weeks of treatment before working again with elephants. Family members of positive individuals will also be tested and treated as determined by public health agencies. TB testing and TB medications are available at no charge in Nepal through government programmes.

In addition, the Plan specifies the development of a TB education programme to minimize risk for elephant handlers and others that come into contact with elephants, including tourists. This programme includes basic information on the disease, how it is spread, and appropriate biosafety practices that should be practised to minimize the possibility of transmission. Handlers of known infected elephants are given additional training and appropriate personal protective gear by the programme.

The programme staff was charged with distributing information for tourists and tour agencies about the Nepal Elephant Tuberculosis Control and Management Action Plan and to assist commercial enterprises to cooperate with the Plan without major disruption to their business. A certification programme was planned in which local elephant tourism agencies and owners could display a certificate of participation in the programme. Subsequent follow-up efforts have introduced reduced working hours and diet diversification for working elephants to support overall health, minimize stress and improve immunity.

5.7 Discussion

Tuberculosis is a complicated disease. Even after decades of efforts by international governmental and non-governmental agencies, it remains one of the most serious global disease issues for humans.

Worldwide, captive elephants are used by people – as draft animals, for processions, in temples, for entertainment in circuses and for education and conservation in zoos. The inherent stigma and fear associated with TB has implications for the owners of captive animals. Upon learning that his elephant has TB, a private owner may sell his elephant to an unsuspecting buyer. Commercial operations such as circuses may experience a loss of revenue from public fear. Stakeholders may lobby against regulations that impact animal movement and business. Perhaps the worst-case scenario would be for infected elephants in range countries to be released into the wild, suffering an untimely death and putting wild animals at risk.

In Nepal, as in many other Asian countries, there is intermingling between humans, domestic livestock and elephants and other wildlife. We know elephants are at risk for human TB but sharing grazing land with cows and buffalo may also put them at risk for bovine TB. If wild elephant bulls breed with infected captive cows, TB could be transmitted to wild elephants. Infected elephants can also pose a risk to other wildlife such as rhinos (see Plate 8).

Nepal was the first Asian elephant range country to acknowledge a TB problem in elephants and to take a proactive approach to address that problem. The collaboration between DNPWC, WWF-Nepal, NTNC, IAAS, ECI, the human health agencies and others was instrumental in developing both the programme and the policy that resulted. Continued collaboration will be important as this programme is updated.

Challenges and next steps

The programme is slowly transitioning to a self-sustaining model and as surveillance continues, it is anticipated that there will be fewer cases. The management of TB in elephants in Nepal and enforcement of the NETCMAP has not been without challenges. Many of these are outlined in the Plan itself and include insufficient technical and managerial capacity, and insufficient financial resources.

There is not always financial and political support to address TB in elephants in a country where TB in humans is still an overwhelming issue. It is expensive to treat an elephant for TB. In Nepal, the private elephant owners have, for the most part, been responsible for the cost of treatment medications for their infected animal; funds to treat government-owned elephants have been provided from international sources. Although sceptical at first, the private owners have come to realize the importance of the programme and its benefits.

Although the documented elephant TB cases have thus far been due to *M. tuberculosis*, the risk of infection with *M. bovis* is unknown. The lack of a TB control programme for domestic species and lack of data regarding prevalence complicates assessing the risk for elephants.

Since 2007, four Nepalese veterinarians have been employed as the TB programme veterinarian. During their tenure, two completed Master's degrees on TB-related topics and two of them are now pursuing PhDs overseas. Another has recently completed a Master's programme on herpes virus infection in elephants and a fourth veterinarian is in a One Health Epidemiology Fellowship programme. The Nepal Elephant Healthcare and TB Surveillance Program has provided knowledge and skills that have enabled these talented individuals to qualify for higher educational opportunities. It is anticipated that these individuals will return to Nepal as the next generation of conservation leaders. The turnover has, however, been challenging for the continuity of the programme.

Measures that enable early detection and prevention of elephant-to-human and human-to-elephant transmission of TB have not been fully realized. While the importance of personal protection has been presented to elephant care staff, it remains a difficult issue. Face masks certified to be protective against TB are not readily available in the country, and cooperation to wear personal protective equipment is often lacking except during post-mortem examinations. From a logistical standpoint, wearing a mask for long periods of time in a high-temperature, high-humidity climate may not be practical, and masks are not always worn even in human medical facilities that care for human TB patients. Policies requiring routine testing of people that maintain close sustained relationships with working elephants have been implemented within government operations, but have not been completely addressed in the private sector.

The government, specifically DNPWC, can be credited with instituting and enforcing policies such as restricting test-positive elephants from participating in large events where elephants intermingle (such as elephant polo, races and festivals), despite limited staffing and resources. However, planned measures to significantly limit new cases, such as certification and systematic testing of elephants entering the country, especially in the private sector where elephants are often hired seasonally and move back and forth between Nepal and India, have not yet been implemented.

Other challenges that have confronted the programme include accessibility of elephants for testing. Government elephants are moved between (often remote) posts and veterinary access has at times been limited. The programme is slated for regular review and renewal. Many of the challenges will have to be addressed in future iterations of the action plan and continued efforts to successfully engage the private sector will need to be strengthened.

Importance of a One Health approach

TB is a classic One Health disease affecting humans, domestic livestock, and wildlife in an ever-narrowing interface. Because of the zoonotic implications, a One Health approach is essential to investigate and manage TB when elephants are involved. A diagnosis of TB can evoke fear and concern among humans, especially in developed countries where it is less common, but also in heavy burden countries where it may have personal implications for elephant owners (income loss) or mahouts (job loss) in addition to personal health concerns. When TB occurs, engaging partners early on and maintaining open communication with stakeholders (which may include the public) are critical to a successful outcome.

Outbreaks that have occurred in zoos and other facilities have demonstrated how collaborative efforts between zoo staff and local or sometimes national health service agencies can effectively address epidemiological, screening, treatment, public relations, and other issues (Oh et al., 2001; Stephens et al., 2013; Murphree et al., 2011).

One Health initiatives have evolved in Nepal in recent years. One such initiative involved the collaboration of organizations in Nepal, the UK and the US and was spearheaded by NTNC and the Zoological Society of London. It targeted the conservation areas and the buffer zones of the Terai and Himalayas with the aim of integrating the human, livestock, wildlife and ecosystem health systems at the interface between environment, species and multi-host diseases. The Nepal Elephant Healthcare and TB Surveillance Program is an obvious fit for this initiative and is now managed under this One Health umbrella.

5.8 Conclusion

- TB is a complicated disease in elephants with political as well as medical challenges.
- Nepal is the first Asian elephant range country to address this problem.
- The Nepal programme has succeeded and is ongoing because stakeholders and partners were brought together early and open communication was maintained.
- When working in another country it is important to engage with local wildlife officials and other stakeholders to fully understand the situation from their perspective and to be aware of limiting factors that may impact the development of viable solutions.
- Veterinary and human health authorities working together with shared goals and a common plan are a formula for success.

References

Abraham, D. and Davis, J. (2008). Revised trunk wash collection procedure for captive elephants in a range country setting. *Gajah*, 28, 53–54.

Angkawanish, T., Wajjwalku, W., Sirimalaisuwan, A., Mahasawangkul, S., Kaewsakhorn, T., Boonsri, K. and Rutten, V.P.M.G. (2010). *Mycobacterium tuberculosis* infection of domesticated Asian elephants, Thailand. *Emerging Infectious Diseases*, 16(12), 1949–1951.

Anon (2008). Tuberculosis may have migrated from humans to cattle, not the reverse. *Science Daily*, www.sciencedaily.com/releases/2008/07/080708092231.htm.

Anon (2010). Guidelines for the control of tuberculosis in elephants. In *Proceedings of 114th Annual Meeting of the United States Animal Health Association*. St Joseph, MO: United States Animal Health Association, pp. 578–639.

Comas, I., Cosolla, M., Luo, T., Borrell, S., Holt, K.E. and Kato-Maeda, M. (2013). Out-of-Africa migration and Neolithic coexpansion of *Mycobacterium tuberculosis* with modern humans. *Nature Genetics*, 45(10), 1176–1184.

DNPWC (2011). *Nepal Elephant Tuberculosis Control and Management Action Plan (2011–2015)*. Government of Nepal, Ministry of Forests and Soil Conservation, Department of National Parks and Wildlife Conservation, Kathmandu, Nepal.

Erwin, P.C. (2004). *Mycobacterium tuberculosis* transmission from human to canine. *Emerging Infectious Diseases*, 10(12), 2258–2259.

Fernando, P. and Pastorini, J. (2011). Range-wide status of Asian elephants. *Gajah*, 35, 15–20.

Fitzgerald, S.D. and Kaneene, J.B. (2013). Wildlife reservoirs of bovine tuberculosis worldwide: hosts, pathology, surveillance, and control. *Veterinary Pathology*, 50(3), 488–499.

Fritsche, A., Engel, R., Buhl, D. and Zellweger, J-P. (2004). *Mycobacterium bovis* tuberculosis: from animal to man and back. *International Journal of Tuberculosis and Lung Diseases*, 8(7), 903–904.

Gairhe, K. (2002). *A Case Study of Tuberculosis in Captive Elephants in Nepal*. Report submitted to Department of National Parks and Wildlife Conservation, Kathmandu, Nepal.

Gavier-Widen, D., Hard Af Segerstad, C., Roken, B., Moller, T., Bolske, G. and Sternberg, S. (2002). *Mycobacterium Tuberculosis Infection in Asian Elephants (Elephas Maximus) in Sweden*. European Association of Zoo and Wildlife Veterinarians 4th Scientific Meeting, Heidelberg, Germany, pp. 165–166.

Greenwald, R., Lyashchenko, O., Esfandiari, J., Miller, M., Mikota, S., Olsen, J.H., Ball, R., Dumonceaux, G., Schmitt, D., Moller, T., Payeur, J.B., Harris, B., Sofranko, D., Waters, W.R. and Lyashchenko, K. P. (2009). Highly accurate antibody assays for early and rapid detection of tuberculosis in African and Asian elephants. *Clinical and Vaccine Immunology*, 16, 605–612.

Isaza, R. and Ketz, C.J. (1999). A trunk wash technique for the diagnosis of tuberculosis in elephants. *Verhandlungsberichte Erkrankungen der Zootiere*, 39, 121–124.

Lewerin, S.S., Olsson, S.L., Eld, K., Roken, B., Ghebremichael, S., Koivula, T., Kallenius, G. and Bolske, G. (2005). Outbreak of *Mycobacterium tuberculosis* infection among captive Asian elephants in a Swedish zoo. *Veterinary Record*, 156(6), 171–175.

Lyashchenko, K.P., Greenwald, R., Esfandiari, J., Mikota, S., Miller, M., Moller, T., Volgelnest, L., Gairhe, K., Robbe-Austerman, S., Gai, J. and Waters, W.R. (2012). Field application of serodiagnostics to identify elephants with tuberculosis prior to case confirmation by culture. *Clinical and Vaccine Immunology*, 19, 1269–1275.

Michalak, K., Austin, C., Diesel, S., Bacon, J.M., Zimmerman, P. and Maslow, J.N. (1998). *Mycobacterium tuberculosis* infection as a zoonotic disease: transmission between humans and elephants. *Emerging Infectious Diseases*, 4, 283–287.

Michel, A.L., Venter, L., Espie, I.W. and Coetzee, M.L. (2003). *Mycobacterium tuberculosis* infections in eight species at the National Zoological Gardens of South Africa, 1991–2001. *Journal of Zoo and Wildlife Medicine*, 34, 364–370.

Mikota, S.K., Peddie, L., Peddie, J., Isaza, R., Dunker, F., West, G., Lindsay, W., Larsen, R.S., Salman, M.D., Chatterjee, D., Payeur, J., Whipple, D., Thoen, C., Davis, D.S., Sedgwick, C., Montali, R., Ziccardi, M. and Maslow, J. (2001). Epidemiology and diagnosis of *Mycobacterium tuberculosis* in captive Asian elephants (*Elephas maximus*). *Journal of Zoo and Wildlife Medicine*, 32(1), 1–16.

Mikota, S.K., Gairhe, K., Giri, K., Hamilton, K., Miller, M., Paudel, S., Lyashchenko, K., Larsen, R.S., Payeur, J., Waters, W.R., Greenwald, R., Dumonceaux, G., Vincent, B. and Kaufman, G.E. (2015). Tuberculosis surveillance of elephants (*Elephas maximus*) in Nepal at the captive-wild interface. *European Journal of Wildlife Research*. 61(2): 221–229.

Moller, T., Roken, B., Petersson, L., Vitaud, C., and Lyashchenko, K. (2005). *Preliminary Results of a New Serological Test for Detection of TB Infection (Mycobacterium tuberculosis) in Elephants (Elephas Maximus and Loxodonta Africanum) – Swedish Case Studies.* Verhandlungsberichte Erkrankungen der Zootiere, 42 Institut fur Zoo-und Wildtierforschung, Berlin, Germany, pp. 173–181.

Murphree, R., Warkentin, J.V., Dunn, J.R., Schaffner, W. and Jones, T.F. (2011). Elephant-to-human transmission of tuberculosis, 2009. *Emerging Infectious Diseases*, 17(3), 366–371.

National Tuberculosis Center (2014). http://nepalntp. gov.np/index.php.

Obanda, V., Poghon, J., Yongo, M., Ngothon, M., Waitiku, K., Makumi, J., Gakuya, F., Osmondi, P., Soriguer, R.C. and Alasaad, S. (2013). First reported case of fatal tuberculosis in a wild African elephant with past human-wildlife contact. *Epidemiology and Infection*, 141, 1476–1480.

Ocepek, M., Pate, M., Žolnir-Dovč, M. and Poljak, M. (2005). Transmission of *Mycobacterium tuberculosis* from human to cattle. *Journal of Clinical Microbiology*, 437, 3555–3557.

Oh, P., Granich, R., Scott, J., Sun, B., Joseph, M., Stringfield, C., Thisdell, S., Staley, J., Workman-Malcolm, D., Borenstein, L., Lehnkering, E., Ryan, P., Soukup, J., Nitta, A. and Flood, J. (2002). Human exposure following *Mycobacterium tuberculosis* infection of multiple animal species in a metropoli-

tan zoo. *Emerging Infectious Diseases*, 8, 1290–1293.

Pandey, G., Dhakal, S., Sadaula, A., KC, G., Subedi, S., Pandey, K.R. and Dhakal, I.P. (2012). Status of tuberculosis in bovine animals raised by tuberculosis infected patients in western Chitwan, Nepal. *International Journal of Infection and Microbiology* 1(2), 49–53.

Perera, B.V.P., Salgadu, M.A., Gunwardena, G.S.P.S., Smith, N.H and Jinadasa, H.R.N. (2015). First confirmed case of fatal tuberculosis in a wild Sri Lankan elephant. *Gajah*, 41, 28–31.

Poudel, A., Maharjan, B., Nakljima, C., Fukushima, Y., Pandy, B.D., Beneke, A. and Suzuki, Y. (2013). Characterization of extensively drug-resistant *Mycobacterium tuberculosis* in Nepal. *Tuberculosis*, 93, 84–88.

Pradhan, N.M.B., Williams, A.C. and Dhakal, M. (2011). Current status of Asian elephants in Nepal. *Gajah*, 35, 87–92.

Stephens, N., Vogelnest, L., Lowbridge, C., Christensen, A., Marks, G.B., Sintchenko, V. and McAnulty, J. (2013). Transmission of *Mycobacterium tuberculosis* from an Asian elephant (*Elephas maximus*) to a chimpanzee (*Pan troglodytes*) and humans in an Australian zoo. *Epidemiology and Infection*, 141, 1488–1497.

WHO (2014). *Global Tuberculosis Report*, www.who.int/ tb/publications/global_report/en.

Wirth, T., Hildebrand, F., Allix-Beguec, C., Wöbeling, F., Kubica, T., Kremer, K., van Soolingen, D., Rüsch-Gerdes, S., Locht, C., Brisse, S., Meyer, A., Supply, P. and Niemann, S. (2008). Origin, spread, and demography of the *Mycobacterium tuberculosis* complex. *PLoS Pathogens*, 4(9), e1000160.

Supplementary materials

Guidelines for the Control of Tuberculosis in Elephants 2008, www.aphis.usda.gov/animal_welfare/downloads/elephant/elephant_tb.pdf

Guidelines for the Control of Tuberculosis in Elephants 2010, http://elephantcare.org/protodoc_files/2015/Elephant TB Guidelines-2010.pdf

Tuberculosis in Elephants: Science, Myths and Beyond! www.aphis.usda.gov/animal_welfare/pg.php?pg=Tuberculosis_in_Elephants

Nepal Elephant Tuberculosis and Control Management and Action Plan (NETCMAP), http://elephantcare.org/protodoc_files/2013/Nepal%20Elephant%20TB%20Control%20and%20Mgt%20Action%20Plan.pdf

chapter 6

Leptospirosis: an emerging health issue in the Asia-Pacific region

Julie M. Collins-Emerson, Jackie Benschop and Stanley G. Fenwick

Abstract

Leptospirosis (also known as Weil's disease, field fever and rat catcher's fever) is a neglected zoonotic disease caused by spirochaete bacteria in the genus *Leptospira*. It is considered both an emerging and a re-emerging disease. Up to 13 different species of *Leptospira* can cause disease in humans and these can be transmitted by both wild and domestic mammals. Most mammalian species can be infected with *Leptospira*; however, some serovars are better adapted to certain host species, including wild rodents and farm livestock. *Leptospira* are typically shed in the urine of the infected host(s), contaminating the environment and subsequently acting as a source of infection for other animals, including humans. In parts of the developing world, the disease most commonly occurs in farmers and in the urban poor, who live in cities with poor sanitary conditions, and outbreaks frequently follow flooding events. In most of the developed world it more commonly occurs in people whose work or recreational pursuits involve spending time in wet areas or on rural land where cases of the disease still occur in livestock. Due to the complex and dynamic ecology of this zoonotic disease, it has been valuable to take a One Health approach when dealing with outbreaks of leptospirosis. In this chapter we present contrasting case studies from New Zealand and Asia to highlight the need for a transdisciplinary approach to investigation, prevention and control.

6.1 Introduction

Leptospirosis is a globally distributed zoonotic disease that is particularly common in the warm, wet conditions found in tropical and subtropical climates (Hartskeerl et al., 2011). It is caused by the spirochaete *Leptospira*. There are currently 21 recognized species of *Leptospira* divided into approximately 300 serovars (KIT, 2014). A number of species are either classified as non-pathogenic or indeterminate in nature (Levett and Haake, 2009). Dual systems of classification are used; one serological, the other based on DNA sequence information. Both schemes have their uses; however, there is little correlation between them, with serologically closely related serovars often falling into more than one leptospiral species by DNA classification.

Most mammalian species can be infected with *Leptospira* (Faine et al., 1999), however, some serovars are better adapted to certain host species than others. In such cases *Leptospira* can cycle within this host population, which acts as a reservoir for the organism. The *Leptospira* colonize the kidneys and are shed in the urine, contaminating the environment and subsequently infecting other animals. Where a serovar is adapted to the host, the disease may be mild or sub-clinical in nature and colonization of the kidneys followed by urinary shedding may be for extended periods of time (Levett and Haake, 2009). In farmed animals this may result in reduced fertility, including abortions, and in suboptimal growth. In less benign serovar/host combinations, the disease is more severe and can be fatal. As the host–serovar combination markedly affects the presentation of the infection, it is sometimes helpful to consider leptospirosis as a collection of diseases.

Due to the difficulties in diagnosing the disease both clinically and in the laboratory, and the fact that this zoonosis is prevalent in developing countries where resources are stretched and surveillance is either poor or absent, the true burden of leptospirosis globally is difficult to ascertain. The most recent global incidence estimate is 1.03 million cases with 58,900 deaths annually, with tropical regions of South and Southeast Asia, Central and South America, Western Pacific and Africa having the highest burdens (Hagan et al., 2013). Leptospirosis is a widespread, neglected disease and one that is both emerging and re-emerging (Hartskeerl et al., 2011).

Leptospirosis can be difficult to diagnose clinically as symptoms can mimic other diseases and it is therefore easily misdiagnosed. In domestic animals leptospirosis is commonly sub-clinical. In humans, disease can be mild (anicteric) or severe (icteric), with the classic Weil's disease being severe and often resulting in jaundice and death. Laboratory diagnostic tests present challenges as different tests are more suitable at various stages of the disease. Although culturing is a gold standard for a definitive diagnosis, there are limited windows of opportunity for culturing the organism from various tissue samples. The use of the host's serological response for diagnostic purposes can also present difficulties when the host is infected with a well-adapted serovar and a strong serological response may not be mounted. The limitations of different tests and the choice of test made at different stages of the disease mean that the disease often can go undiagnosed.

Changes in agricultural land use, human population growth and associated increased urban densities, plus the pressure this places on the zones where human and wildlife populations interface and where climatic changes are trending to the more extreme, all contribute to the dynamic nature of leptospirosis. The increasing frequency of severe weather events associated with changes in climate, such as cyclones and associated flooding, has resulted in outbreaks of leptospirosis in countries such as Nicaragua, Honduras, Fiji and the Philippines. Also, while vaccination programmes can decrease the prevalence of some serovars, this may create an opportunity for other serovars to gain a foothold or for there to be a change in the predominant host reservoir. Given the complex interactions between such factors, the prevalence and distribution of various leptospiral serovars and leptospirosis status worldwide is not static. This dynamism is evidenced by a number of examples such as the rise in severe pulmonary haemorrhagic syndrome seen in South America (Gouveia et al., 2008), newly emergent serovars in American Samoa (Lau et al., 2012) and even in some genomic changes in the bacterium. The reduced size of the *L. borgpetersenii* sv. Hardjo (bovis) genome when compared to other serovars is speculated to represent increasing host adaption coincident with the shedding of genes used mainly for survival in the environment (Bulach et al., 2006).

Integral to the control or management of leptospirosis is the recognition of the interrelatedness of human, animal and environmental health, a concept encompassed by the terms 'One Health' and 'ecohealth'. To highlight how the interaction of human, animal and environmental conditions influences the epidemiology of the disease, two case studies contrasting the different situations in regions of Asia-Pacific will be examined: New Zealand, with a temperate climate; and SE Asia, where the climate is tropical.

6.2   Case study 1: Leptospirosis in New Zealand – a global disease but a local phenomenon.

New Zealand comprises two main islands that are geographically isolated and situated in the southern Pacific Ocean. Its remoteness contributed to it being the last significant land mass to be colonized with the first Polynesian peoples (NZ Māori) estimated to have arrived in significant numbers from around 1300 CE. In addition, it has resulted in a unique native fauna. New Zealand has only two native land mammals; both of which are bats. The ecological niches that are usually occupied by mammals in other parts of the world were instead filled in New Zealand by birds, a number of which are flightless. The first exotic mammals to arrive were rats (*R. exulans*) and the Polynesian dog brought by Māori. Europeans began to arrive in numbers from the very early 1800s and with their settlement came the introduction of production animals such as sheep, cattle, pigs, goats, additional domestic dogs and cats and other introduced mammals such as deer, the Australian possum, the European hedgehog, weasels, stoats and mice. This history has resulted in an unusual situation where there is a very restricted number of pathogenic *Leptospira*

serovars known to be endemic in New Zealand, (*L. interrogans* serovars Pomona, Copenhageni and *L. borgpetersenii* svs. Balcanica [possum variety], Ballum, Hardjo[bovis] and Tarassovi) all of which have arrived with mammals imported relatively recently and many that are domestic. Human leptospirosis in New Zealand is primarily associated with direct or indirect contact with livestock, which act as the largest reservoir for the bacteria. This is a very different situation to that in many other parts of the world where there are large numbers of leptospiral strains circulating in wildlife populations and spilling over into domestic stock and into the human population. This contrast will be explored more fully in the following section that discusses leptospirosis in SE Asia.

New Zealand is a sparsely inhabited country of approximately 4.5 million people with large areas (~40 per cent) developed for pastoral farming of mainly beef and dairy cattle, and sheep, with commercial deer farming introduced in the late 1970s. The first documented case of leptospirosis in New Zealand was identified on a dairy farm in the South Island in 1951 where calves and six dairy farm workers contracted the disease (Bruere, 2003). The outbreak was attributed to serovar Pomona. Leptospirosis continued to be mainly dairy or pig industry-associated until a national vaccination programme (bivalent Pomona/Hardjo vaccine) was introduced at the beginning of the 1980s. This saw a corresponding dramatic decline in reported cases of leptospirosis. Mild cases in people can mimic influenza and hence it frequently goes undiagnosed or misdiagnosed. It is still the most commonly notified, non-foodborne zoonosis in New Zealand and the country has the highest incidence of the disease in humans in the Organisation for Economic Co-operation and Development (OECD).

As much primary produce is exported, the NZ farming sector has become very responsive to market forces in the past few decades.

Initially, commercial deer production was very lucrative and these farms tended to carry deer solely but over time, as the profit margins declined, many farmers changed to mixed-species farming with combinations of sheep, cattle, and deer. Government subsidies that bolstered the rural sector ceased in 1984, resulting in marked changes in farming practices. A formerly strong focus on wool production shifted to that of producing more lamb meat. A boom in dairy profitability since the 1990s has seen a considerable shift from dry stock farming to dairying and has also been responsible for the large numbers of dairy herds being transported from the North Island across the Cook Strait to the South Island to establish new dairying regions. To enable this conversion, large areas of more arid land in the South Island required irrigation and this has had a considerable impact on the environment. A reasonable conjecture is that the introduction of cattle to these areas and the augmented moisture levels in the top layers of soil may well have increased the environmental loading and also improved the survival times of *Leptospira* in this region. The transport of herds between the two main islands presented additional opportunities for *Leptospira* to cross to the South Island either in the cattle host or possibly via rats stowed away on stock trucks. Finally, these factors – plus climatic changes that have occurred in this time, including overall warmer weather and extreme weather events becoming more frequent – are thought to have contributed to a change in the epidemiology of leptospirosis in New Zealand. A change in the prevalence of leptospirosis in various stock classes has been observed in the past few decades. Research carried out in the late 1970s to early 1980s demonstrated a titre prevalence (titre cut point $\geq$ 48) in mixed-aged sheep averaging 20.5 per cent for Hardjo and 4 per cent for Pomona. The very low rate of successful isolation of leptospiral cultures from sheep kidneys was interpreted by the authors as indicating sheep were likely to be sporadically infected by

Leptospira with cattle being the primary hosts (Blackmore et al., 1982). More recent serosurveys, however, indicate that sheep either are or have now become reservoir hosts for Hardjo and Pomona (Dorjee et al., 2008). Deer are also very commonly infected with approximately 75 per cent of herds showing evidence of Hardjo and about 15 per cent with evidence of Pomona infections. Leptospirosis is also highly prevalent in beef cattle (>50 per cent) and approximately 30 per cent of dairy herds were found to be shedding in a recent survey (Heuer et al., 2012). Given sheep, beef cattle and deer are nowadays more frequently run on mixed-species farms, it has raised the question as to whether this practice has influenced the changing epidemiology of the disease in New Zealand. One area of current research is aimed at determining whether there are host-adapted strains of these Hardjo and Pomona or whether it is the same strain of each serovar freely circulating between the various stock classes. The answer is of importance as it will significantly influence the disease management strategies in New Zealand.

The microscopic agglutination test (MAT) has been widely utilized as a diagnostic tool in New Zealand with DNA-based technology more recently included. Given the restricted number of serovars circulating in New Zealand and their particular serogroup affiliations, cross-reactivity between closely related serovars is not the significant issue found in many other countries and serological results are comparatively reliable regarding the identity of the infecting serovar.

In New Zealand, the majority of pork producers house their pigs. The introduction of serological testing of grower herds and vaccination programmes for breeding herds saw a dramatic decline in leptospirosis in commercial pig farms (Heuer et al., 2012). In addition, a certificate of *Leptospira*-free status is required by abattoirs before stock is accepted for slaughter. These practices have resulted in few human cases now linked to commercial pig farming.

The changes in New Zealand farming practices from the early 1970s to 2014 (as discussed previously), possum and rodent control programmes, increased urbanization, population growth and extreme climatic events could be expected to have influenced the dynamics of leptospirosis in the wildlife population. A substantial body of research involving serological surveys and the collection of field isolates from wildlife was conducted in the 1970s and early 1980s. However, current information is lacking. There is some evidence that carriage of serovar Copenhageni is no longer restricted to the brown rat (*R. norvegicus*) populations in the north of the North Island but has drifted south, possibly abetted by mass dairy cattle stock truck movements. Conversion of farming areas from cropping to dairy has also in some cases resulted in additional boundary areas where native bush, which supports wildlife, now interfaces with dairy cattle farms, thus creating opportunity for new infection pressures. Another round of comprehensive research investigating the current status of leptospirosis in New Zealand wildlife is now warranted to inform the understanding of the present day epidemiological landscape.

The demographics of human infection have also changed since the 1970s in that the incidence, serovar prevalence and the occupations most associated with the disease have altered. Traditionally, human infections in New Zealand were caused predominantly by serovars Hardjo (contact with cattle) and Pomona (contact with pigs) and infections, particularly with serovar Hardjo, were mostly anicteric. As mentioned previously, the introduction of vaccination programmes in the dairy and pork industries correlated with a sharp decline in reported human leptospirosis cases in New Zealand. A gradual shift has been observed where human cases are increasingly associated with both farm and abattoir workers. In 2013, of the 59 notified human cases, 22 worked in the meat processing industry and 18 were in farm-associated occupations

accounting for approximately 71 per cent of the cases (ESR, NZ, 2013). Another noted change is the rise in the comparative incidence of the predominantly rodent host serovar, Ballum. In 2011 there were as many human cases of Ballum infection as there were for serovars Hardjo and Pomona (ESR, NZ, 2011). This statistic may have been a result of fewer Hardjo and Pomona infections or indicate a change in the predominant host or the dynamics between the serovars circulating. For example, vaccination programmes against one serovar may create a niche that can be then filled by another serovar. In New Zealand, acute human leptospirosis often presents similarly to influenza (headache, myalgia, chills, fever, nausea) and thus is grossly under- or misdiagnosed. However, more severe cases result in hospitalization and may lead to kidney and liver damage and meningitis. Humans rarely transmit the disease between themselves so, given this, humans can be viewed as 'sentinels' signalling changes in the epidemiology of the disease dynamics in New Zealand.

Given New Zealand's small exposed human population, it would not be financially viable for a company to make a leptospiral vaccine for human use. Furthermore, social acceptance of such a vaccine would be low as management of leptospirosis is viewed primarily as the responsibility of the livestock industry, as this is the main source for human leptospirosis. Prevention or management of human infection is therefore inextricably linked to the infection status of the country's farm animals. The complex interdependence between the environment, domestic animals, humans and wildlife requires a collaborative One Health approach to address the problem. Presently, effective stock vaccination programmes are a key component in preventing or mitigating human leptospirosis in New Zealand.

A One Health approach is evidenced in a functional synergy between medical and veterinary experts working in clinical practice, district health boards, universities and laboratories in New Zealand. This is likely a result of the country having a centralized government, only one veterinary school, two medical schools and a general awareness of the importance of biosecurity and zoonotic diseases. New Zealand embraced a One Health approach to understanding zoonotic disease risks in the early 1980s with the establishment of the Veterinary Human Health Advisory Group under the auspices of the Ministry of Health – Centre for Disease Control, with members from multiple agencies and disciplines from government, academia and the private sector. Current synergistic work on leptospirosis includes joint investigations, publications, research proposals, projects and submissions on policy documents. An example of this multidisciplinary approach is a research proposal on persistent leptospirosis symptoms led by a veterinary epidemiologist and molecular biologist, with the research team comprising a public health epidemiologist and physician, an occupational physician, a clinical psychologist and an economist. Translation of science into policy is further evidenced by the recent (2012) adoption of Polymerase Chain Reaction as a laboratory confirmatory test by the Ministry of Health, the use of local scientific publications to inform Accident Compensation Commission policy (2014) and consultation with scientists in the production of Best Practice Guideline for the Prevention and Control of Leptospirosis for Worksafe NZ (2014).

Beyond scientific collaboration there is also deeply embedded community engagement around this disease that, both in its acute and chronic forms, has had a significant effect on rural communities. An exemplar of this engagement is the relationship between a community group representing farming interests and a university research group. The community group has supported research by fundraising to provide stipend support for university postgraduates and to source funding for leptospirosis research in

sheep and cattle, resulting in the production of a video for farmers on leptospirosis and in the development and maintenance of a leptospirosis website.

6.3 Case study 2: Leptospirosis in South East Asia – a re-emerging disease in an endemic area

In contrast to the situation in New Zealand, where there are limited serovars and a strong link between human disease and farm animals, leptospirosis in SE Asia involves a different epidemiology. Although the disease has been recognized for many years in the region, research has been limited and publications have been largely related to the description of clinical cases. Much of the early literature on leptospirosis came from Malaysia, with the first report of human cases being recorded in 1925 (El Jalii and Bahaman, 2004). Case reports were increasingly documented in the 1950s and 1960s in China, Malaysia and the Philippines, and by military doctors in Vietnam in the 1970s, with a large variety of serovars identified, most linked to rodent reservoirs. In the 1990s, other countries in SE Asia began to progressively report and describe cases of leptospirosis. The disease is thus considered endemic in the region, with multiple wild animal reservoir hosts, but little understanding of the dynamic relationships between domestic and wild animals, humans and the environment exists.

Nevertheless, despite the longstanding endemicity of leptospirosis in the region, the disease is considered to be re-emerging, with severe outbreaks being recorded in Thailand, Malaysia and the Philippines in the past decade (Amilasan et al., 2012; Lim, 2011; Thaipadungpanit et al., 2007). In these countries exposure to contaminated water, whether by occupation (e.g., rice farming); outdoor recreational activities, such as the Eco-Challenge Race in Malaysia (Sejvar et al.,

2003), which included activities such as kayaking, swimming, and caving; or through extreme climatic events causing flooding, such as typhoon Ketsana and tropical storm Parma that hit Manila in the Philippines in 2009), have been strongly linked to disease outbreaks. Additionally, in Thailand an outbreak was linked to the emergence of a particular dominant leptospiral clone (Thaipadungpanit et al., 2007). Two of these above scenarios will be explored in greater depth later in this chapter.

The annual incidence in SE Asia is high, at >10 cases per 100,000 population, during outbreaks and in high exposure risk groups this figure can reach >100 cases per 100,000 (Victoriano et al., 2009). Nevertheless, the true incidence of leptospirosis is likely to be underreported due to poor healthcare systems in many countries in the region and the plethora of other infectious diseases with similar symptoms (dengue, malaria, scrub typhus) (Hartskeerl et al., 2011).

One similarity between the epidemiology in New Zealand and SE Asia is that a large majority of infections are considered to be occupational in origin. However, the occupational risk profiles differ in the two areas. In New Zealand, infections are largely linked to agricultural practices, with abattoir workers and farm workers most at risk, whereas in SE Asia the predominant risk group is people engaged in rice farming, where working barefoot in paddy fields is common and thus exposure to contaminated water is unavoidable. The serovar distribution and clinical disease picture are also markedly different from the situation in New Zealand, with a far wider spectrum of serovars, commonly associated with rodent hosts, causing clinically more severe infections and mortalities in the SE Asia region. Little evidence for links between animal production and leptospirosis exist in SE Asia, with only a limited number of studies carried out in southern Vietnam and Thailand into the role of pigs and other farm animals as potential reservoirs of infection (Boqvist et al., 2005; Suwancharoen et al., 2013). Not surprisingly in these studies the serovars identified were also similar to those found in rodents in other surveys. So until further investigations are carried out, the domestic animal involvement in the epidemiology will remain unconfirmed.

In the humid tropics, leptospires survive for long periods outside the host in water contaminated by animal urine, increasing the chances of infection of those in contact. Thus, as with rice farmers, other occupational and non-occupational groups who come in contact with contaminated water in SE Asian countries also regularly contract leptospirosis. Additionally, the disease in Asia is often associated with extreme climatic events (likely exacerbated by global warming), in particular flooding, with outbreaks following seasonal flooding events commonly reported from many countries in the region (Mendoza et al., 2013; Niwetpathomwat et al., 2005). In Malaysia and Thailand, ecotourism activities such as endurance running and river rafting have also resulted in cases of leptospirosis (Chusri et al., 2012; Sejvar et al., 2003) and in Malaysia survival training of army recruits at a number of rural training centres has resulted in infections and deaths (Lim et al., 2011).

In the following section, two scenarios mentioned earlier in this chapter will be expanded to demonstrate a range of factors involved in the re-emergence of leptospirosis in SE Asia.

6.4 A prolonged outbreak of leptospirosis in Thailand linked to a dominant clone of *Leptospira*

Until 1995 the number of recorded human cases of leptospirosis in Thailand remained relatively low and stable, varying between 50 and 275 per year, and an annual incidence rate of 0.3/100,000 population (Tangkanakul et al.,

2005). Between 1996 and 2003, however, a huge increase in infections was noted, with a peak in 2000 of 14,285 cases, which, given the difficulty in diagnosing the disease, is probably an underestimate. In 2000 the incidence rate was 23.7/100,000 population and the case fatality rate peaked in 1999 at 4.4 per cent. Notable epidemiological and demographic features of the disease showed that it had a distinctive seasonal, occupational and gender association over this period (1996–2003). The leptospirosis season was consistently from June to December, with a peak in September–October, which is the rainy period in Thailand. Eighty per cent of cases were seen in male farmers, 15–45 years old, who are regularly exposed to rat urine and urine-contaminated water. Prior to the epidemic in 1996, the male-to-female ratio was as high as 30:1 in some areas. However, this decreased annually from the start of the epidemic to a low point of 3:1 in the 2000–2003 period. Nevertheless, the majority of cases were still seen in agricultural workers.

The epidemic started in Nakhon Ratchasima province in the north-east of Thailand, preceded by a period of flooding, and by 1999 had spread to 64 provinces in the north-east, north and central regions of the country out of a total of 76 in the country. At the peak of the outbreak in 2000, the highest incidence was seen in the north-east provinces with a rate of 50 cases per 100,000 population recorded.

Evidence from isolates recovered between 2000 and 2005 showed that a single dominant clone, Multilocus Sequence Type ST34 of serovar Autumnalis, was responsible for the majority of human infections in the northeast province of Udon Thani and other parts of Thailand (Thaipadungpanit et al., 2007). This was supported by another study of *Leptospira* isolates recovered during the periods 2001–2002 and 2011–2012, with Autumnalis the major serovar identified in both periods (Thipmontree et al., 2014).

Rodent surveys for *Leptospira* have been carried out since the 1960s and have commonly shown a high prevalence of infection, up to 66 per cent, with serovars the same as those causing human illness. During the outbreak, surveys of rodents were carried out in affected areas and a high prevalence of *Leptospira* infection was demonstrated in a number of species. To determine whether a link could be identified between ST34 and a maintenance host, eight isolates available from rodents captured in northeast Thailand were characterized. Seven strains (from *B. indica* (6) and *B. savilei* (1)), were *L. interrogans* serovar Autumnalis ST34. This confirmed the predominance of the outbreak strain in a maintenance host, which in this case appears to be the bandicoot rat (*Bandicota indica*), commonly found in rice fields throughout Thailand (Tangkanakul et al., 2005; Thaipadungpanit et al., 2007). It was also noted that an increased incidence of infected rats was seen during the rainy season, corresponding to an increase in human cases. Surveys of domestic animals performed in the same period showed a high seroprevalence for *Leptospira*, but with less obvious serovar compatibility with human infections.

Risk factors for leptospirosis were studied by Tangkanakul et al. (2000) and a strong association was seen with walking through water, applying fertilizer, ploughing or removing rice shoots for more than six hours per day. The factors contributing to the outbreak, however, are still largely speculative. These include changing farming practices, climatic and ecological changes, increase in rodent numbers and a raised awareness of the disease in farmers and physicians following publicity and educational campaigns resulting in more notifications. While these could all have played a part, it is thought unlikely that they would have resulted in the dramatic increase in human infections from 1996 to 2000. Thaipadungpanit et al. (2007) have suggested that the introduction of a more bioactive strain, serovar Autumnalis ST34, with a selective advantage in the maintenance host (leading to a higher bacterial load and increased urinary shedding) and a survival advantage in the external environment, such as increased resistance to desiccation, could have triggered the outbreak. The gradual decline in reported incidence since the peak in 2000 could be due to a number of factors including the promotion of safe practices, such as the use of protective footwear and clothing, increased use of laboratory testing and early treatment of mild fevers with doxycycline (Tangkanakul et al., 2005; Thipmontree et al., 2014).

6.5 Occupational and recreational risk factors for leptospirosis in Malaysia

To date, 38 *Leptospira* serovars have been isolated in Malaysia from humans and animals. Infections have been observed in military personnel at rural training centres and the disease is recognized as an occupational hazard for people engaged in agricultural and mining activities. Studies have reported a high enzootic incidence in the domestic animal population (Bahaman et al., 1987; El Jalii and Bahaman, 2004). Outdoor recreational activities have also been associated with leptospirosis in Malaysia, with one of the largest outbreaks reported among participants of an Eco-Challenge race in Sabah in 2000 (Sejvar et al., 2003). Three hundred and four athletes took part in the ten-day endurance race, which involved jungle trekking, kayaking, swimming, caving, climbing and mountain-biking. Many of the athletes became ill on returning home, prompting a public health investigation. Eighty athletes met the case definition for leptospirosis, with 26 of those hospitalized. Risk factors for the disease included kayaking, swimming in the Segama River, swallowing river water and caving. A number of athletes had taken doxycycline during the event and this was identified as a protective factor. Only one positive culture was acquired, and *L. weilii* was identified, a spe-

cies only recovered previously in SE Asia. One possible reason for the high attack rate was the weather, with high rainfall for several months before the event and heavy rain during the event. In addition, athletes all reported cuts and abrasions that may have made them more prone to infection. Since this outbreak, a number of other reports have documented leptospirosis in endurance racers, kayakers and other athletes and recreational groups, and thus leptospirosis needs to be recognized as a cause of fever and illness by public health professionals treating returning travellers who have engaged in these activities.

Other individuals engaged in outdoor recreational activities in Malaysia have also been affected by leptospirosis. In 2010, six people died after exposure to contaminated water in a recreational park near Maran in Peninsular Malaysia. Subsequent investigations found leptospires in water in a recreational lake in Sibu, Sarawak and in a nearby National Service Training Centre (NSTC), resulting in some camps suspending water activities and to the temporary closure of several centres (Lim et al., 2011). In 2011, eight people who had been involved in searching for a drowned boy at a recreational area in eastern Malaysia died of leptospirosis and melioidosis co-infection as a result of exposure to contaminated water (Sapian et al., 2012). Further cases associated with swimming in recreational water parks were documented in the northern state of Kedah, prompting the closure of several picnic areas while investigations were carried out. As Malaysians increasingly use water parks for recreation, the risks of contracting leptospirosis should be noted and appropriate communication methods developed to inform the public.

A serological study of 168 rodents collected from two NSTCs in 2008–2009 found that 17–18 per cent were positive for a range of serovars similar to those affecting humans in Malaysia. The recommendation of the authors was that to prevent leptospirosis in military trainees, control of the rat population in NSTCs is critical (Mohamed-Hassan et al., 2010).

6.6 Conclusion

Leptospirosis is a dynamic, emerging and re-emerging disease of global significance. Two contrasting pictures of the disease have been described; the situation in New Zealand and that in SE Asia. Leptospirosis continues to be a significant public health problem worldwide and management strategies will need to be tailored to individual situations. Given the complex interrelationship between human, animal and environmental health, a One Health or ecohealth approach is required to respond to the challenges. As multiple human, animal and environmental factors are involved in communities where the risk of leptospirosis is high, only a multi-centric, transdisciplinary approach to control will effectively reduce the burden of this disease.

References

Amilasan A.T., Ujiie, M., Suzuki, M., Salva, E., Belo, M.C.P., Koizumi, N., Yoshimatsu, K., Schmidt, W., Marte, S., Dimaano, E.M., Villarama, J.B. and Ariyoshi, K. (2012). Outbreak of leptospirosis after flood, the Philippines, 2009. *Emerging Infectious Diseases*, 18, 91–94.

Bahaman, A.R., Ibrahim, A.L. and Adam, H. (1987). Serological prevalence of leptospiral infection in domestic animals in West Malaysia. *Epidemiology and Infection*, 99, 379–392.

Blackmore, D.K., Bahaman, A.R. and Marshall, R.B. (1982). The epidemiological interpretation of serological responses to leptospiral serovars in sheep. *New Zealand Veterinary Journal*, 30, 38–42.

Boqvist, S., Ho Thi, V.T. and Magnusson, U. (2005). Annual variations in Leptospira seroprevalence among sows in southern Vietnam. *Tropical Animal Health and Production*, 37, 443–449.

Bruere, A.N. (2003). Re: fifty years of leptospirosis research in New Zealand: a perspective. *New Zealand Veterinary Journal*, 51, 44–44.

Bulach, D.M., Zuerner, R.L., Wilson, P., Seemann, T., McGrath, A., Cullen, P.A., Davis, J., Johnson, M., Kuczek, E., Alt, D.P., Peterson-Burch, B., Coppel, R.L., Rood, J.I., Davies, J.K. and Adler, B. (2006). Genome reduction in *Leptospira borgpetersenii* reflects limited transmission potential. *Proceedings of the National Academy of Sciences*, 103, 14560–14565.

Chusri, S., Sritrairatchai, S., Hortiwahul, T., Charoenmak, B. and Silpapojakul, K. (2012). Leptospirosis among river water rafters in Satoon, Southern Thailand. *Journal of the Medical Association of Thailand*, 95, 874–877.

Dorjee, S., Heuer, C., Jackson, R., West, D.M., Collins-Emerson, J.M., Midwinter, A.C. and Ridler, A.L. (2008). Prevalence of pathogenic *Leptospira* spp. in sheep in a sheep-only abattoir in New Zealand. *New Zealand Veterinary Journal*, 56, 164–170.

El Jalii, I.M. and Bahaman, A.R. (2004). A review of human leptospirosis in Malaysia. *Tropical Biomedicine*, 21, 113–119.

ESR, NZ (2011). *Notifiable and Other Diseases in NZ: Annual Report 2011*, https://surv.esr.cri.nz/PDF_surveillance/AnnualRpt/AnnualSurv/2011/2011AnnualSurvRpt.pdf.

ESR, NZ (2013). *Notifiable and Other Diseases in NZ: Annual Report 2013*, https://surv.esr.cri.nz/PDF_surveillance/AnnualRpt/AnnualSurv/2013/2013AnnualSurvRpt.pdf.

Faine, S., Adler, B., Bolin, C. and Perolat, P. (1999). *Leptospira and Leptospirosis*. Melbourne: MediSci.

Gouveia, E.L., Metcalfe, J., Luiza, A.L.F., de Carvalho, A.L.F., Aires, T.S.F., Villasboas-Bisneto, J.C., Queiroz, A., Santos, A.C., Salgado, K., Reis, M.G. and Ko, A.I. (2008). Leptospirosis associated severe pulmonary hemorrhagic syndrome, Salvador, Brazil. *Emerging Infectious Diseases*, 14(3), 505–508.

Hagan, J.E., Costa, F., Calcagno, J., Kane, M., Torgerson, P., Martinez-Silveira, M.S., Stein, C., Abela-Ridder, B. and Ko, A. (2013). Global morbidity and mortality of leptospirosis: a systematic review. In *Proceedings of the 8th International Leptospirosis Society Scientific Meeting*, Fukuoka, Japan.

Hartskeerl, R.A., Collares-Pereira, M. and Ellis, W.A. (2011). Emergence, control and re-emerging leptospirosis: dynamics of infection in the changing world. *Clinical Microbiology and Infection*, 17, 494–501.

Heuer, C., Benschop, J., Stringer, J., Collins-Emerson, J., Sanhueza, J. and Wilson, P. (2012). *Leptospirosis in New Zealand – Best Practice Recommendations for the*

Use of Vaccines to Prevent Human Exposure. A report by Massey University, New Zealand, prepared for the Zealand Veterinary Association.

KIT (2014). *Leptospira* strains archive, www.kit.nl/biomedical-research/product-category/leptospira-strains.

Lau, C.L., Clements, A.C.A., Skelly, C., Dobson, A.J., Smythe, L.D. and Weinstein, P. (2012). Leptospirosis in America Samoa – estimating and mapping risk using environmental data. *PLOS Neglected Tropical Diseases*, 6(5), e1669.

Levett, P.N. and Haake, D.A. (2009). Leptospira species (Leptospirosis). In G.L. Mandell, J.E. Bennett and R. Dolin (eds.), *Mandell, Douglas, and Bennett's Principles and Practice of Infectious Diseases*, 7th edn. Philadelphia: Churchill Livingstone, pp. 241–247.

Lim, J.K., Murugaiyah, V.A., Ramli, A., Abdul Rahman, H., Mohamed, N., Shamsudin, N. and Tan, J.C. (2011). A case study: leptospirosis in Malaysia. *WebmedCentral Infectious Diseases*, 2, WMC002703.

Lim, V.K.E. (2011). Leptospirosis: a re-emerging infection. *Malaysian Journal of Pathology*, 33, 1–5.

Mendoza, M.T., Roxas, E.A., Ginete, J.K., Alejandria, M.M., Roman, A.D., Levritana, K.T., Penamora, M.A. and Pineda, C.C. (2013). Clinical profile of patients diagnosed with leptospirosis after a typhoon: a multicentre study. *Southeast Asian Journal of Tropical Medicine and Public Health*, 44, 1021–1035.

Mohamed-Hassan, S.N., Bahaman, A.R., Mutalib, A.R. and Khairani-Bejo, S. (2010). Serological prevalence of leptospiral infection in wild rats at the National Service Training Centres in Kelantan and Terengganu. *Tropical Biomedicine*, 27, 30–32.

Niwetpathomwat, A., Niwatayakul, K. and Doungchawee, G. (2005). Surveillance of leptospirosis after flooding at Loei Province, Thailand by year 2002. *Southeast Asian Journal of Tropical Medicine and Public Health*, 36(4), 202–205.

Sapian, M., Khairi, M.T., How, S.H., Rajalingam, R., Sahhir, K., Norazah, A., Khebir, V. and Jamalludin, A.R. (2012). Outbreak of melioidosis and leptospirosis co-infection following a rescue operation. *Medical Journal of Malaysia*, 67, 293–297.

Sejvar, J., Bancroft, E., Winthrop, K., Bettinger, J., Bajani, M., Bragg, S., Shutt, K., Kaiser, R., Marano, N., Popovic, T., Tappero, J., Ashford, D., Mascola, L., Vugia, D., Perkins, B., Rosenstein, N. and the Eco-Challenge Investigation Team (2003). Leptospirosis in 'eco-challenge' athletes, Malaysian Borneo, 2000. *Emerging Infectious Diseases*, 9, 702–707.

Suwancharoen, D., Chaisakdanugull, Y., Thanapongtharm, W. and Yoshida, S. (2013). Serological survey of leptospires in livestock in Thailand. *Epidemiology and Infection*, 141, 2269–2277.

Tangkanakul, W., Tharmaphornpil, P., Plikaytis, B.D., Bragg, S., Poonsuksombat, D., Choomkasien, P., Kingnate, D. and Ashford, D.A. (2000). Risk factors associated with leptospirosis in Northeastern Thailand, 1998. *American Journal of Tropical Medicine and Hygiene*, 63, 204–208.

Tangkanakul, W., Smits, H.L., Jatanasen, S. and Ashford, D.A. (2005). Leptospirosis: an emerging health problem in Thailand. *Southeast Asian Journal of Tropical Medicine and Public Health*, 36, 281–288.

Thaipadungpanit, J., Wuthiekanun, V., Chierakul, W., Smythe, L.D., Petkanchanapong, W., Limpaiboon, R., Apiwatanaporn, A., Slack, A.T., Suputtamongkol, Y., White, N.J., Feil, E.J., Day, N.P.J. and Peacock, S.J. (2007). A dominant clone of Leptsopira interrogans associated with an outbreak of human leptospirosis in Thailand. *PLOS Neglected Tropical Diseases*, 1(1), e56.

Thipmontree, W., Suputtmongkol, Y., Tantibhedhyangkul, W., Suttinot, C., Wongswat, E. and Silpasakorn, S. (2014). Human leptospirosis trends: Northeast Thailand, 2001–2012. *International Journal of Environmental Research and Public Health*, 11, 8542–8551.

Victoriano, A.F.B., Smythe, L.D., Gloriani-Barzaga, N., Cavinta, L.L., Kasai, T., Limpakarnjanarat, K., Ong, B.L., Gongal, G., Hall, J., Coulcombe, C.A., Yanagihara, Y., Yoshida, S. and Adler, B. (2009). Leptospirosis in the Asia Pacific region. *BMC Infectious Diseases*, 9, 147–155.

ENVIRONMENTAL COMPLEXITY

chapter 7

Managing marine biosecurity risks: a New Zealand case study

Aurélie Castinel and Grant Hopkins

Abstract

New Zealand is an oceanic nation, comprising two main islands and more than 700 smaller islands and islets. It has an Exclusive Economic Zone of 4.2 million km²; the fifth largest in the world. The marine environment provides a diverse range of habitats for aquatic species, many of which are important for the economy as well as making a contribution to the cultural richness of the country. Due to the complex biodiversity of the ocean ecosystem, a holistic approach is needed when tackling biosecurity challenges. In this chapter we will demonstrate how New Zealand has applied the One Health approach to manage coastal resources.

7.1 Introduction

Primary industries are a major component of New Zealand's economy, with dairy and forestry sectors contributing NZ$17.6 billion and NZ$5.1 billion (respectively) to the country's NZ$231 billion gross domestic product (GDP) in 2013/2014 (MPI, 2014a). Seafood exports consist of wild fisheries and aquaculture, with hoki, rock lobsters and mussels being the most important species exported currently. In recent years, the sector's growth has been driven by aquaculture, especially Chinook salmon (*Oncorhynchus tshawytscha*) and green-lipped mussels (*Perna canaliculus*). In addition to primary industries, tourism contributes significantly to New Zealand's economy (NZ$10.3 billion per annum, or 4 per cent of GDP), with marketing and projected visits relying on a 'clean and green' environment. Because each sector has environmental, economic and cultural ties, taking a holistic approach is needed when tackling challenges, or preparing for them. This has proven to be particularly important in the marine environment, where the One Health concept has been spontaneously applied on many occasions to manage coastal resources.

New Zealand is an oceanic nation, comprising two main islands and more than 700 smaller islands and islets. It has an Exclusive Economic Zone of 4.2 million km²; the fifth largest in the world (Gordon et al., 2010). New Zealand's geological history has shaped the unique biodiversity of this archipelago, and due to its isolation in the

Pacific Ocean, it remains vulnerable to impacts from non-indigenous species. New Zealanders are naturally fond of the outdoors and take great pride in freely enjoying their coastal 'backyard' throughout the year. The cultural importance of the marine environment goes further for the indigenous Māori, who believe there is a fundamental connection between humans and their natural surroundings, known as *kaitiakitanga* (or environmental stewardship). Many Māori associate a healthy ecosystem with a profitable future for their children and following generations (which is reminiscent of the One Health philosophy). The marine environment is the backbone of this nation and its people, and it is extremely difficult, if not impossible, to attribute a monetary value to both its cultural and spiritual values.

Biosecurity is defined by Hewitt et al. (2004) as the 'management of the risks posed by introduced species to environmental, economic, social, and cultural (including spiritual) values'. In order to protect its unique biodiversity and ecosystem health and thus safeguard the aforementioned values, New Zealand has developed pre- and post-border biosecurity systems that are some of the most stringent around the world. Although some pathways are manageable (for example, the importation of aquatic animal products), others – such as biofouling on vessel hulls – remain a huge challenge for regulators. With such diversity of marine users and their respective interests, controlling the marine 'borders' in New Zealand is an ambitious yet critical assignment to maintain the country's unique coastal health. Further, with increasing shipping traffic as a result of globalization and a changing marine environment, biosecurity systems are being put under significant pressure from new and emerging threats.

7.2 What are the risks for New Zealand?

The introduction of marine pest species and disease-causing organisms (hereafter referred to as *pathogens*) can affect a number of sectors and people to varying degrees. Once established, the magnitude of impacts can worsen as a result of natural and human-mediated spread (Forrest et al., 2014). The main pathways for the transfer of marine organisms between international or domestic coastal environments are movements of commercial and recreational vessels (Plate 9). Every year, more than 3,000 international vessels arrive in New Zealand waters, including over 2,000 merchant vessels carrying cargo (Inglis et al., 2010). Vessels can transport organisms or their reproductive propagules (i.e., larvae or spores) in ballast water, in sea chests and other hull recesses and as fouling communities attached to submerged parts of hulls (Hewitt and Campbell, 1999; Inglis et al., 2010). Aquaculture activities and the aquarium trade are other important pathways for the introduction and spread of non-indigenous marine species (MPI, 2011; Fitridge et al., 2012). While international and domestic risk pathways have been well-described for marine pests (Coutts et al., 2003; Minchin and Gollasch, 2003; Minchin, 2007; Acosta and Forrest, 2009; Hopkins and Forrest, 2010; Bell et al., 2011), further work is required for clarifying current risk pathways for pathogens.

Non-indigenous plants, animals and pathogens pose a significant problem to the natural ecology of coastal habitats around the world (Ruiz et al., 2000). New Zealand's marine environment is highly valued and its unique biodiversity makes it even more vulnerable to invasive organisms. To date, approximately 200 non-indigenous marine organisms have been introduced and become established in the country's ports and marinas and in some natural areas (Hayden et al., 2009). A number of invasive species, not already in New Zealand, are deemed a high risk (e.g., the Northern Pacific seastar *Asterias amurensis* and the European shore crab *Carcinus maenas*). However, the behaviour of new invasive organisms can be difficult to predict as their ecology and impact is only known from their native range and other invaded regions (Inglis et al., 2010; Kulhanek et al., 2011). In some instances, introduced species present a lesser impact than anticipated (Simberloff and Gibbons, 2004).

New Zealand has had limited encounters with significant marine pathogens, except for the notifiable parasite *Perkinsus olseni* and an ostreid herpesvirus causing seasonal high mortality in Pacific oysters (see later). However, aquatic diseases should remain a concern, not only for conservation purposes but also for the New Zealand seafood industry. In fact, diseases have become a major limiting factor for aquaculture's growth around the world (Hedrick, 1996; Subasinghe, 2005). Trade of aquatic animals and their products has long been considered the main mode of disease transfer across seas (Renault, 1996; Peeler et al., 2010; Rodgers et al., 2011), but other potential routes may have been overlooked. Although illegal imports cannot be discounted, the only authorized importation of live fish currently allowed in New Zealand is for the aquarium trade, and it is subject to strict quarantine and testing procedures (MPI, 2012). The importation of other potential risk items, such as seafood products and used aquaculture equipment, is the object of stringent biosecurity measures. Less recognized is that biofouling could be another potential pathway for disease transfer: fouling species could either be direct hosts (commercial species; e.g., blue mussels, Pacific oysters) or intermediate hosts (e.g., polychaete worms) for aquatic pathogens (Minchin and Gollasch, 2003; Castinel et al., 2013). Anecdotal reports have linked biofouling molluscs to incursions of exotic diseases into new regions; for example *Ostrea edulis* and the parasite *Bonamia ostreae* (Howard, 1994), but there are currently no studies available to substantiate the associated risk of disease introduction.

Another potential threat is the emergence of aquatic pests and diseases due to changing marine environmental conditions. Warmer climates can modify the behaviour of invasive organisms and their interactions with the environment (Harvell et al., 1999; Sorte et al., 2010), either by increasing host susceptibility to disease (Harvell et al., 1999; Mortensen et al., 2007) or by causing nutrient enrichment favourable to opportunistic agents (Harvell et al., 1999; Johnson et al., 2010). Hence, New Zealand could see the emergence of invasive species or diseases caused by opportunistic pathogens in the future. In addition to causing the emergence of harmful organisms, predictive studies on climate change have indicated that general warming will affect New Zealand coastal ecosystem production, and marine life, from seabirds to fish stock (Nottage et al., 2010).

Harmful algal blooms (HABs) are another emerging issue, for the marine ecosystem and also for public health (Núñez Vázquez et al., 2011; Glibert et al., 2014). The microscopic organisms that cause HABs include common dinoflagellates, cyanobacteria and diatoms. Although blooms have been observed for a long time around the globe, their occurrence is a growing concern for human and animal health, as their epidemiology becomes better understood. New Zealand has developed a performant monitoring system as a warning system to detect specific organisms in water samples before they cause HABs in the marine farming areas (Rhodes et al., 2013). There is also increased awareness amongst industry that movements of gear and stock could transfer microscopic algae responsible for HABs, as it has already been suggested overseas (Hegaret et al., 2008).

7.3 Marine biosecurity in New Zealand: governance and management

In New Zealand, marine biosecurity is regulated across a number of legislative documents. The key regulation is the Biosecurity Act 1993, which is echoed in other documents managing marine resources in general, including the New Zealand Coastal Policy Statement 2010, the Fisheries Act 1996, the Treaty of Waitangi (Fisheries Claims) Settlement Act 1992 and the Resource Management Act 1991 (www.legislation.govt. nz). Local government agencies also have to align their biosecurity policies and strategies with the national legislation to prevent, respond and control organisms declared unwanted under the Biosecurity Act provisions.

The border requirements developed by government to manage the risks of introducing non-indigenous pests and pathogens into New Zealand are supported by risk analyses (e.g., Bell et al., 2011). However, substantial knowledge gaps may hamper these assessments and the government's continuous challenge is to prioritize research needs and allocate the relevant funding to fill those gaps (Hewitt et al., 2004). Biological surveillance activities are one way to improve the general understanding of species occurrence and distribution. For more than a decade, national surveys have been commissioned by government and undertaken by the National Institute of Water and Atmospheric research (NIWA) at major ports and marinas known to be points of entry for international shipping. Marine pest surveillance programmes provide baseline data on non-indigenous marine species distributions, and ideally detect new incursions at a stage where intervention measures are feasible (Morrisey et al., 2014). Surveillance for marine pathogens has been less well-defined and only routinely undertaken in selected shellfish species in key farming regions around New Zealand (Hine, 1997, 2002). Reports of suspected exotic diseases and of unusual mortality events remain the key source of information on New Zealand aquatic animal health (Tana, 2014).

New Zealand is among a long list of countries standing by the International Maritime Organization's (IMO) International Convention for the Control and Management of Ships' Ballast Water and Sediments, adopted in 2004 to minimize the risk of spreading invasive aquatic species in ships' ballast water (IMO, 2004). The New Zealand government has already aligned its biosecurity requirements for ballast water with the Convention (MPI, 2005). Following on from the Convention, the IMO issued risk management guidelines targeting biofouling present on immersed areas of ships, such as the hull, rig pontoons and sea-chests (IMO, 2011). These guidelines are not mandatory but set an example of best practice for the shipping industry in an effort to minimize the risk of international transfer of marine pests.

Accumulation of biofouling on ship hulls remains the main risk pathway for the transloca- tion of marine species (including potential pests) into and within New Zealand (Inglis et al., 2010; Bell et al., 2011). In 2014, the New Zealand government introduced a Craft Risk Management Standard (CRMS) for vessel biofouling, which is aligned with the IMO guidelines. The CRMS sets biofouling management requirements for all vessels entering New Zealand territorial waters (MPI, 2014b). The standard has a four-year vol- untary lead-in period and will come into force in 2018.

New Zealand has made considerable efforts as a nation to keep marine threats under con- trol with pre-border measures. But it also has to anticipate, if not defy the dynamic nature of the marine environment while still enabling various exchanges of people, services and goods com- ing into New Zealand (Plate 10). Even if the government takes the lead on managing inter- national and domestic risk pathways, there is a steady and necessary shift towards increasingly involving stakeholders and the community in controlling the risks within New Zealand.

7.4 Examples of pathway management

Managing international risk pathways –biofouling and oil rigs

The oil and gas (petroleum) industry has gained a significant place in New Zealand's economy in the past decade. Exploration and development of oil and gas fields are continuously undertaken to expand the current production sites mainly located in the Taranaki Basin in the North Island. In addition to holding a petroleum permit, each oil and gas company must comply with New Zealand environmental, health and safety, and hazardous chemicals regulations. For example, a company may be required to apply for resource consent with the local regional council under the Resource Management Act and undertake environmental effects assessments and monitoring, at

its own cost (Taranaki Regional Council, 2013). Each application is different and will be considered by the local authorities on a case-by-case basis. The government is supportive of the petroleum industry in order to attract more investment and develop the full potential of New Zealand's natural resources. However, it must find the right balance between boosting the economy and nurturing the marine environment, and this paradox has been – and will likely remain – a cause of public and political debates within the nation. In addition to the potential environmental disturbances associated with seabed exploration, the mobile structures needed for those activities pose a biosecurity risk for the marine species present in New Zealand.

The number of oil and gas vessels and drilling rigs coming to New Zealand is modest (i.e., two or three per annum) compared to the vast international shipping network that radiates in and out of the main ports (Plate 10). Yet the operational profile of these structures makes them high-risk vectors of marine pests (Hopkins and Forrest, 2010). Rigs can remain idle in one

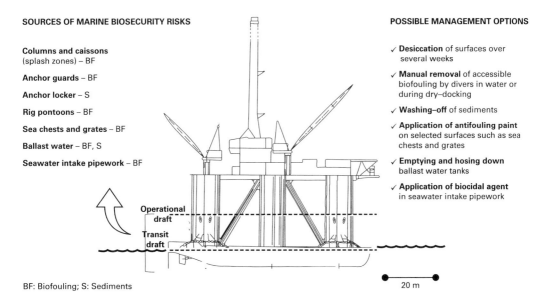

SOURCES OF MARINE BIOSECURITY RISKS

Columns and caissons (splash zones) – BF

Anchor guards – BF

Anchor locker – S

Rig pontoons – BF

Sea chests and grates – BF

Ballast water – BF, S

Seawater intake pipework – BF

Operational draft

Transit draft

BF: Biofouling; S: Sediments

POSSIBLE MANAGEMENT OPTIONS

✓ **Desiccation** of surfaces over several weeks

✓ **Manual removal** of accessible biofouling by divers in water or during dry–docking

✓ **Washing–off** of sediments

✓ **Application of antifouling paint** on selected surfaces such as sea chests and grates

✓ **Emptying and hosing down** ballast water tanks

✓ **Application of biocidal agent** in seawater intake pipework

20 m

Figure 7.1 Examples of sources of marine biosecurity risks on a drilling rig and of risk mitigation measures implemented during recent rig transfers to New Zealand.

location for several weeks or months, facilitating the accumulation of local biofouling species. The petroleum industry has already shown its commitment to meet the new CRMS requirements for biofouling and several companies, from engineers to operations managers, have successfully worked with New Zealand marine scientists to develop effective risk management plans. Thus to produce a biosecurity plan that meets the CRMS and minimizes biosecurity risk to New Zealand, a collaborative effort is required between the owners and operators of the vessels, government and science providers to develop effective and workable solutions. Biofouling mitigation measures have included passive desiccation, manual removal by divers, and dosage of seawater pipes with approved treatments (Figure 7.1).

Managing domestic risk pathways – focus on aquaculture

Once an organism is introduced or emerges as a threat within New Zealand, a number of pathways have the potential to expand its distribution (Castinel et al., 2013; Forrest et al., 2014). Natural spread of marine pests and pathogens is unlikely across long distances due to geographic and hydrodynamic 'firebreaks' (Forrest et al., 2009). However, human activities, such as aquaculture (e.g., via fouled equipment or the stock itself) have a well-documented history of facilitating 'domestic' spread (Forrest and Blakemore, 2006; Peeler et al., 2007).

Marine farming takes place in several areas distributed over New Zealand's main islands, with Chinook salmon (*Oncorhynchus tshawytscha*), green-lipped mussel (*Perna canaliculus*) and Pacific oyster (*Crassostrea gigas*) the main commercial species. Most operations, in particular shellfish farming, require significant transfers of stock and gear across regions. Although the use of hatchery seeds (spat) is gaining momentum in New Zealand, the shellfish industry remains largely dependent on wild-caught spat to supply farms around the country. In the event of an infectious disease circulating in a spat-catching region, the infection could spread very rapidly throughout the industry unless controls were quickly implemented. This was illustrated during the first series of mortality outbreaks involving an ostreid herpes virus (OsHV-1 microvar) in 2010, where movements of barges and equipment from affected areas to other parts of the country may have contributed to exacerbating disease intensity and production losses (Bingham et al., 2013). The index case was never identified.

Some pathogens have been historically deemed important for trade even if they do not noticeably impact the health of their host population. This is the case for the World Organization for Animal Health (OIE)-notifiable parasite *Perkinsus olseni* that has been found in New Zealand clam, cockle and other bivalves for many years (Hine, 1997, 2002) but was only recently found in farmed paua (Māori name for abalone) and in one farmed green-lipped mussel during routine health monitoring (OIE, 2013, 2014). Such findings had to be reported to the OIE to inform trading partners of the novel information. However, in neither case did it prompt the New Zealand government to impose movement controls, as *Perkinsus olseni* is found in wild shellfish around the country. These two events show the importance of routine health surveys to detect new pathogen-host interactions and identify trends in disease emergence over time. It is even more so important given that surveillance of shellfish diseases is currently largely reliant on industry's own monitoring as there is presently no ongoing national surveillance programme.

7.5 Responses to incursions: current state and future directions

Marine biosecurity responses: an integrated approach

There are many factors that could influence the outcome of a biosecurity response; for example, how quickly a pest or pathogen was detected, the number of individuals or affected hosts, their spread potential, the proximity to domestic vectors and the level of support from the community (e.g., recreational users, divers) and stakeholders (e.g., marine farmers, port authorities). Knowledge of the invader is no doubt important to inform decisions about detection and eradication. While incursions by exotic pathogens are most likely to cause noticeable disease outbreaks in naïve animal or plant populations, pest species may be more difficult to detect, especially if they resemble organisms already found on New Zealand shores (e.g., the non-indigenous Chinese mitten crab and the endemic mud crabs).

Given how quickly marine organisms can establish and spread, New Zealand has invested in developing a national biosecurity capability network that can identify and mobilize adequate resources to respond to an incursion as directed by the government. This network includes people with a wide range of specialist skills, from diving to taxonomic diagnostics. It also has a list of scientific experts who have knowledge about marine pest biology, pathology, ecology and even sometimes experience in marine incursion responses. As government-led biosecurity responses follow a generic framework adapted from an international model (Coordinated Incident Management System), it is easy to recruit external technical staff to be part of the response activities. The size and duration of such responses can vary greatly (from weeks to months) in the marine environment, mainly depending on the organism targeted and

the extent of its distribution after first detection. Improvements have been made in the field of preparedness and effective decision-making, with greater consideration given to stakeholders and technical advice from subject matter experts.

Despite the best efforts and intentions, the outcomes of marine biosecurity responses do not always lead to successful eradication of the invasive pest or pathogen. For example, the invasive Mediterranean fanworm (*Sabella spallanzanii*) was discovered in the South Island of New Zealand during surveillance activities and prompted the government to respond to the incursion by eliminating the organism locally (Read et al., 2011). During the local eradication attempt that was achieving considerable reductions in densities, a separate population was also found in a harbour in the North Island (Waitemata Harbour). Eradication attempts at both locations ceased when *Sabella* was subsequently found to be widely distributed in Waitemata Harbour, and long-term management (including surveillance activities) was considered a more sensible option to optimize public resources (Read et al., 2011). This example highlights how difficult decision-making in a biosecurity response can be and that initial assessments need to be revisited many times as events unfold.

Often a marine response consists of local containment and long-term management onsite. This cannot be achieved by the authorities without active support from both the community and the industries impacted by the incursion. A good example is the co-management of the invasive sea squirt *Pyura doppelgangera* in the Northland region. In its native range (Australia), this organism tends to form dense mats; thus it could potentially dominate New Zealand rocky shores and displace some endemic valued species like the green-lipped mussel. Similarly, the impact of *P. doppelgangera* spreading to marine mussel farms could be devastating for New Zealand aquaculture. Accordingly, the mussel industry and government are jointly working to set practical guidelines to prevent further spread of the pest within New Zealand, but the most remarkable aspect of this response is the joint initiative between government agencies and local community members to manually remove the sea squirts from the shores. This is very encouraging for future partnerships in marine biosecurity responses.

Continuing challenges and new directions

Considerable progress has been made to promote biosecurity risk awareness in the marine sector in New Zealand, yet there are ongoing challenges such as uncertainty over the timing and identity of the next invasive pest or disease. This lack of predictability necessitates the development of 'generic' response plans that are adaptable to a range of pests and pathogens. But not all stakeholders see the benefits of being prepared for an event that may never occur. It is, and will always be, challenging to justify preparedness expenditure to industry and the community in the absence of demonstrated impacts. The economic and environmental impacts of marine incursions are typically poorly understood or recorded and can be extremely variable between locations and organisms. Further, both educational work and close engagement between government and stakeholders are essential in order to change risk behaviour in New Zealand.

It is within this spirit that the Biosecurity Act was amended in 2012 to lay out the regulatory framework for the Government Industry Agreement (GIA). This approach (inspired by a similar scheme in Australia) proposes that government and primary industries should work in partnership to achieve the best possible biosecurity outcomes from readiness to response activities. This implies making joint decisions and sharing the cost of the activities while taking into account both the public and industry benefits. The aquaculture industry is one of the potential industry partners in the marine environment (e.g., fisheries could be another candidate) and discussions on a GIA partnership have been initiated. Another way to enhance mutual understanding between stakeholders and the authorities is to organize simulations of incursions and community workshops on biosecurity response challenges in the marine environment. Changing people's perceptions on biosecurity prevention and mobilizing communities to help respond to incursions as a team are the way forward in the marine environment.

While people develop a uniform view of marine biosecurity threats in New Zealand, local regulations also have to be consistent between regions. The Biosecurity Act and the New Zealand Coastal Policy Statement 2010 have given substantial responsibilities to regional councils. In addition to being accountable for managing existing marine pests in their regions, councils are now tasked with developing pathway management plans to reduce the intra- and inter-regional spread of marine pests and diseases that are established in New Zealand. This new mandate may take some time to be effectively developed and implemented.

7.6 Conclusions

Biosecurity is especially complex and challenging in the marine environment. In order to protect its unique biodiversity and ecosystem health, New Zealand has developed some of the most stringent border requirements in the world. It is encouraging to see that government measures are being supported by industries that see the benefits of preserving marine ecosystem health. For instance, oil and gas exploration companies are responding positively to pre-border requirements for managing risk from ballast water and biofouling, and domestic primary industries have an opportunity to take a more active role in preparedness and marine biosecurity responses.

Notwithstanding a solid partnership between government, stakeholders and the community, there are many factors that can influence whether a biosecurity response will reach its objectives or not. Enhancing early detection systems (e.g., through regular marine surveys and active public participation to report suspect exotic organisms and disease outbreaks) is one way to improve post-border risk management. Improving knowledge of marine pests and pathogens, their mode of spread or epidemiology and most importantly their optimum climatic and host range will considerably help in developing effective options to control the invasive organism. Finally, new generations of diagnostic tools are under development, using molecular technologies to identify the species of micro-organisms present on vessel hulls (currently, research in this field is largely government-funded).

Non-indigenous marine pests and emerging diseases have become a reality for New Zealand and a future incursion with serious impacts on the country's environment and economy seems inevitable. While it is crucial to maintain the biosecurity measures currently in place at the border, industries (e.g., shipping, aquaculture and tourism) and the community need to be further involved in controlling critical domestic risk pathways. A 'team approach' is even more important in the marine environment than it is in the terrestrial one. All skills and knowledge, from science to policy, need to be timely pulled together and coordinated to achieve the best results in marine biosecurity risk management. New Zealand is progressively heading in that direction with both industry and the local community increasingly engaged in decisions and response operations. The country's strong experience with biosecurity has shown so far that the problems, as much as the solutions, lie at the crossroad between the use of marine resources, cultural beliefs, regulations and environmental sciences.

References

Acosta, H. and Forrest, B.M. (2009). The spread of marine non-indigenous species via recreational boating: a conceptual model for risk assessment based on fault tree analysis. *Ecological Modelling*, 220, 1586–1598.

Bell, A., Phillips, S., Denny, C., Georgiades, E. and Kluza, D. (2011). *Risk Analysis: Vessel Biofouling*. New Zealand: Ministry of Agriculture and Forestry Biosecurity.

Bingham, P., Brangenberg, N., Williams, R. and van Andel, M. (2013). Investigation into the first diagnosis of ostreid herpesvirus type 1 in Pacific oysters. *Surveillance*, 40(2), 20–24.

Castinel, A., Forrest, B. and Hopkins, G. (2013). *Review of Disease Risks for New Zealand Shellfish Aquaculture: Perspectives for Management*. Prepared for the New Zealand Ministry of Business, Innovation and Employment, Cawthron Report No. 2297.

Coutts, A.D.M., Moore, K.M. and Hewitt, C.L. (2003). Ships' sea-chests: an overlooked transfer mechanism for non-indigenous marine species? *Marine Pollution Bulletin*, 46, 1510–1513.

Fitridge, I., Dempster, T., Geunther, J. and de Nys, R. (2012). The impact and control of biofouling in marine aquaculture: a review. *Biofouling*, 28, 649–669.

Forrest, B.M. and Blakemore, K.A. (2006). Evaluation of treatments to reduce the spread of a marine plant pest with aquaculture transfers. *Aquaculture*, 257, 333–345.

Forrest, B.M., Gardner, J.P.A. and Taylor, M.D. (2009). Internal borders for managing invasive marine species. *Journal of Applied Ecology*, 46(1), 46–54.

Forrest, B., Cahill, P., Newcombe, E. and Taylor, D. (2014). *Marine Pests and Management Priorities for Shellfish Aquaculture*. Prepared for the New Zealand Ministry of Business, Innovation and Employment, Cawthron Report No. 2285.

Glibert, P.M., Icarus Allen, J., Artioli, Y., Beusen, A., Bouwman, L., Harle, J., Holmes, R. and Holt, J. (2014). Vulnerability of coastal ecosystems to changes in harmful algal bloom distribution in response to climate change: projections based on model analysis. *Global Change Biology*, 20, 3845–3858.

Gordon, D.P., Beaumont, J., MacDiarmid, A., Robertson, D.A. and Ahyong, S.T. (2010). Marine biodiversity of Aotearoa New Zealand. *PLOS One*, 5(8), e10905.

Harvell, C.D., Kim, K., Burkholder, J.M., Colwell, R.R., Epstein, P.R., Grimes, D.J., Hofmann, E.E., Lipp, E.K., Osterhaus, A.D.M.E., Overstreet, R.M., Porter, J.W., Smith, G.W. and Vasta, G.R. (1999). Emerging marine diseases – climate links and anthropogenic factors. *Science*, 285, 1505–1510.

Hayden, B.J., Inglis, G.J. and Schiel, D.R. (2009). Marine invasions in New Zealand: a history of complex supply-side dynamics. In G. Rilov and J.A. Crooks (ed.), *Biological Invasions in Marine Ecosystems: Ecological, Management, and Geographic Perspectives*. Berlin: Springer-Verlag, pp. 409–423.

Hedrick, R.P. (1996). Movement of pathogens with the international trade of live fish: problems and solutions. *Revue Scientifique et Technique (International Office of Epizootics)*, 15(2), 523–531.

Hegaret, H., Shumway, S.E., Wikfors, G.H., Pate, S. and Burkholder, J.M. (2008). Potential transport of harmful algae via relocation of bivalve molluscs. *Marine Ecology Progress Series*, 361, 169–179.

Hewitt, C.L. and Campbell, M.L. (1999). Vectors, shipping and trade. In C.L. Hewitt, M.L. Campbell, R.E. Thresher and R.B. Martin (ed.), *Marine Biological Invasions of Port Phillip Bay, Victoria*, Centre for Research on Introduced Marine Pests, Technical Report No. 20.

Hewitt, C.L., Willing, J., Bauckham, A., Cassidy, A.M., Cox, C.M.S., Jones, L. and Wotton, D.M. (2004). New Zealand marine biosecurity: delivering outcomes in a fluid environment. *New Zealand Journal of Marine and Freshwater Research*, 38, 429–438.

Hine, P.M. (1997). Health status of commercially important molluscs in New Zealand. *Surveillance*, 24, 25–28.

Hine, P.M. (2002). Results of a survey on shellfish health in New Zealand in 2000. *Surveillance*, 29, 3–7.

Hopkins, G.A. and Forrest, B.M. (2010). A preliminary assessment of biofouling and non-indigenous marine species associated with commercial slow-moving vessels arriving in New Zealand. *Biofouling*, 26, 613–621.

Howard, A.E. (1994). The possibility of long distance transmission of *Bonamia* by fouling on boat hulls. *Bulletin of the European Association of Fish Pathology*, 14, 211–212.

IMO (2004). *International Convention for the Control and Management of Ships' Ballast Water and Sediments*. International Maritime Organization, www.imo.org/About/Conventions/ListOfConventions/Pages/International-Convention-for-the-Control-and-Management-of-Ships'-Ballast-Water-and-Sediments-(BWM).aspx.

IMO (2011). *Annex 26. Resolution MEPC.207(62) adopted on 15 July 2011. Guidelines for the Control and Management of Ships' Biofouling to Minimize the Transfer of Invasive Aquatic Species*. International Maritime Organization, www.imo.org/blast/blast-DataHelper.asp?data_id=30766.

Inglis, G.J., Floerl, O., Shane, T., Cox, S.L., Unwin, M., Ponder-Sutton, A., Seaward, K., Kospartov, M., Read, G., Gordon, D., Hosie, A., Nelson, W., D'Archino, R., Bell, A. and Kluza, D. (2010). *The Biosecurity Risks Associated with Biofouling on International Vessels Arriving in New Zealand: Summary of the Patterns and Predictors of Fouling*. Prepared for New Zealand Ministry of Agriculture and Forestry Biosecurity New Zealand, NIWA, Christchurch, New Zealand.

Johnson, P.T.J., Townsend, A.R., Cleveland, C.C., Glibert, P.M., Howarth, R.W., McKenzie, V.J., Rejmankova, E. and Ward, M.H. (2010). Linking environmental nutrient enrichment and disease emergence in humans and wildlife. *Ecological Applications*, 20, 16–29.

Kulhanek, S.A., Ricciardi, A. and Leung, B. (2011). Is invasion history a useful tool for predicting the impacts of the world's worst aquatic invasive species? *Ecological Applications*, 21, 189–202.

Minchin, D. (2007). Aquaculture and transport in a changing environment: overlap and links in the spread of alien biota. *Marine Pollution Bulletin*, 55, 302–313.

Minchin, D. and Gollasch, S. (2003). Fouling and ship's hulls: how changing circumstances and spawning events may result in the spread of exotic species. *Biofouling*, 19, 111–122.

MPI (2005). *Import Health Standard For Ships' Ballast Water From All Countries*. New Zealand Ministry for Primary Industries, www.mpi.govt.nz/document-vault/1167.

MPI (2011). *Aquaculture Readiness Data – Phase II*. New Zealand Ministry for Primary Industries Technical Paper No: 2011/68.

MPI (2012). *Pet Biosecurity in New Zealand – Current State of the Domestic Pet Trade System and Options Going Forward*. Information Paper No: 2012/01.

MPI (2014a). *Situation and Outlook for Primary Industries 2014*. New Zealand: Ministry for Primary Industries.

MPI (2014b). *Craft Risk Management Standard: Biofouling on Vessels Arriving to New Zealand*. New Zealand: Ministry for Primary Industries, www.biosecurity.govt.nz/files/regs/ships/crms-biofouling-standard.pdf.

Morrisey, D., Seaward, K. and Inglis, G. (2014). *Marine High-Risk Site Surveillance*. Annual report for all ports and marinas 2013–2014, NIWA, Nelson, New Zealand.

Mortensen, S., Arzul, I., Miossec, L., Paillard, C., Feist, S., Stentiford, G., Renault, T., Saulnier, D. and Gregory, A. (2007). Molluscs and crustaceans. In R.T. Raynard, T. Wahli, I. Vatsos and S. Mortensen (ed.), *Review of Disease Interactions and Pathogen Exchange Between Farmed and Wild Finfish and Shellfish in Europe*. VESO on behalf of DIPNET, Oslo, Norway, pp. 315-446.

Nottage, R.A.C., Wratt, D.S., Bornman, J.F. and Jones, K. (eds.) (2010). *Climate Change Adaptation in New Zealand: Future Scenarios and Some Sectoral Perspectives*. Wellington: New Zealand Climate Change Centre.

Núñez Vázquez, E.J., Lizarraga, I.G., Schmidt, C.J., Tapia, A.C., Cortes, D.J., Sandoval, F.E., Tapia, A.H. and Guzman, J.J. (2011). Impact of harmful algal blooms on wild and cultured animals in the Gulf of California. *Journal of Environmental Biology*, 32, 413–423.

OIE (2013). *OIE Disease Information. Infection with Perkinsus Olseni, New Zealand: Immediate Notification (15/08/2013)*, www.oie.int/wahis_2/public/wahid.php/Reviewreport/Review?page_refer=MapFullEventReport&reportid=13946.

OIE (2014). *OIE Disease Information. Infection with Perkinsus Olseni, New Zealand: Immediate Notification (2/09/2014)*, www.oie.int/wahis_2/public/wahid.php/Reviewreport/Review?page_refer=MapFullEventReport&reportid=15953.

Peeler, E.J., Murray, A.G., Thebault, A., Brun, E., Giovaninni, A. and Thrush, M.A. (2007). The application of risk analysis in aquatic animal health management. *Preventive Veterinary Medicine*, 81, 3–20.

Peeler, E.J., Oidtmann, B.C., Midtlyng, P.M., Miossec, L. and Gozlan, R.E. (2010). Non-native aquatic animal introductions have driven disease emergence in Europe. *Biological Invasions*, 13, 1291–1303.

Read, G.B., Inglis, G., Stratford, P. and Ahyong, S.T. (2011). Arrival of the alien fanworm *Sabella spallanzanii* (Gmelin, 1791) (Polychaeta: Sabellidae) in two New Zealand harbours. *Aquatic Invasions*, 6, 273–279.

Renault, T. (1996). Appearance and spread of diseases among bivalve molluscs in the northern hemisphere in relation to international trade. *Revue Scientifique et Technique Office International des Epizooties*, 15, 551–561.

Rhodes, L., Smith, K.F. and Moisan, C. (2013). Shifts and stasis in marine HAB monitoring in New Zealand. *Environmental Science and Pollution Research*, 20(10), 6872–6877.

Rodgers, C.J., Mohan, C.V. and Peeler, E.J. (2011). The spread of pathogens through trade in aquatic animals and their products. *Revue Scientifique et Technique Office International des Epizooties*, 30, 241–256.

Ruiz, G.M., Rawlings, T.K., Dobbs, F.C., Drake, L.A., Mullady, T., Huq, A. and Colwell, R.R. (2000). Global spread of microorganisms by ships – ballast water discharged from vessels harbours a cocktail of potential pathogens. *Nature*, 408, 49–50.

Simberloff, D. and Gibbons, L. (2004). Now you see them, now you don't! Population crashes of established introduced species. *Biological Invasions*, 6, 161–172.

Sorte, C. J., Williams, S. L. and Zerebecki, R. A. (2010). Ocean warming increases threat of invasive species in a marine fouling community. *Ecology*, 91, 2198–2204.

Subasinghe, R.P. (2005). Epidemiological approach to aquatic animal health management: opportunities and challenges for developing countries to increase aquatic production through aquaculture. *Preventive Veterinary Medicine*, 67, 117–124.

Tana, T. (2014). The Ministry for Primary Industries' animal general surveillance programme. *Surveillance*, 41, 5–8.

Taranaki Regional Council (2013). *Guide to Regulating Oil and Gas Exploration and Development Activities Under the Resource Management Act*. Taranaki: Taranaki Regional Council.

chapter 8

The role of environmental management in snail-borne zoonotic diseases

Patrick Hanington, David C. Hall and William Anyan

Abstract

Snails are gastropod molluscs in which the body can be withdrawn into a spiral shell. There are many different species and they play an important role in balancing the complexity of ecosystems through vegetation control and recycling as well as acting as a food source for invertebrates and vertebrates. Some species also maintain the ecological equilibrium of pond life and other waterways. Snails can also have value as a human food source. However, due to the damage they cause to ornamentals and crops, snails are widely regarded by urban gardeners and agronomists as pests to get rid of. Apart from the damage to plant life, snails can also act as intermediate hosts of zoonotic diseases including a number of pathogenic flukes (trematodes) including intestinal and urinary schistosomiasis and fascioliasis. Due to the fact that these parasites have a complex disease ecology, the development of disease control and prevention guidelines requires the engagement of experts from a number of fields. In this chapter we will examine two case studies of trematode diseases from Africa and Asia, the role of snails in these diseases and the importance of environmental management and interdisciplinary integrated control approaches for achieving sustained control.

8.1 Introduction

Snails play an important role in balancing the complexity of ecosystems through vegetation control and recycling, as a food source for invertebrates and vertebrates including beetles, fireflies, hedgehogs and ducks, and in maintaining the ecological equilibrium of pond life and other waterways. Of course, snails are also valuable as a human food, both cultivated and gathered in their natural habitat. Despite these contributions, snails are widely regarded by urban gardeners and agronomists alike as pests to get rid of due to the damage they cause to ornamentals and crops. Apart from the damage to plant life, snails can also act as intermediate hosts of zoonotic diseases from annoying skin conditions such as swimmer's itch to far more serious diseases caused by pathogenic flukes (trematodes) including intestinal and urinary schistosomiasis and fascioliasis.

Of the more than 18,000 different species of trematode, almost all undergo larval development within a snail (Esch et al., 2002; Littlewood and Bray, 2001). Despite lifecycle variances between different trematode species, the dependence of these parasites on the snail host is absolute, to the point that the geographic ranges of every medically and veterinary relevant trematode is defined by the presence of susceptible snail species (Morgan et al., 2001). In laboratory studies, snail resistance to trematode infection can be experimentally manipulated (Hanington et al., 2010, 2012), and recent examples in field trials indicate that the chances of a schistosome developing to the point of a patent infection (shedding cercariae), within a natural snail is not 100 per cent (Hamburger et al., 2004). Thus, compatibility with the snail host likely serves as a barrier to the propagation of a trematodiasis. Moreover, the spread of many of these diseases into new regions is often prevented simply by an absence of suitable snail hosts. Controlling the snail intermediate host with sustainable methods that consider ecohealth principles is thus a compelling option, not just for countries where drugs and health services may not be available, but also for those countries in which snails are recognized as a valuable element of the ecosystem.

This chapter will look at two regional case studies of trematode diseases from Africa and Asia, the role of snails in these diseases, and the importance of environmental management and integrated control approaches for achieving sustained control.

8.2 Schistosomiasis

The World Health Organization (WHO) regards schistosomiasis as one of the most neglected tropical diseases (WHO, 2015a); it is widely recognized as the second most devastating parasitic disease in the world, following malaria (van der Werf et al., 2003). The WHO estimates that more than 260 million individuals are infected by at least one species of schistosome, resulting in the loss of approximately 3.3 million disability-adjusted life years (DALYs) (Hotez et al., 2014), and it is considered endemic in 78 countries, of which 52 engage in preventive chemotherapy. About half of the 262 million people requiring treatment globally are children; of those, fewer than 15 per cent actually receive treatment (WHO, 2012a). Schistosomiasis is a disease that disproportionately infects and affects impoverished individuals and communities in subtropical and tropical areas. Often, high infection prevalence is found in combination with access to only minimal standards of sanitation, and it is common to find that children bear both the highest prevalence and intensity of infection within a community. Higher prevalence is observed in areas where exposure to fresh water is frequent, and there is also higher parasite burden in infected humans in these regions (Soares Magalhaes et al., 2011).

Recent efforts to control schistosomiasis have been centralized on the application of the single, widely available drug, praziquantel (PZQ), to treat infected people (Hotez et al., 2010; Stothard et al., 2011). This one-dimensional strategy carries with it the obvious risk of widespread development of worms resistant to PZQ (Doenhoff et al., 2009; Lotfy et al., 2015; Melman et al., 2009), a danger that escalates the longer and more extensively it is used. Treatment using the PZQ is effective at clearing adult worms from patients. Eliminating the infection can eventually result in healing of damaged tissue and lesions, provided that reinfection does not occur. Unfortunately, PZQ treatment is often administered irregularly and provides no lasting protection against reinfection. Individuals can be reinfected almost immediately if PZQ is administered prior to peak transmission times, so it is important to acquire information about the transmission dynamics of the infection in a given area (Hotez et al., 2010).

In 2012, the WHO announced an initiative to significantly expand schistosomiasis treatment and control efforts with the vision of eliminating the disease by 2025. While an inspiring and noble call to arms, access to treatment for schistosomiasis was estimated to only reach approximately 8 per cent of those infected in 2008 (WHO, 2011) and 13 per cent in 2013 (WHO, 2015a) leaving around 221 million people without adequate treatment. Complicating the lack of treatment is recent evidence suggesting that PZQ treatment alone will not be sufficient to achieve sustained control, even if accessibility improves (Ross et al., 2015a, 2015b). Moreover, growing concerns about the development of drug resistance to the few anti-schistosome drugs available (Doenhoff et al., 2008; Lotfy et al., 2015; Mwangi et al., 2014; Valentim et al., 2013; Wang et al., 2012), underscores the need for lateral, innovative thinking about schistosome control, outside of the box of traditional chemotherapy alone, including integration of snail control efforts (Adema et al., 2012).

Schistosomiasis in Africa

Globally, there are six species of schistosome associated with human infection: S. mansoni, S. haematobium and S. japonicum are the three species responsible for causing the majority of disease, with S. guineensis, S. mekongi and S. intercalatum being responsible for small pockets of infections in Asia and Africa respectively. Of the main three species, S. haematobium is endemic to Africa, S. mansoni is endemic to Africa and South America (including parts of the Caribbean), and S. japonicum can be found in Asia. By a wide margin, Africa bears the brunt of schistosome infections; 90 per cent of all schistosome-infected persons live in 46 African countries (Barnabas et al., 2012). In Africa, schistosomiasis presents in two general forms that are distinguished by the species of infecting schistosome. Intestinal

schistosomiasis is primarily caused by infection with S. mansoni, and urinary schistosomiasis by infections with S. haematobium.

Schistosoma mansoni – intestinal schistosomiasis

Intestinal schistosomiasis in Africa and South America is caused by S. mansoni, which is considered the most widespread human schistosome. The adult S. mansoni worms typically reside within the small inferior mesenteric blood vessels surrounding the large intestine and caecal region. Male and female worms are found paired, the female worm fitting into the gynaecophoric canal of the male. Each worm pair is able to generate ~300 eggs per day, which are destined to be released into the lumen of the host intestine where they are excreted via the faeces into the environment (Colley et al., 2014).

The geographical distribution of S. mansoni is defined by the presence of snails of the genus *Biomphalaria*. While not all species of *Biomphalaria* are susceptible to S. mansoni infection, the predominant species found in Africa (*B. pfeifferi, B. sudanica, B. alexandrina, B tenagophila, B. straminea*) have all been shown to be compatible with the S. mansoni strains in their locale (Levitz et al., 2013; Moser et al., 2014; Stensgaard et al., 2013).

Schistosoma haematobium – urinary schistosomiasis

Although both S. mansoni and S. haematobium have very similar lifecycles, urinary schistosomiasis is often associated with greater pathology than its intestinal cousin (Rollinson, 2009). S. haematobium adult worms reside within the perivisceral venous plexus. A single female worm can produce hundreds of eggs per day, each of which migrates through basal lamina and tissues into the lumen of the bladder (Krautz-Peterson et al., 2009). If individuals from endemic communities are not treated with PZQ, haematuria (and by proxy infection prevalence) caused by *S. haematobium* can be as high as 100 per cent (Gryseels, 1989; Gryseels et al., 2006). Furthermore, up to 75 per cent of women infected by *S. haematobium* develop irreversible lesions in the vulva, vagina, cervix and uterus, creating long-lasting points of entry for HIV and other sexually transmitted infections. Often infection significantly skews HIV transmission towards females in areas where *S. haematobium* is endemic (Stoever et al., 2009). Despite the importance of urinary schistosomiasis at both individual and population levels, it remains the poorest understood of the three primary schistosome infections of humans from both an epidemiological and pathophysiological point of view (Rollinson, 2009).

Schistosoma haematobium relies on snails of the genus *Bulinus* for its larval development (*B. globosus, B. truncatus, B. forskalii*) being primarily responsible, with numerous less common species also contributing to transmission (Lo, 1972; Mandahl-Barth, 1965). Bulinid snails can be found throughout Africa, and also serve as the intermediate host for a number of animal schistosomes, which complicates identification of *S. haematobium* cercariae. There is growing concern and evidence that *S. haematobium* is able to hybridize with *S. bovis*, a closely related schistosome that infects cattle (Huyse et al., 2009).

Schistosomes and snails

The persistence and tenacity of schistosomiasis in the face of mass-drug administration primarily stems from the reliance of the parasites on freshwater snails for larval development and transmission to humans. Snails are ignored by most current control strategies; however, the importance of snails as a point of control has garnered some attention, and will be discussed in detail later (Adema et al., 2012). Snails become infected by schistosomes following an encounter with one of the free-living stages of the parasite, called a miracidia, which hatches from an egg shed from an infected human. The miracidia penetrates the snail tegument and, providing it is able to establish within the snail, will initiate a program of asexual reproduction that ultimately sees the snail become a home for the larval schistosome, and a 'factory' for the production of the second free-living stage, the cercariae. Snails infected by a schistosome can survive up to year (Mutuku et al., 2014), shedding hundreds of cercariae per day, each of which possesses the potential to initiate new human infections. In the case of *S. haematobium*, it is estimated that a single snail can shed an average of 200 cercariae per day, and up to 1,000 per day in the case of *S. mansoni* (Ayad, 1974; Chu and Dawood, 1970; de Souza et al., 1994; Mutuku et al., 2014). Thus, a single miracidium that infects a snail could theoretically yield up to 365,000 cercariae, and realistically likely results in the production of approximately 20,000 cercariae on average (Ayad, 1974). Epidemiologically, this means that the relationship between excreted eggs/miracidia and infection risk is non-linear, and dramatically amplified by the snail stage of the lifecycle. This is a primary reason why schistosomiasis can persist in an area with only a few infected snails, and that it can be re-established in a short time even when human infections appear to be cleared following treatment (Rollinson et al., 2001).

Animal reservoirs and schistosome hybridization

With the exception of *S. japonicum*, which has been shown to be capable of infecting more than 40 animal hosts following larval development within *Oncomelania sp.* snails (McManus et al., 2009), it is generally thought that *S. mansoni* and *S. haematobium* are exclusive to humans. Sparse evidence exists suggesting that rodents may serve as a possible reservoir host for *S. mansoni*

(Duplantier and Sene, 2000, 2006; Hanelt et al., 2010), and laboratory studies focused on this parasite typically make use of mice as a surrogate host. However, the actual contribution of rodents as a reservoir for *S. mansoni* has yet to be quantified. *S. haematobium* has not been found to infect animal reservoirs naturally. Again, laboratory studies support the fact that hamsters can be used in place of humans for lifecycle maintenance, but the occurrence of naturally occurring infected rodent populations in endemic areas has not been observed. Importantly, *S. haematobium* is closely related to the cattle schistosome *S. bovis*, which also makes use of bulinid snails as an intermediate host. A number of studies have demonstrated that *S. haematobium* and *S. bovis* hybridize, generating a parasite that has been shown to infect humans (Huyse et al., 2009; Webster et al., 2013), but have yet to be found infecting cattle. Whether these hybrids represent a true zoonotic schistosome capable of infecting both humans and cattle as a definitive host is currently under investigation; this would represent a significant issue for current control efforts. The presence of these two closely related parasite species in the same water body results in an increased likelihood of both parasite species co-infecting a host, allowing for mating between the two species to occur, and thus a high potential for hybridization in either human or cattle (Huyse et al., 2009; Southgate et al., 1998).

Hybridization between *S. haematobium* and *S. bovis* presents a significant issue for future control and prevention of human schistosomiasis in areas where both species are present. Although hybridization has been conclusively demonstrated between these two species (Huyse et al., 2009; Webster et al., 2010), little is understood regarding the mechanics of hybridization. The host in which hybridization occurs is unknown, the infectivity profile of the hybrid species is poorly understood, and to date, hybrid parasites have only been isolated from humans. Thus, we do not know anything about the epidemiology of this hybrid-induced infection and disease it causes. However, what is certain is that hybrid *S. haematobium-S. bovis* parasites represent a public health threat that has expanded beyond the handful of studies that have identified these parasites in pockets of Africa. In 2014–2015, *S. haematobium* along with hybrids were found to be responsible for an outbreak of urinary schistosomiasis in Corsica, France (Berry et al., 2014; Boissier et al., 2015; Calavas and Martin, 2014; de Laval et al., 2014), where a suitable snail host, *B. truncatus*, is endemic.

Environmental management and schistosome transmission

Sanitation

The lifecycle of schistosomes makes measurement of the impact from improved sanitation on schistosomiasis challenging to assess (Grimes et al., 2014, 2015). Schistosomes do not follow a faecal–oral infection route that is common to other water- and excreta-transmitted diseases, instead it is contact with infested water that must be reduced. Thus, with respect to schistosomiasis, prevention of water contamination by both schistosomes and snails is an important consideration of any sanitation initiative. Given the importance of snails to the amplification of schistosomiasis, it is just as important to devise means to reduce snail host presence or infection prevalence as it is to reduce excreta contamination. While the importance of improved sanitation and hygiene practices in regions where schistosomiasis is endemic is unquestionable, there are a number of integrated control approaches that appear to have a meaningful impact on schistosome transmission.

Water recreation areas

There are a number of activities, both recreational and vocational, that require contact with fresh water, and thus represent a risk of schistosome transmission. Some of these practices (for example, swimming, laundry, bathing, sand collecting, fishing and car washing) present unavoidable risks if undertaken in natural freshwater bodies. While the practices themselves may be essential aspects of life, where they are undertaken could be altered to reduce risks. In studies where practices such as bathing, laundry and swimming were moved from transmission sites by providing washing sinks, showers and swimming pools, and chemotherapy was provided, the prevalence of both *S. haematobium* and *S. mansoni* declined over a decade (Pitchford, 1966, 1970a, 1970b). These initial studies were reinforced by examples from St Lucia, where the inclusion of swimming pools, showers and laundry facilities significantly lowered *S. mansoni* infection incidence compared to control communities (Jordan, 1977, 1988; Jordan et al., 1975, 1978; Jordan and Unrau, 1978), and Ghana, where the installation of a water recreation area significantly reduced the number of school children infected by *S. haematobium* (Kosinski et al., 2011, 2012).

Application of molluscicides

Chemical control of snail populations has been a commonly used approach to interrupt the schistosome lifecycle by effectively removing the snail intermediate hosts from the environment (reviewed in King and Bertsch, 2015). Since the 1950s, niclosamide has been the most commonly used molluscicide. Following a screen of more than 20,000 compounds for toxicity against *B. glabrata*, niclosamide became preferred over other chemicals such as copper sulphate and sodium pentachlorophenate for snail control (Andrews et al., 1982). It has a low toxicity for humans and agricultural animals, is relatively stable when exposed to ultraviolet light, displays persistent lethal effects on snails for up to 24 hours, and achieves more than 90 per cent snail mortality at concentrations lower than 1ppm (~1mg per litre) (Foster et al., 1960).

Mollusciciding was a popular strategy for schistosomiasis control prior to the advent and initiation of oral chemotherapy, which was anticipated as being a more effective means to controlling the disease (Christie et al., 1980). Because of its popularity, however, there are a number of examples of well-designed mollusciciding strategies that demonstrate that with proper knowledge it can be an effective means to achieve a sustained reduction in schistosome transmission. Important considerations include a sound biological understanding of the snail population and possible off-target effects on fish, amphibians and other aquatic organisms, environmental factors that may impact application approaches or distribution of the chemical, and epidemiological aspects of disease transmission timing, rates and risk-associated behaviours (King and Bertsch, 2015). In examples where these impacting factors have been investigated, drastic declines in relevant snail population numbers have been reported within as little as three years (Brazil) (Barbosa and Costa, 1981), and human infection prevalence declined from 22 per cent to 4.3 per cent compared to 22 per cent to 20 per cent in control (non-molluscicided areas) within a five-year span (St Lucia) (Sturrock et al., 1974). Examples from Egypt demonstrated a clear reduction in the prevalence of both *S. haematobium* (22.8 per cent to 8.3 per cent in seven-year-old children) and *S. mansoni* (8.5 per cent to 1.9 per cent in seven-year-old children) in children aged one to seven from areas treated with molluscicide over a four-year span (1962–1965), compared to adjacent areas not treated (*S. haematobium*, 18 per cent to 21.4 per cent; *S. mansoni*, 6.4 per cent to 13.4 per cent in seven-year-old children) (Dawood et al., 1966; Farooq et al., 1966).

From the examples of mollusciciding successes, a number of noteworthy observations have been made that highlight strengths and drawbacks of this approach to schistosome transmission control. While snail populations can be significantly reduced by molluscicide application, they are also able to rebound rapidly if molluscicide pressure is removed or relaxed. Furthermore, there are numerous environmental variables that can influence success such as water chemistry and movement, temperature, vegetation and organic sediments. Thus, while success can be achieved, it requires thoughtful design and skilled implementation in order to yield meaningful impacts in schistosomiasis in an area.

Biological control – snail predators

The use of snail predators (either introduced or native) has been a suggested method for snail population control for a number of years. Initially, the North American crayfish *Procambarus clarkii*, which was introduced to East Africa as an aquacultural animal around 1970, was shown to significantly reduce the number of *B. pfeifferi* from controlled enclosures (Hofkin et al., 1991, 1992; Mkoji et al., 1999). These findings paralleled field experiments that also demonstrated that snails kept in unprotected enclosures in habitats where *P. clarkii* was present fared poorly when compared to snails kept in similar enclosures, but in habitats where crayfish were not present (Hofkin et al., 1992; Mkoji et al., 1999). While these initial demonstrations of a possible method for the biological control of schistosome-transmitting snails did not develop much traction as a control strategy when first proposed in the early 1990s, it has recently experienced a resurgence in interest. Evidence supporting *P. clarkii* as a means to control snails and schistosomiasis in Egypt confirmed the initial studies suggesting this species of crayfish may serve as a natural means to suppress snail populations

relevant to schistosome transmission (Khalil and Sleem, 2011). More recently, a number of high-profile studies, focused on a river prawn species native to Africa, *Machrobrachium vollenhoveni*, have demonstrated that restoration of the prawn to its native habitat reduces snail populations and also schistosome transmission (Savaya Alkalay et al., 2014; Sokolow et al., 2014, 2015). Underpinning these investigations are actual initiatives, such as Projet-Crevette, to integrate prawn aquaculture into schistomiasis control efforts, restoring prawns to their native freshwater ranges, thereby providing both a means to reduce snail populations as well as a local food and economic resource.

A case study: schistosomiasis in Ghana

Schistosomiasis remains one of the most widespread neglected tropical diseases (NTDs), and its impact is felt most significantly in the countries of Africa where it is firmly entrenched. Ghana, has the third highest prevalence of schistosome infections in Africa (Hotez and Kamath, 2009), and was one of the first African countries to implement a National Integrated Control Program for Neglected Tropical Diseases (Yirenya-Tawiah et al., 2011a). Both *S. mansoni* and *S. haematobium* are endemic throughout the country (Bosompem et al., 2004), and continue to pose a significant public health problem in spite of numerous efforts that have been put in place for control. Epidemiological data on the two forms of the disease were first documented between 1952 and 1955, revealing that 20 per cent of Ghana's total population suffered from urogenital schistosomiasis at some point in their lives (Edwards and McCullough, 1954). Following the construction of the Akosombo dam that created Lake Volta, there was increase in schistosomiasis prevalence and further spread of the disease necessitating control measures that could not be sustained over the years (Paperna, 1970; Scott et al., 1982).

Over the past decade, extensive epidemiological surveys and field studies that focus on schistosomiasis have been carried out in Ghana. From these reports, the prevalence of *S. haematobium* is estimated to range between 10 per cent and 60 per cent (Bosompem et al., 2004; Yirenya-Tawiah et al., 2011a, 2011b), and the prevalence of *S. mansoni* ranges between 10 per cent and 90 per cent (Aboagye and Edoh, 2009; Abonie, 2013; Aryeetey et al., 2000b; Nsowah-Nuamah et al., 2001; Scott et al., 1982). Higher prevalence is observed in areas where exposure to fresh water is frequent, and there is also higher parasite burden in infected humans in these regions, with many of the infected individuals passing more than 100 eggs per 10ml of urine (Soares Magalhaes et al., 2011). Studies over the years have revealed an alarming situation with schistosomiasis in infants a few months old (Bosompem et al., 2004), and significant morbidity in adults through the use of ultrasound and bio-markers for early detection of bladder cancer (Shiff et al., 2006). A recent study on schistosomiasis in reproductive age females has also shown involvement of female genital schistosomiasis (FGS) and potential co-infections with sexually transmitted diseases (STIs) (Yirenya-Tawiah et al., 2011a).

Children ranging in age from five to 14 years old are the primary infected demographic, often displaying the highest infection intensity and prevalence in a community, from as low as 43 per cent to as high as 100 per cent across the country, a fact the defines Ghana's current control approach; school-based administration of PZQ once per year (Fentiman et al., 2001; Gryseels et al., 2006). School-based urinary schistosomiasis treatment programmes significantly improve a number of qualitative and quantitative metrics of child health. The mean height, weight and haemoglobin levels (g/L) of children enrolled in school were all statistically higher (and thus

better) than age-matched controls not enrolled in the programme (Fentiman et al., 2001). Despite these successes, school-based mass drug administration has significant flaws. Children not attending school fail to receive treatment, and studies reveal that greater than 20 per cent of school-aged children not in school miss treatment (Fentiman et al., 2001). In fact, of the 20 per cent not attending school (59 per cent male, 41 per cent female), 66 per cent were found to have *S. haematobium* infections (compared to 34 per cent of school-enrolled children). There was also a significant difference in parasite burden; children not attending school excreted 41 eggs/10ml of urine, compared to 15 eggs/10ml in children enrolled in the program (Fentiman et al., 2001). Additionally, school-based treatment programmes ignore the infected adults in the community, who are only likely to report when the acute symptoms are very severe (van der Werf et al., 2004).

In Ghana, the distribution and spread of schistosomiasis has been influenced by water development projects like the construction of the Akosombo dam in 1964, and later the Kpong dam on the Volta River in 1981, as well as the Weija dam in 1979 on the Densu River and irrigation systems (Aryeetey et al., 2000a; Shiff et al., 2006). The sudden reduction in the flow rate of these reservoirs provided a large floodplain ideal for snail colonization and hence promoted the spread of both urinary and intestinal schistosomiasis in the country. The normal activities of fisherman, which include movement by water between interconnected communities, continued the spread of the disease to areas previously free from infection, and there has been an increase in prevalence and intensity of schistosomiasis nationwide. Another hydroelectric dam, the Bui dam, was completed in 2013, and resettling communities in the catchment areas has been undertaken with much more care and consideration of possible schistosome transmission than was the case in previous

Table 8.1

Disease	Infectious agent	Important snail intermediate hosts	Acquired by consuming[a]	Natural final host(s)	Human illness	Countries with documented cases[b]
Schistosomiasis			Skin penetration when exposed to cercariae in water			
Intestinal	Schistosoma mansoni Schistosoma japonicum Schistosoma mekongi Schistosoma intercalatum	Biomphalaria spp. Oncomelania spp. Oncomelania spp. Bulinus spp.	Humans ~40 animal hosts	Acute flu-like illness (Katayama Fever), chronic fatigue, granuloma formation in liver.	
Urinary	Schistosoma haematobium Schistosoma bovis	Bulinus spp. Bulinus spp.		Humans Cattle	Haematuria, urogenital lesions.	
Foodborne Trematode Zoonoses						
Clonorchiasis	Clonorchis sinensis	Melanoides spp. Parafossarulus manchourichus	Fresh/brackish water fish (raw, fermented, poorly cooked)	Dogs, fish-eating carnivores	Inflammation and fibrosis of hepatic biliary tissue, cholangiosarcoma.	CN, JA, VN
Fascioliasis	Fasciola hepatica Fasciola gigantica	Lymnaea spp. Fossaria spp.	Aquatic vegetables (poorly cooked)	Sheep, cattle, other herbivores	Hepatic inflammation, fibrosis, blockage, jaundice.	CA, CH, KO, LA, TH, VN
Heterophydiasis	Heterophyes heterophyes Heterophyes nocens Haplorchis pumilio Haplorchis taichui	Bithynia fuchsiana Melanoides tuberculate Angulyagra polyzonata	Fresh/brackish water fish (raw, fermented, poorly cooked)	Cats, fish-eating carnivores	Intestinal irritation, chronic diarrhoea, nausea; myocardial and cerebral granuloma.	KO, LA, TH, VN
Opisthorchiasis	Opisthorchis viverrini, Opisthorchis felineus	Bithynia spp.	Fresh/brackish water fish (raw, fermented, poorly cooked)	Cats, fish-eating carnivores	Inflammation and fibrosis of hepatic biliary tissue, cholangiosarcoma.	CA, CH, JA, KO, LA, TH, VN
Paragonimiasis	Paragonimus spp.	Semisulcospira spp. Brotia spp. Melanopides spp. Tricula spp.	Crustaceans (raw, poorly cooked)	Cats, dogs, other crustacean-eating carnivores	Chronic cough, chest pain, dyspnoea, fever; migration to cerebral locations.	CH, JA, LA, TH, VN

Compiled by the authors from numerous sources referenced in this chapter.
a Fish and crustaceans are considered secondary hosts containing larval stages of the parasite.
b CA = Cambodia, CH = China, JA = Japan, KO = South Korea, LA = Lao PDR, TH = Thailand, VN = Vietnam

projects. However, without appropriate research and expert management and/or intervention, the dynamic interactions between schistosome parasites, host snails and human hosts in the new dam area could lead to an explosion of schistosomiasis transmission in Western Ghana.

Displacement of individuals and communities, as well as migratory activities of specific populations, have all contributed to different species of schistosome and snail hosts coexisting in areas where they had not previously overlapped. This has resulted in the mixing of *S. haematobium* strains, and *S. haematobium* and *S. mansoni* species in infected people (Abonie, 2013; Chu et al., 1978). Currently, it appears as though the prevalence of *S. mansoni* infections in Ghana is increasing likely in part because its *Biomphalaria spp.* snail vectors are rapidly colonizing new areas that were initially noted for *S. haematobium* infections only. Where suitable snail hosts for *S. mansoni* and *S. haematobium* overlap, there is higher prevalence of *S. mansoni* infections than *S. haematobium* infection (Abonie, 2013). Additionally, preliminary evidence suggests that cattle herdsmen presenting eggs in their urine with morphological characteristics of *S. haematobium* are, upon molecular assessment by PCR, more closely related to *S. bovis*, than *S. haematobium*, reinforcing the concern over hybridization between these two schistosome species (Abonie, 2013). These situations call for the need to investigate possible hybridization and/or parthenogenesis between *S. haematobium* globosus strain and *S. haematobium* truncatus strain, *S. mansoni* and *S. haematobium* species, as well as *S. haematobium* and *S. bovis* species that can now all be found overlapping in distribution in endemic areas. As mentioned previously, these hybridization events may have significant implications for infectivity, fecundity, pathogenicity and future approaches to treatment and control.

8.3 Foodborne trematodiases in Vietnam

In much of Asia, the primary form of infection with trematodes is foodborne, in contrast to the majority of cases in Africa in which infection is usually from direct contact with the parasite in water. This section explores the situation in Vietnam and other parts of Asia where infection occurs through consumption of raw or poorly cooked aquatic species including fish and vegetables grown or washed in contaminated water. The result of infection without treatment can be prolonged liver and lung disease that is often not diagnosed, compromising not only the patient's ability to work and function normally in society but also increasing the burden on healthcare delivery systems.

Foodborne trematode ecology

Globally, there are four primary foodborne trematodes that require the freshwater snail as a primary host (WHO, 2015b). These are *Clonorchis spp.*, *Opisthorchis spp.*, *Fasciola spp.* and *Paragonimus spp.* Although not all require a secondary host, the final host is always mammalian, including humans. In cases of clonorchiasis and opisthorciasis, the secondary host is usually fish; the secondary host in paragonimiasis is usually a crustacean such as shrimp or crab. Fascioliasis is the only foodborne trematodiasis that does not typically involve a secondary host; patients are usually directly infected when consuming poorly cooked vegetables such as water morning glory and watercress raised in or washed in contaminated water such as an unclean local pond inhabited by snails.

Fasciola spp. – including *F. hepatica* and *F. gigantica* – have been reported as the major foodborne trematodes of Asia including China, Lao PDR and Vietnam (WHO, 1995; WHO and FAO, 2004). The other three primary foodborne trematodes noted above have also been reported by researchers from many parts of Asia in the past three decades (Rhee et al., 1988; De et al., 2003; Chai, 2005; Chai et al., 2005a, 2005b; Tesana, 2005; Yoshida, 2005; Nguyen et al., 2012; Anh et al., 2014). It is difficult to find reports that indicate well-researched prevalence rates, but the relative frequency of reporting of the burden of various trematode species does seem to have shifted in the past two decades.

While *Fasciola spp.* is still noted as a worry in Vietnam and a neglected disease in general (Tolan, 2011), recent research suggests that greater concern from an ecological perspective might be directed at trematodes from the *Heterophydae* family in Lao PDR, Thailand, and Vietnam (Chi et al., 2008; Chontananarth and Wongsawad, 2013; Clausen et al., 2012, 2015; Hung et al., 2013, 2015). Reasons for the increase in reported findings of *Heterophyidae* are unclear, although several authors suggest increased involvement of farmers in aquaculture plays a role. Thu et al. (2007) document one of the first reports of fish-borne trematodes of the *Heterophyidae* family in Vietnam. Chi et al. (2008) found a high level of fish-borne trematodes in farm-raised fish although the prevalence in humans was very low. They note that the rarity of earlier investigations which makes it difficult to conclude when *Heterophyidae* might have started to increase in prevalence in farm-raised fish in Vietnam.

8.4 The role of integrated agriculture in foodborne trematodiases in Vietnam

Aquaculture has become increasingly important in integrated small-scale farming systems in Vietnam in the past two decades. Aquaculture is a key element of the VAC system (named after the Vietnamese words for garden, fishpond and cattle shed), an integrated agricultural system that incorporates crops, aquaculture and livestock production. This small-scale agricultural system has been promoted by the Vietnam government as a sustainable agricultural system that generates food and income for poor farmers while recycling waste products within the system (Hop, 2003).

However, as aquaculture production has increased in Vietnam, an unexpected and certainly unintended consequence seems to have been the negative externality of increased risk of fish-borne zoonotic trematodes (FZTs) in fish due to the integration in the VAC system. As animal and sometimes human manure is recycled in the system, relying on this as a mechanism for waste disposal, as well as providing supplementary food and promoting algal growth for fish, increases the likelihood of FZT eggs present in the aquatic environment. This in turn increases the number of snail hosts, enhances merazoite transmission to fish, and ultimately facilitates infection back again to dogs, cats, livestock, and humans. Chi et al. (2008) outline this scenario examining data from Nghe An Province in Northern Vietnam, noting the reservoir in dogs, cats and pigs is more important to sustaining the parasite lifecycle than is the human reservoir. Research by Hung et al. (2015) has also indicated the important role of cats and dogs in sustaining FZT infections.

The problem of FZTs presents a challenge to advocates of integrated small-scale sustainable agricultural production. The disposal of animal and human excreta, which contain trematode eggs, in fishponds clearly contributes to sustaining the infection in fish and humans. Eliminating this activity from the otherwise highly sustainable integrated agricultural system would substantially help to reduce the cycle of infection in humans and animals, but this presents another problem. What to do with the build-up of animal and human waste? Putting manure on crops instead of in ponds is one solution but this requires a method for storage that does not result in runoff. Other options include pre-drying manure to the extent that parasite eggs do not survive or storing waste in a communal biogas system (i.e., composting of waste) or possibly treating the manure with molluscicides before placement into fishponds. Solutions to this problem that do not jeopardize sustainability of the VAC system have not been found in the literature; this is an area in need of further agricultural systems research.

Although treatment of the human host alone is clearly not a full solution, it is important to consider the WHO stance on FZT control, particularly as it makes sustainability of the VAC system more challenging. The WHO (2012b) has outlined a detailed roadmap for the control and possible eradication of neglected tropical diseases before 2020, including trematode diseases. The WHO strategy outlines five intervention strategies of which preventive chemotherapy is promoted as the most important. Other strategies include vector (snails?) control and improving water and sanitation. Accurate diagnosis including species identification as well as improved knowledge of disease prevalence are also needed. The chemotherapy approach typically refers to mass drug administration, which has greatly reduced the human burden of trematode diseases, most particularly schistosomiasis in Africa. For many health professionals, chemotherapy is also a principal method of choice for eradication and control of trematode diseases (Keenan et al., 2013). However, where environmental factors play a vital role in maintaining intermediate hosts, the cost and sustainability of drug administration to humans as a primary control technology has been challenged (Lima dos Santos and Howgate, 2011). Because of the nature of the VAC system in Vietnam and the presence of the snail host in agricultural and canal water, rice paddies and fishponds, environmental control of the snail vector will also be essential to controlling FZT parasite burden in reservoir hosts.

8.5 One Health options for change

A number of elements have an impact on the problem of emerging zoonotic trematodes within the VAC system in Vietnam and these make this a challenging One Health problem. The VAC system offers food and income solutions for poor rural families, thus addressing social equity, while encouraging sustainability of agricultural resources in a community-based system, all part of an ecohealth approach. Furthermore, due to the multidisciplinary nature of the elements of the problem (e.g., human and animal health are compromised, expertise is required on agricultural systems as well as an understanding of snail ecology and parasitology, and change will require proficiency in rural communication and education), a One Health approach is appropriate.

In this section we do not advocate for a particular solution, but instead point to the factors of the problem that seem most compelling while placing sustainability of the VAC system into jeopardy. These elements include:

- use of animal and human waste in fishponds, which recycles trematode eggs;
- presence of dogs and cats around VAC farmsteads as well as the inclusion of livestock in the VAC system, which can act as an intermediate host for FZT parasites;
- consumption of fish from VAC ponds without proper cooking;
- use of water from irrigation canals and rice paddies that may contain infected snails or FZT eggs, reinfecting snails in the VAC ponds;
- prohibitive cost of molluscicide or other pesticide treatments as well as potential toxicity to fish and environmental damage.

Evidence from Clausen et al. (2013, 2015) researching methods of reducing FZT burden in the VAC system in Vietnam addressed some of these elements, noting that mass drug treatment alone will not significantly impact on the risk of FZTs due to consuming infected fish. Their recommendations for an integrated parasite management control programme included lowering of snail populations and reducing trematode egg contamination in fish nursery ponds as well as targeting control in dogs and cats and avoiding introduction of untreated canal water, which resulted in more than a 90 per cent significant reduction in metacercariae in fish from ponds following an integrated parasite management approach.

Policy options to support integrated parasite management methods for FZT control while not disrupting the benefits of the VAC system would benefit from consideration of a One Health approach to solutions. Solutions relying on single methodologies or without transdisciplinary consultation are unlikely to be sustainable or widely adopted for reasons of cost, practicality and lack of insight to the complexity of the problem. An integrated supportive policy would consider low-cost treatment options of manure, use of filtration or treatment methods in irrigation and canal water to prevent snail introduction, education programmes advocating revised community-based VAC methods, communication of the public health hazards associated with consuming raw fish and vegetables grown in ponds or feeding fish waste to pets and livestock, modification of pond and canal banks, and pond drainage and treatment for snails. In short, targeting FZT parasites requires a widely integrated approach that addresses not just the health of humans and animals but also considers health and management of the environmental factors.

8.6 Conclusions

The complex disease ecology of trematodiases makes them ideal diseases to approach with a One Health framework in mind. It is true for most diseases caused by digenean trematodes that an integrated approach to prevention and control is necessary, and that inclusion of the human, animal and ecosystem aspects of each disease must be considered if sustained control is to be achieved. Additionally, because these diseases typically affect individuals and communities pressured by numerous co-infections and weight of poverty, it is essential that community needs be considered when attempting comprehensive disease prevention and control programmes. Since all human trematodiases are considered to be neglected diseases, it is also important to recognize the need for increased recognition by local governments and health authorities, and significant attention from the global community to facilitate more comprehensive drug interventions to alleviate human suffering and to provide a foundation for environmental and veterinary management, and to improve our general understanding of these parasites by supporting research. While the costs often associated with integrated control approaches are often significant (and can be inhibitory), it is important to recognize that basic improvements in sanitation and farming techniques, access to clean and safe water for drinking, occupations and recreation, as well as fostering an understanding of the value of ecosystem health, are improvements that would significantly improve health and reduce the burden of a number of diseases in areas endemic for trematodiases. Shifting away from the one-dimensional, drug administration approach to control, towards integration and improved understanding of these diseases is essential for long-term control. Lessons learned from the above examples illustrate the value of taking a One Health approach to disease prevention and control.

References

Aboagye, I. and Edoh, D. (2009). Investigation of the risk of infection of urinary schistosomiasis at Mahem and Galilea communities in the Greater

Accra region of Ghana. *West African Journal of Applied Ecology*, 18(1), 39–45.

Abonie, S., (2013). *Impact of Concurrent Schistosoma Mansoni and S. Haematobium Infections on Schistosomiasis Demographics and Pathology in an Endemic Community in Ghana*. Thesis, University of Ghana.

Adema, C.M., Bayne, C.J., Bridger, J.M., Knight, M., Loker, E.S., Yoshino, T.P. and Zhang, S.M., (2012). Will all scientists working on snails and the diseases they transmit please stand up? *PLOS Neglected Tropical Diseases*, 6, e1835.

Adenowo, A.F., Oyinloye, B.E., Ogunyinka, B.I. and Kappo, A.P., (2015). Impact of human schistosomiasis in sub-Saharan Africa. *Brazilian Journal of Infectious Diseases*, 19, 196–205.

Andrews, P., Thyssen, J. and Lorke, D. (1982). The biology and toxicology of molluscicides, Bayluscide. *Pharmacololgy & Therapeutics*, 19, 245–295.

Anh, L.T.N., Thanh, D.T.H., Hoan, D.H., Thuy, D.T., Khong, N.V. and Anderson, N. (2014). The transmission of *Fasciola spp.* to cattle and contamination of grazing areas with *Fasciola* eggs in the Red River Delta region of Vietnam. *Tropical Animal Health and Production*, 46(4), 691–696.

Anon (2015). Schistosomiasis: number of people treated worldwide in 2013. *Weekly Epidemiological Record*, 90, 25–32.

Aryeetey, M.E., Wagatsuma, Y., Yeboah, G., Asante, M., Mensah, G., Nkrumah, F.K. and Kojima, S. (2000a). Urinary schistosomiasis in southern Ghana: 1. Prevalence and morbidity assessment in three (defined) rural areas drained by the Densu river. *Parasitology International*, 49, 155–163.

Aryeetey, M.E., Wagatsuma, Y., Yeboah, G., Asante, M., Mensah, G., Nkrumah, F.K. and Kojima, S. (2000b). Urinary schistosomiasis in southern Ghana: 1. Prevalence and morbidity assessment in three (defined) rural areas drained by the Densu river. *Parasitology International*, 49, 155–163.

Ayad, N. (1974). A short review of the epidemiology of schistosomiasis in Africa. *Egyptian Journal of Bilharziasis*, 1, 9–27.

Barbosa, F.S. and Costa, D.P.P. (1981). A long-term schistosomiasis control project with molluscicide in a rural area of Brazil. *Annals of Tropical Medicine and Parasitology*, 75, 41–52.

Barnabas, B., Aliyu, M., Gbate, M., Obi, P. and Attairu, A. (2012). Survey of schistosomiasis and other intestinal helminthiases among school-aged children in Agaie, Niger State, Nigeria. *Journal of Pharmaceutical and Biomedical Sciences*, 15.

Berry, A., Mone, H., Iriart, X., Mouahid, G., Aboo, O., Boissier, J., Fillaux, J., Cassaing, S., Debuisson, C., Valentin, A., Mitta, G., Theron, A. and Magnaval, J.F. (2014). *Schistosomiasis haematobium*, Corsica, France. *Emerging Infectious Diseases*, 20, 1595–1597.

Boissier, J., Mone, H., Mitta, G., Bargues, M.D., Molyneux, D. and Mas-Coma, S. (2015). Schistosomiasis reaches Europe. *Lancet Infectious Diseases*, 15, 757–758.

Bosompem, K.M., Bentum, I.A., Otchere, J., Anyan, W.K., Brown, C.A., Osada, Y., Takeo, S., Kojima, S. and Ohta, N. (2004). Infant schistosomiasis in Ghana: a survey in an irrigation community. *Tropical Medicine International Health*, 9, 917–922.

Calavas, D. and Martin, P.M. (2014). Schistosomiasis in cattle in Corsica, France. *Emerging Infectious Diseases*, 20, 2163–2164.

Chai, J.Y. (2005). Intestinal trematode infections in Korea. *Asian Parasitology*. 1: 79–102.

Chai, J.Y., Murrell, K.D. and Lymbery, A.J. (2005a). Fish-borne parasitic zoonoses: status and issues. *International Journal for Parasitology*, 35, 1233–1254.

Chai, J.Y., Park, J.H., Han, E.T., Guk, S.M., Shin, E.H., Lin, A., Kim, J.L., Sohn, W.M., Yong, T.S. and Eom, K.S. (2005b). Mixed infections with *Opisthorchis viverrini* and intestine flukes in residents of Vientiane municipality and Saravane province in Lao. *Journal of Helminthology*, 79, 283–298.

Chi, T.T.K., Dalsgaard, A., Turnbull, J. F., Tuan, P.A., and Murrell, K.D. (2008). Prevalence of zoonotic trematodes in fish from a Vietnamese fish-farming community. *Journal of Parasitology*, 94(2), 423–428.

Chontananarth, T. and Wongsawad, C. (2013). Epidemiology of cercarial stage of trematodes in freshwater snails from Chiang Mai province, Thailand. *Asian Pacific Journal of Tropical Biomedicine*, 3, 237–243.

Christie, J.D., Prentice, M.A. and Barnish, G. (1980). Control of schistosomiasis by mollusciciding. *American Journal of Tropical Medicine & Hygiene*, 29, 323–324.

Chu, K.Y. and Dawood, I.K. (1970). Cercarial production from Biomphalaria alexandrina infected with Schistosoma mansoni. *Bulletin of the World Health Organization*, 42, 569–574.

Chu, K.Y., Kpo, H.K. and Klumpp, R.K. (1978). Mixing of Schistosoma haematobium strains in Ghana. *Bulletin of the World Health Organization*, 56, 601–608.

Clausen, J.H., Madsen, H., Murrell, K.D., Thi, V.P., Manh, H.N., Viet, K.N. and Dalsgaard, A. (2012). Relationship between snail population density and infection status of snails and fish with zoonotic trematodes in Vietnamese carp nurseries. *PLOS Neglected Tropical Diseases*, 6, e1945.

Clausen, J.H., Madsen, H., Murrell, K.D., Bui, T.N., Nguyen, N.T., Do, B.T., Anh, L.N.T., Manh, H.N. and Dalsgaard, A. (2013). The effectiveness of different intervention strategies for the prevention of zoonotic metacercariae infection in cultured fish. *Aquaculture*, 416–417, 135–140.

Clausen, J.H., Madsen, H., Van, P.T., Dalsgaard, A. and Murrell, K.D. (2015). Integrated parasite management: path to sustainable control of fishborne trematodes in aquaculture. *Trends in Parasitology*, 31, 8–15.

Colley, D.G. and Secor, W.E. (2014). Immunology of human schistosomiasis. *Parasite Immunology*, 36, 347–357.

Colley, D.G., Bustinduy, A.L., Secor, W.E. and King, C.H. (2014). Human schistosomiasis. *Lancet*, 383, 2253–2264.

Dawood, I.K., Dazo, B.C. and Farooq, M. (1966). Large-scale application of Bayluscide and sodium pentachlorophenate in the Egypt-49 project area: evaluation of relative efficacy and comparative costs. *Bulletin of the World Health Organization*, 35, 357–367.

De, N.V., Murrell, K.D., Cong, L.D., Cam, P.D., Chau, L.V., Toan, N.D. and Dalsgaard, A. (2003). The food-borne trematode zoonoses of Vietnam. *Southeast Asian Journal of Tropical Medicine and Public Health*, 34, 12–35.

de Laval, F., Savini, H., Biance-Valero, E. and Simon, F. (2014). Human schistosomiasis: an emerging threat for Europe. *Lancet*, 384, 1094–1095.

de Souza, C.P., Araujo, N., Jannotti-Passos, L.K. and Guimaraes, C.T. (1994). Production of Schistosoma mansoni cercariae by Biomphalaria glabrata from a focus in Belo Horizonte, Minas Gerais. *Revista do Instituto de Medicina Tropical de São Paulo*, 36, 485–489.

Doenhoff, M.J., Cioli, D. and Utzinger, J. (2008). Praziquantel: mechanisms of action, resistance and new derivatives for schistosomiasis. *Current Opinion in Infectious Diseases*, 21, 659–667.

Doenhoff, M.J., Hagan, P., Cioli, D., Southgate, V., Pica-Mattoccia, L., Botros, S., Coles, G., Tchuem Tchuente, L.A., Mbaye, A. and Engels, D. (2009). Praziquantel: its use in control of schistosomiasis in sub-Saharan Africa and current research needs. *Parasitology*, 136, 1825–1835.

Duplantier, J.M. and Sene, M. (2000). Rodents as reservoir hosts in the transmission of Schistosoma mansoni in Richard-Toll, Senegal, West Africa. *Journal of Helminthology*, 74, 129–135.

Duplantier, J.M. and Sene, M. (2006). Rodents as definitive hosts of Schistosoma, with special reference to S. mansoni transmission. In S. Morand, B.R. Krasnov and R. Poulin (eds.), *Micromammals and Macroparasites: From Evolutionary Ecology to Management*, Berlin: Springer, pp. 527–543.

Edwards, E.E. and McCullough, F.S. (1954). Studies on the life cycles of Schistosoma haematobium and S. mansoni in the Gold Coast. *Annals of Tropical Medicine and Parasitology*, 48, 164–177.

Esch, G.W., Barger, M.A. and Fellis, K.J. (2002). The transmission of digenetic trematodes: style, elegance, complexity. *Integrative and Comparative Biology*, 42, 304–312.

Farooq, M., Hairston, N.G. and Samaan, S.A. (1966). The effect of area-wide snail control on the endemicity of bilharziasis in Egypt. *Bulletin of the World Health Organization*, 35, 369–375.

Fentiman, A., Hall, A. and Bundy, D. (2001). Health and cultural factors associated with enrolment in basic education: a study in rural Ghana. *Social Science and Medicine*, 52, 429–439.

Foster, R., Teesdale, C. and Poulton, G.F. (1960). Trials with a new molluscicide. *Bulletin of the World Health Organization*, 22, 543–548.

Grimes, J.E., Croll, D., Harrison, W.E., Utzinger, J., Freeman, M.C. and Templeton, M.R. (2014). The relationship between water, sanitation and schistosomiasis: a systematic review and meta-analysis. *PLOS Neglected Tropical Diseases*, 8, e3296.

Grimes, J.E., Croll, D., Harrison, W.E., Utzinger, J., Freeman, M.C. and Templeton, M.R. (2015). The roles of water, sanitation and hygiene in reducing schistosomiasis: a review. *Parasit Vectors*, 8, 156.

Gryseels, B. (1989). The relevance of schistosomiasis for public health. *Annals of Tropical Medicine and Parasitology*, 40, 134–142.

Gryseels, B., Polman, K., Clerinx, J. and Kestens, L. (2006). Human schistosomiasis. *Lancet*, 368, 1106–1118.

Hamburger, J., Hoffman, O., Kariuki, H.C., Muchiri, E.M., Ouma, J.H., Koech, D.K., Sturrock, R.F. and King, C.H. (2004). Large-scale, polymerase chain reaction-based surveillance of *Schistosoma haematobium* DNA in snails from transmission sites in coastal Kenya: a new tool for studying the dynamics of snail infection. *American Journal of Tropical Medicine & Hygiene*, 71, 765–773.

Hanelt, B., Mwangi, I.N., Kinuthia, J.M., Maina, G.M., Agola, L.E., Mutuku, M.W., Steinauer, M.L.,

Agwanda, B.R., Kigo, L., Mungai, B.N., Loker, E.S. and Mkoji, G.M. (2010). Schistosomes of small mammals from the Lake Victoria Basin, Kenya: new species, familiar species, and implications for schistosomiasis control. *Parasitology*, 137, 1109–1118.

Hanington, P.C., Forys, M.A., Dragoo, J.W., Zhang, S.M., Adema, C.M. and Loker, E.S. (2010). Role for a somatically diversified lectin in resistance of an invertebrate to parasite infection. *Proceedings of the National Academy of Sciences USA*, 107, 21087–21092.

Hanington, P.C., Forys, M.A. and Loker, E.S. (2012). A somatically diversified defense factor, FREP3, is a determinant of snail resistance to schistosome infection. *PLOS Neglected Tropical Diseases*, 6, e1591.

Hofkin, B.V., Mkoji, G.M., Koech, D.K. and Loker, E.S. (1991). Control of schistosome-transmitting snails in Kenya by the North American crayfish Procambarus clarkii. *American Journal of Tropical Medicine & Hygiene*, 45, 339–344.

Hofkin, B.V., Hofinger, D.M., Koech, D.K. and Loker, E.S. (1992). Predation of Biomphalaria and non-target molluscs by the crayfish Procambarus clarkii: implications for the biological control of schistosomiasis. *Annals of Tropical Medicine and Parasitology*, 86, 663–670.

Hop, L.T. (2003). Programs to improve production and consumption of animal source foods and malnutrition in Vietnam. *Journal of Nutrition*, Supplement, S4006–S4009.

Hotez, P.J. and Kamath, A. (2009). Neglected tropical diseases in sub-saharan Africa: review of their prevalence, distribution, and disease burden. *PLOS Neglected Tropical Diseases*, 3, e412.

Hotez, P.J., Engels, D., Fenwick, A. and Savioli, L. (2010). Africa is desperate for praziquantel. *Lancet*, 376, 496–498.

Hotez, P.J., Alvarado, M., Basanez, M.G., Bolliger, I., Bourne, R., Boussinesq, M., Brooker, S.J., Brown, A.S., Buckle, G., Budke, C.M., Carabin, H., Coffeng, L.E., Fevre, E.M., Furst, T., Halasa, Y.A., Jasrasaria, R., Johns, N.E., Keiser, J., King, C.H., Lozano, R., Murdoch, M.E., O'Hanlon, S., Pion, S.D., Pullan, R.L., Ramaiah, K.D., Roberts, T., Shepard, D.S., Smith, J.L., Stolk, W.A., Undurraga, E.A., Utzinger, J., Wang, M., Murray, C.J. and Naghavi, M. (2014). The global burden of disease study 2010: interpretation and implications for the neglected tropical diseases. *PLOS Neglected Tropical Diseases*, 8, e2865.

Hung, N.M., Madsen, H. and Fried, B. (2013). Global status of fish-borne zoonotic trematodiasis in humans. *Acta Parasitologica*, 58, 231–258.

Hung, N.M., Dung, D.T., Anh, N.T.L., Van, P.T., Thanh, B.N., Ha, NV., Hien, H.V. and Canh, L.X. (2015). Current status of fish-borne zoonotic trematode infections in Gia Vien district, Ninh Binh province, Vietnam. *Parasites & Vectors*, 8, 21.

Huyse, T., Webster, B.L., Geldof, S., Stothard, J.R., Diaw, O.T., Polman, K. and Rollinson, D. (2009). Bidirectional introgressive hybridization between a cattle and human schistosome species. *POS Pathogens*, 5, e1000571.

Jordan, P. (1977). Schistosomiasis – research to control. *American Journal of Tropical Medicine and Hygiene*, 26, 877–886.

Jordan, P. (1988). Schistosomiasis can be prevented. *World Health Forum*, 9, 104–106.

Jordan, P. and Unrau, G.O. (1978). Simple water supplies to reduce schistosomiasis. *Tropical Doctor*, 8, 13–18.

Jordan, P., Woodstock, L., Unrau, G.O. and Cook, J.A. (1975). Control of Schistosoma mansoni transmission by provision of domestic water supplies. A preliminary report of a study in St Lucia. *Bulletin of the World Health Organization*, 52, 9–20.

Jordan, P., Bartholomew, R.K., Unrau, G.O., Upatham, E.S., Grist, E. and Christie, J.D. (1978). Further observations from St Lucia on control of Schistosoma mansoni transmission by provision of domestic water supplies. *Bulletin of the World Health Organisation*, 56, 965–973.

Keenan, J.D., Hotez, P.J., Amza, A., Stoller, N.E., Gaynor, B.D., Porco, T.C. and Lietman, T.M. (2013). Elimination and eradication of neglected tropical diseases with mass drug administrations: a survey of experts. *PLOS Neglected Tropical Diseases*, 7(12), e2562.

Khalil, M.T. and Sleem, S.H. (2011). Can the freshwater crayfish eradicate schistosomiasis in Egypt and Africa? *Journal of American Science*, 7, 457–462.

King, C.H. and Bertsch, D. (2015). Historical perspective: snail control to prevent schistosomiasis. *PLOS Neglected Tropical Diseases*, 9, e0003657.

Kjetland, E.F., Leutscher, P.D. and Ndhlovu, P.D. (2012). A review of female genital schistosomiasis. *Trends Parasitology*, 28(2), 58–65.

Kosinski, K.C., Crocker, J.J., Durant, J.L., Osabutey, D., Adjei, M.N. and Gute, D.M. (2011). A novel community-based water recreation area for schistosomiasis control in rural Ghana. Journal of Water Sanitation and Hygiene for Development, 1, 259–268.

Kosinski, K.C., Adjei, M.N., Bosompem, K.M., Crocker, J.J., Durant, J.L., Osabutey, D., Plummer,

J.D., Stadecker, M.J., Wagner, A.D., Woodin, M. and Gute, D.M. (2012). Effective control of *Schistosoma haematobium* infection in a Ghanaian community following installation of a water recreation area. *PLOS Neglected Tropical* Diseases, 6(7), e1709.

Krautz-Peterson, G., Ndegwa, D., Vasquez, K., Korideck, H., Zhang, J., Peterson, J.D. and Skelly, P.J. (2009). Imaging schistosomes in vivo. *FASEB Journal*, 23, 2673–2680.

Levitz, S., Standley, C.J., Adriko, M., Kabatereine, N.B. and Stothard, J.R. (2013). Environmental epidemiology of intestinal schistosomiasis and genetic diversity of Schistosoma mansoni infections in snails at Bugoigo village, Lake Albert. *Acta Tropica*, 128, 284–291.

Lima dos Santos, C.A.M. and Howgate, P. (2011). Fishborne zoonotic parasites and aquaculture: a review. *Aquaculture*, 318: 253–261.

Littlewood, D.T.J. and Bray, R.A. (2001). Interrelationships of the Platyhelminthes. *Systematics Association Special Volume Series*, 60, i–xii, 1–356.

Lo, C.T. (1972). Compatibility and host-parasite relationships between species of the genus Bulinus (Basommatophora: Planorbidae) and an Egyptian strain of Schistosoma haematobium (Trematoda: Digenea). *Malacologia*, 11, 225–280.

Lotfy, W.M., Hishmat, M.G., El Nashar, A.S. and Abu El Einin, H.M. (2015). Evaluation of a method for induction of praziquantel resistance in Schistosoma mansoni. Pharmaceutical Biology, 53, 1214–1219.

Mandahl-Barth, G. (1965). The species of the genus Bulinus, intermediate host of Schistosoma. *Bulletin of the World Health Organization*, 33, 33–44.

McManus, D.P., Li, Y., Gray, D.J. and Ross, A.G. (2009). Conquering 'snail fever': schistosomiasis and its control in China. *Expert Review of Anti-Infective Therapy*, 7, 473–485.

Melman, S.D., Steinauer, M.L., Cunningham, C., Kubatko, L.S., Mwangi, I.N., Wynn, N.B., Mutuku, M.W., Karanja, D.M., Colley, D.G., Black, C.L., Secor, W.E., Mkoji, G.M. and Loker, E.S. (2009). Reduced susceptibility to praziquantel among naturally occurring Kenyan isolates of Schistosoma mansoni. *PLOS Neglected Tropical Diseases*, 3, e504.

Mkoji, G.M., Hofkin, B.V., Kuris, A.M., Stewart-Oaten, A., Mungai, B.N., Kihara, J.H., Mungai, F., Yundu, J., Mbui, J., Rashid, J.R., Kariuki, C.H., Ouma, J.H., Koech, D.K. and Loker, E.S. (1999). Impact of the crayfish Procambarus clarkii on Schistosoma haematobium transmission in Kenya. *American Journal of Tropical Medicine and Hygiene*, 61, 751–759.

Morgan, J.A., Dejong, R.J., Snyder, S.D., Mkoji, G.M.

and Loker, E.S. (2001). Schistosoma mansoni and Biomphalaria: past history and future trends. *Parasitology*, 123, S211–S228.

Moser, W., Greter, H., Schindler, C., Allan, F., Ngandolo, B.N., Moto, D.D., Utzinger, J. and Zinsstag, J. (2014). The spatial and seasonal distribution of Bulinus truncatus, Bulinus forskalii and Biomphalaria pfeifferi, the intermediate host snails of schistosomiasis, in N'Djamena, Chad. *Geospatial Health*, 9, 109–118.

Mutuku, M.W., Dweni, C.K., Mwangi, M., Kinuthia, J.M., Mwangi, I.N., Maina, G.M., Agola, L.E., Zhang, S.M., Maranga, R., Loker, E.S. and Mkoji, G.M. (2014). Field-derived *Schistosoma mansoni* and Biomphalaria pfeifferi in Kenya: a compatible association characterized by lack of strong local adaptation, and presence of some snails able to persistently produce cercariae for over a year. *Parasitic Vectors*, 7, 533.

Mwangi, I.N., Sanchez, M.C., Mkoji, G.M., Agola, L.E., Runo, S.M., Cupit, P.M. and Cunningham, C. (2014). Praziquantel sensitivity of Kenyan Schistosoma mansoni isolates and the generation of a laboratory strain with reduced susceptibility to the drug. *International Journal of Parasitology Drugs Drug Resistance*, 4, 296–300.

Nguyen, S.T., Nguyen, D.T., Nguyen, T.V., Huynh, V.V., Le, D.Q., Fukuda, Y. and Nakai, Y. (2012). Prevalence of *Fasciola* in cattle and of its intermediate host Lymnaea snails in central Vietnam. *Tropical Animal Health and Production*, 44, 1847–1853.

Nsowah-Nuamah, N.N., Mensah, G., Aryeetey, M.E., Wagatsuma, Y. and Bentil, G. (2001). Urinary schistosomiasis in southern Ghana: a logistic regression approach to data from a community-based integrated control program. *American Journal of Tropical Medicine & Hygiene*, 65, 484–490.

Paperna, I. (1970). Study of an outbreak of schistosomiasis in the newly formed Volta lake in Ghana. *Z Tropenmed Parasitol*, 21, 411–425.

Pitchford, R.J. (1966). Findings in relation to schistosome transmission in the field following the introduction of various control measures. *South African Medical Journal*, 40(S40), 41–46.

Pitchford, R.J. (1970a). Control of bilharziasis by rural management. *Central African Journal of Medicine*, Supplement, 31–33.

Pitchford, R.J. (1970b). Further observations on bilharzia control in the Eastern Transvaal. *South African Medical Journal*, 44, 475–477.

Rhee, J.K., Lee, S.B. and Kim, P.G. (1988). The wormicidal substances of freshwater fish on *Clonorchis sinensis*. VII. The effect of linoleic acid and ethyl linoleate on parasite viability. *Korean Journal of Parasitology*, 26, 175–178.

Rollinson, D. (2009). A wake up call for urinary schistosomiasis: reconciling research effort with public health importance. *Parasitology*, 136, 1593–1610.

Rollinson, D., Stothard, J.R. and Southgate, V.R. (2001). Interactions between intermediate snail hosts of the genus Bulinus and schistosomes of the Schistosoma haematobium group. *Parasitology*, 123, S245–S260.

Ross, A.G., Olveda, R.M., Chy, D., Olveda, D.U., Li, Y., Harn, D.A., Gray, D.J., McManus, D.P., Tallo, V., Chau, T.N. and Williams, G.M. (2015a). Can mass drug administration lead to the sustainable control of schistosomiasis? *Journal of Infectious Diseases*, 211, 283–289.

Ross, A.G., Olveda, R.M. and Li, Y. (2015b). An audacious goal: the elimination of schistosomiasis in our lifetime through mass drug administration. *Lancet*, 385, 2220–2221.

Savaya Alkalay, A., Rosen, O., Sokolow, S.H., Faye, Y.P., Faye, D.S., Aflalo, E.D., Jouanard, N., Zilberg, D., Huttinger, E. and Sagi, A. (2014). The prawn Macrobrachium vollenhovenii in the Senegal River basin: towards sustainable restocking of all-male populations for biological control of schistosomiasis. *PLOS Neglected Tropical Diseases*, 8, e3060.

Scott, D., Senker, K. and England, E.C. (1982). Epidemiology of human Schistosoma haematobium infection around Volta Lake, Ghana, 1973–75. *Bulletin of the World Health Organization*, 60, 89–100.

Shiff, C., Veltri, R., Naples, J., Quartey, J., Otchere, J., Anyan, W., Marlow, C., Wiredu, E., Adjei, A., Brakohiapa, E. and Bosompem, K. (2006). Ultrasound verification of bladder damage is associated with known biomarkers of bladder cancer in adults chronically infected with Schistosoma haematobium in Ghana. *Transactions of the Royal Society of Tropical Medicine and Hygiene*, 100, 847–854.

Soares Magalhaes, R.J., Biritwum, N.K., Gyapong, J.O., Brooker, S., Zhang, Y., Blair, L., Fenwick, A. and Clements, A.C. (2011). Mapping helminth co-infection and co-intensity: geostatistical prediction in Ghana. *PLOS Neglected Tropical Diseases*, 5, e1200.

Sokolow, S.H., Lafferty, K.D. and Kuris, A.M. (2014). Regulation of laboratory populations of snails (*Biomphalaria and Bulinus* spp.) by river prawns, *Macrobrachium* spp. (Decapoda, Palaemonidae): implications for control of schistosomiasis. *Acta Tropica*, 132, 64–74.

Sokolow, S.H., Huttinger, E., Jouanard, N., Hsieh, M.H., Lafferty, K.D., Kuris, A.M., Riveau, G., Senghor, S., Thiam, C., N'Diaye, A., Faye, D.S. and De Leo, G.A. (2015). Reduced transmission of human schistosomiasis after restoration of a native river prawn that preys on the snail intermediate host. *Proceedings of the National Academy of Science USA*, 112, 9650–9655.

Southgate, V.R., Jourdane, J. and Tchuente, L.A. (1998). Recent studies on the reproductive biology of the schistosomes and their relevance to speciation in the Digenea. *International Journal of Parasitology*, 28, 1159–1172.

Stensgaard, A.S., Utzinger, J., Vounatsou, P., Hurlimann, E., Schur, N., Saarnak, C.F., Simoonga, C., Mubita, P., Kabatereine, N.B., Tchuem Tchuente, L.A., Rahbek, C. and Kristensen, T.K. (2013). Large-scale determinants of intestinal schistosomiasis and intermediate host snail distribution across Africa: does climate matter? *Acta Tropica*, 128, 378–390.

Stoever, K., Molyneux, D., Hotez, P. and Fenwick, A. (2009). HIV/AIDS, schistosomiasis, and girls. *Lancet*, 373, 2025–2026.

Stothard, J.R., Sousa-Figueiredo, J.C., Betson, M., Green, H.K., Seto, E.Y., Garba, A., Sacko, M., Mutapi, F., Vaz Nery, S., Amin, M.A., Mutumba-Nakalembe, M., Navaratnam, A., Fenwick, A., Kabatereine, N.B., Gabrielli, A.F. and Montresor, A. (2011). Closing the praziquantel treatment gap: new steps in epidemiological monitoring and control of schistosomiasis in African infants and preschool-aged children. *Parasitology*, 138, 1593–1606.

Sturrock, R., Barnish, G. and Upatham, E.S. (1974). Snail findings from an experimental molluscicid-ing programme to control Schistosoma mansoni transmission on St Lucia. *International Journal for Parasitology*, 4, 231–240.

Tesana, S. (2005). Opisthorchiasis in Thailand. *Asian Parasitology*, 1, 113–121.

Thu, N.D., Loan, L.T.T., Dalsgaard, A. and Murrell, K.D. (2007). Survey for zoonotic and intestinal trematode metacercariae in cultured and wild fish in An Giang Province, Vietnam. *Korean Journal of Parasitology*, 45, 45–54.

Tolan, R.W. (2011). Fascioliasis due to *Fasciola hepatica* and *Fasciola gigantica* infection: an update on this 'neglected' neglected tropical disease. *Laboratory Medicine*, 42, 107–116.

Valentim, C.L., Cioli, D., Chevalier, F.D., Cao, X., Taylor, A.B., Holloway, S.P., Pica-Mattoccia, L.,

Guidi, A., Basso, A., Tsai, I.J., Berriman, M., Carvalho-Queiroz, C., Almeida, M., Aguilar, H., Frantz, D.E., Hart, P.J., LoVerde, P.T. and Anderson, T.J. (2013). Genetic and molecular basis of drug resistance and species-specific drug action in schistosome parasites. *Science*, 342, 1385–1389.

van der Werf, M.J., de Vlas, S.J., Brooker, S., Looman, C.W., Nagelkerke, N.J., Habbema, J.D. and Engels, D. (2003). Quantification of clinical morbidity associated with schistosome infection in sub-Saharan Africa. *Acta Tropica*, 86, 125–139.

van der Werf, M.J., de Vlas, S.J., Landoure, A., Bosompem, K.M. and Habbema, J.D. (2004). Measuring schistosomiasis case management of the health services in Ghana and Mali. *Tropical Medicine & International Health*, 9, 149–157.

Wang, W., Wang, L. and Liang, Y.S. (2012). Susceptibility or resistance of praziquantel in human schistosomiasis: a review. *Parasitology Research*, 111, 1871–1877.

Webster, B.L., Rollinson, D., Stothard, J.R. and Huyse, T. (2010). Rapid diagnostic multiplex PCR (RD-PCR) to discriminate Schistosoma haematobium and S. bovis. *Journal of Helminthology*, 84, 107–114.

Webster, B.L., Diaw, O.T., Seye, M.M., Webster, J.P. and Rollinson, D. (2013). Introgressive hybridization of Schistosoma haematobium group species in Senegal: species barrier break down between ruminant and human schistosomes. *PLOS Neglected Tropical Diseases*, 7, e2110.

WHO (1995). *Control of Foodborne Trematode Infections*. WHO Technical Report Series No. 849, Geneva: World Health Organization.

WHO (2011). Schistosomiasis. *Weekly Epidemiological Record*, 9, 73–80.

WHO (2012a). Schistosomiasis: population requiring preventive chemotherapy and number of people treated in 2010. *Weekly Epidemiological Record*, 27 January.

WHO (2012b). *Accelerating Work to Overcome the Global Impact of Neglected Tropical Diseases: A Roadmap for Implementation*. Geneva: World Health Organization.

WHO (2015a). *Schistosomiasis*. WHO Fact Sheet No. 115.

WHO (2015b). *Foodborne Trematodiases*. WHO Fact Sheet No. 368.

WHO and FAO (2004). *Joint WHO/FAO Workshop On Foodborne Trematode Infections In Asia*. Hanoi, Vietnam, 26–28 November.

Yirenya-Tawiah, D., Amoah, C., Apea-Kubi, K.A., Dade, M., Ackumey, M., Annang, T., Mensah, D.Y. and Bosompem, K.M. (2011a). A survey of female genital schistosomiasis of the lower reproductive tract in the volta basin of ghana. *Ghana Medical Journal*, 45, 16–21.

Yirenya-Tawiah, D., Abdul Rashid, A., Futagbi, G., Aboagye, I. and Dade, M. (2011b). Prevalence of snail vectors of schistosomiasis in the Kpong Head Pond, Ghana. *West African Journal of Applied Ecology*, 18, 39–45.

Yoshida, Y. (2005). *Clonorchis sinensis* and clonorchiasis in Japan. *Asian Parasitology*, 1, 27–33.

chapter 9

Transdisciplinary collaboration for wildlife conservation: a practitioner's perspective

Richard Jakob-Hoff

Abstract

People are, by nature, a social species with strong territorial affinities. Mindful of this, a challenge to the application of a One Health approach is finding ways of working across disciplinary, social and individual boundaries while respecting and acknowledging what each of us brings to the table. There is something about the appeal of wild animals that brings out the most generous part of people's nature and makes this a little easier. Unlike domestic animals, or even people, it seems that wild animals have a natural appeal to people from all cultures and most walks of life. There is often a sense that helping wildlife feels like a contribution to the common good. Consequently wildlife health concerns provide a natural focus for cross-disciplinary collaboration in which people are prepared to put aside their differences and this can be instructive in applying the transdisciplinary approach to other branches of the health sciences. By way of illustration, in this chapter I have included a number of case studies that draw on my personal experience of collaborating across disciplines as a wildlife veterinarian – all with the objective of helping wildlife in need.

9.1 Introduction

What do we mean by 'transdisciplinary' collaboration? In the context of One Health, the transdisciplinary approach involves individuals from multiple disciplines combing their knowledge and skills to address complex health-related problems that involve the interaction of human, animal and environmental factors. When transdisciplinary teams work effectively the members learn from each other, expand their individual understanding of the problem and increase the likelihood of gaining new insights into the problem at hand. This makes for some really interesting discussions that are not without their challenges, but which hold the promise of great rewards. This collaborative and integrative approach is essential to the study of wildlife disease where relevant information, knowledge and skills are often missing or scattered among a variety of specialists. In the field of wildlife conservation there is, added to this need, a sense of urgency as the drivers of species population decline, including disease, continue to push species towards extinction. Consequently, if we are to change this pattern, we have to abandon old habits of working in silos and, instead, reach out to anyone who can help us make the difference needed before it's too late.

9.2 Background

Losing sight of the whole

In the past 150 years or so, the rate at which we've been able to acquire information and build on our scientific understanding of the world has been exponential. In the biological sciences, as elsewhere, new disciplines and sub-disciplines have mushroomed as ever-more sophisticated tools and methods for detailed investigations have developed. Examples include the study of animal or human behaviour (e.g., ethology, psychology, psychiatry), body structure (e.g., anatomy, histology, surgery), function (e.g., physiology, biomechanics) or the workings of individual organ systems (e.g., gastroenterology, urology, endocrinology), cells (e.g., cell biology, oncology), the chemical reactions within those cells (e.g., biochemistry, immunology, pharmacology) or the multitude of organisms living on or within larger organisms (e.g., microbiology, virology, parasitology). It's very hard, when immersed in one or even a few of these disciplines, to keep sight of the bigger whole – whether this is the whole living organism or the social group, population or ecosystem of which it is a part.

Reconnecting the parts

As we know, in biology and all living systems, there is an inherent level of complexity that means that the whole is never just the simple sum of the parts. (Hit your finger with a hammer and the way your body and mind respond won't just be isolated to your finger!) Change one part of any biological system – a living body, a rainforest, a pond or the atmosphere – and there will be repercussions, often unanticipated, that affect other parts of that system.

As human populations expand and modify the landscapes around them there is, inevitably, a shift in the balance of interactions between the living and non-living components of those landscapes as the whole system tries to restabilize itself (Walker and Salt, 2006). Under these circumstances, microorganisms capable of causing disease but previously isolated and in balance with their ecosystem, may find opportunities to spread and multiply in new hosts who lack the immune defences acquired from previous exposure.

The One World, One Health movement was initiated in 2004, at a symposium in New York City, in response to a growing awareness and concern about the transmission of diseases between humans, domestic animals and wildlife (WCS, 2015). The organizers felt that, to fully understand and address the factors driving the increasing emergence of diseases crossing species boundaries, we had to find ways to reintegrate disciplines and break down the artificial boundaries that have arisen between specialists. Cook et al. (2004) put it like this:

> It is clear that no one discipline or sector of society has enough knowledge and resources to prevent the emergence or resurgence of diseases in today's globalized world. No one nation can reverse the patterns of habitat loss and extinction that can and do undermine the health of people and animals. Only by breaking down the barriers among agencies, individuals, specialties and sectors can we unleash the innovation and expertise needed to meet the many

serious challenges to the health of people, domestic animals, and wildlife and to the integrity of ecosystems. Solving today's threats and tomorrow's problems cannot be accomplished with yesterday's approaches. We are in an era of 'One World, One Health' and we must devise adaptive, forward-looking and multidisciplinary solutions to the challenges that undoubtedly lie ahead.

The transdisciplinary approach is not new

During my research for this chapter I came across the concept of 'ako' that I think captures both the intent and the reward of this type of collaboration. This term is embedded in the teaching practices of Māori, the Polynesian people who were the first to populate New Zealand some 800 years ago.[1] 'Ako' describes the teacher–student relationship as a collaboration between pupil and teacher in which both learn from each other (Anon, 2009).

Many of our greatest thinkers were characterized by broad interests that allowed them to think outside the box. This included pioneers of Western science and medicine, such as Hippocrates (460–375 BCE) and Aristotle (384–322 BCE) who laid the foundations for the medical and veterinary sciences and John Hunter (1728–1793), the father of modern surgery (Dunlop and Williams, 1996). Charles Darwin, who dropped out from his medical studies, was renowned for his broad interests. His development of the theory of evolution through natural selection was influenced as much by the economic theories of Thomas Malthus, the biogeographic observations of the mathematician Georges Louis Leclerc and the geological theories of Charles Lyell as by his personal observations of the natural world (Jenkins, 1978).

Although my contributions to science are much less impressive, I have always been fasci-

nated by the natural world around me and driven by an insatiable thirst to learn more. As a very unpromising student, I began my working life at 16 years old, as a zookeeper at Whipsnade Zoo in England. Some years later I was fortunate enough to spend two years working for one of my childhood heroes, the naturalist and conservation pioneer Gerald Durrell. Home-schooled and running wild on the Greek island of Corfu, young Gerry was infatuated with the animals he encountered in his island paradise. Like his brother, Lawrence, he became a talented and engaging writer able to convey the wonder he experienced while accurately describing both the physical features and personalities of the animals he brought home and studied, much to the consternation of his family (Durrell, 1956)! Given his unconventional upbringing, it's not surprising that he became such an innovative thinker. In 1959, on the British Channel Island of Jersey, he was the first to develop a zoo that was solely committed to conservation. It was here, ten years later, that I learnt from him some of the most fundamental rules of effective wildlife conservation:

1. It's not enough to be an individual interested in, and passionate about conserving wild animals. On your own you can at best, learn a little about a small number of animals.
2. Zoos can, at best, preserve animals in the short term. To conserve wildlife in the long term you need secure, large populations in the wild, preferably several populations at several sites, with some interchange between them.
3. The knowledge, skills and commitment of a large number of people with a very wide range of expertise, working together over a sustained period of time, is essential.

9.3 My story – why I became a transdisciplinarian

Ultimately I went back to school to study veterinary medicine with the aim of applying this discipline to the care and conservation of wild animals. Later, as a vet working in a zoo, I had to be the ultimate medical generalist with a working knowledge of the biology and diseases of a wide range of animal species. Identifying, managing and preventing a disease in a sick animal, whether in the zoo or in the field, has to include consideration of the animal's interactions with its environment including any other animals and people in close proximity. This is the basic concept underlying the practice of conservation medicine (Aguirre et al., 2012), a discipline closely aligned to the One Health movement. As a generalist, my depth of understanding in all but a small number of areas of special interest is inevitably limited so I've often found myself faced with health challenges where I needed the help of specialists with knowledge and skills outside my own. Zoonotic diseases – those diseases that can be transmitted between people and animals – are a special case where there is a common interest between the veterinary and human medical professions. People doctors tend to be concerned most about diseases like highly pathogenic avian influenza (HPAI or 'bird flu') or severe acute respiratory syndrome (SARS) where animals are the main reservoir and humans the 'victim'. But there are also many so-called 'reverse zoonoses', such as measles in gorillas (Epstein and Price, 2009) and tuberculosis in elephants (Michalak et al., 1998) where people are the primary reservoirs and other species the 'victims' of disease. Often, when I first reach out to medical specialists they are taken slightly aback but, invariably, once they see how they could be of help, enthusiastically offer their services, more often than not waiving their charges and keen to 'have a go'! After all, given the chance, what gynaecologist wouldn't want to apply their specialist knowledge and skills to an orang-utan or a chimpanzee? (See the box 'Lucy the chimp' for a simple example.)

The three case studies selected for this chapter illustrate how transdisciplinary collaboration has been essential to address the complexity of each case and enabled the implementation of practical steps to advance the conservation of the species. The kiwi story (Case study 1) had the potential to be catastrophic for the conservation management of these unique birds and, potentially, threatened the nation's cattle industry but was rapidly resolved through the cooperation and collaboration of an international group of specialists. The story of 'Mrs Bones' the black stilt or *kaki* (Case study 2), illustrates on a much more intimate scale, the welfare and conservation benefits of transdisciplinary collaboration for this critically endangered species. Wildlife conservation and environmental issues, however, are more often than not controversial, involving a wide range of people (stakeholders) with an equally wide range of perspectives. The approach taken to the Tasmanian devil conservation planning workshop (Case study 3) features a process used to help groups of passionate people work effectively towards a common conservation goal.

> ### Lucy the chimp
>
> Sometimes it's an individual animal that needs the combined help of veterinary and medical specialists.
>
> In 2001 Lucy, at 26 years of age, was the matriarch of the chimp family at Auckland Zoo. She had two sons, Lucifer (aged 13) and Luca (aged eight) and was the partner of Mike (28), the alpha male. Suzie (37) and Sally (31), two post-reproductive females made up the rest of the group. The chimp facilities at Auckland Zoo were only just

adequate for this number of chimps and so breeding was being controlled through contraception of Lucy. The long-acting contraceptive (etonogestrel, Implanon® Merck, Sharp and Dohme) prevented ovulation but not the signs of oestrus at 5–6-week intervals. Despite this, she was often not receptive to Mike's amorous advances and tensions ran high at these times – with Mike venting his frustrations by attacking Lucy and other members of the group. Various changes in husbandry and, on occasion, testosterone-suppressant drugs, all failed to stop this behaviour and I was increasingly called to patch up bite wounds. The problem was that Lucy's method of contraception, while effective, still allowed her to display the 'come-on' signs of oestrus but not with enough desire to mate and satisfy Mike. Discussions with other zoo vet colleagues and a look through the literature failed to find a tried and true method of handling such a situation in a way that didn't harm the overall group bonds. The solution we ultimately came up with was to remove the hormone implant and insert an intrauterine device (IUD). Used as a method of contraception by women for many years, this device acts as a physical contraceptive without affecting the normal cycle of reproductive hormones. Having no experience in placing such a device I grabbed the Yellow Pages, rang the first name in the list of gynaecologists and obstetricians and the conversation went something like this:

Dr John Anderson's office, how can I help you?

Good morning, my name is Richard Jakob-Hoff. I'm a veterinarian at the Auckland Zoo and wondered if I could have a word with Dr Anderson on a professional matter.

[Slight pause] Oh good morning. Is he expecting a call from you?

No, but is he available? It will only take five minutes.

Just a moment [a few bars of Beethhoven's ninth while the call is put on hold]. . . Putting you through.

Hello John Anderson here. How can I help you?

Hello John, my name is Richard Jakob-Hoff. I'm a vet at Auckland Zoo and need to place an IUD in a chimp. I've never done it before and wondered if you would help?

[Very long pause . . . then, suspiciously] You are joking aren't you?

No, not at all. The hormonal contraceptive I'm using now is causing all sorts of adverse social dynamics in the chimp group so I want to try a physical form of contraception. Only I've never placed an IUD before and so wondered if you could be there when I have her under anaesthetic to show me how to do it?

Well, yes, OK, I suppose I could do that. Have a chat with my receptionist and she can organize a time.

Oh that's great! Just one thing, I have a very limited budget – how much will you be charging?

Oh that's OK – I think we can waive my fee on this occasion.

Thank you so much – that's very generous of you!

And so, it came to pass. Lucy was duly anaesthetized and, after removing the hormonal implant, the IUD was placed in her cervix with Dr Anderson's guidance. For his part, he was fascinated to see how similar the reproductive anatomy of the chimp was to that of his more familiar human clients and that the anaesthetic drugs and instruments we used to monitor Lucy's vital signs were virtually identical to those used for people. He appreciated this rather rare opportunity to apply his knowledge and skills to such an exotic animal and was equally generous with his help when needed on subsequent occasions. For my part, I also gained some extra knowledge and a new skill by combining my veterinary medical training with his human medical training.

9.4 Case studies

Case study 1: Biosecurity and the discovery of a 'new' parasite of kiwi

What would you do if you received a package from someone you had never met, sent from the other side of the world and, when you opened it, it contained a piece of glass broken in seven pieces but tantalizingly labelled 'Kiwi'? That was the experience of Dr Mike Peirce in England when the package arrived in his mail, postmarked 'New Zealand'.

Kiwi (*Apteryx* spp.) are considered by many to be the national emblem of New Zealand. There are five species (www.kiwisforkiwi.org/about-kiwi), although most of my personal experience has been with the brown kiwi, *Apteryx mantelli*, which is restricted to the country's North Island. To look at, kiwi are rather nondescript birds, about the size of a small chicken that, because they are shy and nocturnal, nobody ever sees! But, under this plain exterior lives a bird capable of the extraordinary feats of laying the biggest egg compared to body size of any bird, growing up with virtually no parental care, walking every-where (because they are flightless) and using its sense of smell to find invertebrates doing their best to escape detection underground! They are only found in New Zealand and were once widely distributed but are now confined to fragments of suitable habitat (DOC, 2015). As a ground-dwelling, flightless bird, kiwi are especially susceptible to predation by introduced carnivores, including dogs, cats, stoats, ferrets and weasels. Although secretive and nocturnal, kiwi have a distinctive smell that makes them

easy for these animals to track and, other than a feisty disposition and sharp claws, they have little with which to defend themselves. This is especially so for chicks who hatch in an advanced stage of development (fully feathered and with the features of a miniature adult) and, as men-tioned, receive very little in the way of parental care after the first couple of weeks. As a result, in areas where predators are uncontrolled they only have a 10 per cent chance of survival (Robertson et al., 2010). Consequently the Department of Conservation (DOC), as part of its kiwi recovery strategy (Holtzapfel et al., 2008), has enlisted the help of zoos and wildlife parks in a scheme designed to give these chicks a head start in life (Colbourne et al., 2005). Called Operation Nest Egg (ONE), it works like this: using spe-cially trained dogs, DOC rangers find nesting kiwi and monitor their nests. When they esti-mate the chicks are close to hatching, the eggs are removed and taken to a participating site to complete their incubation and hatch in a safe environment. Here they are cared for until they are self-feeding and rapidly gaining weight (3–4 weeks), at which time they are transferred to a predator-free 'crèche' island that has suitable habitat and a plentiful supply of invertebrate food. When fully grown, some 12–18 months later, they are recaptured and released near their site of origin. This has been found to increase survival in predator-controlled sites from 10 per cent to 83 per cent (Robertson et al., 2010).

In November 1999, as senior veterinarian at Auckland Zoo, I examined two young kiwi chicks that had been brought to the zoo as part of the ONE programme. As they had already hatched under the parent bird (it's not always possible for rangers to predict the exact hatch date), they were covered in ticks. These external parasites are commonly found on kiwi with rangers referring to them as 'cattle ticks' on the assumption that cattle, which often graze in close proximity to kiwi habitat, are the source. These chicks, however, were clearly unwell: feverish, lethargic and with a dry plumage. On examination of a blood smear, taken as part of my health screen, I found a number of parasites within the circulating red blood cells (Plate 11). As they were unfamiliar to me I took photographs and sent the images to parasitologist colleagues in Hawaii and Australia. They referred me to Dr Mike Peirce, who is a world authority on avian blood parasites. Soon after, he faxed me an excited note to say he would like to confirm his preliminary identification by directly examining a blood smear. And so it was that my carefully packaged glass slide with blood smear arrived in his mail in several pieces. Undaunted, Mike grabbed his superglue and carefully pieced the fragments together, keen to get his first glimpse of a kiwi (albeit a very small part)! Having scanned the smear he could then say with some confidence that, as he'd thought, this was a species of *Babesia*, a blood parasite, transmitted by ticks and capable of causing serious illness in cattle and dogs with clinical signs similar to those seen in these kiwi chicks (Plate 11).

The disease babesiosis can be fatal in cattle, dogs and other species and no *Babesia* parasites had previously been identified in New Zealand. Consequently the Ministry of Agriculture and Fisheries (now Ministry of Primary Industries), took this very seriously and launched an investigation to find out if kiwi could, in fact, be acting as a reservoir of this pathogen for domestic animals. Fortunately, it was quickly established by Dr Allen Heath, an expert in identification of external parasites, that the so-called 'cattle ticks' found on kiwi were, in fact, *Ixodes anatis*, a species with a narrow host range, largely confined to kiwi. Subsequent further surveillance of

free-ranging kiwi found the parasite in low numbers in the blood of 12/26 (46 per cent) healthy birds (Peirce et al., 2003). Given this, we now believe it likely that this parasite has been part of the kiwi's microflora for a long time but not previously found because very few blood smears from kiwi had been examined before.

This episode involved the input of parasitologists in four countries together with epidemiologists, domestic and wildlife veterinarians, wildlife biologists, laboratory technicians as well as government conservation and agricultural compliance departments and funding agencies. Their collaboration allowed us to quickly resolve a potential biosecurity threat and establish a basis for assessing the risk to wild populations of kiwi from exposure to parasites carried by captive-raised birds. Another outcome was that it revealed the need to increase the country's diagnostic capability for avian blood parasites and, subsequently, with funds from the Ministry of Agriculture and Fisheries (now MPI), I was able to commission Dr Peirce to run a national training workshop for veterinary haematologists at the Auckland Zoo's New Zealand Centre for Conservation Medicine (www.aucklandzoo.co.nz/sites/explore-the-zoo/zoo-precincts/NZCCM).

The original kiwi chicks fortunately recovered with some supportive care after removing their heavy burden of ticks (which were the main reason for their anaemia) and were subsequently placed on a crèche island to complete their growth.

Case study 2: 'Mrs Bones' the extraordinary black stilt

'Mrs Bones' was a female kakī or black stilt (*Himantopus novaezelandiae*) – a critically endangered endemic wader – who, in 2000, having been startled, collided with the mesh of her aviary at the Department of Conservation's captive breeding facility in New Zealand's South

Island. The result was a fracture of the upper bill that prevented her feeding. By the time she was noticed she had already lost weight and that is how she came to be known as 'Mrs Bones' (E. Sancha, pers. comm., 2015). Not only was this an immediate welfare concern for Mrs Bones but, as one of the most prolific breeders, she was hugely important for the recovery of this critically endangered species. The birds' carer, Emily Sancha, phoned me in Auckland (as a veterinary advisor to the Department), for advice and faxed a diagram of the fractured upper bill. Given the position of the fracture, I thought there was a good chance of a successful repair but it would need to be done quickly to allow the bird to feed and prevent any secondary complications. I wasn't able to leave my post at Auckland Zoo so Emily contacted a dental surgeon and a veterinarian in the nearby township of Geraldine. They enthusiastically took up the challenge and, with some guidance from a diagram I provided, the dentist repaired the fracture while the veterinarian managed the general anaesthetic. Mrs Bones was able to feed almost immediately, put the meat back on her bones (see Plate 12), and went on to produce a further 32 chicks over the next four years. This was not only a nice demonstration of a transdisciplinary collaboration but a remarkable example of how important a single bird can be to the survival of its species. In her 12-year lifetime, Mrs Bones produced an extraordinary 68 chicks! (www.scoop.co.nz/stories/GE0201/S00014.htm).

Case study 3: Devil's in the detail: working with multiple stakeholders

Tasmanians have historically had divided attitudes and opinions on the so-called Tasmanian devil (*Sarcophilus harrisii*), a carnivorous marsupial native to their island state.

Extinct on mainland Australia for a very long time – estimates vary from 500 years (Owen and Pemberton, 2005) to 3,000 years (Hunter et al., 2015) – the Tasmanian devil is the largest remaining carnivorous marsupial in Australia, with a range restricted to the state of Tasmania. Even in this last stronghold, the devil has long been considered 'vermin' by some sectors of the population and persecuted through poisoning, shooting and trapping. Named for its fearsome nocturnal screams rather than its actual propensity to do harm, the Tasmanian devil generally avoids contact with people and provides a similar ecosystem service in cleaning up dead carcases as vultures and other scavengers do elsewhere.

In 1996, a Dutch wildlife photographer, Christo Baars, first observed devils in the northeast of the state with large, tumorous growths on their faces (Owen and Pemberton, 2005). Subsequently named devil facial tumour disease (DFTD), this consistently fatal condition rapidly spread through the once abundant devil population driving a population decline of some 60 per cent over little more than a decade (McCallum, 2008). Investigators found that the tumours are unique to this species, infectious and transmitted from animal to animal by biting – something the animals do during courtship and mating. As the animals range widely to seek out mates, the spread of this disease is independent of the population density and therefore has the potential to drive this species to extinction (CBSG, 2008).

The gross appearance of this condition (Plate 13) and the associated widespread publicity, evoked a groundswell of public sympathy both within and outside Tasmania. Although the immediate concern was for the future survival of this iconic species, there were wider public health concerns. With the disappearance of this effective scavenger, rotting carcases became increasingly abundant (estimates of up to 100 tons/day) providing increased breeding sites for flies and a source of food for feral cats, dogs and foxes (www.tassiedevil.com.au/tasdevil.nsf).

The first meeting of experts to discuss this disease in detail was held in 2003 amid considerable political tensions that reflected the continuing, unresolved division of social and political views on the animal. A government-supported Save the Tasmanian Devil programme was initiated in the same year with a steering committee to coordinate research and rescue efforts. Alongside research into the disease and methods of treating or preventing it, an urgent need to establish an 'insurance' population of uninfected animals was identified by the group. In 2008, the committee sought the help of the IUCN-SSC[2] Conservation Breeding Specialist Group (CBSG) to facilitate a planning workshop (CBSG, 2008).

The CBSG provides a conservation planning approach that creates an objective and collaborative environment using expert knowledge and thoughtful group facilitation. As a neutral body, its workshop facilitators engage experts and stakeholders in systematically identifying and addressing key issues and developing focused solutions and measurable action plans (CBSG, 2015). Founded in 1979 by Dr Ulysses (Ulie) Seal, a charismatic scientist with a background in biochemistry and psychology, this organization has since honed its planning and facilitation tools and processes in more than 500 workshops in 67 countries involving conservation programmes for 240 species to date (www.cbsg.org). A key discovery has been that some 80 per cent of the knowledge needed to make informed conservation planning decisions has not been published and is either not available or is only documented in notes, reports and unfinished manuscripts or is in the heads of individuals.

How the CBSG came about is instructive and described by Westley et al. (2007) in their excellent book *Getting to Maybe: How the World is Changed*. Working on cancer research, Ulie's broader interests found him investigating tiger reproduction at the Minnesota Zoo. Westley et al. described the way he combined his psychological and scientific knowledge to address the key issues of the time:

He noticed the multiple stakeholders associated with wildlife (e.g. zoo curators, field ecologists, hunters, scientists, government agencies, NGOs) and that each had their own agenda and perspective and were unwilling to share their data. Attitudes about how species should be managed were often polarized. Arguments were based on beliefs and attitudes rather than knowledge and settled by power and resources rather than reason. He helped these people to contribute their knowledge and skills more effectively to conservation of threatened species by 1) developing a global database in which to pool relevant wildlife information to inform decision-making and minimize adverse inbreeding effects in small populations and 2) establishing the CBSG and designing workshop processes that would equalize power, putting zoo directors, wildlife managers, scientists and NGO activists on the same footing.

(Westley et al., 2007, p. 103)

He spent 'a lot of time developing relationships with people in power whose decisions were critical for the implementation of workshop recommendations [and] he avoided funding from 'big international agencies' to ensure that the work of CBSG was not compromised by external agendas' (Westley et al., 2007, p. 124).

In 2008, the CBSG Population and Habitat Viability (PHVA) workshop on Tasmanian devils was held in Hobart, the island state's capital. Forty people participated and pooled their knowledge and expertise in relevant research, wildlife biology, captive management, species recovery planning, legislation and permitting, government liaison, population modelling, conservation medicine and disease risk analysis. Perspectives were also contributed by members of Tasmania's aboriginal community.

Significantly the request for facilitation of this workshop by CBSG had come from the

Tasmanian government in the form of the Minister of Primary Industries and Water. A core principle of CBSG is that its services are provided at the invitation of the decision-makers whose support is needed to implement key recommendations arising from the workshop. Wherever possible these individuals participate in the workshop and are involved in the consensus decision-making of the group. In this way, all recommendations are 'owned' by the workshop participants and not CBSG. This increases the likelihood that the agreed action plan will be implemented.

The PHVA process involves the participants in coming to consensus around a common goal for the workshop and developing a 'working agreement' that defines how they will conduct themselves. Key topics are identified and individuals self-select to join the group they can best contribute to or have greatest interest in. Once or twice daily these groups reassemble into plenary and share the results of their deliberations to allow for cross-pollination of ideas.

My role was to facilitate the discussion on disease risks involved in the movement of animals between the various sites that would accommodate the members of the uninfected insurance populations. This sub-group included veterinarians, virologists, immunologists and pathologists with experience in working with Tasmanian devils as well the state government's chief veterinary officer (CVO) and a veterinary representative from the Save the Tasmanian Devil steering committee. I find facilitating a group like this is very much like conducting an orchestra, except the music is made up by the players as we go! For me it's an exhausting and yet joyful experience to nurture the discussion, keep it on track, see the lights go on as new insights arise and witness the group putting aside all concerns except the common goal of conserving a species. I could tell our job was done when, after identifying the disease risk priorities and developing protocols to manage them, the CVO gratefully said that,

had we not done this, he would have had to do it himself and he couldn't have done such a good job on his own!

Some four years later the insurance population had reached its goal of 500 disease-free individuals incorporating 98 per cent of the known genetic diversity and jointly managed by 26 zoos and wildlife parks, with other individuals held in three big 'free-range exclosures' and one offshore island (www.tassiedevil.com.au/tasdevil.nsf). Research continues with some recent breakthroughs in developing a vaccine that may help to protect what remains of the free-living population (Kreiss et al., 2015).

9.5 Conclusion – practising transdisciplinary collaboration

So what does it take to bring people together from a wide range of disciplines to pool their knowledge and set aside natural tendencies to guard their 'patch' or firmly held positions? To open themselves up to the possibilities of widening their horizons and discovering the child within that is naturally curious and unattached to a single view of the world?

First, you need a common interest or goal and be able to articulate it together in a language that everyone involved understands.

Second, you need to approach your potential collaborators with respect, curiosity and openness to perspectives and ideas that may be different to your own.

Third, for group discussions, the use of tools and processes like those developed by the CBSG (Case study 3) can lead to truly new thinking. Sometimes the most exciting and unexpected insights can arise when the group mind gets truly engaged and transcends each individual's capabilities. I can wish nothing more for you the reader than to experience this at least once in your life.

Final word

The final word goes to Gerald Durrell, the great naturalist who inspired so many of us including my own career path. In the introduction to his book *The Amateur Naturalist* (1982, co-authored with his wife, Lee Durrell) he waxes lyrical with the following advice, which Darwin and many of the great thinkers, past and present, would, I think, wholly endorse:

> Our planet is beautifully intricate, brimming over with enigmas to be solved and riddles to be unravelled . . . A naturalist must keep an open mind and be interested in many things, although he may specialize in one particular subject . . . so go out and greet the world with curiosity and delight, and enjoy it.
>
> (Durrell and Durrell, 1982)

Endnotes

1 www.teara.govt.nz/en/history/page-1.
2 International Union for the Conservation of Nature-Species Survival Commission, a global body with almost 1,300 government and non-government members and more than 15,000 volunteer experts in 185 countries, www.iucn.org.

References

Aguirre, A.A., Tabor, G.M., Ostfeld, R.S. (2012). Conservation medicine: ontogeny of an emerging discipline. In A.A. Aguirre, R.S. Ostfeld and P. Daszak (eds.), *New Directions in Conservation Medicine: Applied Cases of Ecological Health*. Oxford: Oxford University Press, pp. 3–16.

Anon (2009). *Te Aho Arataki Marau– Kura Auraki Te Reo Māori: Curriculum Guidelines for Teaching and Learning Te Reo Māori in English-medium Schools: Years 1–13*. Wellington: Ministry of Education.

CBSG (2008). *Tasmanian Devil PHVA Final Report*. Apple Valley, MN: IUCN/SSC Conservation Breeding Specialist Group.

CBSG (2015). *Conservation Breeding Specialist Group*, www.cbsg.org/about-cbsg/history.

Colbourne, R., Bassett, S., Billing, T., McCormick, H., McLennan, J., Nelson, A. and Robertson H. (2005). The development of Operation Nest Egg as a tool in the conservation management of Kiwi. *Science for Conservation*, 259. Department of Conservation.

Cook, R.A., Karesh, W.B. and Osofsky, S.A. (2004). *Conference Summary One World, One Health: Building Interdisciplinary Bridges to Health in a Globalized World*, www.oneworldonehealth.org/2004.

DOC (2015). *Department of Conservation*, www.doc.govt.nz/nature/native-animals/birds/birds-a-z/kiwi.

Dunlop, R.H. and Williams, D.J. (1996). *Veterinary Medicine: An Illustrated History*. St Louis: Mosby.

Durrell, G. (1956). *My Family and Other Animals*. London: Penguin Books.

Durrell, G. and Durrell, L. (1982). *The Amateur Naturalist: A Practical Guide to the Natural World*. London: Hamish Hamilton Ltd.

Epstein, J.H. and Price, J.T. (2009). The significant but understudied impact of pathogen transmission from humans to animals. *Mount Sinai Journal of Medicine*, 76, 448–455.

Holtzapfel, S., Robertson, H.A., McLennan, J.A., Sporle, W.A., Hackwell, K. and Impey, M. (2008). *Kiwi (Apteryx spp.) Recovery Plan: 2008–2018*. Threatened Species Recovery Plan 60. Department of Conservation.

Hunter, D.O., Britz, T., Jones, M. and Letnic, M. (2015). Reintroduction of Tasmanian devils to mainland Australia can restore top-down control in ecosystems where dingoes have been extirpated. *Biological Conservation*, 191, 428–435.

Jenkins, A.C. (1978). *The Naturalists: Pioneers of Natural History*. London: Book Club Associates, Webb and Bower Ltd.

Kreiss, A., Brown, G.K., Tovara ,C., Lyons, A.B. and Woods, G.M. (2015). Evidence for induction of humoral and cytotoxic immune responses against devil facial tumor disease cells in Tasmanian devils (*Sarcophilus harrisii*) immunized with killed cell preparations. *Vaccine*, 33(26), 3016–3025.

McCallum, H. (2008). Tasmanian devil facial tumour disease: lessons for conservation biology. *Trends in Ecology and Evolution*, 23(22), 631–637.

Michalak, K., Austin, C., Diesel, S., Bacon, M.J., Zimmerman, P. and Maslow, J.N. (1998). *Mycobacterium tuberculosis* infection as a zoonotic disease: transmission between humans and elephants. *Emerging Infectious Diseases*, 4, 283–287.

Owen, D. and Pemberton, D. (2005). *Tasmanian Devil: A Unique and Threatened Animal*. London: Natural History Museum.

Peirce, M.A., Jakob-Hoff, R.M. and Twentyman, C. (2003). New species of haematozoa for apterygidae in New Zealand. *Journal of Natural History*, 37, 1797–1804.

Robertson, H.A.,Colbourne, R.M., Graham, P.J., Miller P.J. and Pierce, R.J. (2010). Experimental management of Brown Kiwi *Apteryx mantelli* in central Northland, New Zealand. *Bird Conservation International*, 21(2), 207–220.

Walker, B.H. and Salt, D.A. (2006). *Resilience Thinking: Sustaining Ecosystems and People in a Changing World*. Washington, DC: Island Press.

WCS (2015) *Wildlife Conservation Society*, www.wcs.org/conservation-challenges/wildlife-health/wildlife-humans-and-livestock/one-world-one-health.aspx.

Westley, F., Zimmerman, B. and Quinn Patton, M., (2007). *Getting to Maybe: How the World is Changed*. Toronto: Vintage Canada, Random House of Canada Ltd.

chapter 10

Climate change and vector-borne diseases – North America

Kathryn Berger and Susan C. Cork

Abstract

The emergence of vector-borne diseases in formerly unaffected regions of the world is one of the many consequences of environmental change. It is recognized that even small changes in climate, land use and other natural and anthropogenic factors can have an impact on the reproduction, survival and competence of potential arthropod disease vectors. Subsequently, these changes influence the risk of disease emergence and transmission within and between human and animal populations. In this chapter we examine the global spread of selected zoonotic vector-borne diseases and the importance of taking a 'One Health' approach using Lyme disease in North America as our key case study.

10.1 Introduction

The ecology of diseases transmitted by arthropod vectors is complex and their geographic distribution is subject to constant change. This can be caused by a number of factors, including, but not limited to: (1) a change in the habitat of either the vector or vertebrate host; (2) the introduction and establishment of competent vector arthropods to new geographic regions; or (3) the introduction of the pathogen through host movement from a region where a disease is endemic and established within native vector populations (Sellers, 1980; Sellers and Maarouf, 1993; Mirzaian et al., 2010; Gubbins et al., 2010; Ducheyne et al., 2007). As a result of these and other factors, along with changes in climate and land use, the risk of a vector-borne disease occurring in a specific region must be reassessed on a regular basis. Climatic variables are known to play a key role in determining the distribution of arthropod vectors and whether or not a pathogen can be readily transmitted by these vectors to susceptible vertebrate hosts (Sellers and Maarouf, 1993). Climate change has been directly linked to changes in the distribution of a number of important pathogens and their vectors worldwide. Over the past few decades there have been a number of examples where arthropod-borne pathogens have been detected in previously unaffected regions (Sellers, 1980). These include the spread of West Nile virus (WNV) across

North America in the late 1990s, the appearance of *Aedes albopictus* mosquitoes in Italy and the subsequent detection of Chikungunya virus (Bonilauri et al., 2008), the establishment of endemic cycles of Dengue in Latin America (Jelinek, 2009), and the recent expansion of Lyme disease in Ontario, Canada (Ogden et al., 2014a). Many vector-borne diseases can be considered zoonotic, i.e., transmitted from animals to humans, and are best controlled using an integrated One Health approach. This involves a collaborative, multidisciplinary effort to address the many risks that originate at the animal–human–environment interface. To effectively tackle vector-borne diseases, a One Health approach requires the engagement of an array of professionals including specialists such as entomologists, epidemiologists and disease experts as well as human and animal health professionals. In many cases, additional research is required to fully understand the ecology of vector-borne diseases and to provide the baseline data needed to establish targeted and cost-effective vector and disease surveillance programmes. Due to the complexity of vector-host-pathogen dynamics, disease modelling has proved especially challenging, making it hard to extrapolate observations from one region to another (Zuliani et al., 2015). It is also difficult to apply experimental findings to the natural setting. The integration of science and research into public and animal health policy is essential for the development of effective disease intervention programmes and this should be done alongside well-planned education and public awareness campaigns. The One Health approach, and the need to integrate science into policy, is well-illustrated in how regulatory authorities dealt with WNV as it spread across North America and during the more recent outbreaks of Lyme disease in eastern Canada.

10.2 The emergence of West Nile virus (WNV) in North America

West Nile virus is a flavivirus transmitted by a number of different mosquito vectors and the natural reservoir hosts are thought to be wild water birds, such as herons and egrets. The key mosquito vectors can vary from region to region with *Culex* spp. being especially important in North America (Diaz-Badillo et al., 2011). Additionally, there is significant variation in species susceptibility to West Nile virus that makes it difficult to predict the likely impact of the disease on wild bird populations (Perez-Ramirez et al., 2014). A wide range of mammalian hosts can also be infected including horses and humans (Lanciotti et al., 2002). Mosquitoes become infected with WNV when they feed on infected wild birds. The virus can circulate for a few days in the blood, and eventually gets into the mosquito's salivary glands. During later blood meals (when mosquitoes bite), the virus may be injected into humans and other vertebrates, where it can multiply. However, this transfer from avian to mammalian hosts depends on the predominant species of mosquitoes present because many mosquito species prefer either avian or mammalian hosts (Takken and Verhulst, 2013). The virus can also be transmitted through contact with infected blood or other tissues, but this is uncommon. Human infection is most often the result of bites from infected mosquitoes (WHO, 2011). More recently, equine cases in North America have largely been controlled using vaccination. Human cases can be mild and are often not reported.

In North America, WNV gained importance after the first outbreak was observed in exotic birds at the New York Bronx Zoo in the late 1990s. These first cases were identified by a zoo veterinarian and were followed by cases of encephalitis in humans in New York City during the summer of 1999 (Asnis et al., 2001). The disease was subsequently attributed to an introduction of a lineage 1 strain WNV, which had formerly been isolated in sub-Saharan Africa (Gubler, 2007). The most likely origin of the virus causing the initial outbreaks in New York was through introduction from the Middle East from infected wild birds. Consecutive phylogenetic comparisons of the strain isolated from a Chilean flamingo in the New York Zoo demonstrated a high homology to an isolate from an outbreak in geese in Israel in 1998 (Lanciotti et al., 1999, 2002). After the initial outbreak, the virus successively spread westward throughout Canada and the United States (US), killing a large number of wild birds and causing clinical disease in humans and horses.

WNV spread to Ontario, eastern Canada in 2001 (Drebot et al., 2003), but the first human case of the disease in western Canada was not reported until 2002. This case was detected in Alberta, although it was later linked to the patient's travel to the US. In 2003, when the provinces of Saskatchewan and Alberta faced numerous outbreaks in humans and horses, the disease was considered endemic. During the outbreak, WNV was also detected in birds and arthropod vectors, especially *Culex* spp., during routine surveillance. After the detection of a large number of human cases in Ontario in 2002 (394 reported cases), WNV subsequently spread to the Prairie provinces (Alberta, Saskatchewan and Manitoba). In the course of this western shift, two distinct disease peaks were observed: the first in 2003 (143 human cases in Manitoba, 974 in Saskatchewan and 275 in Alberta) and the second in 2007 (587 human cases in Manitoba, 1456 in Saskatchewan and 320 in Alberta). Between years of very high incidence, the virus was seemingly maintained at a low prevalence with anywhere between three (Manitoba in 2004) and 61 (Saskatchewan in 2005) cases reported in humans (PHAC, 2008). The northernmost evidence of WNV in horses in Alberta was observed in Grande Prairie, a municipality in the northern Albertan foothills region, where a seropositive case had been diagnosed in 2007

(PHAC, 2008). The introduction of an extensive vaccination campaign in horses against WNV, as well as enhanced mosquito control in Canada and the US has resulted in a fall in reported cases of the disease, although there are still sporadic reports in both humans and horses. It is likely that the virus is still maintained in its natural reservoirs. WNV has since spread as far south as Central America and Argentina (Artsob et al., 2009). In British Columbia, the first isolation of WNV from arthropods (ten cases) and from clinical disease in three humans and three horses occurred in 2009 (BCCDC, 2014). This added the westernmost Canadian province to the list of endemic regions for WNV.

The rapid spread of WNV across North America prompted the development and implementation of numerous surveillance systems by the responsible governmental agencies in both the US and Canada. Public health and animal health agencies were encouraged to work together to ensure the development of seamless disease prevention and control recommendations for the public. In Canada, these were implemented at a provincial level and consisted of (1) the establishment of a mosquito surveillance programme; (2) the mandatory notification of human disease cases; (3) serological surveys in horses, and in most provinces, either an active or a passive WNV monitoring programme in wild birds. Sentinel chickens were used to detect new waves of virus, while passive surveillance of wild birds, especially dead corvids (e.g., crows and magpies), was undertaken in conjunction with wildlife agencies. During the peak of the disease epidemic in wild birds there was significant public concern in some parts of eastern Canada where populations of once common corvid species had been decimated. The establishment of comprehensive disease surveillance networks provided detailed epidemiological data at both the provincial and national level.

In the US there was recently enhanced surveillance for WNV in Texas, and a number of other states, due to the resurgence of clinical cases triggered by a wet and warm summer in 2012. Elsewhere across the US the number of cases has remained low since the early outbreaks. In Canada, there has been less investment in WNV surveillance in recent years, due largely in part to the decrease in human cases. Additionally, public health efforts to increase awareness and education on minimizing the exposure to mosquito bites, increasing larval control efforts and horse vaccination campaigns have vastly improved the ability to deal with and maintain low levels of infection. Passive surveillance of corvid and other wild bird deaths is still undertaken by wildlife agencies such as the Canadian Wildlife Health Cooperative (CWHC, 2005). Currently there have been only sporadic cases of WNV reported in humans and horses in 2012–2014 and background mosquito surveillance is still in place in some provinces. Throughout the disease control and prevention campaign there was a focus on public education, especially the avoidance of mosquito bites. Routine mosquito surveillance for WNV has since been discontinued in most municipalities in Canada due partly to the expense and logistical challenges involved and also due to the fact that mosquito control using larvicides and other measures in towns has reduced the public health risk. The spread of WNV across North America since the late 1990s required a rapid coordinated effort to develop and implement effective disease prevention and control plans. It is a good example of the success of taking a One Health approach with timely and appropriate engagement of both human and animal health agencies as well as experts in entomology, virology, epidemiology and environmental sciences. Although it is well-recognized that the disease has most likely not disappeared, there is currently less focus on it compared to other emerging diseases in the region. This is in contrast to Lyme disease, which seems to be a growing problem, especially in parts of eastern Canada.

10.3 Lyme disease in Canada – a case study

Lyme disease is caused by the bacterium *Borrelia burgdorferi* and transmitted by the bite of infected ticks of the genus *Ixodes*. These ticks primarily feed on small mammals and birds, which act as wildlife reservoirs for the pathogen. Humans are accidental hosts for *B. burgdorferi*, and contract Lyme disease from the bite of an infected tick. In humans, the disease is often referred to as the 'summer flu' characterized by fever, muscle aches, fatigue, swollen lymph nodes and joint pain, with the peak of cases occurring late spring through summer. If left untreated, the infection can progress into advanced arthritic and neurological problems.

Lyme disease is distributed in northern temperate regions worldwide, and is the most common vector-borne disease in North America. *Ixodes pacificus* (western blacklegged tick) is the main vector along the Pacific coast of the US, and is responsible for Lyme disease transmission west of the Rocky Mountains. *Ixodes scapularis* (blacklegged tick) is found along the eastern seaboard of the continent, and is the primary vector of *B. burgdoferi* and Lyme disease in the region. This case study will focus on *I. scapularis* as it poses the greatest threat for three reasons: (1) its geographic distribution in the north-eastern and upper Midwestern US coincides with the highest concentration of human populations; (2) infection rates of *I. scapularis* are high (often exceeding 20 per cent) in this region; and (3) together with the *B. burgdoferi* pathogen, its geographical distribution is expanding into areas not previously considered Lyme-endemic.

The Intergovernmental Panel on Climate Change (IPCC) has reported that the number of human Lyme disease cases in Canada is already on the rise and that *I. scapularis* populations will continue to spread following climate-determined trajectories (IPCC, 2013). Migratory birds and warmer temperatures have played a large role in

Lyme disease headlines

'US Lyme disease cases vastly underreported: CDC' – Department of Health and Human Services (2013)

Lyme disease made headlines in the summer of 2013, when the Centers for Disease Control and Prevention (CDC) announced that approximately 300,000 people are diagnosed with Lyme disease in the US each year. This number is roughly ten times greater than prior CDC estimates based solely on reported cases (CDC, 2013). Using an array of reporting sources to determine the number of people diagnosed on an annual basis, these new estimates confirmed Lyme disease as a significant public health threat in the US and underlined the need for an established surveillance programme to improve awareness and prevention.

'Climate change may spread Lyme disease' – B. Mole, *Science News* (2014)

In only a few decades *I. scapularis* has expanded its territory beyond its historical range across the north-eastern US and into south-eastern Canada (Ogden et al., 2008). Lyme disease incidence has increased in known endemic areas and has spread into regions previously considered pathogen-free. Climate change model simulations have shown that warmer temperatures spreading northward between 1971 and 2010 corresponded with the tick's geographic expansion (Ogden et al., 2014b). Scientists project a further northward range expansion of the vector within Canada, which sits at the northern edge of the vector's current distribution (Brownstein et al., 2005; Ogden et al., 2006, 2008).

'Lyme disease experts fear disease explosion' – A. Favaro, *CTV News* (2012)

Lyme disease was virtually unheard of in Canada until the 1980s, when it was identified at Long Point and Point Pelee, Ontario, the southernmost points of the Canadian border, just 40 miles southeast of Detroit (CBC News, 2013). Until 1997, the tick populations of Long Point and Point Pelee were the only reproducing populations known in Canada (Lindsay et al., 1998). Over the past 30 years, however, *I. scapularis* has become established in every Canadian province except for Alberta and Saskatchewan. Conducive habitat, high densities of suitable hosts and rodent reservoirs are already widespread in these heavily populated areas of Canada where *I. scapularis* has already become established – creating an ideal situation for Lyme disease expansion, if climate conditions continue to permit it (Ogden et al., 2006).

carrying tick vectors into Canada from endemic hotspots in the US, with a tenfold increase of tick populations over the past 20 years (Ogden et al., 2014a). In 2009, the Public Health Agency of Canada (PHAC) added Lyme to a list of nationally reportable diseases, underscoring the importance of the disease and the public health threat it poses to Canada (PHAC, 2013).

How has Lyme disease spread so rapidly throughout North America in such a relatively short period of time? Which preventative measures can be taken to reduce the risk of exposure to Lyme disease? Gaining a better understanding of the multifaceted ecological components that play a role in the ecology of this disease can provide answers to these questions. Increased knowledge of Lyme disease dynamics will help formulate predictive models to identify areas at greatest risk for tick encounter and disease transmission.

Tick lifecycle

The primary vector of Lyme disease in the northeastern and upper midwestern US is the tick *I. scapularis* (Plate 14). Despite the presence of *I. scapularis* in the southern states, its feeding habits and potential reservoir hosts available in the area make disease transmission less likely. Lyme disease is maintained within a complex cycle characterized by small mammals and birds serving as reservoirs and white-tailed deer (*Odocoileus virginianus*) promoting vector abundance. Blacklegged ticks go through four lifecycle stages: (1) egg; (2) six-legged larva; (3) eight-legged nymph; and (4) adult. This process generally takes two years to complete and requires a blood meal to progress into the next stage of the lifecycle. Eggs hatch into larvae, which emerge pathogen-free in August. At any further stage (i.e., larva, nymph or adult) ticks may acquire *B. burgdoferi*, the causative agent of Lyme disease, from an infected host. Both larval and nymphal stages find a suitable host (generally small mammals or birds) and take a blood meal. Once adults, ticks feed for several days and mate on large mammals, primarily white-tailed deer. Deer play an important role in spreading Lyme disease as they are able to move larger distances than the ticks can travel themselves.

Nymph-stage *I. scapularis* are the primary culprits of disease transmission, since they are most active during the late spring and summer, corresponding with peak of human activity outdoors (i.e., hiking, camping) in prime tick habitat (Plate 15). No bigger than the size of a poppy seed, these nymphal ticks are difficult to identify. In areas where Lyme disease is endemic, 20 per cent of blacklegged ticks may be positive for the spirochete bacterium (Diuk-Wasser et al., 2012), increasing the probability of acquiring the disease when spending time outdoors.

Ticks are arthropods, which means they are ectothermic (cold-blooded) organisms relying on the surrounding environment to regulate their body temperature. Therefore, climatic conditions play an influential role in the lifespan of a tick and on its potential disease transmission. Weather conditions influence vector survival and reproduction, habitat suitability, tick population dynamics and intensity, and temporal pattern of tick activity throughout the season. In addition, climate also affects the transmission of *B. burgdoferi* by altering its rates of survival and reproduction within the tick vector. Climatic conditions, however, are just one of the many factors that influence vector distribution and disease transmission, with land use, preventative measures/surveillance and host density also playing key roles.

To summarize, throughout each stage of their lifecycle, blacklegged ticks are required to quest for a host and a blood meal. If a tick is unable to successfully acquire a blood meal, it may die of starvation (Rodgers et al., 2007). While ticks do experience high rates of mortality, they are relatively unaffected by predators or pathogens. During each questing experience, the tick is exposed to a number of natural elements that might prevent its successful transition. It has been well-recognized that environmental factors such as temperature and humidity play a considerable role in tick survival and activity (Vail and Smith, 1998). In particular, unfed blacklegged ticks are susceptible to desiccation if unable to intake enough water from the moisture in the atmosphere.

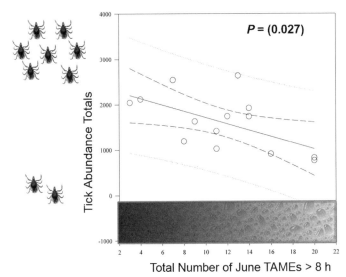

Figure 10.1 Linear relationship between total TAMEs in June and seasonal tick abundance totals (adapted from Berger et al., 2014).

A number of studies have examined environmental factors that could be used to trigger an early warning system for Lyme disease (Killilea et al., 2008). Laboratory studies have shown significant nymphal blacklegged tick mortality if continuously exposed to < 82 per cent relative humidity for > 8 hours (Rodgers et al., 2007). These periods of suboptimal relative humidity, termed tick-adverse moisture events (TAMEs) were found to be good predictors of inter-annual tick abundance (Berger et al., 2014) (Figure 10.1). Few available estimates suggest that roughly 10 per cent of the total *I. scapularis* population is questing at any given time (Daniels et al., 2000), meaning these suboptimal events will likely have their greatest impact on ticks questing at or near the top of the leaf litter surface where the ticks are more exposed to suboptimal conditions. If, however, TAMEs were to occur early and often enough in the lifespan of the tick, they may deplete more than 10 per cent of the questing populations. Researchers have found that an accumulation of these adverse events may lead to significantly lower seasonal nymphal abundance totals (Berger et al., 2014). These findings allow for the potential application of readily available measures of atmospheric moisture to provide near real-time estimates of tick activity.

The identification of potential environmental and climatic factors influencing the density and behaviour of *I. scapularis* is essential to understanding the basic biological and ecological processes of the disease vector. The development of a biologically-based ecological model will allow for more accurate predictions of vector expansion and provide a critical component in the development of public health policy.

Tick surveillance methods

Sampling of nymphal ticks consists of flannel dragging through leaf-litter in order to capture a count of questing ticks over a set distance or time of exposure (Plate 16). In areas where the disease is endemic, an entomological index can provide a good estimate of human risk for Lyme disease (Mather et al., 1996). Ticks can also be surveyed by counts acquired from small mammals and bird captures. Infected companion animals pose a minimal threat to humans, but do provide a pathway for introduction of ticks into the domestic environment. For this reason, companion animals may act as 'sentinel' animals for monitoring the risk of Lyme disease to humans.

Since its addition to the list of reportable diseases in Canada in 2009, a nationwide surveillance programme has been implemented even in areas where tick populations have not yet been fully established. Due to the immense size of the country, performing a systematic field surveillance campaign would be impractical, if not impossible. Instead, governmental agencies associated with both human and animal health are requesting the submission of blacklegged ticks found on humans and companion animals for further identification and testing. Ticks submitted to these agencies will help determine what kind of tick was submitted and whether it was capable of carrying *B. burgdorferi*. Additionally, it will help to determine the presence and distribution of ticks that transmit Lyme disease. This kind of passive surveillance will be able to detect both adventitious and established tick populations, but will need active surveillance efforts (e.g., standardized drag-sampling through leaf litter) to differentiate between the two. Passive surveillance data gathered from these voluntarily submitted blacklegged tick samples will allow for the earlier identification of areas where ticks may be soon become established. Alternatively, active surveillance using a systematic sampling scheme and standardized field methods would be used to determine if reproducing blacklegged tick populations have already become established. Repeated active surveillance efforts within the same study areas will confirm the presence of an established vector, indicating a Lyme disease endemic area. Lyme disease risk maps developed using current knowledge on the ecological constraints limiting blacklegged tick survival will assist in guiding active surveillance efforts and provide a resource for health professionals for improved diagnosis. This successful interagency approach between provincial authorities and public health

officials has improved surveillance and identified areas where Lyme disease is emerging and populations may be at risk. Likewise, incorporating medical practitioners into the surveillance programme has improved the knowledge of vector distribution and enhanced the capacity for rapid diagnosis and treatment, as well as the development of prevention and disease control efforts. These combined efforts display how Canadian public health officials have successfully applied a One Health approach to identify the emerging risk posed by Lyme disease.

10.4 Summary and conclusions

In order to monitor and predict outbreaks of zoonotic vector-borne disease, active disease surveillance that targets both hosts and arthropod vectors is necessary, along with the integration of disease reports from human and animal cases. The latter requires good communication and a shared set of goals and objectives between public health, animal health and environmental authorities. When done well, this collaborative One Health approach can be highly effective in dealing with emerging and re-emerging diseases of zoonotic concern. Data gathered from active human and animal disease surveillance can also be used to inform the development of risk assessments. However, to make sense of the data gathered, it is essential to understand the dynamic ecology of the specific disease and the associated vectors involved, along with the factors that determine whether or not a vector will be competent to transmit the disease of interest under the prevailing environmental conditions. The density of the vector population, the virulence of the pathogen and the immune status of prospective hosts will also be relevant with respect to predicting the extent and severity of any disease outbreak. Such studies require the engagement of appropriate subject specialists within the One Health team (e.g., medical doctors, veterinarians, entomologists, ecologists, statisticians, ecological modellers, risk analysts, policymakers, etc.).

Both WNV and Lyme disease are good examples of emerging vector-borne diseases that have been tackled using a One Health approach. Both are influenced by a wide range of factors related to human, animal and ecosystem health. The current method used by Canadian public health officials to reduce the risk of Lyme disease transmission to humans demonstrates how a One Heath approach can be implemented across multiple governmental agencies and disciplines. Enhanced blacklegged tick surveillance will help to improve current maps of vector distribution, while ecological modellers will identify potential human populations at risk. Collaboration between scientists, physicians and veterinarians will enhance disease knowledge, improving efficiency in diagnosis and treatment. Additionally, this partnership will provide public health officials with improved information on disease surveillance, prevention and vector control.

With regard to the development of disease distribution models for WNV, knowledge of vector ecology and the interplay between the vector and the viral pathogen is essential. Temperature and humidity have a significant influence on vector abundance and vector seasonality as well as the presence of suitable wetland habitats. Even small changes in temperature over short periods of time, such as the ones detected recently in north western Canada, could have a considerable impact on the transmission rates of WNV. Therefore, although the current rates of infection are low, ongoing surveillance and disease monitoring is essential.

To develop effective surveillance and disease control programmes for vector-borne diseases, One Health experts must consider arthropod vector population dynamics (e.g., abundance, seasonal activity, length of breeding season, vector development), host population dynamics (e.g., abundance, diversity, host biology and migra-

tion patterns) and environmental conditions (e.g., suitable habitat, weather, potential effects of climate change) that will generate favourable circumstances for disease transmission and human populations at risk. A well-designed surveillance programme is important in order to identify where vector populations have become established, and subsequently to facilitate risk forecasts for human and animal hosts. The identification of potential risk areas is fundamental to prioritize areas for vector control and prevention efforts.

References

Alberta Health Services (2008). www.health.alberta.ca/health-info/WNv-evidence.html.

Artsob, H., Gubler, D.J., Enria, D.A., Morales, M.A., Pupo, M., Bunning, M.L. and Dudley, J.P. (2009). West Nile virus in the New World: trends in the spread and proliferation of West Nile virus in the Western Hemisphere. *Zoonoses and Public Health*, 56, 357–369.

Asnis, D.S., Conetta, R., Waldman, G. and Teixeira, A.A. (2001). The West Nile virus encephalitis outbreak in the United States (1999–2000): from Flushing, New York, to beyond its borders. *Annals of the New York Academy of Sciences*, 951, 161–171.

BCCDC (2014). *British Columbia Centre for Disease Control*, www.bccdc.ca/dis-cond/a-z/_w/WestNileVirus/default.htm.

Berger, K.A., Ginsberg, H.S., Dugas, K.D., Hamel, L.H. and Mather, T.N. (2014). Adverse moisture events predict seasonal abundance of Lyme disease vector ticks (*Ixodes scapularis*). *Parasites and Vectors*, 7, 181.

Bonilauri, P., Bellini, R., Calzolari, M., Angelini, R., Venturi, L., Fallacara, F., Cordioli, P., Angelini, P., Venturelli, C., Merialdi, G. and Dottori, M. (2008). Chikungunya virus in *Aedes albopictus*, Italy. *Emerging Infectious Diseases*, 14(5), 852–854.

Brownstein, J.S., Holford, T.R. and Fish, D. (2005). Effect of climate change on Lyme disease risk in North America. *EcoHealth*, 2, 38–46.

CBC News (2013). Lyme Disease: Tiny Tick, Big Problem, www.cbc.ca/news/health/lyme-disease-tiny-tick-big-problem-1.1325529.

CDC (2013). *CDC Provides Estimate of Americans Diagnosed with Lyme Disease Each Year*, www.cdc.gov/media/releases/2013/p0819-lyme-disease.html.

CWHC (2005). *Canadian Wildlife Health Cooperative*, www.cwhc-rcsf.ca.

Daniels, T.J., Falco, R.C. and Fish, D. (2000). Estimating population size and drag sampling efficiency for the blacklegged tick (Acari: Ixodidae). *Journal of Medical Entomology*, 37(3), 357–363.

Department of Health and Human Services (2013). *US Lyme Disease Cases Vastly Underreported: CDC*, www.womenshealth.gov/news/healthday/en/2013/aug/19/679369.html.

Diaz-Badillo, A., Bolling, B.G., Perez-Ramirez, G., Moore, C.G. and Martinez-Munoz, J.P. (2011). The distribution of potential West Nile virus vectors, *Culex pipiens pipiens* and *Culex pipiens quinquefasciatus* (Diptera: Culicidae), in Mexico City. *Parasites & Vectors*, 4, 70.

Diuk-Wasser, M.A., Hoen, A.G., Cislo, P., Brinkerhoff, R., Hamer, S.A., Rowland, M., Cortinas, R., Vourc'h, G., Melton, F., Hickling, G.J., Tsao, J.I., Bunikis, J., Barbour, A.G., Kitron, U., Piesman, J. and Fish, D. (2012). Human risk of infection with *Borrelia burgdorferi*, the Lyme disease agent, in eastern United States. *American Journal of Tropical Medicine and Hygiene*, 86(2), 320–327.

Drebot, M.A., Lindsay, R., Barker, I.K., Buck, P.A., Fearon, M. and Hunter, F (2003). West Nile virus surveillance and diagnostics: a Canadian perspective. *Canadian Journal of Infectious Diseases*, 14(2), 105–114.

Ducheyne, E., De Deken, R., Bécu, S., Codina, B., Nomikou, K., Mangana-Vougiaki, O., Georgiev, G., Purse, B.V. and Hendickx, G. (2007). Quantifying the wind dispersal of *Culicoides* species in Greece and Bulgaria. *Geospatial Health*, 1(2), 177–189.

Favaro, A. (2012). Lyme disease experts fear disease explosion. *CTV News*, www.ctvnews.ca/health/health-headlines/lyme-disease-experts-fear-disease-explosion-1.846229.

Gubbins, S., Szmaragd, C., Burgin, L., Wilson, A., Volkova, V., Gloster, J. and Gunn, G.J. (2010). Assessing the consequences of an incursion of a vector-borne disease I. Identifying the feasible incursion scenarios for bluetongue in Scotland. *Epidemics*, 2(3), 148–154.

Gubler, D.J. (2007). The continuing spread of West Nile virus in the Western Hemisphere. *Clinical Infectious Diseases: An Official Publication of the Infectious Diseases Society of America*, 45(8), 1039–1046.

IPCC (2013). *Impacts, Adaptation, and Vulnerability. Part B: Regional Aspects*. Contribution of Working Group II to the Fifth Assessment Report of the Intergovernmental Panel on Climate Change. Cambridge: Cambridge University Press.

Jelinek, T. (2009). Trends in the epidemiology of dengue fever and their relevance for importation to Europe. *Euro Surveillance: Bulletin Européen Sur Les Maladies Transmissibles/European Communicable Disease Bulletin*, 14(25), www.ncbi.nlm.nih.gov/pubmed/19555595.

Killilea, M.E. (2008). Spatial dynamics of Lyme disease: a review. *EcoHealth*, 5(2), 167–195.

Lanciotti, R.S., Roehrig, J.T., Deubel, V., Smith, J., Parker, M., Steele, K., Crise, B., Volpe, K.E., Crabtree, M.B., Scherret, J.H., Hall, R.A., MacKenzie, J.S., Cropp, C.B., Panigrahy, B., Ostlund, E., Schmitt, B., Malkinson, M., Banet, C., Weissman, J., Komar, N., Savage, H.M., Stone, W., McNamara, T. and Gubler, D.J. (1999). Origin of the West Nile virus responsible for an outbreak of encephalitis in the northeastern United States. *Science*, 286(5448), 2333–2337.

Lanciotti, R.S., Ebel, G.D., Deubel, V., Kerst, A.J., Murri, S., Meyer, R., Bowen, M., McKinney, N., Morrill, W.E., Crabtree, M.B., Kramer, L.D. and Roehrig, J.T. (2002). Complete genome sequences and phylogenetic analysis of West Nile virus strains isolated from the United States, Europe, and the Middle East. *Virology*, 298(1), 96–105.

Lindsay, R., Artsob, H. and Barker, I. (1998). Distribution of *Ixode pacificus* and *Ixodes scapularis* reconcurrent babesiosis and Lyme disease. *Canadian Communicable Disease Report*, 24, 121–122.

Mather, T.N., Nicholson, M.C., Donnelly, E.F. and Matyas, B.T. (1996). Entomological index for human risk of Lyme disease. *American Journal of Epidemiology*, 144(11), 1066–1069.

Mirzaian, E., Durham, M.J., Hess, K. and Goad, J.A. (2010). Mosquito-borne illnesses in travellers: a review of risk and prevention. *Pharmacotherapy*, 30(10), 1031–1043.

Mole, B. (2014). Climate change may spread Lyme disease. *Science News*, www.sciencenews.org/article/climate-change-may-spread-lyme-disease.

Ogden, N.H., Maarouf, A., Barker, I.K., Bigras-Poulin, M., Lindsay, L.R., Morshed, M.G., O'Callaghan, C.J., Ramay, F., Waltner-Toews, D. and Charron, D.F. (2006). Climate change and the potential for range expansion of the Lyme disease vector *Ixodes scapularis* in Canada. *International Journal of Parasitology*, 36(1), 63–70.

Ogden, N.H., St-Onge, L., Barker, I.K., Brazeau, S., Bigras-Poulin, M., Charron, D.F., Francis, C.M., Heagy, A., Lindsay, L.R., Maarouf, A., Michel,

P., Milord, F., O'Callaghan, C.J., Trudel, L. and Thompson, R.A. (2008). Risk maps for range expansion of the Lyme disease vector, *Ixodes scapularis*, in Canada now and with climate change. *International Journal of Health Geographics*, 7, 24.

Ogden, N.H., Koffi, J.K., Pelcat, Y. and Lindsay, L.R. (2014a). Environmental risk from Lyme disease in central and eastern Canada: a summary of recent surveillance information. *Canadian Communicable Disease Report*, 40(5), 74–82.

Ogden, N.H., Radojevic, M., Wu, X., Duvvuri, V.R., Leighton, P.A. and Wu, J. (2014b). Estimated effects of projected climate change on the basic reproductive number of the Lyme disease vector *Ixodes scapularis*. *Environmental Health Perspectives*, 122(6), 631–638.

Perez-Ramirez, E., Llorente, F. and Jimenez-Clavero, M.A. (2014). Experimental infections of wild birds with West Nile virus. *Viruses*, 6, 752–781.

PHAC (2008). *West Nile Virus*, www.phac-aspc.gc.ca/id-mi/westnile-virusnil-eng.php.

PHAC (2013). *Public Health Reminder: Lyme Disease*, www.phac-aspc.gc.ca/phn-asp/2013/lyme-0730-eng.php.

Rodgers, S.E, Zolnik, C.P. and Mather, T.N. (2007).

Duration of exposure to suboptimal atmospheric moisture affects nymphal blacklegged tick survival. *Journal of Medical Entomology*, 44(2), 372–375.

Sellers, R.F. (1980). Weather, host and vector – their interplay in the spread of insect-borne animal virus diseases. *The Journal of Hygiene*, 85, 65–102.

Sellers, R.F. and Maarouf, A.R. (1993). Weather factors in the prediction of Western equine encephalitis epidemics in Manitoba. *Epidemiology and Infection*, 111, 373–390.

Takken, W. and Verhulst, N.O. (2013). Host preferences of blood-feeding mosquitoes. *Annual Review of Entomology*, 58, 433–453.

Vail, S.G. and Smith, G. (1998). Air temperature and relative humidity effects on behavioral activity of blacklegged tick (Acari: Ixodidae) nymphs in New Jersey. *Journal of Medical Entomology*, 35(6), 1025–1028.

WHO (2011). *West Nile Virus Fact Sheet*, www.who.int/mediacentre/factsheets/fs354/en.

Zuliani, A., Massolo, A., Lysyk, T.,Johnson, G., Marshall, S., Berger, K. and Cork, S.C (2015). Modelling the northward expansion of *Culicoides sonorensis* (Diptera Ceratopogonidea) under future climate scenarios. *PLOS One*, 10(8), e0130294.

chapter 11

Monitoring wildlife health for conservation and food security in the Canadian North: a case study from the Sahtu settlement area in the Northwest Territories

Anja M. Carlsson, Alasdair M. Veitch, Richard Popko, Stephanie Behrens and Susan J. Kutz

We need to meet everything with our mind and our hearts, to do things together without prejudice. Wildlife, environment, everything works together. We don't know what our future holds, it's important that we protect for the future . . . the land is our livelihood. We need it for future generations; there are lots of resources in our land, so there is going to be a lot of development. It is really important that we work together. . . I really like the suggestions that we work together. It really makes me happy.

Alfred Taniton, elder from Déline, NWT, speaking in Norman Wells, NWT, October 2002

Abstract

Wildlife plays an integral role in the lives of people across the Canadian North, and in particular for Aboriginal Canadians. Several northern wildlife species are critical sources of food for northerners, serve as a focus of cultural traditions and generate economic activity for northern communities. Arctic Canada is currently undergoing significant changes due to accelerated climate warming and anthropogenic disturbances, which threaten the persistence of wildlife populations, food security and traditional ways of life. Monitoring and managing wildlife health is, therefore, a top priority for the continued wellbeing of northerners. In this chapter we use a case study to illustrate how a community-based monitoring approach, combined with broad interagency collaboration (government, co-management and university) and outreach, can facilitate knowledge exchange and build community capacity for wildlife health monitoring. We describe the evolution and outcomes of the Sahtu community-based monitoring of wildlife health programme that was established in 2003 in response to community concerns about wildlife health, conservation, food safety and youth preparedness for the future. For ten years, wildlife biologists, veterinarians, and graduate students have worked with youth, subsistence harvesters, government wildlife managers and community leaders in the Sahtu Settlement Area in the Northwest Territories, Canada, to engage youth in science, to incorporate local and traditional knowledge about wildlife health into wildlife management and research, and to promote community-based wildlife health monitoring. The programme also engaged community members and the regional wildlife co-management board in wildlife health research and resulted in the publication of peer-reviewed papers, the discovery of new parasites and the development of new tools for wildlife health education and monitoring. By using a community-based approach, local people and communities who depend on species such as caribou and moose for their livelihood, became active members of the monitoring and research process. Hunters are the 'eyes on the land' and are in a unique position to observe and interpret changes as they happen. Hunters also hold a wealth of traditional knowledge that can contribute to an integrated view of individual and population health. Simultaneous engagement of Aboriginal youth serves to provide the foundations and stimulate interest in wildlife health and management, and ultimately promotes the engagement of these same youth in wildlife research, management and policy in the future.

11.1 Introduction

One could argue that there is true embodiment of 'One Health' in the Canadian North. Here wildlife species are not only integral components of ecosystems but are also the cornerstone of human societies (Metlofte, 2013). Northern Aboriginal peoples have lived together with, and depended on, wildlife on the land, in the waters and in the sky since time immemorial. Wildlife provide a critical source of food, clothing and income, are a focus for cultural activities and are important for the socioeconomic and physical health of many people around the Arctic. Food security across the Arctic is generally low, with off-reserve Aboriginal households experiencing food insecurity at double the rate compared to Canadian households. Today, the food systems of northern Aboriginal people are characterized by a mixed diet of harvested food from the land and imported food sold in stores (Statistics, 2009; Council of Canadian Academics, 2014). In an environment where store-bought food is often prohibitively expensive and fresh produce is typically far from fresh because of the great distances it has to be transported, the availability of sustainable and healthy wildlife populations as a source of affordable, safe and high-quality food is a priority (Wesche and Chan, 2010; Meakin and Kurvits, 2009; Council of Canadian Academics, 2014). Therefore, healthy wildlife populations are essential for ecosystem and cultural integrity, economic development, food safety and food security across the Canadian North.

Today a range of disturbances threatens the health and sustainability of wildlife across the Canadian North. Climate change is substantially altering these ecosystems (Post et al., 2013) leading to invasion and transmission of parasites and emergence of new diseases (Kutz et al., 2005, 2013b; Laaksonen et al., 2010). The northward movement of humans with their pets and livestock, increased tourism and increasing shipping traffic also threaten to transport new pathogens into naïve arctic ecosystems (Davidson et al., 2011). In addition, other anthropogenic disturbances such as increased exploration and development of renewable (e.g., tourism) and non-renewable (oil, gas and minerals) resources across the Arctic are potentially significant stressors to northern wildlife and this can negatively impact population viability (Gamberg et al., 2005; Wasser et al., 2011; Fisk et al., 2005; Post et al., 2013). It follows that effective mechanisms to determine the current status of wildlife health are essential in order to anticipate and, when appropriate, mitigate threats to wildlife sustainability, while at the same time ensuring food safety and security for northerners. We suggest that strong levels of community engagement, youth empowerment, cross-cultural education, broad interagency collaborations and an interdisciplinary approach are essential components to achieve long-term monitoring of wildlife health to ensure healthy people and healthy animals for generations to come.

11.2 Monitoring in the Arctic and Subarctic

In the Arctic and Subarctic, accessing the data necessary to monitor and understand the health status of wildlife populations can be difficult for scientists and wildlife managers. Here, small communities are widely scattered over a vast landscape and travel and other logistical costs are high. Weather is often unpredictable and harsh, and access to wildlife can be hampered both by logistical constraints and transboundary issues, thus compounding the difficulties of monitoring wildlife species. Due to many of these complications, there has been limited information

available on the health status of wildlife in the Canadian North. Without knowledge of pathogen diversity and distribution, body condition, stress levels and other health indices (i.e., knowing the baselines) it is difficult to track changes over time and hard to make informed decisions with respect to wildlife management and public health. By using a community-based approach, incorporating traditional and local knowledge, and engaging subsistence hunters in sample collection and submission, the logistical difficulties, high costs and transboundary issues of bringing scientists in to do fieldwork can, to some extent, be circumvented. Additionally, by engaging communities in the research process, an entirely new body of knowledge, steeped in tradition, experience and personal reflections, can be accessed and applied.

11.3 Community-based monitoring of wildlife health in the Sahtu Settlement Area, Northwest Territories

In this section we discuss the evolution, implementation, and outcomes of a long-term community-based wildlife health monitoring (WHM) programme, established in 2003 in response to community demand, in the Sahtu Settlement Area of Canada's Northwest Territories (NT) (Kershaw, 2005 & Brook et al, 2009). This WHM programme began with the identification of community concerns at a regional workshop held in Norman Wells, NT, in 2002. To address these concerns a team was assembled, consisting of university researchers, government employees, co-management boards (boards established by the land-claim agreements that are responsible for managing renewable resources, where half of the members are nominated by Aboriginal land claim organizations, and the other half by federal and territorial governments) and community renewable resource councils. This lead to activities such

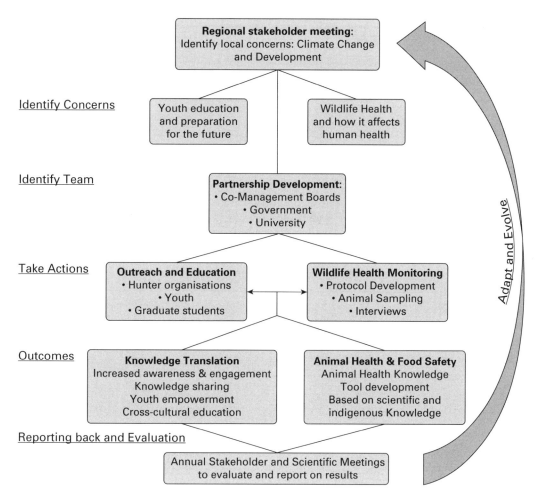

Figure 11.1 Flow chart of key activities in the community-based wildlife health monitoring programme. The programme began in response to community concerns about wildlife health and over the years has evolved and adapted to address new concerns as they arise.

as outreach and wildlife health monitoring, with outcomes reported back to the communities on an annual basis. In these meetings, feedback from local stakeholders was used to adapt the wildlife health monitoring programme to evolving needs (Figure 11.1).

Impetus and establishment of the programme

In 2002, a workshop co-hosted by the Department of Environmental and Natural Resources (ENR), government of the NWT (GNWT) and the Sahtu Renewable Resource Board (SRRB) brought together representatives from all five communities in the Sahtu (Figure 11.2) with the aim of determining research and monitoring needs as they relate to wildlife and the environment.

The Sahtu Settlement Area

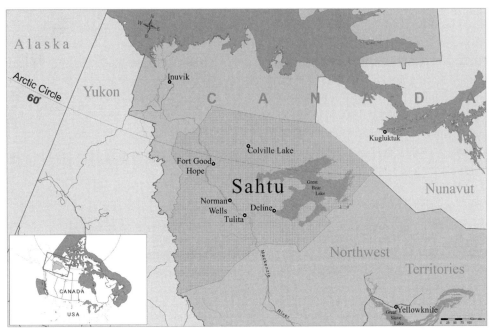

Figure 11.2 Map of the Sahtu Settlment Area, Northwest Territories Canada. Created by P. Spencer, Sahtu GIS, GNWT

The Sahtu Settlement Area (SSA) was established in the Northwest Territories, Canada, in 1993 through a land-claim agreement between the Sahtu Dene and Métis (as represented by the Sahtu Secretariat Incorporated) and the governments of Canada and the Northwest Territories. The Sahtu lies in the centre of the NWT and encompasses an area of 283,988km² and includes the Mackenzie Mountains, the Mackenzie River and Mackenzie River Valley, and Great Bear Lake. It includes the communities of Déline, Tulita, Norman Wells, Fort Good Hope and Colville Lake (Kershaw, 2005). In a 2012 census, 74 per cent of 2,680 Sahtu residents identified as Aboriginal. In the Sahtu, people rely heavily on subsistence hunting and country foods dominate the diet for more than 60 per cent of Sahtu residents (Statistics, 2009). The SSA is home to a wide variety of important ungulate species, including barren-ground and woodland caribou (*Rangifer tarandus* ssp.), moose (*Alces alces gigas* and *A. a. andersoni*), muskoxen (*Ovibos moschatus moschatus*) and Dall's sheep (*Ovis dalli dalli*). These species are important sources of food through subsistence hunting, they generate economic activity through hunting and tourism, and they are critical for the maintenance of many cultural traditions (Kershaw, 2005). Wildlife, fisheries and forest management in the Sahtu is the joint responsibility of the Sahtu Renewable Resources Board, which is a wildlife co-management board of public government that was set up under the Sahtu Dene and Métis Comprehensive Land Claim Agreement to be the 'main instrument of wildlife management in the settlement area', and the government of the Northwest Territories, Department of Environment and Natural Resources.

Government and university-based scientists were present to provide background information and additional support as requested. Community participants highlighted the impact of climate change and increasing exploration and development of oil, gas and mineral resources in the area as major issues influencing food safety, food security and cultural activities. In particular, they voiced concern about the impacts on wildlife health and consequent impacts on human health. They also emphasized a major concern that youth were not gaining the necessary knowledge and experience to help them to deal with these changes in the future. Community members also expressed a keen interest in having a more active role in wildlife health monitoring and research (Brook et al., 2009).

> Alfred was saying there is no doctor for the wildlife when the wildlife get sick, we need to preserve our wildlife. A long time ago it was not like that because our land was not disturbed, but now it's different. Now we are becoming aware of all these things happening. We need to educate our children, so they know how to preserve wildlife and fish.
>
> Andrew John Kenny, elder from Déline, NWT (translated from North Slavey), Norman Wells, NWT, October 2002

In response to these concerns, the community-based monitoring of wildlife health programme was initiated as a collaborative endeavour between ENR, SRRB and university-based researchers. The objective of the programme was to work with local hunters and youth to maintain an ongoing wildlife health monitoring and education programme that was responsive to the changing needs of the community and the changing health issues that emerge in wildlife (Brook et al., 2009).

Initial aims of the programme included:

- Sharing knowledge about wildlife biology, management, wildlife health and wildlife disease.
- Youth engagement in science.

- Building community capacity for wildlife health monitoring.
- Establishing field methods that could be used for community-based monitoring.
- Establishing baselines of body condition and pathogen diversity and prevalence (or exposure) in caribou and moose.
- Providing a manageable, sustainable and cost-effective means of monitoring health and condition of key wildlife species in the long term.

The initial programme included community workshops and classroom visits and these evolved to incorporate traditional knowledge, community-based wildlife health monitoring and training opportunities for university students (in research and knowledge exchange) and targeted research projects (see Figure 11.1). Communities involved in monitoring varied over time depending on the wildlife issues of concern; however, school outreach occurred in all schools in the five communities every year (barring weather or other unforeseen circumstances) (Table 11.1) (Brook et al., 2009).

11.4 Outreach and education

Youth engagement

Responding to the communities' wishes to engage youth in science and wildlife health, the programme provided interactive presentations to students from kindergarten to grade 12 through annual school visits (2003–2012) in all five communities. Each year had a different wildlife theme (see Table 11.1), intended to highlight topical issues relevant to the ecology and health of local wildlife species and to present possible career options, such as what becoming a veterinarian or wildlife biologist entails. Hands-on participation by students was always encouraged. For the older students, activities included

Table 11.1 Annual education themes for the Sahtu youth engagement programme (adapted from Brook et al., 2009)

Year	Local students	Biological theme	Veterinary theme
2003	~400	What is a biologist?	What is a veterinarian?
2004	464	Trap line ecology and management	Lynx anatomy
2005	457	Ecology of marten	CSI (crime scene identification)
2006	466	Ecology of snowshoe hares and barren-ground caribou population cycles	Disease of caribou and hare
2007	401	Bird migration	Bird disease (West Nile virus, avian influenza)
2008	250*	Ecology of wolves, foxes and coyotes	Dog health, welfare and safety, wild–domestic interactions
2009	258*	Ecology of muskoxen	Health of muskoxen
2010	Est. 450	Winter ticks and barren-ground caribou herd population declines and management options	Winter ticks
2011	267*	Ecology of wolverines and biology of aquatic insects	Moose health
2012	Est. 400	Responsible hunting	Caribou anatomy

*Severe cold weather caused school closures or examinations occurring in some schools

dissections and data collection from locally important wildlife species, while younger students were engaged in activities such as drawing and games that focused on wildlife health. In addition to training youth of the Sahtu, graduate students and postdoctoral students that participated in the programme gained unique opportunities for active learning and cross-cultural experiences in northern research, outreach and the logistics of winter travel and life (Brook et al., 2009).

Workshops on wildlife health and management

Between 2003 and 2005, annual workshops for the local Renewable Resources Councils (RRCs) were held in each of the communities; however, attendance at these was variable. In subsequent years, workshops were offered as requested by the community or were co-arranged in response to specific wildlife health concerns (e.g., 'ghost' or hairless moose due to heavy infestation of winter ticks). In addition, research results were presented during the annual meetings of the SRRB where representatives from all five communities (Tulita, Norman Wells, Fort Good Hope, Déline and Colville Lake) gathered together with wildlife managers and scientists to share wildlife management and research needs and results. During these workshops, updates on research methods, study findings and an overview of common diseases of local wildlife and food safety were presented. Local perceptions and interpretation of findings were also sought (Brook et al., 2009). It was through these workshops and direct interactions with hunters and RRCs that feedback on study design and data interpretation was acquired and local priorities and concerns were brought to light.

This approach takes time but when done well it results in a valuable collaboration with the community in which the work done is relevant and useful to local stakeholders as well as to researchers and policymakers.

Community insights and feedback helped the research programme to evolve, and later lead to targeted studies and changes in methodology (Brook et al., 2009). Occasionally, more targeted consultations were conducted within communities to discuss specific research programmes or results. For example, there was a meeting in three of the communities to discuss the naming of a new lungworm from caribou and muskoxen that was first discovered in the Sahtu. This was named *Varestrongylus eleguneniensis*, where '*elegu nene*' indicates 'cold land' in North Slavey, the language of the Sahtu Dene and Métis, and the Latin ending '*ensis*' means 'from', thus the worm is 'from the cold land' (Kutz et al., 2007; Verocai et al., 2014). Additional meetings were also held in select communities to discuss the development of a community-based moose-monitoring programme in Fort Good Hope.

Interviews

Although local ecological knowledge was informally exchanged and recorded in workshops, meetings and casual encounters, a more formal documentation was done in 2005 as part of a broader project that also included nearby regions in the NWT and Nunavut (Kutz, 2007). Thirty-one experienced harvesters and elders from all Sahtu communities participated in focus group interviews aimed at documenting knowledge of past and current distribution of diseases in caribou, moose, muskoxen and Dall's sheep (Brook et al., 2009). Additionally, in 2006, wildlife health monitors were interviewed about wildlife health. This was done by using an existing questionnaire developed by the Arctic Borderlands Ecological Knowledge Co-op (ABEKC). The

ABEKC uses this community-based interview process in other regions of the Arctic to gather local information on an annual basis (Eamer, 2006). The questionnaire was modified to be relevant to the Sahtu situation and used to interview five active wildlife health monitors. This process resulted in substantial additional insights into the condition, behaviour and land-use patterns of the targeted species, as well as a much broader sharing of knowledge and observations on other ecosystem components and how they played into the daily lives of the wildlife health monitors.

Participation in community harvests

By invitation from the community of Colville Lake, the programme was expanded into the field setting and university researchers and graduate students participated in the annual Horton Lake community barren-ground caribou harvest in 2007 and 2008 (Plate 17). This hunt occurs at the treeline north of Great Bear Lake and provided a great opportunity to work together with caribou hunters while on the land. The experience provided an opportunity to share knowledge, train hunters and graduate students in sample collection, and interact with youth about science. The community harvest also provided the opportunity to work together with a local videographer and culminated in the production of a caribou sampling and disease video (Brook et al., 2009; Kutz et al., 2013c). A similar, but smaller hunt with researcher participation occurred in 2009 in the Mackenzie Mountains with the community of Fort Good Hope. In 2013, researchers also participated in the Caribou Flats community mountain woodland caribou harvest in the central Mackenzie Mountains by invitation of the community of Tulita. This was in response to community wishes to monitor impacts of ongoing liquid and shale oil exploration along the Front Range of the Mackenzie Mountains as well as in the central Mackenzie River Valley. The collection also established baselines for mountain woodland caribou, an ecotype of the woodland subspecies that had not previously been sampled as part of the WHM programme. Participation in the hunt provided the opportunity to connect with community members and harvesters in Tulita, who had previously had little involvement in the monitoring programme.

11.5 Wildlife health monitoring and research

Hunter training

Initially, caribou and moose hunters interested in becoming wildlife health monitors that were recommended by community RRCs were trained by a wildlife veterinarian to collect samples according to standardized protocols; the type of training can broadly be divided into three approaches; (1) a combination of 'classroom' and hands-on sessions, (2) 'classroom' sessions only and (3) working with hunters on-the-land during harvest. For the first approach, harvesters were shown pictures of visibly recognizable caribou and moose diseases and were given an overview of the project. They were then trained to collect data and samples by demonstration using a freshly killed caribou. The importance of recording sample data on standard forms was also highlighted and emphasized. In subsequent years, when caribou were not in the near vicinity and herd numbers were down dramatically, training was done solely through 'classroom' sessions using digital slide presentations and props to illustrate sampling methods. The third approach was for members of the research team to work together with harvesters during the community hunts. This provided the opportunity to share knowledge and to train interested individuals in sample collection as they were butchering caribou and moose. Overall, the hands-on approaches were better than the 'classroom' approach and resulted in higher-quality samples and more productive interactions and collaborations.

Throughout the years of the monitoring and research programme there were additional training sessions and meetings to recruit new wildlife health monitors and renew contacts with existing monitors. This was achieved through formal and informal meetings as outlined previously. In addition to the in-person training sessions, the caribou sampling and disease video produced in collaboration with communities was widely distributed in the Sahtu and beyond as an educational resource to be used, in combination with in-person instruction, for demonstrating how and why to collect samples. These resources are still available, and used, today.

Sampling kits and datasheets

Caribou and moose sampling involved recording data (i.e., body condition score, location of harvest, age and sex of animal, and pregnancy status) from individual animals as well as collection of specific organs and body parts. A collection kit originally consisted of a small field clipboard with datasheets, sampling diagrams, and pre-labelled sample collection bags. The sampling protocol was designed to be comprehensive and to maximize the amount of information gained while minimizing time and effort for harvesters. The data and samples requested were selected to provide data on age, disease, physiological condition, short and long-term nutritional status, and maternal investment in reproductive fitness (Carlsson et al., 2015; Kutz et al., 2013a) (Table 11.2). To improve the ease of sample collections and the quality of the samples, the structure of the collection kits was modified throughout the programme in response to feedback from hunters. Changes included visual representation of collection methods, reduction in the amount

Table 11.2 Samples collected by wildlife health monitors and the information that each sample provides on animal body condition, disease or contamination (Kutz et al., 2013a)

Sample collected	Animal health information
Hunter Observations	
Location	Herd origin and range
Age	Estimated age of animal
Sex	Sex of animal
Back fat depth	Body condition
Body condition	Overall body condition
Abnormalities: Specifically, white spots or cysts on liver, eye, skin on legs, testicles, and joints	Presence of parasites and other diseases
Warble larvae count	Level of warble larvae infection
Lower Jaw	
Morphometrics	Body size
Marrow fat	Body condition
Tooth eruption and tooth wear	Age class
Incisor I cementum	Age
Premolars and molars	Enamel defects indicating stress during enamel development
Lower left hind leg (metatarsus)	
Skin and subcutaneous	Parasites (*Besnoitia, Onchocerca, Setaria microfilaria*), Hoof deformities and foot rot
Morphometrics	Body size
Marrow fat content	Body condition
Feces	Genetics, fecal glucocorticoids (stress), parasites, bacteria, and viruses that are shed in feces
Blood on filter paper	Serology for various pathogens
Kidney	Contaminants
Kidney + fat	Riney kidney fat index for body condition
Liver	Contaminants
Testicles	Confirmation of sex, Infectious diseases: e.g., *Brucella suis, Besnoitia tarandi*
Hide/Skin + hair Hair	Ectoparasites: Warble fly larvae, winter ticks, lice, hair glucocorticoids (stress)
Abnormalities	Unusual diseases
Lungs	Lungworms, *Echinococcus*

of information requested, and switching from datasheets to tags only (Plate 18).

Once samples were collected, the kits were submitted to the local RRC office and subsequently collected and then processed (Carma, 2008; Kutz et al., 2013a). For each completed sample kit, harvesters were compensated for the time and effort taken to collect the sample and the loss of meat/hide that would otherwise have been used for food or to make clothing and tools. Compensation was in the form of a gift card, a cheque or gas credit, and was distributed by the local RRC office or ENR. The cash value of the reimbursement varied during the course of the programme depending on the size of the sample kit, the time and effort needed to collect the samples and input from the programme participants and RRCs.

Targeted empirical research

During the course of the WHM programme, several needs-specific studies were done. Conceptualization of these studies was driven by concerns of local hunters, elders and wildlife managers, and the need for easier and more efficient sampling protocols (Carlsson et al., 2015). Notable studies included: the evaluation of the effectiveness of blood on filter paper strips for caribou disease surveillance (Curry, 2012); winter tick range expansion in moose and possibly caribou (Kashivakura, 2013); dental enamel hypoplasia as a measure of stress (Wu et al., 2012); and the caribou anatomy initiative (www.ucalgary.ca/caribou/CaribouAnatomy.html). For the purpose of these studies, more targeted sampling, sometimes with reduced sample kits but with more animals sampled, was often performed.

Examples of needs-specific studies

Winter tick range expansion

Wildlife biologists in the Sahtu began hearing about and seeing evidence of winter ticks on moose (in some cases severe infestation) in the mid-1990s. During our community meetings and planned focus group interviews, hunters and elders of the Sahtu also expressed concern about the recent appearance of the winter tick, *Dermacentor albipictus*, in the southern areas of the region. Larvae of winter tick attach to moose and caribou in the fall and then moult twice to become adult ticks on the same animal by late winter. The ticks can cause severe itching, hair loss and blood loss as they feed and grow. Community and wildlife managers' concerns about range expansion of the tick resulted in a Master's of Science project at the University of Calgary (Cynthia Kashivakura) to investigate the range expansion. During this time, the WHM programme was expanded to target moose hide sampling in all communities. Hide samples from the neck, shoulder and the base of the tail from harvested moose were collected by wildlife health monitors and tested for presence of winter tick (Kashivakura, 2013).

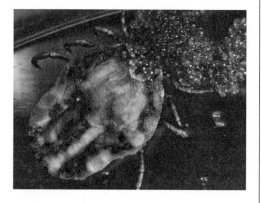

Figure 11.3 Female winter tick laying eggs (courtesy of Cynthia Kashivakura).

Blood on filter paper for caribou disease surveillance

Blood samples can provide substantial information on animal health through testing for exposure to a variety of pathogens, or using molecular techniques to detect the presence of specific pathogens. However, collecting blood samples in the field is challenging, particularly under harsh weather conditions and remote settings (Curry, 2009). To circumvent this problem, University of Calgary PhD student Pat Curry tested the lab accuracy and field implementation of filter paper strips for blood sampling. Filter paper blood sampling requires that the hunters soak the paper in clean blood shortly after the animal is killed during the butchering process and then store the papers in an envelope that is then either frozen or dried. In the laboratory, these strips are soaked in a solution to elute the blood out of the paper and then standard serological assays can be performed (Curry et al., 2014b).

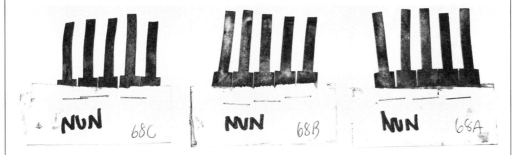

Figure 11.4 Filter paper strips fully saturated with blood (courtesy of Patricia Curry).

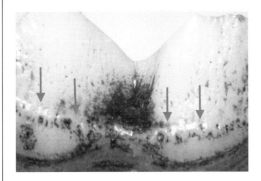

Figure 11.5 Caribou molar with a linear dental enamel lesion indicated by arrows (courtesy of Jessica Wu).

Dental enamel lesions as indicators of stress

Defects in the enamel of the teeth can be caused by chronic stress that occurs during the development of that enamel. Once the defects appear, they are permanent markers of that stress and can be observed years later. To determine if caribou can get these defects, University of Calgary undergraduate veterinary student Jessica Wu engaged wildlife health monitors and asked them to collect jaws from all caribou harvested that year, not just the 20 animals that were routinely sampled, in order to increase the sample size (Wu et al., 2012).

11.6 Outcomes of the wildlife health monitoring programme

To protect this land, we need to collect the baseline information. We've learned how to collect information from the land, and we can use that when oil companies come here. After they leave, we can do another study and find out what has changed. That's how we learn about the effects of these oil and gas and mineral companies. The studies that we do are for our people, our young people, our future generations.

Michael Neyelle, Déline, NWT (currently (2015) chairperson, Sahtu Renewable Resources Board) (SRRB, 2014)

Sample collections

Sample size

From 2004 to 2014, a total of 423 samples from moose and caribou were collected by wildlife health monitors in the Sahtu (Figure 11.6) (Carlsson et al., 2015). Sampling had a known bias in that hunters are most likely to take the healthiest looking animals. However, this bias was assumed to be consistent across the years. The data/samples collected most often were recordings of location of harvest (391/423), the metatarsal (372/423), date of collection (year and month) (370/423), and the sex of the animal (338/423). Those collected least often were other hunter observations on the condition of the animals harvested.

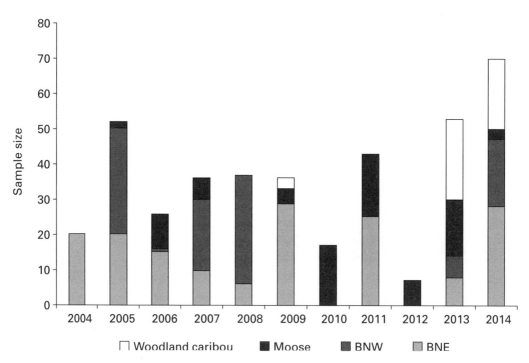

Figure 11.6 Number of barren-ground caribou (Bluenose-West and Bluenose-East herds), boreal woodland caribou, mountain woodland caribou and moose samples collected between 2004 and 2014 in the community-based monitoring of wildlife health programme.

Sample quality

Sample size and quality varied among years and among hunters, but quality generally improved over the years with ongoing feedback (to and from researchers) that modified the kit structure and contents. Sample sizes and quality varied for a number of reasons, including but not limited to, decline in barren-ground caribou numbers, accessibility, hunting patterns, funding and researcher presence (Carlsson et al., 2015). For example:

- Collections occurred year-round and did not consistently target the same sex. Most caribou were collected from January to April and during fall community hunts, and from 2006 onward wildlife managers and the SRRB encouraged a switch to a male-only harvest to allow the declining barren-ground caribou populations to recover, leading to variability in sample sizes.
- Research based on community interests increased sample sizes. If the community was interested in the issue, more samples were generally collected, as was the case with the winter tick study (see 2010 and 2011 increase in moose samples in Figure 11.6). Additionally, a dedicated researcher (e.g., the graduate student working on winter ticks) increased contact time with the community, which resulted in contagious enthusiasm for the sampling.
- Funding and availability of dedicated personnel influenced the number of collected samples. For example, in 2012, there was reduced funding to support the programme and this was reflected in reduced numbers of samples from that year (see Figure 11.6). In contrast, during the winter tick study, increased funding and dedicated programme personnel increased community interest in the study.
- Researchers' participation in community hunts increased quantity and quality of samples.

Targeted studies, with smaller sample kits, usually lead to higher sample submission. For example, the dental enamel lesion and winter tick studies were positively received and sample collection was very successful.

Additional data and sample quality concerns included: data not being recorded (e.g., back fat not measured), different scoring criteria for hunter observations of body condition and incorrect collection of samples. These problems were reduced by: providing a visual instruction sheet; simplifying the data collection; and following up with hunters to more clearly explain the sampling and data collection. Finally, the importance of personal interaction and in-person training became very clear. Although there are good written protocols and a hunter training video for correct sample collection and processing (Carma, 2008), these could not replace personal communication, demonstrations and time on-the-land with harvesters (Carlsson et al., 2015).

Overall, reliable data and reasonable samples sizes were obtained for serology (filter papers), parasitology and stress hormones (feces and metatarsals), contaminants and age. In particular, the use of filter papers to collect blood for serology was well-accepted and a great tool for community-based wildlife health monitoring (Curry et al., 2011, 2014a, 2014b). Body condition measures were less reliable because the two most important measures, back-fat and kidney fat, were not recorded or sampled consistently (Carlsson et al., 2015).

New discoveries

Perhaps one of the greatest benefits of the WHM programme from a science perspective was the serendipitous discovery of several new pathogens for the region. Noteworthy are the discoveries in caribou of a previously unknown lungworm,

Varestrongylus eleguneniensis, the species name was derived from the North Slavey language after consultation with elders. In moose, a nematode parasite, the 'leg worm', *Onchocerca cervipedis*, was discovered, demonstrating a new geographic record and a broader distribution than previously known (Verocai et al., 2012).

In addition to investigations driven by scientific interests, observation by hunters and elders communicated during the course of the programme brought other wildlife diseases of concern to the forefront of research and monitoring. In particular, there was concern in the southern part of the region about moose with hair loss, signs usually associated with the infestation of *Dermacentor albipictus*, the winter tick. As a result of the moose study conducted in 2010–2011, the winter tick was found to be present in moose in the south, but extremely rare further north (e.g., Fort Good Hope) (Kashivakura, 2013); however, in recent years there are increasing reports of the tick in the Fort Good Hope area as well. The Sahtu lies beyond the previously known northern limit for the distribution of winter tick, and the recent studies and observations suggest that the ticks' geographical range is expanding quite rapidly (Kashivakura, 2013; Kutz et al., 2009). In light of the rapid changes that are occurring in the Arctic, continued monitoring of all three emerging parasites – leg worm, lungworm and winter tick – is a priority.

New tools

The development of filter paper blood sampling for use in serology was very successful. Interviews with hunters demonstrated that this is a relatively easy technique to use in the field (Curry, 2012), and filter papers were generally submitted properly and consistently by the hunters. Lab and field experiments demonstrated that filter papers were reliable for serology using

standard ELISA tests (Curry, 2009, 2012; Curry et al., 2011, 2014a, 2014b). This technique is now being implemented much more broadly across North America for hunter-based sampling of wildlife (Kutz et al., 2012).

The dental enamel hypoplasia study concluded that caribou can get dental enamel defects as a result of 'stress', and that these defects could potentially be used as retrospective indicators of herd health and proactive indicators of herd trajectory (Wu et al., 2012).

In collaboration with communities, the programme contributed to the design of an online tool for teaching and learning and exchanging knowledge about caribou: the *Rangifer* Anatomy Atlas (www.ucalgary.ca/caribou). These resources were used extensively during the youth programme to teach anatomy and responsible hunting as well as being an online resource for other programmes implementing caribou sampling. Similarly, the caribou sampling and disease video was also a great teaching tool developed through collaborations with communities and provides information on caribou disease and sampling as well as illustrating traditional methods of harvesting and butchering and youth engagement in science.

Traditional ecological knowledge

Workshops, meetings and structured interviews produced a wide range of new information that complemented empirical research. Focus group interview participants indicated that they were noticing changes in caribou health. In particular, there had been an increase in the number of cases of 'green slimy wet stuff' under the skin (Kutz, 2007) and an increasing number of moose with poor coats and hair loss. Formal interviews with WHM participants in 2006, using the ABEKC interview form, were particularly interesting. Some of the notable observations were:

- Caribou migrated to calving ground early.
- Caribou really skinny – cows and bulls both.
- No calves returning to calving grounds.
- Snow crusty, caribou turned back.
- Hooves worn.
- Lots of frogs.
- Swallows gone.
- Gulls – nesting in town last two years.
- Geese – flying high, couldn't hunt.

WHM and focus group participants also emphasized the need for more discussions between scientists and community members about wildlife health, with a particular and critical need to focus on the younger generation (Brook et al., 2009).

11.7 Discussion

The Sahtu community-based monitoring of wildlife health program was established in 2003 in response to community concerns about wildlife and human health, conservation, food safety and security, and youth preparedness for the future. For ten years, government biologists, veterinarians and graduate students travelled to all the schools of the Sahtu, providing interactive educational opportunities to youth, including elders and local knowledge when possible. The programme outcomes have not been formally evaluated; however, limited youth and teacher interviews, anecdotal reports, 'yearbook' quotes and general feedback suggests that the youth outreach component of the programme was successful in engaging youth in science. With respect to wildlife health and research, community representatives expressed a desire for a wildlife health monitoring programme in which they were involved in the planning, implementation and interpretation. In many ways these desires have been met and the WHM programme has demonstrated that community-based monitoring can be successful for obtaining some

baseline indices and also for targeted research studies (Carlsson et al., 2015).

Monitoring has been defined as 'the systematic measurement of variables and processes over time', and assumes that 'there is a specific reason for that collection of data' (Spellerberg, 2005). Spellerberg (2005) summarized the main reasons to undertake monitoring. These are: (1) to provide basic knowledge about an unknown ecological system; (2) to provide accurate scientific data to policymakers and managers; (3) to understand trends over time; and, finally, (4) to provide early detection of potentially harmful effects. The Sahtu programme has met many of these monitoring objectives. The programme has provided basic knowledge of health and pathogen diversity for caribou and moose (1), and for some health indicators, the sample sizes are adequate for evaluating trends (3). The programme detected 'new to us' pathogens and documented range expansion of others (4). All data have been provided to government wildlife agencies and local and regional wildlife co-management boards to be used in policy and wildlife management (2). The programme has further contributed to responsive research projects and peer-reviewed publications.

There are many different models for community-based monitoring, with different degrees of community involvement. Danielsen et al. (2009) provide a good overview and assess strengths and weaknesses of different types of monitoring. In brief, they discuss five categories ranging from externally driven, professionally executed monitoring with no involvement of local stakeholders to autonomous local monitoring, with no involvement of external agencies (Danielsen et al., 2009). From the perspective of being 'community-based', the Sahtu WHM programme sits in Danielsen et al.'s third category, 'collaborative monitoring with external data interpretation, where the design and data analysis is undertaken by external scientists and local people are responsible for data collection and local management and decision-making'. The initial impetus for the programme was driven by community concerns, and community members have been active partners in data collection, and to some extent in the interpretation. The university (an external entity) has been responsible for the majority of grant applications, data analysis and collaborative interpretation, while the regional co-management board, together with the government, makes the management decisions. The different organizations and local communities have collaborated in all parts of the research process. For the programme to continue in a meaningful capacity, long-term commitment from communities, researchers and local government institutions is essential. Ultimately, the goal is for this programme to move to a 'category 4' 'collaborative monitoring with local data interpretation, where local stakeholders are involved every step of the way and external scientists only provide advice and training'. In line with this, other authors have suggested that 'collaborative governance' structures for community-based monitoring may yield more decision-making power and have better likelihood of influencing conservation efforts than other types of monitoring, although governance structure alone does not provide a recipe for success and other factors play key roles as well (Conrad and Hilchey, 2011; Conrad and Daoust, 2008).

In addition to providing robust scientific outcomes, programmes such as the WHM programme also serve to foster positive relationships between researchers, government and co-management boards, and communities, including youth in schools. Involving local stakeholders in the programme has the potential to improve co-management strategies by building trust and improving communication. Several studies have reported that the interaction between managers, researchers and users, at the local level, independent of formal administrative structures, is key to acceptance of management plans and suc-

cessful collaborations (Klein et al., 1999; Kofinas et al., 2003; Russell et al., 2013). Communities need a forum in which to share their knowledge with researchers and managers, and managers and researchers need to make sure that results are disseminated within communities, including with school students where possible. Employing local people to collect data and running programmes from a local agency improves access to stakeholders, increases interaction time between managers and stakeholders, improves the opportunities for knowledge exchange and builds trust between managers and users (Klein et al., 1999; Kofinas et al., 2003). To some degree, the Sahtu programme has contributed to fostering these types of exchanges and has created a space where researchers, managers and communities can interact with a common goal.

The annual visits to all grade schools by a multifaceted team was key to engaging young people in the Sahtu in issues that affect locally important wildlife, teaching them about possible science careers and wildlife monitoring and management methods. Over the course of many years of school visits, the biologists and veterinarians became well-known among students and staff in the schools, and visits were eagerly anticipated. These visits helped to 'put a face' on scientists and the work they conducted within the Sahtu, and elsewhere, helping to create bonds and understanding that can have ramifications well into the future, when students become community leaders and regular subsistence harvesters themselves.

In conclusion, perhaps the most important point to note is that, by using a community-based monitoring approach to conduct health monitoring, local communities who depend on caribou for their livelihood become active members of the monitoring and research process. Simultaneous engagement of youth, through interactive school-based programmes and on the land, serves to provide the foundations and stimulate interest in wildlife health and management, and ultimately promotes the future engagement of these same youth in wildlife research, management and policy. The multi-agency (government, co-management and university) collaboration in wildlife health monitoring demonstrated through the Sahtu programme, serves as a strong model for promoting information exchange and effective action in wildlife conservation and management and helping to promote food safety and security. Hunters are the 'eyes on the land'; they are in a unique position to observe changes when they happen and hold traditional knowledge that can contribute to an integrated view of individual and population health.

> Finally things are happening. We need the research people to come into the communities, at least one or two, because we want to have input into what is being discussed. It's good to see all these people participating here. So let's continue going forward, we settled the land claim so it is important that we have input into preserving our wildlife and the environment, we need to work together and talk things out. The communication today is just starting and we need to continue going forward from today because the industry is coming. The elders always got us prepared for future impact. I am satisfied with the process here, this will help us with the future . . . we need to work together, we don't want anything happening on the land without the consultation . . . We need to say thank you to each other and have input with each other. Thank you for listening.
>
> Alfred Taniton, elder from Déline, NWT in Norman Wells, NWT, October 2002

References

Brook, R.K., Kutz, S.J., Veitch, A.M., Popko, R.A., Elkin, B.T. and Guthrie, G. (2009). Fostering community-based wildlife health monitoring and research in the Canadian North. *Ecohealth*, 6, 266–278.

Carlsson, A.M., Kutz, S.J., Popko, R., Veitch, A.M., Behrens, S., the Sahtu Renewable Resources Board and Sahtu Renewable Resource Councils (2015). *Community-Based Monitoring of Wildlife Health in the Sahtu Settlement Area: A Synthesis of the Program, 2002–2014*. Report prepared for the Sahtu Renewable Resources Board and the Department of Environment and Natural Resources, Government of the Northwest Territories.

Carma (2008). *Rangifer Health and Body Condition Monitoring Protocols Level 1 and 2*. Circumarctic Rangifer Monitoring and Assessment Network, www.caff.is/resources/field-protocols.

Conrad, C.C. and Hilchey, K.G. (2011). A review of citizen science and community-based environmental monitoring: issues and opportunities. *Environmental Monitoring and Assessment*, 176, 273–291.

Conrad, C.T. and Daoust, T. (2008). Community-based monitoring frameworks: increasing the effectiveness of environmental stewardship. *Environmental Management*, 41, 358–366.

Council of Canadian Academics (2014). *Aboriginal Food Security in Northern Canada: An Assessment of the State of Knowledge*. Ottawa: Council of Canadian Academics.

Curry, P.S. (2009). Caribou herds and arctic communities: exploring a new tool for caribou health monitoring. *Arctic*, 62, 495–499.

Curry, P.S. (2012). *Blood on Filter Paper for Monitoring Caribou Health: Efficacy, Community-Based Collection and Disease Ecology in Circumpolar Herds*. PhD, University of Calgary.

Curry, P.S., Elkin, B.T., Campbell, M., Nielsen, K., Hutchins, W., Ribble, C. and Kutz, S.J. (2011). Filter-paper blood samples for Elisa detection of Brucella antibodies in caribou. *Journal of Wildlife Diseases*, 47, 12–20.

Curry, P.S., Ribble, C., Sears, W. C., Hutchins, W., Orsel, K., Godson, D., Lindsay, R., Dibernardo, A. and Kutz, S.J. (2014a). Blood collected on filter paper for wildlife serology: detecting antibodies to Neospora caninum, West Nile virus, and five bovine viruses in Rangifer tarandus subspecies. *Journal of Wildlife Diseases*, 50(2), 297–307.

Curry, P.S., Ribble, C., Sears, W.C., Orsel, K., Hutchins, W., Godson, D., Lindsay, R., Dibernardo, A., Campbell, M. and Kutz, S.J. (2014b). Blood collected on filter paper for wildlife serology: evaluating storage and temperature challenges of field collections. *Journal of Wildlife Diseases*, 50(2), 308–321.

Danielsen, F., Burgess, N.D., Balmford, A., Donald, P.F., Funder, M., Jones, J.P.G., Alviola, P., Balete, D.S., Blomley, T.O.M., Brashares, J., Child, B., Enghoff, M., Fjeldså, J.O.N., Holt, S., Hübertz, H., Jensen, A.E., Jensen, P.M., Massao, J., Mendoza, M.M., Ngaga, Y., Poulsen, M.K., Rueda, R., Sam, M., Skielboe, T., Stuart-Hill, G., Topp-Jørgensen, E. and Yonten, D. (2009). Local participation in natural resource monitoring: a characterization of approaches, *Conservation Biology*, 23, 31–42.

Davidson, R., Simard, M., Kutz, S.J., Kapel, C.M.O., Hamnes, I.S. and Robertson, L.J. (2011). Arctic parasitology: why should we care? *Trends in Parasitology*, 27, 239–245.

Eamer, J. (2006). Keep it simple and be relevant: the first ten years of the Arctic Borderlands Ecological Knowledge Co-op. In W.V. Reid, F. Berkes, T. Wilbanks and D. Capistrano (eds.), *Bridging Scales and Knowledge Systems: Concepts and Applications in Ecosystem Assessment (Millennium Ecosystem Assessments)*. Washington, DC: Island Press.

Fisk, A.T., De Wit, C.A., Wayland, M., Kuzyk, Z.Z., Burgess, N., Letcher, R., Braune, B., Norstrom, R., Blum, S.P., Sandau, C., Lie, E., Larsen, H.J.S., Skaare, J.U. and Muir, D.C.G. (2005). An assessment of the toxicological significance of anthropogenic contaminants in Canadian Arctic wildlife. *Science of the Total Environment*, 351, 57–93.

Gamberg, M., Braune, B., Davey, E., Elkin, B., Hoekstra, P.F., Kennedy, D., Macdonald, C., Muir, D., Nirwal, A., Wayland, M. and Zeeb, B. (2005). Spatial and temporal trends of contaminants in terrestrial biota from the Canadian Arctic. *Science of the Total Environment*, 351, 148–164.

Kashivakura, C. K. (2013). *Detecting Dermacentor albipictus (Packard, 1869), the Winter Tick, at the Northern Extent of its Distribution Range: Hunter Based Monitoring and Serological Assay Development*. MSc, University of Calgary.

Kershaw, R. (ed.) (2005). *The Sahtu Atlas: Maps and stories from the Sahtu Settlement Area in Canada's Northwest Territories*, Sahtu GIS Project.

Klein, D.R., Moorehead, L., Kruse, J. and Braund, S.R. (1999). Contrasts in use and perceptions of biological data for caribou management. *Wildlife Society Bulletin*, 27, 488–498.

Kofinas, G., Lynn, P., Russell, D., White, R., Nelson, A. and Flanders, N. (2003). Towards a protocol for community monitoring of caribou body condition. *Rangifer*, 23(S14), 43–22.

Kutz, S.J. (2007). *An Evaluation of the Role of Climate Change in the Emergence of Pathogens and Diseases in Arctic and Subarctic Caribou Populations. Climate Change Action Fund, Project A760*. Calgary, Alberta: Research Group for Arctic Parasitology (RGAP), Faculty of Veterinary Medicine, University of Calgary.

Kutz, S.J., Hoberg, E.P., Polley, L. and Jenkins, E.J. (2005). Global warming is changing the dynamics of Arctic host-parasite systems. *Proceedings of the Royal Society Biological Sciences Series B*, 272, 2571–2576.

Kutz, S.J., Asmundsson, I., Hoberg, E.P., Appleyard, G.D., Jenkins, E.J., Beckmen, K., Branigan, M., Butler, L., Chilton, N.B., Cooley, D., Elkin, B., Huby-Chilton, F., Johnson, D., Kuchboev, A., Nagy, J., Oakley, M., Polley, L., Popko, R., Scheer, A., Simard, M. and Veitch, A. (2007). Serendipitous discovery of a novel protostrongylid (Nematoda: Metastrongyloidea) in caribou, muskoxen, and moose from high latitudes of North America based on DNA sequence comparisons. *Canadian Journal of Zoology/Revue Canadienne De Zoologie*, 85, 1143–1156.

Kutz, S.J., Jenkins, E.J., Veitch, A.M., Ducrocq, J., Polley, L., Elkin, B. and Lair, S. (2009). The Arctic as a model for anticipating, preventing, and mitigating climate change impacts on host-parasite interactions. *Veterinary Parasitology*, 163, 217–228.

Kutz, S.J., Ducrocq, J., Curry, P., Russell, D. and Gunn, A. (2012). *Widespread Wildlife Health Assessment in the Arctic: The CARMA Model*. Lyon: Wildlife Disease Association.

Kutz, S.J., Ducrocq, J., Cuyler, C., Elkin, B., Gunn, A., Kolpashikov, L., Russell, D. and White, R.G. (2013a). Standardized monitoring of Rangifer health during International Polar Year. *Rangifer*, 33, 91–114.

Kutz, S.J., Checkley, S., Verocai, G.G., Dumond, M., Hoberg, E., Peacock, R., Wu, J., Orsel, K., Seegers, K., Warren, A. and Abrams, A. (2013b). Invasion, establishment, and range expansion of two protostrongylid nematodes in the Canadian Arctic. *Global Change Biology*, 19, 3254–3262.

Kutz, S.J., Checkley, S., Verocai, G.G., Dumond, M., Hoberg, E.P., Peacock, R., Wu, J.P., Orsel, K., Seegers, K., Warren, A.L. and Abrams, A. (2013c). Invasion, establishment, and range expansion of two parasitic nematodes in the Canadian Arctic. *Global Change Biology*, 19, 3254–3262.

Laaksonen, S., Pusenius, J., Kumpula, J., Venalainen, A., Kortet, R., Oksanen, A. and Hoberg, E. (2010). Climate change promotes the emergence of serious disease outbreaks of filarioid nematodes. *Ecohealth*, 7, 7–13.

Meakin, S. and Kurvits, T. (2009). Assessing the Impacts of Climate Change on Food Security in the Canadian Arctic. Ottawa: GRID-Arendal.

Metlofte, H. (2013). *CAFF 2013. Arctic Biodiversity Assessment: Status and Trends in Arctic Biodiversity*, Akureyri: Conservation of Arctic Flora and Fauna, Arctic Council.

Post, E., Bhatt, U., Bitz, C., Brodie, J., Fulton, T.L., Hebblewhite, M., Kerby, J., Kutz, S.J., Stirling, I. and Walker, D.A. (2013). Ecological consequences of sea-ice decline. *Science*, 341, 519–524.

Russell, D., Svoboda, M. Y., Arokium, J. and Cooley, D. (2013). Arctic Borderlands Ecological Knowledge Cooperative: can local knowledge inform caribou management? *Rangifer*, 33, 71–78.

Spellerberg, I.F. (2005). *Monitoring Ecological Change*, Cambridge: Cambridge University Press.

SRRB (2014). *At Home on the Land: Sahtu Cross-Cultural Research Camp at Stewart Lake*. Sahtu Renewable Resources Board.

Statistics (2009). *2009 NWT Community Survey*.

Verocai, G.G., Lejeune, M., Beckmen, K.B., Kashivakura, C.K., Veitch, A.M., Popko, R.A., Fuentealba, C., Hoberg, E.P. and Kutz, S.J. (2012). Defining parasite biodiversity at high latitudes of North America: new host and geographic records for Onchocerca cervipedis (Nematoda: Onchocercidae) in moose and caribou. *Parasites & Vectors*, 5, 242.

Verocai, G.G., Kutz, S.J., Simard, M. and Hoberg, E.P. (2014). *Varestrongylus eleguneniensis* sp. n. (Nematoda: Protostrongylidae): a widespread, multi-host lungworm of wild North American ungulates, with an emended diagnosis for the genus and explorations of biogeography. *Parasites & Vectors*, 7, 149–189.

Wasser, S.K., Keim, J.L., Taper, M.L. and Lele, S.R. (2011). The influences of wolf predation, habitat loss, and human activity on caribou and moose in the Alberta oil sands. *Frontiers in Ecology and the Environment*, 9, 546–551.

Wesche, S.D. and Chan, H.M. (2010). Adapting to the impacts of climate change on food security among Inuit in the western Canadian Arctic. *EcoHealth*, 7, 361–373.

Wu, J.P., Veitch, A., Checkley, S., Dobson, H. and Kutz, S.J. (2012). Linear enamel hypoplasia in caribou (Rangifer tarandus groenlandicus): a potential tool to assess population health. *Wildlife Society Bulletin*, 36, 554–560.

chapter 12

Using One Health to benefit animals: the case of declining sockeye salmon

Craig Stephen

Abstract

Sockeye salmon are the most economically important of the six species of salmon found in British Columbia. They have sustained Aboriginal communities for thousands of years and have been a major economic resource for coastal communities as well as being key to both marine and freshwater ecosystems. A population crash in 2009 was preceded by a decade's decline in population numbers and three consecutive years of a closed fishery. As a result of concerns over the population decline, the Canadian government established the Cohen Commission into the Decline of Fraser River Sockeye Salmon and charged it with determining the causes for the unexpected and precipitous drop in the number of returning sockeye salmon. In this chapter we explore the application of a One Health approach to examine the complex problem of population decline in this iconic species.

12.1 Introduction

Because there is no universal definition of One Health, the term has been defined and used in a wide variety of ways. There are, however, two general 'types' of One Health (Figure 12.1). The first is reminiscent of veterinary public health and focuses on detecting, managing or eliminating hazards to people that arise in animals or the environment. This can be termed the 'anthropocentric hazards model of One Health'. Most often, people are the beneficiaries of this approach. Projects that strive to detect and eliminate zoonotic pathogens in animals before they

impact public health serve as an example. The second type of One Health can trace its roots to the *Ottawa Charter for Health Promotion* (Anon, 1986). This approach advocates for reciprocal care of the health of people, animals and the environment and can be termed the 'socioecological model'. It strives to co-manage the determinants of health, seeking to achieve mutual benefits for people, animals and their shared environment. Projects that work to promote environmentally sustainable livestock production for poverty reduction are examples of this model.

Regardless of the type, most One Health investments and associated activities have been

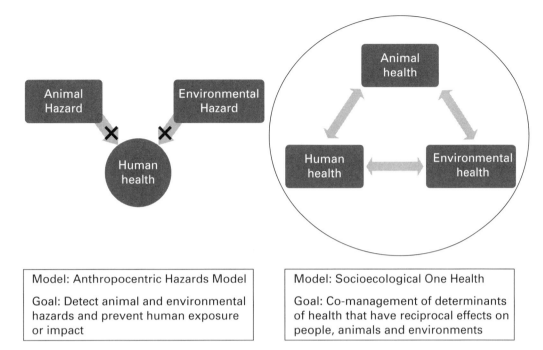

Figure 12.1 Two conceptual models of One Health.

preoccupied with improving human health outcomes as their primary goal. But the triad of interactions between animals, environments and people lacks directionality. Just as animals and environments influence human health, people and environments affect animal health, and animals and people impact their environments. This chapter explores how the socioecological model of One Health has utility for working on issues where the primary goal is to protect and maintain animal health while simultaneously caring about people and the environment.

12.2 The case

In 2009, 1.5 million sockeye salmon (*Oncorhynhus nerka*) returned to the Fraser River in British Columbia, Canada. Pre-season estimates for the return had anticipated that 10.5 million fish would come back to the river to spawn. Later that

year, the Canadian government established the Cohen Commission into the Decline of Fraser River Sockeye Salmon (hereafter called the Commission) and charged it with determining the causes for the unexpected and precipitous drop in the number of returning sockeye salmon.

The population crash of 2009 was preceded by a decade's decline in population numbers and three consecutive years of a closed fishery. The Fraser River had historically produced more salmon than any single river in the world. Sockeye salmon have been prized by fishers and consumers and have been the most economically important of the six species of salmon found in British Columbia. Sockeye salmon have sustained Aboriginal communities for thousands of years, have been a major economic resource for coastal communities and are key to both marine and freshwater ecosystems.

An overview of the lifecycle of sockeye salmon provides the context needed to understand the case and the Commission's conclusions (Figure

12.2). Pacific salmon are anadromous, meaning that they spend part of their life in freshwater and part in the ocean. Fraser River sockeye typically have a 3–5-year lifecycle. Adults, which can measure up to 86cm in length and weigh an average of 3.6kg, return to their natal streams to deposit and fertilize eggs in gravel beds. There are hundreds of such streams throughout the massive Fraser River watershed and salmon are faithful to their stream of birth. The eggs develop over the winter and hatch in the spring after about five months of incubation. Three months later, the juveniles move into lakes and live there for one to two years before migrating to the ocean. At about 20 months after spawning, the juveniles begin undergoing physiological changes to adapt to saltwater. This serves as a cue for outmigration to the ocean; a trip that can range from 40 to 1,200km, depending on the location of their nursery lake. The ocean movements of Fraser River sockeye is the least-understood part of their life but they are known to swim up into the Gulf of Alaska and forage for two to three years before returning as adults to their natal stream. Normally, only a very small proportion of eggs return as adults. The salmon's lifecycle covers many habitats distributed over thousands of kilometres, exposing them to a wide suite of hazards and challenges.

After 18 months and hundreds of public submissions, numerous scientific reports and weeks of hearings, the Commission generated a list of possible attributing causes of the sockeye salmon's decline (Table 12.1). Upon reviewing the evidence Justice Cohen, the lead of the Commission, concluded that the idea of a single event or stressor leading to the decline was appealing but improbable (Cohen, 2012a). Rather, the decline had to be seen as the result of the cumulative effects of these multiple interacting factors for which there is much uncertainty and complexity. Rather than investing or managing single factors in isolation, the judge saw the wisdom in trying to create a system that helps the salmon cope with the many interacting hazards that they encounter over their life course. The Commission astutely recognized that to preserve the positive contributions salmon made to the welfare of people and their critical ecological role, there was a need to manage human effects on salmon and help the salmon become more resilient to environmental change.

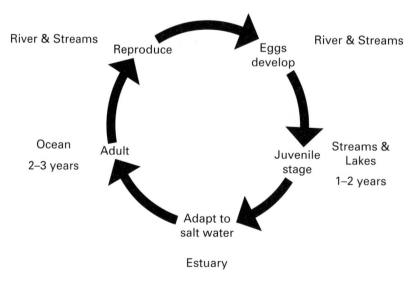

Figure 12.2 The sockeye salmon lifecycle.

Table 12.1 Abbreviated list of possible contributing causes to the decline of Fraser River sockeye salmon presented through public submissions and expert reports to the Cohen Commission into the Decline of Fraser River Sockeye Salmon (Cohen, 2012b)

Theme	Category	Examples
Effects in the river watershed	Habitat loss and alteration	Forestry Urbanization Mining Gravel extraction
	Water diversion and use	Groundwater use Hydroelectric dams
	Pollution	Wastewater Pulp mill effluent Pesticides Other point and non-point source contaminants
	Ecological interactions	Interaction with fish released from government enhancement facilities Naturally occurring disease Predation
	Climate change	Water near lethal temperature Change in parasite/pathogen dynamics
Effects in the marine environment	Water quality and pollution	Harmful algae blooms Point and non-point source contaminants
	Ecological interactions	Interaction with fish released from government enhancement facilities Naturally occurring disease Predation Change in marine food abundance
	Salmon farms	Disease interactions
	Climate change	Alterations in migration timing

The case of the Fraser River sockeye salmon illustrates the general fate of salmon in western North America. Approximately half of all populations in Washington, Oregon and California in the United States of America are under threat of extinction (Healey, 2009). In British Columbia, 142 runs have gone extinct since the mid-twentieth century and nearly half of the remaining commercially important populations are at high risk (Healey, 2009). There is broad consensus that recovery of Pacific salmon cannot be achieved without fostering their resilience to social and environmental pressures (Bisson et al., 2009).

12.3 Resilience as the future of salmon health

One of the major distinctions between the anthropocentric and socioecological models of One Health is that one focuses on hazards and diseases and the other focuses on resilience and health. Fish health, like a majority of wildlife health work, typically deals with the detection and response to infectious or parasitic diseases; a situation that has been re-enforced by the anthropocentric focus of One Health on animals as sources of emerging infection (Stephen, 2014). The socioecological health model is based on the premise that no single factor can explain differences in health status between populations.

Despite the growing prominence of resilience and sustainability as defining features of wildlife health (Deem et al., 2008; Hanisch et al., 2012), the concept has yet to be widely adopted in fish health. Resilience in socioecological systems includes concepts of adaptability and the capacity to persist in the face of disturbance or hazards. Until recently, fish health research has been largely restricted to laboratory studies of pathological mechanisms or clinical diagnostics that served to identify single hazards and their impacts on individual fish. Although one way to promote resilience may be to buffer populations by reducing their exposures to hazards, so little is known about the role of disease in fish population health or about how to effectively reduce exposure of wild fish to hazards, that a hazards-focused approach to stopping salmon declines cannot be well-founded in evidence. Government agencies responsible for salmon management, researchers and other stakeholders are struggling with meeting social expectations for salmon health in the absence of a definition of health that can simultaneously address social expectation and ecological needs and uncertainties. They are looking for ways to wed social sciences with cumulative impact assessment to generate the necessary research findings to manage salmon health as a product of socioecological interactions rather than investing exclusively in detecting hazards that cannot practically be managed in free-ranging marine species.

The idea that salmon could be sustained by removing some hazards and obstacles to reproduction motivated the development of extensive hatchery systems in countries rim-

ming the North Pacific Ocean. Public or private interests built hatcheries that could protect eggs and juvenile fish from predation and bad environments, optimize the size and timing of releases into natural waters to improve growth and survival, and select spawning partners; all to optimize salmon production. Their goal has been to compensate for excessive mortality due to multiple hazards – such as dams, habitat loss, harvesting or disease – by maximizing the numbers of fish put into the ocean. They have been so successful that hatchery fish often outnumber truly wild salmon in their ocean environments. Take Oregon, for example, where 80 per cent of salmon in the Columbia River are of hatchery origin (Bottom et al., 2009). But, their effects on genetic diversity, ecological competition with truly wild fish and disease transmission has led many to believe that hatcheries are now one of the major threats to salmon (Rand et al., 2012). The involvement of people in the triad of human–animals–environment must, therefore, involve more than trying to compensate for poor health or population declines through new technological interventions. A socioecological approach works to foster the capacity of populations or ecosystems for self-repair to support human uses or expectations.

The failure of past approaches to salmon health and management to pay attention to the relationships that bind salmon, people, other animals and environments has undermined the development of socioecological approaches. The Commission revealed that not only have fish disease management programmes not interacted with programmes dealing with population management, but also that programmes dealing with freshwater management were separate from those dealing with the saltwater phase of their lifecycle, each of which were isolated from habitat programmes, aquaculture management and pollution control. The push towards specialization in education and legislation had subdivided our knowledge and control of a salmon's life to such an extent that influences across the salmon's life courses were disconnected to the point that a comprehensive view of risks or causes of population decline were elusive at best. It was recognized as early as 1996 that the fragmentation of responsibilities and mismatch between how we studied salmon and how they lived severely undermined salmon conservation (Bottom et al., 2009).

One of the scientific reports to the Commission (Stephen et al., 2011) dealt exclusively with the impact of hatcheries on wild Fraser River sockeye salmon. A key recommendation of that report was to reorganize programmes so that salmon health was not a science of the parts but rather a science of the whole. The goal would be to 'get ahead of the curve' to inspire or sustain action in the absence of a threat or to prepare populations to resist multiple, uncertain or unknown risks. An overall recommendation of the Commission was to make it someone's job to try to pull together the various elements and information needed to think about and manage sockeye salmon health from a cumulative effects perspective. A primary role for this person would be to break down barriers and facilitate collaboration toward conservation.

12.4 Ways forward

In the 'real world', salmon are confronted with numerous interacting factors influencing health and disease outcomes. Emerging diseases, pollution, climate change, habitat loss, harvest, predation and other threats happen concurrently rather than in isolation. It seems reasonable, therefore, to ask whether an interdisciplinary approach to a single problem, such the anthropocentric hazards model of One Health, is sufficient to protect salmon health in a sustainable way in a world faced with unprecedented social and environmental change; and whether salmon health research and management needs

to evolve from an interdisciplinary field to one that is 'interprobleminary' (Stephen et al., 2015) – an approach that examines the interactions and implications of multiple problems occurring simultaneously in a place or population.

In a world of concurrent problems, unique solutions for each problem is neither feasible nor effective (Fried et al., 2012), and we may fail to find the 'levers' to pull to keep populations healthy if we retain an interdisciplinary approach to a single problem rather than thinking of the interactions of hazards, determinants of health and populations in a shared social and physical space. Moreover, if we remain fixated on discovering the 'scientific laws of health' to predict impacts rather than use One Health as a tool to solve health problems, we get farther behind. We must conclude that prediction may be futile if we accept that (1) health is the capacity to adapt to, respond to or control life's challenges and changes (Stephen, 2014); (2) health is the result of interacting biological, social and environmental determinants that affect the capacity to cope with change; and (3) there is significant ambiguity and uncertainty at the human–animal–environment interface.

The goal of an 'interprobleminary' approach is not to build more and more complex models to predict the next hazard, but rather to build robustness against negative events that occur and be able to exploit positive ones. Achieving success in an 'interprobleminary' approach will require researchers to act as information brokers who can connect specialized pools of knowledge. The socioecological approach requires us to think not of problems in terms of species or pathogens but rather in terms of the shared biophysical and social space in which everyday health occurs and focus on those conditions that influence their capacity to cope with the multiple interacting problems.

12.5 Conclusions

This case illustrates that animals can be the primary focus on One Health thinking and not just be considered as source of hazards to people. It further demonstrates how effective management of animal health problems requires simultaneous consideration of human, environmental and animal factors. The socioecological approach advocated for in this case is somewhat atypical for One Health and veterinary medicine. It is more familiar in environmental sustainability and human health promotion. However, the approach has been recommended as a strategy against emerging infectious diseases (Stephen et al., 2015), and for linking human development and aquaculture (Burns et al., 2014). It has been applied to the challenge of controlling vectorborne diseases in situations of extreme poverty (Hecker et al., 2014), management of wildlife zoonoses (Nishi et al., 2002) and for identifying policy priorities for avian influenza (Stephen et al., 2010). A problem-focused approach to One Health that aims to promote health as opposed to manage diseases will undoubtedly benefit from this type of thinking. The looming challenges of climate change, depletion of ecological services and exponentially growing human population suggest that achieving animal, environmental and human health by separate science, policies and actions is impossible. The ideal of One Health recognizes that our historic approach to dealing with health is poorly suited to the challenges that will confront us in the next century. The socioecological model of One Health is a critical step in bringing animal health out of a reductionist single hazard focussed approach pursued largely in clinics and laboratories and into a broader holistic, multicausal approach embedded in the real world.

References

Anon (1986). *Ottawa Charter for Health Promotion*, www.euro.who.int/en/publications/policy-documents/ottawa-charter-for-health-promotion-1986.

Bisson, P.A., Dunham, J.B. and Reeves, G.H. (2009). Freshwater ecosystems and resilience of Pacific salmon: habitat management based on natural variability. *Ecology & Society*, 14(1), 45

Bottom, D.L., Jones, K.K., Simenstad, C.S. and Smith, S.L. (2009). Reconnecting social and ecological resilience in salmon ecosystems. *Ecology and Society*, 14(1), 5.

Burns, T., Stephen, C. and Wade, J. (2014) A scoping analysis of peer reviewed literature about linkages between aquaculture and human development outcomes. *Ecohealth*, 11(2), 227–240.

Cohen B. (2012a). *The Uncertain Future of Fraser River Sockeye. Vol 3. Recommendations, Summary, Process.* Report of the Commission of Inquiry into the Decline of Fraser River Sockeye Salmon. Ottawa: Public Works and Government Services Canada.

Cohen B. (2012b). *The Uncertain Future of Fraser River Sockeye. Vol 2. Causes of the Decline.* Report of the Commission of Inquiry into the Decline of Fraser River Sockeye Salmon. Ottawa: Public Works and Government Services Canada.

Deem, S.L., Parker, P.G. and Miller, R.E. (2008). Building bridges: connecting the health and conservation professions. *Biotropica: The Journal of Tropical Biology & Conservation*, 40(6), 662–665.

Fried, L.P., Piot, P., Frenk, J.J., Flahault, A. and Parker, R. (2012). Global public health leadership for the twenty-first century: towards improved health of all populations. *Global Public Health*, 7(S1), S5–S15.

Hanisch, S.L., Riley, S.J. and Nelson, M.P. (2012). Promoting wildlife health or fighting wildlife diseases: insights from history, philosophy, and science. *Wildlife Society Bulletin*, 36(3), 477–482.

Healey, M.C. (2009). Resilient salmon, resilient fisheries for British Columbia, Canada. *Ecology & Society*, 14(1), 2.

Hecker, K., el Kurdi, S., Joshi, DD. and Stephen, C. (2014). Using network analysis to explore if professional opinions on Japanese Encephalitis risk factors in Nepal reflect a socio-ecological system perspective. *Ecohealth*, 10(4), 415–422.

Nishi, J.S., Stephen, C. and Elkin, B.T. (2002). Implications of agriculture and wildlife policy on management and eradication of bovine tuberculosis and brucellosis in free ranging Wood Bison in northern Canada. In E.P.J. Gibbs and B.H. Bokma (eds.), *The Domestic Animal/Wildlife Interface: Issues for Disease Control, Conservation, Sustainable Food Production, and Emerging Diseases*. New York: Annals of the New York Academy of Sciences, pp. 1–9.

Rand, P.S., Berejikian, B.A., Bidlack, A., Bottom, D., Gardner, J., Kaeriyama, M., Lincoln, R., Nagata, M., Pearsons, T.N., Schmidt, M., Smoker, W.W., Weitkamp, L.A. and Zhivotovsky, L.A. (2012). Ecological interactions between wild and hatchery salmonids and key recommendations for research and management actions in selected regions of the North Pacific. *Environmental Biology of Fishes*, 94(1), 343–358.

Stephen C. (2014). Towards a modernized definition of wildlife health. *Journal of Wildlife Disease*, 50(3), 427–430.

Stephen, C., Ninghui, L., Zhang, L. and Yeh, F. (2010). Animal health policy principles for highly pathogenic avian influenza: shared experience from China and Canada. *Zoonoses and Public Health*, 58(5), 334–342.

Stephen, C., Stitt, T., Dawson-Coates, J. and McCarthy, A. (2011). *Assessment of the Potential Effects of Diseases Present in Salmonid Enhancement Facilities on Fraser River Sockeye Salmon*. Report to the Cohen Commission into the Decline of Sockeye Salmon in the Fraser River.

Stephen, C., Berezowski, J. and Misra, V. (2015). Surprise is a neglected aspect of emerging infectious disease. *Ecohealth*, 12(2), 208–211.

chapter 13

Marine animal health in a changing Arctic

Sandra Black, Padraig Duignan,
Japatee Akeeagok and Stephen Raverty

Abstract

The polar regions are experiencing environmental changes at an unprecedented rate, related to climate change and anthropogenic activity. This chapter will introduce the reader to responses occurring at all biotic levels in the Arctic and to scientific inquiry exploring links between environmental change and those responses. A One Health approach employing interdisciplinary research and cooperation is illustrated through an ongoing investigation of an unusual mortality event in ice seals of the Western Arctic.

13.1 Introduction

Climate change related to anthropogenic activities is changing the 'landscape' within which all life forms on earth exist. The 2014 Fifth Assessment report (AR5) of the Intergovernmental Panel on Climate Change states:

> Human influence on the climate system is clear, and recent anthropogenic emissions of greenhouse gases are the highest in history. Recent climatic changes have had widespread impacts on human and natural systems.

There is a rapidly growing body of scientific literature replete with examples of the effects of climate change within natural systems. These impacts appear to be occurring at amplified levels in the Arctic, where sea ice loss is augmenting atmospheric warming at a rate two to three times the global mean (Kumar et al., 2010; Stroeve et al., 2012a). The 2013 report of the International Panel on Climate Change Working Group I states: 'Multiple lines of evidence support very substantial Arctic warming since the mid 20th century.' All organisms in the Arctic from the smallest phytoplankton and deepest benthic invertebrates to the charismatic megafauna are being impacted (Wassmann et al., 2011; Post et al., 2013). However, changes are not always predictable or uniform and the perturbations of natural and human systems may well create unique conditions bringing not only exceptional challenges but also opportunities (Prowse and Furgal, 2009). How some of these changes are currently impacting Arctic wildlife and ecosystems, as well as the indigenous people who depend on them, is the subject of this chapter.

The most visible changes in Arctic marine ecosystems are those in the realm of snow and ice – the *cryosphere*. The decreasing extent of sea ice cover as measured at the end of the melt season in September is a trend that has accelerated significantly in the first decade of the twenty-first century. Warmer autumn temperatures in the Arctic reflect the increased global temperatures in all seasons from greenhouse gas forces. This leads to later ice formation in the autumn, thinner spring ice, decreased albedo or reflectance of solar energy and more open water in September creating a self-sustaining cycle of escalation (Stroeve et al., 2012b). In numbers, this translates to an average annual increase in the melt season of 20 days over the past 30 years (Markus et al., 2009). Not only is Arctic sea ice decreasing in extent, but it is also losing

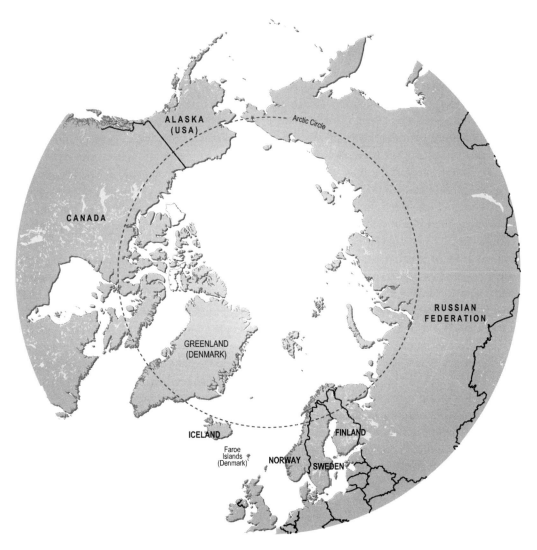

Figure 13.1 The Arctic Ocean and surrounding lands.

volume, as the percentage of thicker multiyear ice declines and is replaced by thinner first-year ice that forms and melts annually (Comiso, 2012). These trends have been strongest in the western Arctic (Chukchi, Siberian and Beaufort Seas). Observational studies and models predict that the Arctic will become seasonally ice-free by the middle of this century if greenhouse gas emissions continue to increase (Stroeve et al., 2012a).

13.2 Direct and indirect impacts of climate change on Arctic plankton and fish species

Sea ice represents a major biome, providing substrate for phyto- and zooplankton and habitat for a diversity of vertebrates. Since the end of the twentieth century, more than two million square kilometres of sea ice has been lost (Kinnard et al., 2011). Presence and thickness of ice affects the physical factors of light penetrance and temperature, which directly influence primary productivity. Increased melting also decreases ocean salinity, and may relate to physical changes in current and upwelling activity. Earlier ice retreat has been associated with changes in the timing of phytoplankton blooms, particularly for species that are pelagic rather than ice-associated (Ji et al., 2013). Phytoplankton are the primary food source for zooplankton grazing species such as *Calanus glacialis* (a marine copepod), providing high-quality fatty acids in two spring peaks that coincide with periods of reproduction and growth of offspring for *Calanus* (Søreide et al., 2010). Temporal asynchrony between phytoplankton blooms and zooplankton production is likely to have negative consequences for the latter and at higher trophic levels.

While the ecosystem effects of many observed changes are not fully known, changing conditions in the Arctic Ocean may favour some organisms but harm others. One such observa-

tion involves a decrease in nutrient availability in the water column as it has become warmer and less saline. This has been associated with an alteration in the ratio of small to large phytoplankton. Picoplankton are very small and are more effective at acquiring nutrients and photons, while more resistant to sinking in the water column than larger nanoplankton. In recent years, increasing numbers of picoplankton and decreasing numbers of nanoplankton have been recorded in the western Canadian Arctic (Li et al., 2009). In the eastern Canadian Arctic archipelago on the other hand, eutrophication, associated with sea ice loss and changes in vertical mixing, has increased primary productivity (Ardyna et al., 2011). With decreased snow cover and sea ice thickness, and increased spring melt ponds on the ice surface, there is more light transmission through ice, and in many areas, a coincident increase in primary productivity below the ice, an area previously little studied (Palmer et al., 2013). The ecological consequences of changes in the phenology, biodiversity and structure of phytoplankton communities are still largely unknown, particularly for higher trophic levels. We do know that to propose a hypothesis of a match-mismatch between prey productivity and predator energy need, both must have a high level of seasonality, and predator abundance must be controlled in a bottom-up manner (Moline et al., 2008). Marked seasonality is a hallmark of polar species, and the potential for adverse consequences of these changes is therefore high.

In terms of economics, and as we consider the potential effects of climate change at higher trophic levels, potential shifts in the distribution and productivity of fish stocks are of increasing concern and interest. While small fisheries have been operating for the past 30 years in some communities, the prediction that the Arctic Ocean will soon be ice-free throughout the summer fuels speculation about future economically viable fisheries in these waters (Ashley, 1993).

Cheung et al. (2009) analysed the current and projected physical changes in the world's oceans using *bioclimate envelope analysis*, and predicted future colonization of the Arctic Ocean by temperate and Subarctic fish. In the Bering Sea, benthic water temperature has increased significantly since 1982 and is the variable most closely associated with the distribution of deep water fish. Concurrently, there has been a northwards shift in latitudinal distribution for 46 Bering Sea taxa, indicating that change is occurring at the level of community, not just individual species (Mueter and Litzow, 2008). How this will play out with the restructuring of predator–prey dynamics at the highest trophic levels is as yet unknown. In an analysis of 17 potentially commercial Subarctic species, Hollowed and others (2013) looked at species vulnerability as a sum of exposure and sensitivity to climate-induced change and the adaptive capacity of the species. Based on these models, six species including polar cod and Bering flounder have a high likelihood of moving to and colonizing the Arctic Ocean. Invasion of predatory ground fish may result in greater predation pressure on lower trophic levels, again with ecosystem-wide impacts that are difficult to predict (Mueter and Litzow, 2008). Arctic cod are currently the only fish found with amphipod communities at the floe edge – the melting edge of Arctic cryopelagic systems, or those systems consisting of ice and open ocean. This small fish constitutes a critical lipid rich food source for apex Arctic predators (Lønne and Gulliksen, 1989). One speaker at the 2013 Alaska Sea Grant Wakefield Symposium on responses of Arctic marine ecosystems to climate change, quipped that polar bears (and by definition all Arctic marine predators) are simply 'repackaged Arctic cod'. Thus, changes to Arctic fish communities may have significant repercussions for Arctic predators.

13.3 Direct and indirect impacts of climate change on Arctic marine avian and mammalian species

Black guillemots (*Cepphus grille mandtii*) are piscivorous Subarctic and Arctic nesting birds dependent on ice-associated prey in the northern portion of their range, where seasonal ice scour reduces near-shore demersal species. Breeding colonies are concentrated in areas on the north coast of Alaska where sea ice has typically remained close to the shore for much of the melt season (Moline et al., 2008). During the nesting season, adults fly out in a radius of 30–40km to feed at the floe edge, largely on Arctic cod. A clutch of two eggs is usual, and when food supplies are high, most pairs raise and fledge both chicks. From hatch to fledging, chicks increase tenfold in weight over 35 days. That was how it was for millennia. Now, increasing temperatures, earlier melt seasons and increasing distances from shore to the foraging grounds have forced the birds to shift their prey to the less energy-rich sculpin (order Scorpaeniformes) because they can be found closer to the nesting colonies. Consequently, the colonies have contracted as the overworked parents struggle to raise only one chick (Moline et al., 2008).

Among the ice seals, the ringed seal (*Pusa hispida*) is one of the smallest and most widespread through the Arctic with a circumpolar distribution and ranging into the North Atlantic and North Pacific Oceans (Smith and Hammill, 1981). It is the mainstay of polar bears, but they are also eaten by walrus, Greenland sharks, killer whales and Arctic foxes. In addition, they are a key species for northern communities as a source of pelts and meat for people and their dogs. However, it is one of the most ice-obligate seals, with pregnant females giving birth to a single pup in a lair they excavate in snow overlying the thick pack ice or land-fast ice that provides shelter from the elements and predators alike. The minimum snow depth for use by whelping ringed seals is 20cm. Hetzel and others (2012) project that areas with adequate snow depth will decrease by 70 per cent before the end of the twenty-first century. Without these lairs the tiny pups, usually around 5kg at birth, would have little chance of survival. Harp seals (*Pagophilus groenlandicus*) also rely on ice platforms for pupping. If no ice is available they have been observed to shift away from traditional whelping areas; however, in these seasons of poor ice availability, pup mortality is high (Stenson and Hammill, 2014). Reduction in suitable breeding and haul-out habitat for ringed seals, harp seals and their pinniped kin (bearded, spotted, ribbon and hooded seals and walrus) will greatly impact recruitment through lack of suitable breeding habitat and increased vulnerability to predators and will likely increase contact rates both among conspecifics and between species. For a species like the ringed seal that prefer some personal space, this could be a source of chronic stress, decreased immune response and increased disease incidence and severity. Increased levels of contact between different species may also facilitate the transmission of pathogens to new hosts precipitating unusual mortality events. MacCracken (2012) describes the effects of diminishing extent and duration of sea ice habitats on walrus (*Odobenus rosmarus*) behaviour. As sea ice declines, some walrus, particularly those in the western Arctic, are finding themselves stranded far from food sources or hauled out on shore in vastly increased numbers; both situations may create population stress and increased disease susceptibility, whereas shore-crowding may also increase disease transmission and death from trampling and increased predation.

While ringed seals may be a keystone species in the Arctic ecosystem, the polar bear (*Ursus maritimus*) has become the poster child for climate change in the region. As with the ringed seal, the polar bear is dependent on snow and ice (Stirling 1988; Stirling and Derocher, 1993). Females give birth in snow dens and most of their diet is derived directly from the ocean during the winter months. They prey predominantly on ice seals and walrus but will opportunistically take ice-entrapped cetaceans, sea birds and scavenge beach-cast whale carcasses. The polar bear range is circumpolar, with the most southerly population on the western shores of Hudson Bay, Canada. There is considerable debate among the scientific community and among indigenous people as to how and whether polar bears are being impacted by climate change. At higher latitudes, traditional hunters say that polar bears are as numerous as ever and are in good body condition (Voorhees et al., 2014). The same is not true for the western Hudson Bay population. Stirling and others (1999) presented the first conclusive evidence from data collected through the 1980 and 1990s that progressive warming of April to June temperatures were causing earlier ice break-up, forcing bears to spend more time fasting ashore. Synthesis of several studies shows that female body mass, number of cubs per litter, cub survival and number of independent yearlings decreased while the mean birth interval increased from the 1960s to the present, and these changes are statistically associated with the earlier spring melt (Stirling and Derocher, 2012). Similar marked declines in population size (up to 40 per cent) driven by high cub and juvenile mortality have also recently been reported for the southern Beaufort Sea (Rode et al., 2010). However, rates of change are not the same through the polar bear range and complex mathematical modelling of future climate change on survivorship and fecundity of bears from the Western Hudson Bay and those from Lancaster Sound show non-linear effects of temperature increase on both key indices (Molnar et al., 2010). This research is focused on the effects of climate change on sea ice cover and how that will affect length of fast (ice-free period when bears have little access to their normal prey) and contact rates between breeding age males and females. What is not yet fully understood is the effect that stress and malnutrition will have on immune response, disease resistance and health status. Certainly the negative effects of pollution on the health of adults and particularly suckling cubs is of concern as greater levels of lipophilic toxic chemicals circulate in animals metabolizing fat stores when body condition decreases (Sonne, 2010; Stirling and Derocher, 2012). Jensen and others (2010) link climate change related increasing water temperatures with a doubling in the observed exposure levels of polar bears in the Svalbard region to the parasite *Toxoplasma gondii*. These findings raise many questions about the health of polar bear populations in coming decades. Will endemic diseases and parasites have a greater impact on malnourished bears? Will stressed bears be more susceptible to pathogens from southern latitudes introduced through contact with brown (grizzly, *Ursus arctos horribilis*) bears or through predation on unusual prey such as sea birds or terrestrial animals? (Plate 19) Will the lack of extensive sea ice result in higher contact rates between the remaining polar bears and promote disease transmission? Will the hybridization of polar bears with grizzly bears lead to a genetic change with unknown consequences?

Many factors influence emergence, transmission and persistence of infectious diseases in populations. The ecology of the host species is an obvious influence and for seasonally or temporally aggregated species such as ice seals, or highly social species such as narwhal (*Monodon monoceros*) or belugas (*Delphinapterus leucas*), it is apparent how highly infectious agents such as viruses can transmit from the infected to susceptible members of the group. The social dynamics of harbour seals (*Phoca vitulina*) was identified as a risk factor in the propagation of two massive phocine distemper virus (PDV) epidemics in Western Europe in the 1988 and 2002 (Harwood and Hall, 1990; Hall et al., 2006; Harkonen et al., 2006). Interestingly, this virus was shown to be endemic in harp seals of the Canadian eastern Arctic and European Arctic (Markussen and Have, 1992; Duignan et al., 1997, 2014). Spillover into the North Sea is thought to have precipitated the European epidemics following environmental perturbations in the Arctic that drove virus-carrying harp seals south. If relatively minor and short-term perturbations could precipitate such events, what could the major long-term changes wrought by climate change do for the ecology of infectious diseases? Of concern is the fact that until the early years of this century, there was no evidence for PDV in the huge pinniped populations in the Bering, Chukchi and Siberian Seas or in the North Pacific (Osterhaus and Vedder, 1988; Duignan et al., 1995a; Hanni et al., 2003; Burek et al., 2005; Zarnke et al.. 2006). Then in 2006, an unusual mortality event (UME) was declared for northern sea otters (*Enhydra lutris kenyoni*) in the Western Aleutian Islands and mid-central Alaska. Subsequent investigations of these animals and surveys of several pinniped species around Alaska found evidence of PDV infection by serology and molecular diagnostic techniques (Goldstein et al., 2009; Duignan et al., 2014). Genetically the virus was very similar to that isolated from the North Atlantic. So, where did the virus come from? Why had there been no mass mortality of seals as in Europe when the seals present in Alaskan waters were known to be naïve? In 2004 and 2005, immediately preceding the sea otter deaths, the extent of sea ice cover in summer was particularly low (Goldstein et al., 2009). So while there are no concrete answers yet, it is tempting to speculate that the opening of the Northwest Passage has facilitated the east-to-west dispersal of marine mammals. We already know this is happening for narwhal as these have now been observed as far west as Victoria Island well beyond their previous range (www.nunatsiaqonline), so it is conceivable that seals may also be shifting their ranges along the Arctic coast.

Resident cetaceans in the Arctic are equally vulnerable to the introduction of potentially lethal viruses such as *Cetacean morbillivirus* (CeMV), the cetacean equivalent of PDV. This virus is endemic among many odontocete species of the North Atlantic (Duignan et al., 1995b; Van Bressem et al., 2001), and has been the cause of major epidemics among dolphins on the US Atlantic coast, Gulf of Mexico, Mediterranean, North and Black Seas, and around Australia (Van Bressem et al., 2014). However, to date, there is no evidence for infection in either belugas or narwhal from the Canadian Arctic (Duignan et al., 1995b; Nielsen et al., 2000). The retreat of the north polar ice cap in recent years has seen a marked shift in the northern distribution of some of species known to harbour CeMV (Duignan et al., 1995b). One such species, the killer whale, (*Orcinus orca*) is now a regular summer visitor north of 70°N, where they actively seek out narwhal and belugas as prey (Higdon et al., 2012).

Other potential disease concerns are arising not because of host animal movement, but due to changes in the environment. *Vibrio parahaemolyticus* is a potentially pathogenic bacterium that thrives when water temperatures are above 15°C, and salinities are lower than 28ppm. Prior to 2004, this bacterium had only been reported once from southern Alaska as generally the water there is too cold. In recent years however, Goertz and others (2013), report isolating pathogenic strains of *V. parahaemolyticus* from several sea otters, a harbour porpoise (*Phocoena phocoena*) and a beluga whale sampled in several different Alaskan locations. As the biological and physical characteristics of Arctic marine environments change, the distribution and pathogenicity of many disease agents will shift concurrently (Baker-Austin et al., 2012).

Not all population health issues will arise from pathogens and toxicants. Mortalities of hundreds of narwhal have occurred many times because of ice entrapment. These events are potentially associated with climate change-related increases in winter ice cover trends and predictability (Laidre and Heide-Jørgensen, 2005), delayed freeze-up (Laidre et al., 2011) as well as anthropogenic noise such as that associated with seismic exploration techniques (Heide-Jørgensen et al., 2013). Access to narwhal for subsistence hunting is improving harvest success in some communities related to decreases in the presence of spring ice (Nielsen, 2009). Both of these changes may have negative population impacts that could exceed the ability of narwhal populations to respond, however, the magnitude is not yet clear. Attempts at modelling these and other effects under different climate scenarios projected biomass changes at all trophic levels in the Hudson Bay marine ecosystem. Under every scenario tested, narwhal biomass fell 50–75 per cent below that observed in 1970, indicating that current hunting pressures will not be sustainable as the effects of climate change accumulate (Hoover et al., 2013).

As change is already so advanced in the Arctic, the focus of current research is no longer to establish baselines but rather to try and predict potential tipping points, vulnerability and resilience in species and systems, and in conducting benchmark studies (Post et al., 2009; Burek et al., 2008). Consequently, convincing examples of how the ecology of the Arctic is adapting in the face of climate warming are being recorded. While it is difficult to predict the potential for resilience in higher vertebrate species, the fossil record has examples of species that survived past climate change events, albeit changes less rapid than the current one (Moritz and Agudo, 2013). Species vulnerability to climate change is affected by the rate of change both at the means and extremes, and by their ability to respond behaviourally, physiologically and genetically (Moritz and Agudo, 2013). As an example, the highly ice-associated narwhal has evolved morphologically and physiologically to forage with physical endurance and prolonged diving ability, operating near the limits of its aerobic capacity (Williams et al., 2011). So much so in fact that it was thought to have lost its evolutionary plasticity in the face of changing environment and prey dynamics. Recently, however, stable isotope analysis of narwhal skin found a level of diversity in prey selection within different populations, which suggests an unexpected level of adaptability (Watt et al., 2013).

13.4 Health assessments of Arctic marine animals

While measuring changes in biological parameters such as population size and reproductive success is relatively straightforward, assessing the overall health of individuals and populations is more challenging. There is a paucity of health-related studies, or baseline information for many Arctic species. When considering any population, wildlife or otherwise, the definition of health should be very general as Stephen (2014) proposes: the cumulative result of an array of recent and past biotic and abiotic factors on the animal or species. Individual animal health depends on an intricate interplay between the environment, toxicant burdens, immune status, pathogen load, energy availability in body stores and available food, and behavioural stress. Any deviations in biological parameters can therefore be considered as measures of changes in health, positive and negative. More traditional methods of inquiry yield important information about the presence or absence of disease-causing organisms or factors. Necropsy of hunted or stranded animals can provide a general assessment of health based on gross pathology as well as samples for culture of potentially pathogenic bacteria, viruses or fungi. Histopathology provides information on organ health while molecular methods identify the presence of pathogens. Blood samples collected from live captured or freshly harvested animals can be used to look for serological evidence of exposure to selected diseases such as morbilliviruses. One of the richest fields in the literature explores the accumulation of persistent organic pollutants and heavy metals such as mercury in Arctic marine species, although less is known of the health effects associated with their presence.

Tracking developing trends in Arctic wildlife health and ecology is important for modelling effects on the food security of Arctic residents, who access many of these species through hunting and fishing activities (Wesche and Chan, 2010). There are other modalities that can offer a potential health index from easily collected samples such as skin. Assessing the health of Arctic marine species can be very challenging due to remoteness and severe weather, so techniques that can provide health information from easily collected and archived samples are extremely valuable in this context. Apprill and others (2014) found that the bacterial microbiome of the skin of humpback whales (*Megaptera novaeangliae*) undergoes measurable changes that correspond to conditions of declining fitness. Their conclusions suggest that these techniques may provide a health index for marine mammals. Skin can also be used for quantifying proteins, which are expressed in conditions of stress in marine mammals (Southern et al., 2002).

Hormones associated with stress, such as cortisol, can be measured in blubber and hair, tissues that accumulate and store hormones over time periods measured in months. In belugas, for example, blubber samples collected and archived between 1981 and 2010, provided high-quality results showing that levels of cortisol in blubber were higher in animals experiencing significant stress, such as an ice entrapment (Trana et al., 2015). Thus, the use of microbiomes, stress-related proteins and stress hormone monitoring can serve as broad measures of population health over time, particularly in areas such as the Arctic marine ecosystem, where adverse change is evident.

Health assessments on any species should also include traditional knowledge, information collected and assimilated by Aboriginal peoples for centuries. In Western science, we have stock questions we ask about disease entities in animals, or suspected disease entities. We ask: where did the pathogen come from? How did it get to the infected site in the body? What damage is it causing? What are the health effects associated with its presence? However, there is one question that we rarely ask: why is the pathogen there? What purpose might it serve its host?

Let's consider a possible health issue: when we have the opportunity to conduct a necropsy on a narwhal in the high Arctic, almost every whale will have small nematode worms present in the head sinuses. Our cause-and-effect thinking leads us to label this as a parasitic infection, which we believe will likely have negative consequences for the host. Further, we describe these nematode infestations as a state of ill-health, although there is no information in this little-studied species that would lead us to conclude that the parasites are harmful to the whale's health. The numbers of nematodes and thus the severity of the infection appear to be greater in juvenile animals than in adults. From our Western scientific point of view, this is believed to be because of an increased and more effective immune response in the adult whales when compared to the more immunologically naïve juveniles. This leads to a decrease in the numbers of parasitic nematodes as an animal ages and becomes more immunologically competent.

Northern Inuit people are observing changes in their environment, such as slumping permafrost near the coast. Their concerns and observations are tied to local and traditional knowledge, and may differ from those of the scientific community. There is rich potential for exchange and comparison as we seek to fully understand ecosystem changes and effects of climate change. There are excellent documentary projects that explore the challenges facing northern communities in the face of environmental change (see Appendix). When we look to the traditional knowledge of the Inuit, to their ways of knowing about the animals that live around them, they tell us *why* the nematodes are always seen in the ears of the narwhal, a species that has formed part of their diet and culture for generations. In a marine world, surrounded by potential predators such as polar bears and killer whales, and to weather conditions favouring the formation of ice or challenging wave conditions, narwhal must be both wary and wily to survive. The 'why' of these nematode infestations has always been understood in this way: the presence of the worms moving in the ear sinuses keeps the whale alert, the movement of these parasites reminds the whale to be constantly vigilant and watching for danger in its environment. By looking at the presence of the nematode infection through that lens, one could deduce that the larger number of worms in a juvenile whale balance out the lack of experience a young animal has, thereby keeping it on 'high alert' as it moves through its environment. As a whale gets older and has more experience and knowledge in its environment, it requires less reminders, less worms moving in the sinuses to remain appropriately vigilant in order to survive the conditions of life in the Arctic Ocean. Perhaps the one-sided parasitic assumption we make about these nematodes might be better described as a commensal relationship, when we consider them in this way. One Health thinking encourages us to use every available perspective when describing health in an individual or population.

13.5 Case study: Alaskan pinniped and walrus unusual mortality event, 2011–2012

In the summer of 2011, traditional hunters in the Arctic and Bering regions of Alaska reported sick seals with skin ulcers and unusual behaviour.

Abnormal hair growth and hair loss in ringed seals has been observed historically, but the severity of skin and mucosal involvement, coupled with neurologic signs were unprecedented (Plate 20). Close to 300 cases were reported in the first year and initially involved ringed seals, although spotted, ribbon and bearded seal cases were subsequently detected. Reports of similar but more generalized skin lesions and some associated mortality in walruses were observed during the same time period in Alaska, while similar cases in ice seals were seen in both the eastern and western Canadian Arctic, eastern Russia and Japan (Stimmelmayr, 2014).

Seals of all age classes and both sexes were represented. Lethargy and lack of evasive behaviour or flight response were observed in about one-third of cases, and respiratory signs included nasal discharge and dyspnoea. Skin lesions were variable and ranged from mild alopecia or abnormal hair retention in some animals to erosions and ulceration and vasculitis with secondary or opportunistic infections in others. In phocids, the lesions were on the flippers, face, head, axillae and mucocutaneous junctions. Lung oedema, friable livers, enlarged hearts with areas of degeneration and necrosis, oedematous lymph nodes and thymic atrophy were also noted (Burek and Raverty, 2012; Stimmelmayr, 2014).

Walrus were less severely affected. Juvenile and sub-adult animals that had died from other causes such as trampling, often had widely disseminated skin papules, erosions and ulcers with associated bleeding on head, neck, flippers and trunk in otherwise normal healthy animals (NOAA, 2014b).

Periodically between 1998 and 2012, alopecia has been reported in sub-adult polar bears from Alaska, and particularly in animals from the Prudhoe Bay area, with peaks of incidence in 1999 and 2012 (Atwood et al., 2015). Affected bears were malnourished with thinning of the hair on the neck and shoulders and nodules and crusting on ears, lips and conjunctiva. While the cause of this condition is as yet unresolved, histological examination of skin biopsies confirmed that the lesions are distinct to those observed in Alaskan phocids and walrus (NOAA, 2012; Atwood et al., 2015).

Ice seals and walrus are important subsistence food sources and cultural icons for northern communities, and Aboriginal hunters were the first to observe affected animals. Some hunters shot obviously sick seals to relieve suffering without butchering or using the pelt and meat from affected animals; whereas others fed meat from affected seals to dogs to assess the potential risk of disease exposure and infection to humans. Traditional knowledge from community elders confirmed that the severity of both skin lesions were more severe than any previously recognized (Castrodale, 2012).

Due to the unprecedented and simultaneous development of clinical disease in ring and other ice seals, as well as walrus, in December of 2011 an unusual mortality event (UME) was declared through the United States National Oceanic and Atmospheric Administration (NOAA) and Fish and Wildlife Service (USFWS), establishing a multi-agency investigation lead by the NOAA and the USFWS, including Alaskan and Canadian native and Aboriginal communities, scientists and officials from several Alaska state and federal US and Canadian agencies, government diagnostic and reference laboratories.

Working case definitions were developed in consultation with native hunters and collaborators and relied on field, clinical and pathologic observations. Skin erosions and ulcerations were associated with dermal vasculitis, infarction and superficial bacterial and fungal colonization and proliferation (Burek and Raverty, 2012). Based on initial histopathology, infectious agents such as viruses, bacteria or fungi were prime differentials. External factors that interrupt normal moulting were also considered, as well as allergic or autoimmune diseases caused by exposure to novel environmental allergens or irritants.

Potential effects of changing food web dynamics were investigated. Finally, the potential contribution of environmental factors such as ultraviolet exposure, freshwater effluents, pH, temperature and salinity of seawater, harmful algal blooms and toxins and the presence of Fukushima radionuclides were all considered.

Although conventional microbiology yielded predominantly mixed bacterial isolates *Streptococcus phocae* was isolated from many affected seals. The contribution of this microbe to lesions is unknown. Attempted virus isolation, electron microscopy and advanced molecular sequencing were pursued, but no consistent pathogens were identified (Burek and Raverty, 2012). A few animals were seropositive for *Leptospira* sp., phocid Herpesvirus and *Brucella* sp. and likely represent pre-existing background levels in the population. Based on extrapolation from other marine mammal species, many other specific pathogens were ruled out, including calicivirus, influenza A, morbillivirus, picornavirus, papillomavirus, poxvirus, para poxvirus, vesicular stomatitis virus, foot and mouth disease virus and many others (NOAA, 2014a).

Heavy metal levels were determined in postmortem case material and efforts to validate hormonal assays for both seals and walrus are underway with the expectation to measure levels of thyroid and other hormones involved with moulting. Other factors which can affect healthy skin, hair coats and moulting (trace minerals, vitamins A, E and some B vitamins) were assessed in both healthy and affected seals (NOAA, 2013).

With the Fukushima power plant meltdown in Japan in March 2011, radiation exposure was also a consideration. However, there were no radiomimetic lesions and levels of Cesium-134 and Cesium-137 were elevated relative to the 1990s, but were within the typical background range for Alaska (NOAA, 2013).

From 2009 to 2011, large blooms of algae with the capability of elaborating natural toxins were documented in Kotzebue Sound using satellite imaging and substrate analysis. As the mucocutaneous lesions were suggestive of photosensitization, analyses for several potential algal toxins were conducted. Microcystin immunohistochemistry revealed only very low levels in the liver of one of four seals examined (NOAA, 2013) and domoic acid and saxitoxin assays were conducted but no toxic levels were found. These toxins are more typically associated with algae found in subtropical and temperate regions, but are increasingly found in Arctic waters and in screened marine mammal tissues from northern latitudes.

Solar radiation may have contributed to the development of skin lesions. Coincident with the UME, there was a hole detected in the atmospheric ozone layer over the Bering Strait area. Sunburn lesions have been previously described in cetaceans, particularly relating to stranding events (Kritzler, 1952).

While no definitive cause for the UME has yet been identified from diagnostic and epidemiological research efforts, the collaborative nature of the investigations and its massive scope are instructive. Native community involvement, public health initiatives and international collaboration have all been important components of this investigation. In this UME and in future ecosystem perturbations, indigenous marine mammals of Arctic waters will continue to act as valuable sentinel of ecosystem change.

It is likely that an environmental component contributed either directly or indirectly to the development of clinical disease in ringed seals and walrus. Lack of appropriate environmental cues to initiate a normal moult cycle, inappropriate substrate associated with hauling ashore, persistent stressors and elevated stress hormones that interfere with normal shedding of hair are all considerations. Additional factors may include increased energy expenditure to forage offshore without the benefit of ice floes, leaving animals in a negative energy balance and more susceptible to disease. The most severely affected animals appeared to be immunosuppressed and debilitated, suffering from secondary opportunistic infections. However, preliminary review of environmental data indicates that 2011, the year the UME started, was fairly representative of the changes being observed throughout the Arctic with continued retreat of sea ice, warming ocean temperatures, increased ice algae, jellyfish and less predictable weather (Stimmelmayr, 2014).

Changes in environmental factors coincident to the disease outbreak and mortality also need to be considered. Sea ice changes have been measured in the Bering and Chukchi seas over the past several decades, with decreased summer ice, and increasing rate of spring ice retreat through the Bering Strait. This has resulted in a decrease in available ice for hauling out, resting and as platforms for foraging. The deleterious effects of this change in available ice on both walrus and heavily ice-associated seals such as the ringed seal can be expected to be higher than in species with less dependence on ice platforms.

13.6 Conclusion

It is clear that climate change has already had significant measurable impact on Arctic ecosystems affecting all biota from picoplankton to humans and the largest marine predators. However, this is an ecosystem in relatively rapid transition and the complex interactions between the different abiotic and biotic elements are far from understood. What is clear is that the traditional scientific approach is unlikely to provide the insights needed to model and predict the probable outcomes resulting from the emerging interactions that will inevitably arise as temperatures rise and ecosystem communities change in response. An interdisciplinary approach exemplified by the One Health paradigm involving a wide range of expertise from biomedical sciences, earth sciences and social sciences, and the custodians of traditional knowledge will be needed to conduct research, develop models and formulate recommendations that will inform the international community and relevant policymakers to safeguard critical polar habitats and the food security and health of all its inhabitants.

Climate change and northern communities documentary information

www.peopleofafeather.com
http://tvo.org/story/polar-sea-unprecedented-look-northwest-passage

References

Apprill, A., Robbins, J., Eren A.M., Pack, A.A., Reveillaud, J., Mattila, D., Moore, M., Niemeyer, M., Moore, K.M.T. and Mincer, T. (2014). Humpback whale populations share a core skin bacterial community: towards a health index for marine mammals? *PLOS One*, 9, 1–17.

Ardyna, M., Gosselin, M., Michel, C., Poulin, M. and Tremblay, J.É. (2011). Environmental forcing of phytoplankton community structure and function in the Canadian High Arctic: contrasting eutrophic and oligotrophic regions. *Marine Ecology Progress Series* 442, 37-57.

Ashley, B.D. (1993). Community economic impact of commercial fisheries development in Canada's eastern Arctic: The Pangnirtung winter turbot fishery. PhD dissertation, Simon Fraser University (Canada), Proquest, UMI Dissertations Publishing. MM91265.

Atwood, T., Peacock, E., Burek-Huntington, K., Shearn-Bochsler, V., Bodenstein, B., Beckmen, K., and Durner, G. (2015). Prevalence and spatio-temporal variation of an alopecia syndrome in polar bears (*Ursus maritimus*) of the southern Beaufort Sea. *Journal of Wildlife Diseases* 51 (1), 48-59.

Baker-Austin, C., Trinanes, J.A., Taylor, N.G.H., Hartnell, R., Siitonen, A. and Martinez-Urtaza. (2012). Emerging *Vibrio* risk at higher latitudes in response to ocean warming. *Nature Climate Change* 3, 73-77.

Burek, K. and Raverty, S. (2012). Working Group 1: Laboratory analyses. In Goertz, C.E.C ed. *Proceedings of the Arctic Pinniped Disease Investigation Workshop*, Alaska Marine Science Symposium, 10-11.

Burek, K.A., Gulland, F.M., Sheffield, G., Beckmen, K.B., Keyes, E., Spraker, T.R., Smith, A.W., Skilling, D.E., Evermann, J.F., Stott, J.L., Saliki, J.T. and Trites, A.W. (2005). Infectious disease and the decline of Steller sea lions (*Eumetopias jubatus*) in Alaska, USA: Insights from serologic data. *Journal of Wildlife Disease* 41, 512–524.

Burek, K.A., Gulland, M.D. and O'Hara, T.M. (2008). Effects of climate change on marine mammal health. *Ecological applications* 18, s126-s134.

Castrodale, L. (2012). Public Health and food security perspective. In Goertz, C.E.C. ed. *Proceedings of the Arctic Pinniped Disease Investigation Workshop*, Alaska Marine Science Symposium, 7-8.

Cheung, W.W.L., Lam, V.W.Y., Sarmiento, J.L., Kearney, K, Watson, R. and Pauly, D. (2009). Projecting global marine biodiversity impacts under climate change scenarios. *Fish and Fisheries* 10, 236-248.

Comiso, J.C. (2012). Large decadal decline of the Arctic multiyear ice cover. *Journal of Climate* 25, 1176-1193.

Duignan, P.J., Saliki, J.T., St Aubin, D.J., Early, G., Sadove, S., House, J.A., Kovacs, K. and Geraci, J.R. (1995a). Epizootiology of morbillivirus infection in North American harbor seals (*Phoca vitulina*) and gray seals (*Halichoerus grypus*). *Journal of Wildlife Disease*, 31, 491–501.

Duignan, P.J., House, C., Geraci, J.R., Early, G., Copeland, H.G., Walsh, M.T., Bossart, G.D., Cray, C., Sadove, S., St. Aubin, D.J. and Moore, M. (1995b). Morbillivirus infection in two species of pilot whales (Globicephala sp.) from the western Atlantic. *Marine Mammal Science*, 11, 150–162.

Duignan, P.J., Nielsen, O., House, C., Kovacs, K.M., Duffy, N., Early, G., Sadove, S., St Aubin, D.J., Rima, B.K. and Geraci, J.R. (1997). Epizootiology of morbillivirus infection in harp, hooded, and ringed seals from the Canadian Arctic and western Atlantic. *Journal of Wildlife Disease*, 33, 7–19.

Duignan, P.J., Van Bressem, M.F., Baker, J.D., Barbieri, M., Cosgrove, K.M., De Guise, S., de Swart, R.L., Di Guardo, G., Dobson, A., Duprex, W.P., Early, G., Fauquier, D., Goldstein, T., Goodman, S.J., Grenfell, B., Groch, K.R., Gulland, F., Hall, A., Jensen, B.A., Lamy, K., Matassa, K., Mazzariol, S., Morris, S.E., Nielsen, Rotstein, D., Rowles, T.K., Saliki, J.T., Siebert, U., Waltzek, T. and Wellehan, J.F.X. (2014). Phocine distemper virus: current knowledge and future directions. *Viruses*, 6, 5093–5134.

Goertz, C.E.C., Walton, R., Rouse, N., Belovarac, J., Burek-Huntington, K., Gill, V., Hobbs, R., Xavier, C., Garrett, N. and Tuomi, P. (2013). *Vibrio parahemolyticus* in Alaska marine mammals. In F.J. Mueter, D.M.S. Dickson, H.P. Huntington, J.R. Irvine, L.A. Logerwell, S.A. MacLean, L.T. Quakenbush and C. Rosa (eds.), *Responses of Arctic Marine Ecosystems to Climate Change*. Alaska: Alaska Sea Grant, University of Alaska Fairbanks.

Goldstein, T., Mazet, J.A., Gill, V.A., Doroff, A.M., Burek, K.A. and Hammond, J.A. (2009). Phocine distemper virus in northern sea otters in the Pacific Ocean, Alaska, USA. *Emerging Infectious Disease*, 15, 925–927.

Hall, A.J., Jepson, P.D., Goodman, S.J. and Harkonen, T. (2006). Phocine distemper virus in the North and European Seas: data and models, nature and nurture. *Biological Conservation*, 131, 221–229.

Hanni, K.D., Mazet, J.A., Gulland, F.M., Estes, J., Staedler, M., Murray, M.J., Miller, M. and Jessup, D.A. (2003). Clinical pathology and assessment of pathogen exposure in southern and Alaskan sea otters. *Journal of Wildlife Disease*, 39, 837–850.

Harkonen, T., Dietz, R., Reijnders, P. Teilman, J., Harding, K., Hall, A., Brasseur, S., Siebert, U., Goodman, S.J., Jepson, P.D, Rasmussen, T.D. and Thompsom, P. (2006). The 1988 and 2002 phocine distemper virus epidemics in European harbour seals. *Diseases of Aquatic Organisms*, 68, 115–130.

Harwood, J. and Hall, A. (1990). Mass mortality in marine mammals: its implications for population dynamics and genetics. *Trends in Ecology and Evolution*, 5, 254–257.

Heide-Jørgensen, M.P., Hansen, R.G., Westdal, K., Reeves, R.R. and Mosbech, A. (2013). Narwhals and seismic exploration: is seismic noise increasing the risk of ice entrapments? *Biological Conservation*, 158, 50–54.

Hetzel, P.J., Zhang, X., Bitz, C.M., Kelly, B.P. and Massonet, F. (2012). Projected decline in spring snow depth on Arctic sea ice caused by later autumn open ocean freeze-up this century. *Geophysical Research Letters*, 39, L17505.

Higdon, J.W., Hauser, D.D.W. and Ferguson, S.H. (2012). Killer whales (*Orcinus orca*) in the Canadian Arctic: distribution, prey items, group size and seasonality. *Marine Mammal Science*, 28, E93–E109.

Hollowed, A.B., Planque, B. and Loeng, H. (2013). Potential movement of fish and shellfish stocks from the sub-Arctic to the Arctic Ocean. *Fisheries Oceanography*, 22, 355–370.

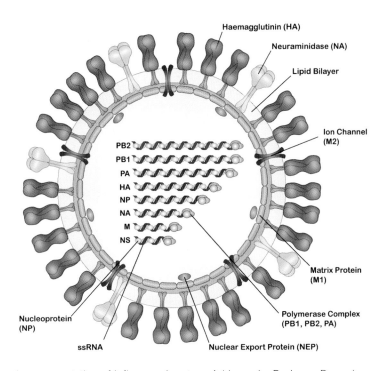

Plate 1 Schematic representation of influenza virus type A (drawn by Dr Jenny Draper).

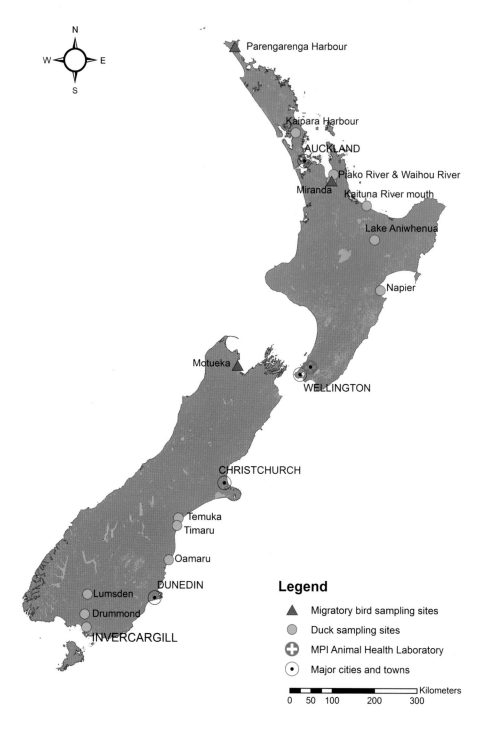

Plate 2a New Zealand sites where birds were captured for sample collection 2004–2013 (courtesy of Dr Thomas Rawdon, Investigation & Diagnostic Centre, Ministry for Primary Industries, Wallaceville, New Zealand).

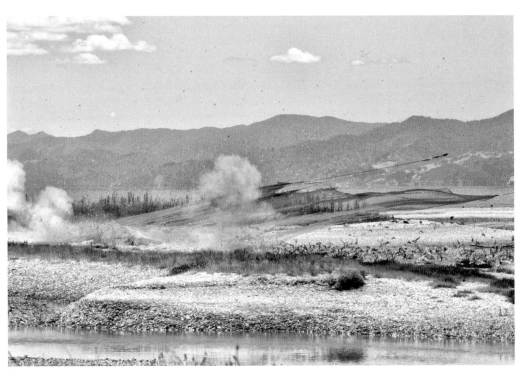

Plate 2b Shorebirds are caught in a cannon net. These birds are banded by ornithological and conservation agencies to assist with population monitoring. The birds are sampled before being released (courtesy of Anna Deverall).

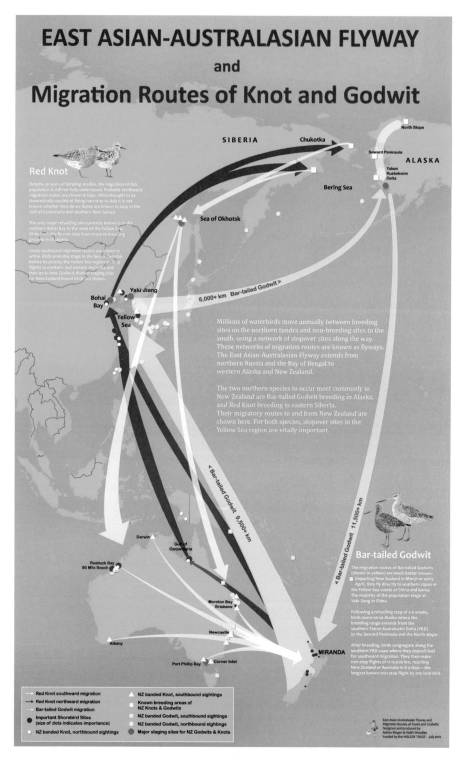

Plate 3 East Asian-Australasian Flyway and Shorebird Site Network (courtesy of Miranda Shorebird Centre).

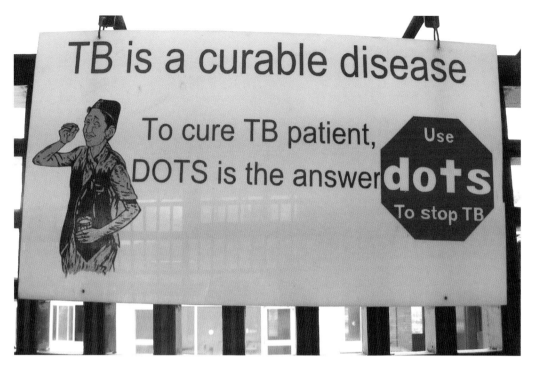

Plate 4 Sign outside of the Nepal National Tuberculosis Center. Nepal instituted a Directly Observed Therapy Short Course (DOTS) programme in 1996.

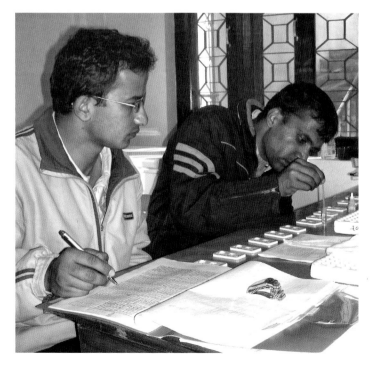

Plate 5 Nepal veterinarians, Dr Jeewan Thapa (left) and Dr Sarad Paudel (right) performing serological testing for TB at the National Trust for Nature Conservation.

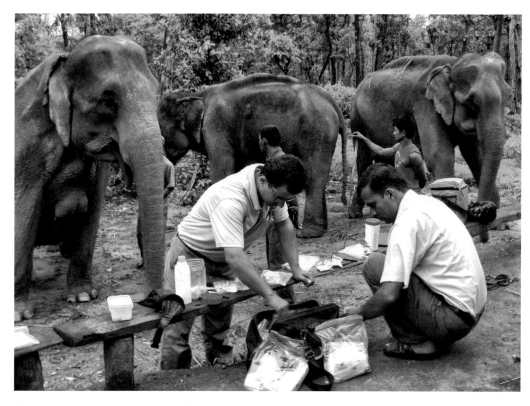

Plate 6 Nepal veterinarians, Dr Jeewan Thapa (left) and Dr Sarad Paudel (right) preparing TB medications.

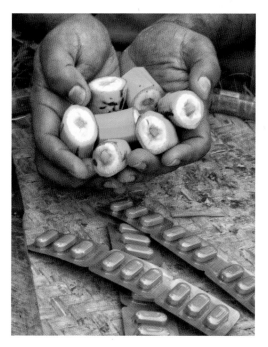

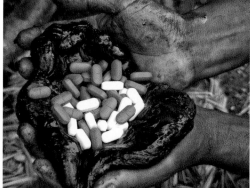

Plate 7a–b Elephants have a well-developed sense of taste and administering oral medications can be challenging. Pills are often hidden in fruit (a) or molasses (b) to disguise the bitter taste.

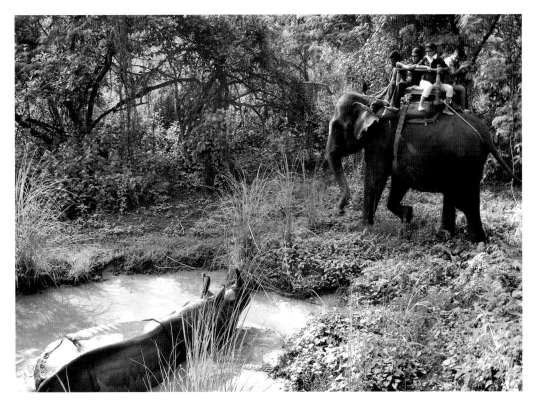

Plate 8 Elephants come into close contact with other native wildlife such as rhinos during elephant-back safaris, popular in Nepal. If elephants used for tourism activities such as this are infected with TB, there is potential for the disease to be transmitted to other wild species.

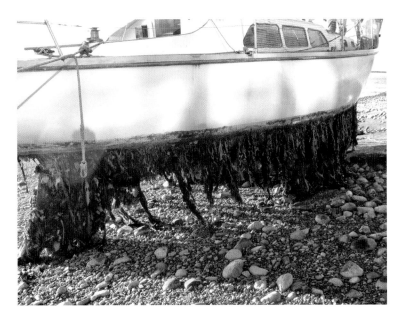

Plate 9 Yacht with a heavily fouled hull, including the invasive Japanese kelp (*Undaria pinnatifida*) and colonial tunicate *Didemnum vexillum* (courtesy of the Cawthron Institute).

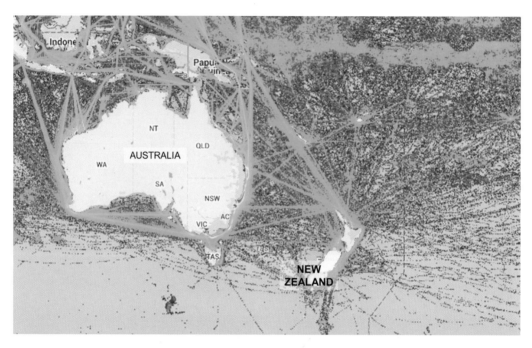

Plate 10 Screenshot of shipping routes in and out of New Zealand. The vast majority of the traffic comes from passenger and cargo vessels (map adapted from marinetraffic.com, December 2014).

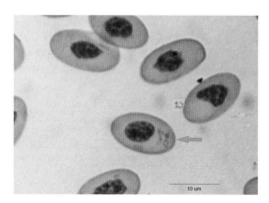

Plate 11 *Babesia kiwiensis* (arrow) in a kiwi red blood cell (× 1000, Leishman's stain) (courtesy of Auckland Zoo).

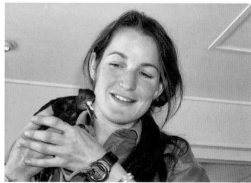

Plate 12 Emily Sancha holds the black stilt, 'Mrs Bones' following her successful fracture repair (courtesy of Fairfax Media NZ/The Press).

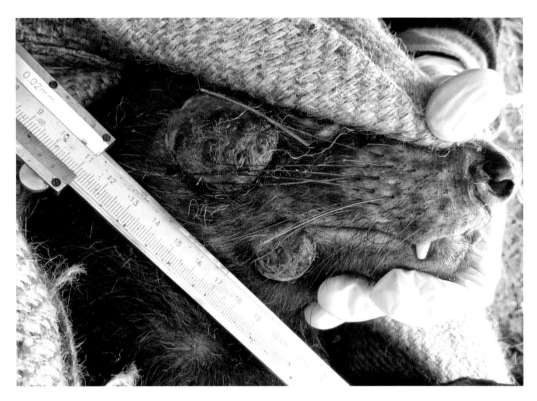

Plate 13 Tasmanian devil with fleshy growths typical of devil facial tumour disease (courtesy of Sarah Doornbusch).

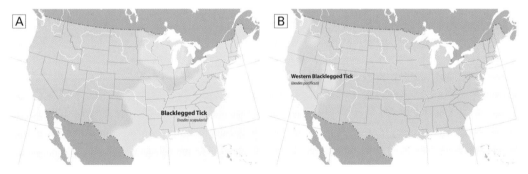

Plate 14a–b Geographic distribution of *Ixodes scapularis* (A) and *Ixodes pacificus* (B) within the United States (courtesy of the Centers for Disease Control and Prevention).

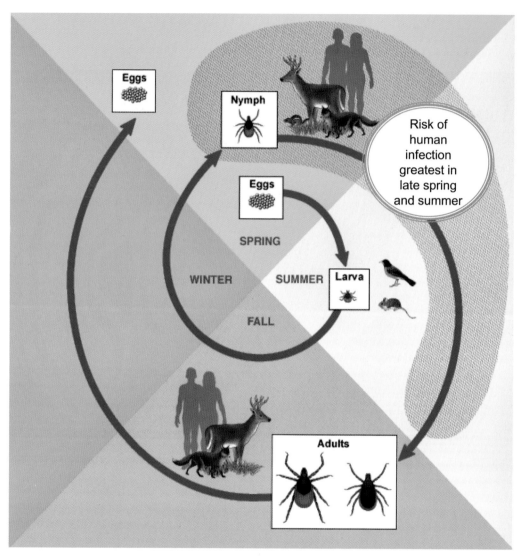

Plate 15 Lifecycle of *Ixodes scapularis* (courtesy of the Centers for Disease Control and Prevention).

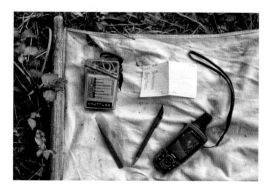

Plate 16 Tools and resources for sampling (courtesy of Dr Kathryn Berger).

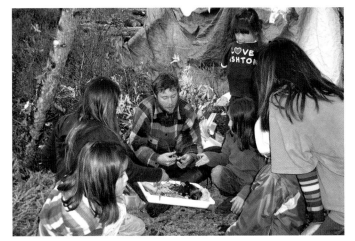

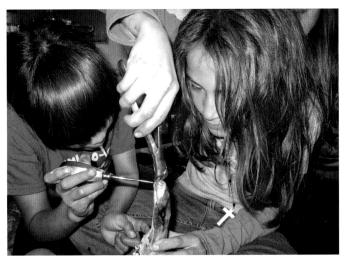

Plate 17 Engaging with youth on-the-land: (a) A university graduate student participates in a community hunt and shows Colville Lake youth how to sample caribou; (b) Youth try their hands at extracting incisor teeth from a caribou jaw.

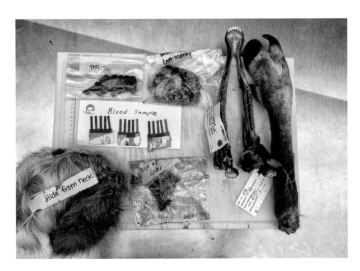

Plate 18 A complete caribou health monitoring sample kit.

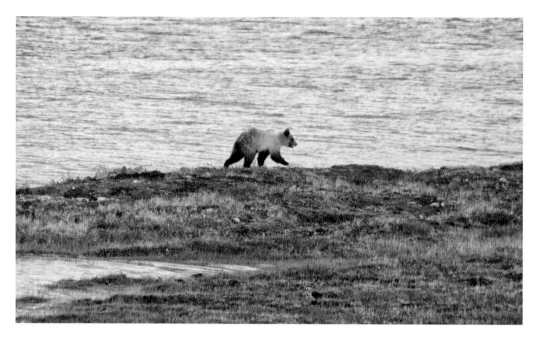

Plate 19 Grizzly bear well above treeline south of Qingaut (Bathurst Inlet) Nunavut 65.916679N; −108.363060W in August 2014 (courtesy of Johann Wagner, Canadian High Arctic Research Station).

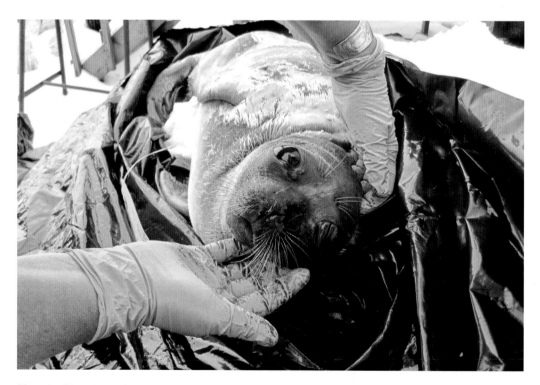

Plate 20 Ringed seal from Alaska showing typical skin lesions (courtesy of R. Stimmelmayr).

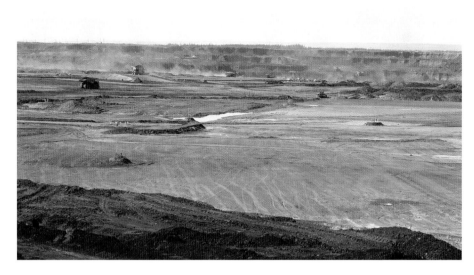

Plate 21 Open-pit mine in the Alberta oil sands.

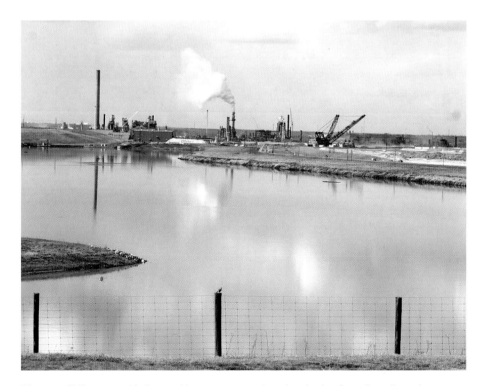

Plate 22 Tailings pond in front a bitumen processing plant in the Canadian oil sands.

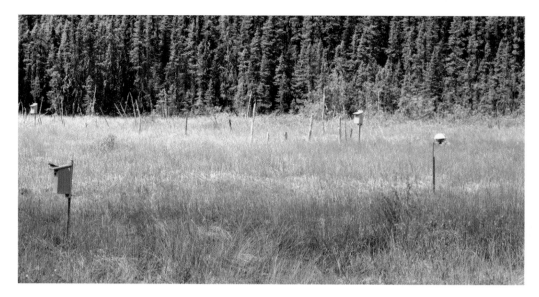

Plate 23 Artificial nest boxes for breeding pairs of tree swallows in a reference site in northern Alberta.

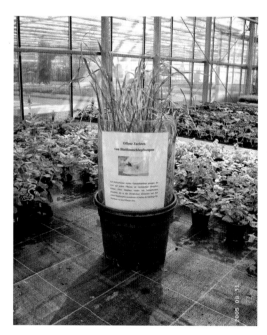

Plate 24 A 'banker plant' or open-rearing system for maintaining beneficial insects. Banker plants support biological control agents in greenhouse systems by providing them to be introduced pre-emptively prior to the development of key crop pests. Courtesy of Dr. Petra Christiansen-Weniger of BorbyControl, Germany).

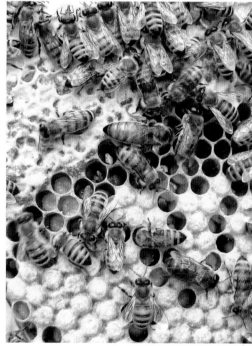

Plate 25 Honey bees are valuable pollinators of horticultural crops. They are responsible for the production of about one third of the food consumed in Western societies (courtesy of Ernesto Guzman-Novoa).

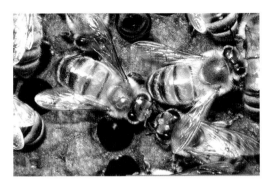

Plate 26 The parasitic mite *Varroa destructor* is one of the main culprits of winter colony losses (courtesy of Ricardo Anguiano).

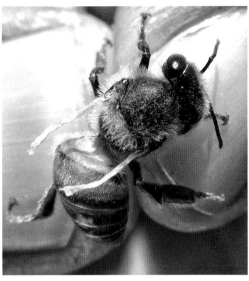

Plate 27 Worker bee with damaged wings as a result of deformed virus infection (courtesy of Ricardo Anguiano).

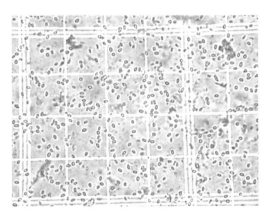

Plate 28 *Nosema ceranae* spores seen under a microscope (400 ×). This microsporidian fungus has been linked to CCD cases (courtesy of Ernesto Guzman-Novoa).

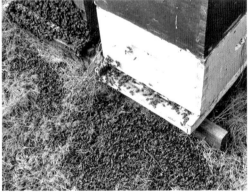

Plate 29 Dead bees in front of hive entrances as a result of pesticide poisoning (courtesy of Nicholas Calderone).

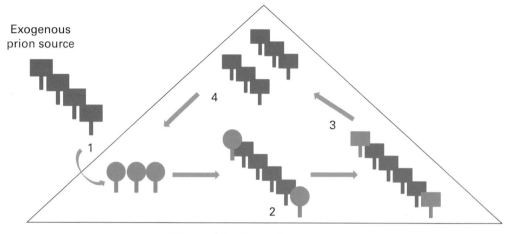

Exogenous prion source

Prion replication in host organism

Plate 30 Prion replication in an infected host organism. (1) Prions are taken up, e.g., orally, by a certain host species. (2) PrP^{Sc} interacts with endogenously expressed PrP^{C}. Thereby, a conformational change is induced and PrP^{C} adopts the PrP^{Sc} conformation (3). Growing aggregates of PrP^{Sc} can disassemble into smaller units (4) and can serve as templates for the conversion of further PrP^{C} molecules.

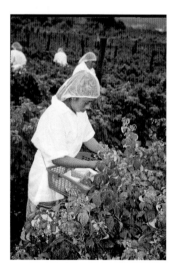

Plate 31 Direct contamination of fresh produce from infected farm workers.

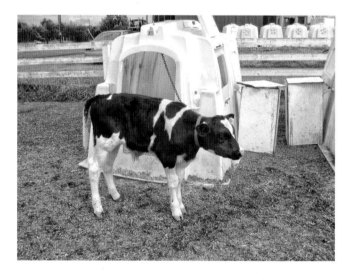

Plate 32 Cattle and other livestock (especially young animals) are important reservoirs for *Cryptosporidium* and *Giardia*.

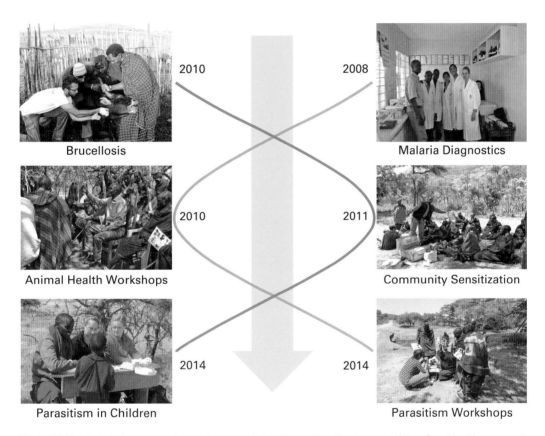

2010

2008

Brucellosis

Malaria Diagnostics

2010

2011

Animal Health Workshops

Community Sensitization

2014

2014

Parasitism in Children

Parasitism Workshops

Plate 33 Parallels in human and veterinary medicine illustrating the impact of the One Health approach (courtesy of Frank van der Meer).

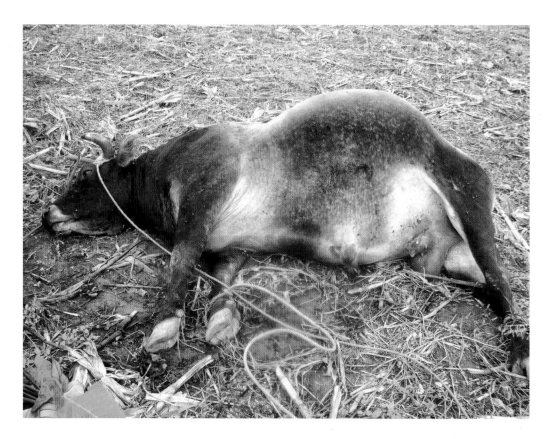

Plate 34a–b Animal cases of anthrax are typically reported as sudden death due to toxaemia. Subclinical cases are rarely observed in ruminants and the first indication that the cause of death is anthrax is the bloated carcass with bloody discharges from the nose and rectum.

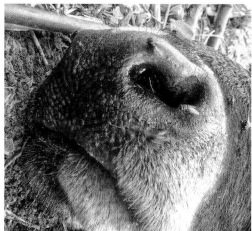

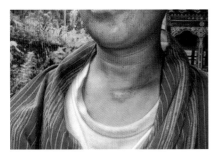

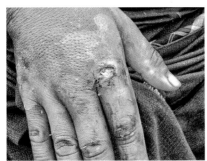

Plate 35a–b Human cases of anthrax reported during the outbreak. The cutaneous form of the disease in humans typically appears as black eschars or scabs on the limbs, neck and face.

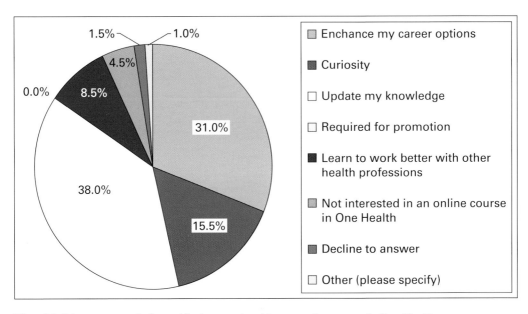

Plate 36 Primary reason indicated for interest in taking an online course in One Health.

Hoover, C., Pitcher, T.J. and Christensen, V. (2013). Effects of hunting, fishing and climate change on the Hudson Bay marine ecosystem: II. Ecosystem model future projections. *Ecological Modelling*, 264, 143–156.

Jensen, S.K., Aars, J., Lydersen, C., Kovacs, K.M. and Asbakk, K. (2010). The prevalence of *Toxoplasma gondii* in polar bears and their marine mammal prey: evidence for a marine transmission pathway? *Polar Biology*, 33, 599–606.

Ji, R., Jin, M. and Varpe, R. (2013). Sea ice phenology and timing of primary production pulses in the Arctic Ocean. *Global Change Biology* 19, 734–741.

Kinnard, C., Zdanowicz, C.M., Fisher, D.A., Isaksson, E., de Vernal, A. and Thompson, L.G. (2011). Reconstructed changes in Arctic sea ice over the past 1,450 years. *Nature*, 479, 509–512.

Kritzler, H. (1952). Observations on the pilot whale in captivity. *Journal of Mammalogy*, 33, 321–334.

Kumar, A., Perlwitz, J., Eischid, J., Quan, X., Xu, T., Zhang, T., Hoerling, M., Jha, B. and Wang, W. (2010). Contribution of sea ice loss to Arctic amplification. *Geophysical Research Letters*, 37, L21701.

Laidre, K.L. and Heide-Jørgensen, M.P. (2005). Arctic sea ice trends and narwhal vulnerability. *Biological Conservation*, 121, 509–517.

Laidre, K.L., Heide-Jørgensen, M.P., Stern, H. and Richard, P. (2011). Unusual narwhal ice entrapments and delayed autumn freeze-up trends. *Polar Biology*, 35, 149–154.

Li, W.K.W., McLaughlin, F.A., Lovejoy, C. and Carmack, E.C. (2009). Smallest algae thrive as the Arctic Ocean freshens. *Science*, 326, 539.

Lønne, O.J. and Gulliksen, B. (1989). Size, age and diet of Polar cod *Boreogadus saida lepechin 1773* in ice covered waters. *Polar Biology*, 9, 187–192.

MacCracken, J.G. (2012). Pacific walrus and climate change: observations and predictions. *Ecology and Evolution*, 2, 2072–2090.

Markus, T., Stroeve, J.C. and Miller, J. (2009). Recent changes in sea ice melt onset, freezeup, and melt season length. *Journal of Geophysical Research*, 114, C12024.

Markussen, N.H. and Have, P. (1992). Phocine distemper virus infection in harp seals (*Phoca groenlandica*). *Maine Mammal Scence*, 8, 19–26.

Moline, M.A., Karnovsky, N.J., Brown, Z. Divoky, G.J., Frazer, T.K., Jacoby C.A., Torres, J.J. and Fraser W.A. (2008). High latitude changes in ice dynamics and their impact on polar marine ecosystems. *Annals of the New York Academy of Sciences*, 1134, 267–319.

Molnar, P.K., Derocher, A.E., Thiemann, G.W. and Lewis, M.A. (2010). Predicting survival, reproduction and abundance of polar bears under climate change. *Biological Conservation*, 143, 1612–1622.

Moritz, C. and Agudo, R. (2013). The future of species under climate change: resilience or decline? *Science*, 341, 504–508.

Mueter, F.J. and Litzow, M.A. (2008). Sea ice retreat alters the biogeography of the Bering Sea continental shelf. *Ecological Applications*, 18, 309–320.

Nielsen, M.R. (2009). Is climate causing the increasing narwhal (*Monodon monoceros*) catches in Smith Sound, Greenland? *Polar Research*, 28, 238–245.

Nielsen, O., Stewart, R.E.A., Measures, L., Duignan, P. and House, C. (2000). A morbillivirus antibody survey of Atlantic walrus, narwhal and beluga in Canada. *Journal of Wildlife* Disease, 36, 508–517.

NOAA (2012). *Polar Bears in Alaska Observed with Patchy Hair Loss and Other Skin Lesions*, www.usgs.gov/newsroom/article_pf.asp?ID=3162.

NOAA (2013). *Northern Pinnipeds Unusual Mortality Event (UME)*, http://alaskafisheries.noaa.gov/protectedresources/seals/ice/diseased/ume_update 0413.pdf.

NOAA (2014a). *Northern Pinnipeds Unusual Mortality Event: Update 2014*, https://alaskafisheries.noaa.gov/protectedresources/seals/ice/diseased/ume_factsheet0214.pdf.

NOAA (2014b). Northern Pinnipeds Unusual Mortality Event: Unusual Mortality Event Closes for Pacific Walruses Due to Lack of New Cases, http://alaskafisheries.noaa.gov/protectedresources/seals/ice/diseased/ume_factsheet0514.pdf.

Osterhaus, A.D. and Vedder, E.J. (1988). Identification of virus causing recent seal deaths. *Nature*, 335, 20.

Palmer, M.A., van Dijken, G.L., Mitchell, B.G., Seegers, B.J., Lowry, K.E., Mills, M.M. and Arrigo, K.A. (2013). Light and nutrient control of photosynthesis in natural phytoplankton populations from the Chukchi and Beaufort seas, Arctic Ocean. *Limnology and Oceanography*, 58, 2185–2205.

Post, E., Forchhammer, M.C., Bret-Harte, M.S., Callaghan, T.V., Christensen, T.R., Elberling, B, Fox, A.D., Gilg, O., Hik, D.S., Høye, T.T., Ims, R.A., Jeppesen, E, Klein, D.R., Madsen, J, McGuire, A.D., Rysgaard, S., Schindler, D.E., Stirling, I., Tamstorf, M.P., Tyler, N.J.C., van der Wal, R., Welker, J., Wookey, P.A., Schmidt, N.M. and Aastrup, P. (2009). Ecological dynamics across the Arctic associated with recent climate change. *Science*, 325, 1355–1358.

Post, E., Bhatt, U.S., Bitz, C.M., Brodie, J.F., Fulton, T.F, Hebblewhite, M., Kerby, J., Kutz, S.J., Stirling, I.

and Walker, D.A. (2013). Ecological consequences of sea ice decline. *Science*, 341, 519–524.

Prowse, T.D. and Furgal, C. (2009). Northern Canada in a changing climate: major findings and conclusions. *Ambio*, 38, 290–292.

Rode, K.D., Amstrup, S.C. and Regehr, E.V. (2010). Reduced body size and cub recruitment in polar bears associated with sea ice decline. *Ecological Applications*, 20, 768–782.

Smith, T.G. and Hammill, M.O. (1981). The ecology of the ringed seal, *Phoca hispida*, in its fast ice breeding habitat. *Canadian Journal of Zoology*, 59, 966–981.

Sonne, C. (2010). Health effects from long-range transported contaminants in Arctic top predators: an integrated review based on studies of polar bears and relevant model species. *Environment International*, 36, 461–491.

Søreide, J.E., Leu, E., Berge, J. Graeve, M. and Falk-Petersen, S. (2010). Timing of blooms, algal food quality and *Calanus glacialis* reproduction and growth in a changing Arctic. *Global Change Biology*, 16, 3154–3163.

Southern, S., Allen, A. and Kellar, N. (2002). *Molecular Signature of Physiological Stress Based on Protein Expression Profiling of Skin*. Administrative Report No. LJ-02-27, NMFS, Southwest Fisheries Science Center, California.

Stenson, G.B. and Hammill, M.O. (2014). Can ice seals adapt to habitat loss in a time of climate change? *ICES Journal of Marine Science*, 71, 1977–1986.

Stephen, C. (2014). Towards a modernized definition of wildlife health. *Journal of Wildlife Diseases*, 50(3), 427–430.

Stimmelmayr, R. (2014). Update on a new disease syndrome in ice seals and Pacific walrus in the Arctic. In K.M. Kovacs (ed.), *Circumpolar Ringed Seal (Pusa hispida) Monitoring*. Norway: Norwegian Polar Institute.

Stirling, I. (1988). *Polar Bears*. Ann Arbor: University of Michigan Press.

Stirling, I. and Derocher, A.E. (1993). Possible impacts of climate warming on polar bears. *Arctic*, 46, 240–245.

Stirling, I and Derocher, A.E. (2012). Effects of climate warming on polar bears, a review of the evidence. *Global Change Biology*, 36, 2694–2706.

Stirling, I., Lunn, N.J and Iacozza, J. (1999). Long term trends in the population ecology of polar bears in western Hudson Bay in relation to climatic change. *Arctic*, 52, 294–306.

Stroeve, J.C., Kattsov, V., Barrett, A., Serreze, M.C., Pavlova T., Holland, M. and Meier, W.N. (2012a). Trends in Arctic sea ice extent from CMIP5, CMIP3 and observations. *Geophysical Research Letters*, 39, L16502.

Stroeve, J.C., Serreze, M.C., Holland, M.M., Kay, J.E., Malanik, J. and Barrett A.P. (2012b). The Arctic's rapidly shrinking sea ice cover: a research synthesis. *Climatic Change*, 110, 1005–1027.

Trana, M.R., Roth, J.D., Tomy, G.T., Anderson, W.G. and Ferguson, S.H. (2015). Influence of sample degradation and tissue depth on blubber cortisol in beluga whales. *Journal of Experimental Marine Biology and Ecology*, 462, 8–13

Van Bressem, M.F., Waerebeek, K.V., Jepson, P.D., Raga, J.A., Duignan, P.J., Nielsen, O., Beneditto, A.P.D., Siciliano, S., Ramos, R., Kant, W., Peddemors, V., Kinoshita, R., Ross, P.S., Lopez-Fernandez, A., Evans, K., Crespo, E. and Barrett, T. (2001). An insight into the epidemiology of dolphin morbillivirus worldwide. *Veterinary Microbiology*, 81, 287–304.

Van Bressem, M.F., Duignan, P.J., Baynard, A., Barbieri, M., Colegrove, K.M., De Guise, S., Di Guardo, G., Dobson, A., Domingo, M., Fauquier, D., Fernandez, Goldstein, T., Grenfell, B., Groch, K.R., Gulland, F., Jensen, B.A., Jepson, P.D., Hall, A., Kuiken, T., Mazzariol, Marrois, S.E., Nielsen, O., Raga, J.A., Rowles, T.K., Saliki, J., Sierra, E., Stephens, N., Stone, B., Tomo, I., Wang, J., Waltzek, T. and Wellehan, J.F.X. (2014). Cetacean morbillivirus: Current knowledge and future directions. *Viruses*, 6, 5145–5148.

Voorhees, H., Sparks, R., Huntington, H.P. and Rode, K.D. (2014). Traditional knowledge about polar bears (*Ursus maritimus*) in northwestern Alaska. *Arctic*, 67, 523–536.

Wassmann, P., Duarte, C.M., Agust, S. and Sejr, M.K. (2011). Footprints of climate change in the Arctic marine ecosystem. *Global Change Biology*, 17, 1235–1249.

Watt, C.A., Heide-Jørgensen, M.P. and Ferguson, S.H. (2013). How adaptable are narwhal? A comparison of foraging patterns among the world's three narwhal populations. *Ecosphere* 4, 1–15.

Wesche, S.D. and Chan, H.M. (2010). Adapting to the impacts of climate change on food security among Inuit in the western Canadian Arctic. *EcoHealth*, 7, 361–373.

Williams, T.M., Noren, S.R. and Glenn, M. (2011). Extreme physiological adaptations as predictors of climate change sensitivity in the narwhal, *Monodon monoceros. Marine Mammal Science*, 27, 334–349.

Zarnke, R.L., Saliki, J.T., Macmillan, A.P., Brew, S.D., Dawson, C.E., Ver Hoef, J.M., Frost, K.J. and

Small, R.J. (2006). Serologic survey for *Brucella* spp., phocid herpesvirus-1, phocid herpesvirus-2, and phocine distemper virus in harbor seals from Alaska, 1976–1999. *Journal of Wildlife Disease*, 42, 290–300.

chapter 14

Avian wildlife as sentinels of environmental disruption

Judit E.G. Smits and Luis A. Cruz-Martinez

Abstract

For the many scientists involved in studies encompassing ecosystem health, ecology, animal health and environmental sustainability, wildlife are the logical choice of biota that provide a reliable reflection of the capacity of their particular habitats to support free-living life. Fish, birds and terrestrial mammals have all been the subjects of ecosystem-level investigations. In terrestrial habitats, birds are one important class of vertebrates recognized as sensitive indicators of the health and productivity of the local environments that they inhabit.

14.1 Introduction

The unique structure and physiology of the avian respiratory system makes it more sensitive to air quality and airborne toxicants than similarly sized mammals. However, the majority of studies involving environmental health focus on food- and waterborne problems. The different orders of birds represent a huge range of food webs, from nectar-dependent humming birds, to seed-eating granivores, herbivores, insectivores, piscivores and carnivores. Birds that forage higher in the food web reflect the quantity and quality of the flora and fauna that make up that food web. Particularly during the breeding season, there is much that can be learned about the balance of food chain diversity and productivity within relatively definable areas.

This is because during incubation and rearing of the offspring, adult birds forage primarily within a fairly defined radius to meet the demands of their rapidly developing nestlings. Adults may be affected to greater or lesser degrees by physical, social, biological and toxicological challenges during their migrations and on the wintering grounds. In contrast, we can be confident that the nestlings reflect the locally available food items, contaminants and other stressors. Although for some compounds there may be maternal transfer of the female's contaminant burden to the egg, this represents an ever-decreasing proportion as the offspring grows. For non-migratory birds, the adults as well as young-of-the-year, provide valuable insights into the 'health' of their habitats that reflect ecosystem function.

The cases described in this chapter, provide two distinct examples of anthropogenically driven challenges that have overarching and detrimental impacts on local ecosystems. We present methods of investigating the problem or threat to specific, sentinel wild avian species. The studies seek to define more thoroughly the nature and extent of the costs to 'One Health', which, by definition, encompasses the wellbeing of animals including invertebrates and humans, as well as the diversity of the vegetation, quality of water and productivity of the land. Those effects detected in the wildlife that are the subjects of our investigations, give us meaningful insight into the environmental and human costs of the ecosystem disruption.

> Often in the scientific literature the terms '(bio)indicator', '(bio)monitor' and 'sentinel' are used interchangeably. There is a distinction, however; indicator and monitoring species are those that can be examined to flag the presence and biological effects of contaminants in their environment (Stahl, 1997). In contrast, a sentinel species refers to 'an animal system used to identify potential health hazards to other animals or humans' (National Research Council, 1991).

14.2 Background

Bioindicators of environmental stressors

In recent years, with growing concerns about climate change and human-imposed impacts on ecosystem integrity, several taxa have been offered in the scientific literature as potential bioindicators of environmental stress or ecosystem disruption as a result of large-scale industrial activities worldwide. For example, epiphytic moss (*Hypnum cupressiforme*) and oak tree bark (*Quercus* spp.) have been studied in Romania to assess atmospheric deposition of trace elements from industrial emissions, road traffic and agriculture in Romania (Cucu-Man, 2013); the lettuce plant (*Lactuca sativa*) has been used as a bioindicator of toxic discharge from industrial wastewater effluent (Charles et al., 2011); lichens are widely used to test the air quality as a prerequisite requirement of environmental impact assessments (EIA) for developing industrial plants (Conti and Cecchetti, 2001). Similarly, ichthyofauna has served to evaluate the environmental quality from industrial facilities and cargo terminals in an Amazon estuary in Brazil (Viana and Lucena Frédou, 2014).

Because of the highly visible and widely enjoyed presence of wild birds, population numbers are relatively well-established, having been recorded and shared by bird banding societies on a global scale. Birds as sentinels of ecosystem health can reflect changes in habitat quality. Exposure to chemical contaminants may directly affect health of individuals, whereas habitat degradation would have indirect impacts by imposing chronic stress that exacerbates susceptibility to infectious and parasitic diseases, or that could require behavioural changes. Avian-based research on the biological impacts of environmental change often focuses on the breeding period. This allows endocrinological, behavioural and developmental factors related to population health to be observed over a concentrated timespan. Animals higher in the food web will reflect cumulative effects of multiple stressors. Such features make birds important subjects for evaluating environmental health in areas of concern.

Birds have been widely studied in many parts of the world to detect and assess environmental disruption resulting from agrochemicals, mine tailings, oil and gas extraction, and other industrial activities. For more than 2,000 years, humans have released Hg into the environment. Mercury has been released through production of dye (the red pigment, HgS, or cinnabar), from mining of elemental Hg, from smelting to recover gold and silver, from pulp and paper production, and it is actively cycled through the food chain and environmental compartments from microbial activation of elemental Hg after flooding of land (Wiener et al., 2003). Marsh wrens (*Cistothorus palustris*) were studied as bioindicators for mercury (Hg) deposition in wetlands in the United States (Hartman et al., 2013), kingfishers (*Alcedo atthis*) were investigated near an intensive electronic waste recycling depot in China (Mo et al., 2013), tree swallow (*Tachycineta bicolor*) nestlings have been widely studied as bioindicators of industrial contaminants, such as those related to waste water treatment and pollutants released from oil and gas extraction activities in Canada (Dods et al., 2005; Smits et al., 2005b; Cruz-Martinez et al., 2015) and higher trophic-level species such as birds of prey are commonly studied as well (Bowerman et al., 1994; Smits et al., 2002; Smits and Fernie, 2013).

To be valuable sentinels for studying ecosystem disruption, there are specific characteristics that an avian species must have (Hollamby et al., 2006; Burger, 2006). For example, they must be physiologically or behaviourally sensitive enough that exposure to a stressor (including contaminants) elicits a measurable response or a biological effect. A remarkable example of an animal as a sentinel for human health was the use of canaries in coalmines. Canaries would die or become clinically ill at low concentrations of methane and carbon monoxide inside coalmines, and whereas these low concentrations would not affect miners as rapidly, the build-up of these gases would have lethal effects on humans as the concentrations increased. Therefore, canaries acted as an early warning system indicating that miners should evacuate before they were at significant risk (Brown et al., 1997; Stahl, 1997).

The sentinel animals must be present (1) in sufficient numbers (2) in the particular area of

Table 14.1 Characteristics and methods for studying birds as sentinels of ecosystem disruption

Biological	Methodological
✓ Provides an early warning	✓ Provide cost-effective sampling and testing
✓ Widely spread, common, with well-known biology	✓ Restricted home range
✓ Sensitive to stressors so that the biological responses can be measured	✓ Logistically feasible for obtaining sufficient sample sizes
✓ Complement other sentinel and bioindicator systems	✓ Feasible to study in both captive and field settings

Table created from data described by Burger et al. (2006), Hollamby et al. (2006) and Basu et al. (2007).

interest (3) during given times; sampling should ideally be cost-efficient and practical; and it is generally most effective if the species is appealing to policymakers and to the general public (e.g., falcons versus vultures).

Disease in wildlife

'Disease' refers to any impairment of normal physiological or social function, which may be precipitated by infectious organisms, or a range of non-infectious causes such as nutritional, genetic, stress-related, hormonal or toxic factors. Environmental pollutants may play a primary or secondary role in disease.

The study of disease in wildlife requires good observation, deserves investigation and, in some cases, interventions. Some wildlife managers feel that some level of disease in free-ranging populations is normal and that it plays a role in maintaining balanced population levels. These managers suggest that we should not interfere with natural processes that function to maintain the balance of nature. We would argue that this perspective ignores increasingly important issues resulting from anthropogenic interference with the environment. Humans have had a profound influence in changing the environment through deforestation, poor agricultural practices, urban sprawl, industrial expansion, etc. that has led to changes in habitat, availability and quality of resources, and population density. It has introduced new, invasive species and has transported disease agents around the world (Aguirre and Tabor, 2008).

Wildlife has inherent value and also offers recreational and economic opportunities. Besides bird-watching and the interests of naturalists and ecologists, there is another major consideration; the economic value of publically owned wildlife. In the interest of having healthy game animals, we must determine as efficiently as possible the significance of lesions or disease conditions found in hunted or 'found-dead' wildlife so that we can make sound decisions on disposal and determine what actions we may recommend. In particular, we often need to establish whether urgent disease intervention measures are required, or whether it is simply an individual animal problem.

Disease is much more than death or physical disability. We must not assume that a 'normal' parasite burden or other common diseases are not important to individuals or populations. Although subclinical disease may not be apparent, the host always pays a price for harbouring parasites and microorganisms that live, grow, and reproduce at the expense of the host (e.g., ectoparasitism and survival during inclement weather in tree swallows (Gentes et al., 2006), breeding success of male sage grouse on the lek (Wobeser, 1994)). Environmental contaminants, even at low levels, can cause immunosuppression (Nain et al., 2011; Fairbrother et al., 2004). Indirect impacts of environmental damage that result in diminishing food resources can lead to poor body condition and reduced fitness. For example, fields sprayed with chemical insec-

ticides that successfully control a grasshopper infestation have, at the same time, taken away the major dietary items of burrowing owls living in that area that feed heavily on grasshoppers.

Ecosystem damage from animal agriculture

Agriculture in developed and developing countries can be a major source of environmental damage. There are two primary ways in which this degradation occurs. One is a result of agrochemicals used to enhance crop production; for example, through the use of herbicides to control competitive plant species, plus insecticides and fungicides, meant to limit the crop losses from pest infestations. The other is through livestock management practices that are unsustainable from an ecosystem health point of view.

In Western countries where intensive livestock production is the norm, i.e., in most areas except in very arid regions, commercial concentrations of poultry, swine and cattle yield effluents that contaminate surface and ground water sources. Increasingly, pharmaceuticals are becoming routine management tools used in intensively raised livestock (Henderson and Coates, 2009). Medicated feed is used to control coccidiosis, organic arsenicals are formulated to enhance growth particularly in poultry and swine production, and hormonal implants are used to improve feed conversion and growth rate by suppressing reproductive behaviour. During the Great Depression in North America, desperate agricultural practices of trying to raise animals and crops on dry, delicate, unproductive land lead to the devastation of vast areas of the Midwest as the disturbed soil blew away (Faber and O'Connor, 1988). These days, many regions of the world are still suffering from desertification from overgrazing, or overharvesting of plants that would otherwise be stabilizing the soil, practices that are largely driven by the same economically rooted problems of poverty (Geist and Lambin, 2004; Davis, 2005). In other areas, environmental degradation is driven through complacence or ignorance. In the Great Plains regions of Canada and United States, it is not difficult to detect rangeland that has been severely overgrazed. In other areas, marginal, delicate, native prairie land has been developed for unsuitable crops driven by political pay-offs in the form of subsidies and guaranteed insurance for failed crops (Riemer, 2005). These areas have historically been used for extensive grazing, because it was recognized that they could never be productive under cultivation because of insufficient rainfall, or because the soil simply cannot not support crops. This is especially evident in the south-eastern corner of Alberta where the endangered sagebrush habitat has largely disappeared due to fragmentation by agricultural crops and extensive oil and gas industry activity (Walker et al., 2007). The Greater Northern Sage grouse (*Centrocercus urophasianus*) that formerly inhabited this entire region with counts of 400 to 500 males in the mid-1980s, are critically endangered there now with only 13 male animals being found displaying on the breeding grounds in a recent survey (AB-SRD, 2013; Dale Eslinger, senior wildlife biologist, Alberta Fish and Wildlife Division, pers. comm., 2011).

The ideas introduced here will be further illustrated in the following case studies.

14.3 Case study 1: oil sands of northern Alberta, Canada and effects on health of wild birds

The Canadian oil sands in northern Alberta are under western Canada's boreal forest. They represent the source of more than 170 billion barrels of recoverable oil making these reserves the second largest in the world (Government of Alberta, 2013). The crude oil here, known as bitumen, is a thick mixture of hydrocarbons, sand, clay, dissolved metals such as lead (Pb), mercury (Hg), arsenic (As) and vanadium (V), and gases such as hydrogen sulphide (H_2S), nitrogen (N_2) and methane (Czarnecki et al., 2005; Simpson et al., 2010). Recovery of bitumen is done by one of two approaches depending on the depth of the deposits. Open-pit mining (Plate 21) is used for the shallow oil deposits and involves clearing the land, shovelling the sands from the ground and transporting the sands to processing plants where hot water and several solvents are added to extract the oil from the sands. The water used in this process is referred to as oil sands processed water because it contains toxic substances. This contaminated water is stored in large dykes called tailings ponds (Plate 22), where detoxification occurs over time (Gosselin et al., 2010).

To recover crude oil from the shallow bitumen deposits of the Athabasca oil sands, the land has to be cleared first, then large electric shovels dig the sands that are transported on large diesel trucks (heavy haulers) to the processing plants.

Oil sands processed water cannot be returned to the river from where it was originally taken and therefore it is stored in large ponds. Many bird species reside around this industrial site including American kestrels, like the one perched on the fence post in Plate 22.

For the deeper deposits, a process called *in situ* is used and it consists of hot water and steam injection into the ground for releasing the bitumen from the substrate. From these deposits, bitumen is pumped through a series of pipeline networks to processing plants for further refinement of the crude oil (Percy, 2013).

The development of the oil sands is occurring at a fast pace and through both recovery processes, immense amounts of energy and water are being used (Giesy, 2010). Environmental concerns exist because of greenhouse emissions, intense water use and contamination associated with processing (Schindler, 2010). Most of the toxicological research in the oil sands region has focused on aquatic contaminants with little attention being given to airborne contaminants beyond measuring concentrations. Because of this gap in knowledge, the Joint Canada-Alberta Implementation Plan for Oil Sands Monitoring, a collaborative research effort, was established in 2011 for conducting field studies on wild birds (tree swallow nestlings) as sentinels for effects from emissions from the oil sands industry. This collaboration included academia (University of Calgary), an agency from the Canadian federal government (Environment Canada) and industry that lease land in the oil sands region (Shell Canada Ltd. and Syncrude). For this project, several variables were measured to comprehensively assess the birds' health. Together, these biological responses were used as proxies to determine how contaminants emitted from the mining and upgrading activities on the industrial sites affected the birds.

For this multiyear study, nest boxes for tree swallows were erected at two previously mined,

reclaimed sites on the oil sands, and a reference site in the same region. Passive air monitors were set up underneath and adjacent to the boxes (Plate 23).

The air monitors have a filtering membrane that adheres specific air contaminants as air passively flows through.

To help determine the contribution of contaminants from sources other than air, water samples were collected from the water bodies adjacent to the nest box sites. Air contaminants were higher at the oil sands sites for NO_2, SO_2, volatile organic compounds (VOCs) and polycyclic aromatic compounds (PACs) (> fivefold) (Figure 14.1). Although some differences were noted, overall the contaminants measured in the water samples were similar among the industrial and reference sites (Figure 14.2).

As noted in Table 14.2, the results show evidence of biological costs associated with exposure to the air pollutants. It is important to note that the birds have the capacity to compensate for such costs. In this situation, the

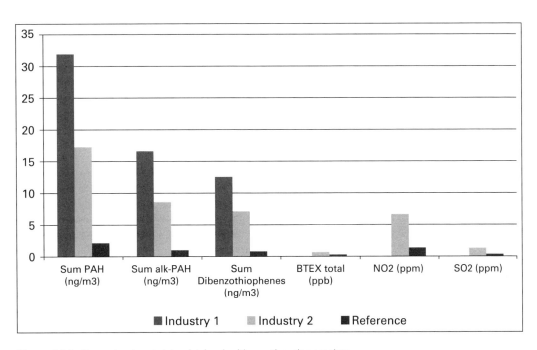

Figure 14.1 Air contaminant data obtained with passive air samplers.

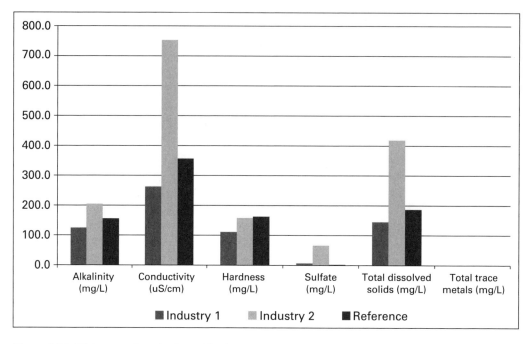

Figure 14.2 Water sampling at adjacent body waters.

Table 14.2 Physiological responses used to evaluate the effect of oil sands-related emissions on wild birds (tree swallow nestlings)

Endpoints	Nestlings from industrial sites compared to reference nestlings
Detoxification efforts	Increased hepatic enzymes (EROD induction)[1] Reduced liver mass
Immune responses	Decreased T-lymphocyte response[2] Reduced mass of bursa of Fabricius[3] Similar spleen mass No histological alterations in the bursa of Fabricius or spleen
Endocrine response (stress)	No significant differences in feather corticosterone levels
Thyroid function	Altered histological anatomy of the thyroid gland[4]
Body condition	Smaller body mass (gr)/wing length (mm) ratio

1 EROD = ethoxyresorufin-0-deethylase. This assay detects a family of hepatic enzymes when increased (induction) after the exposure to several contaminants.
2 Measured by the phytohemagglutinin (PHA) skin test.
3 All B-lymphocytes are produced in the bursa of Fabricius early in birds' development.
4 Unpublished findings

functional changes observed in the immune system (such as the decreased response of T lymphocytes) were subtle and did not progress into structural alterations that would have been evident on histology. In addition, simple and readily collectable data such as morphometric evaluations (body mass, wing length and internal organ mass) provide important baseline data. In this study, the physical data provided valuable insight, although when not evaluated in conjunction with other more sensitive toxicological responses, can offer misleading reassurance of 'no effect'. The findings from this study are especially biologically relevant considering the nestlings are preparing for the post-fledgling period. Even subclinical compromise of physiological functions or increased energy expenditure for detoxification can occur during the critical fledgling period. This is the period of greatest attrition in the life history of passerines (Witter et al., 1994). Survival may be compromised, resulting in low recruitment of birds into the breeding population, which has potentially long-term consequences.

There are several important questions to consider when faced with scenarios of potential impacts on wild birds from industrial activities. Knowledge of the population and habitat is crucial, therefore:

- Are tree swallows in their natural habitat?
- Are tree swallow populations increasing, decreasing or stable?
- Are there changes in the diversity of other fauna normally associated with that habitat?

From the variables and responses that can be examined in wild bird species,

- Is finding contaminants in the birds' tissue indicative of a health impact?
- How would you differentiate if the birds are being sub-clinically affected or are compensating for the impact?
- If you determine a population level impact from industrial activities, what would be the next steps for attempting to remedy such impact?

In the above case, there are many stakeholders involved from academia (researchers, graduate and undergraduate students), industry (managers, technicians, consultants) and government (researchers, managers, administrative staff); therefore,

- Are there stakeholders relevant to this case that were not included? (Is public engagement needed?)
- Which group (s) should be in charge of communicating the results to the scientific community and the general public?
- What challenges do you envision in such large collaborative efforts?
- How would you prevent biased participations from any of the stakeholder groups?
- Who should be responsible for funding such projects?

In conclusion, studying the effects of contaminants from industrial developments on avifauna can provide meaningful information for environmental management. We suggest that combining data from avian species with data collected from other potential bioindicator species (e.g., mammals, invertebrates, lichens), would add valuable information for policy decision-making processes. Bird populations residing near to industrial developments, such as breeding tree swallow populations in the Canadian oil sands region, are valuable sentinels of environmental health and are good models for studying the long-term impacts of contaminants on biota.

14.4 Case study 2: Desertification of a region and a disease outbreak among birds

Fuerteventura and Lanzarote are two small desert islands primarily made up of steppe habitat, in the Canary Islands. Biologists have been studying the ecosystems on these islands for decades (Donázar et al., 2002; Illera, 2001; Medina et al., 2004) with increasing efforts focused on the ecology and conservation of several species of birds, many of which are endangered or threatened. Studies have included ecology and conservation of several species of passerines, as well as columbiformes (Medina et al., 2004), houbara bustards (Carrascal et al., 2008) and vultures (Donázar et al., 2002). The work described here was the first recognition of an epizootic of poxvirus infection in passerine species on these desert islands.

In the course of banding desert passerines, ornithologists detected that a high proportion had proliferative lesions on their legs and occasionally on their faces. They recruited a veterinarian to help unravel the findings, which ended up being remarkable on several accounts; the diseased birds were exclusively from two of the four species we were trapping, often in the

same nets and on the same properties (Smits et al., 2005a).

All collections were made around farmyards in the steppe habitats where the principal livestock is dairy goats, although domestic sheep, chickens, pigeons, peafowl, ducks, camels and donkeys were also present on small holdings throughout the study area. Both islands have a dry climate with annual precipitation of approximately 111mm in Fuerteventura and 162mm in Lanzarote. Wild birds congregate in large flocks in and around the farms for feeding on grains provided to the goats and poultry, as well as on worms living in the manure.

Common species in this habitat are the Spanish sparrow *Passer hispaniolensis*, the trumpeter finch *Bucanetes githagineus amantum*, the short-toed lark *Calandrella rufescens polatzeki* (both subspecies of which are endemic to the Canary Islands) and Berthelot's pipit *Anthus bertelotti* which has a circum-Mediterranean distribution.

It is relevant to the situation being described here to have background information on the natural history of the species involved. The short-toed lark is a species of desert steppe. A study was carried out to determine the response of short-toed larks to available and apparently richer vegetation. In areas in which steppe habitat represented at least 50 per cent of the region, with improved pastures adjacent to the open steppe areas, larks did not use the enriched pasture area.

Berthelot's pipit is endemic to Europe, found only on the Canary Islands, Madeira and the Savage Islands. It shows a preference for dry, open areas scattered with bushes, grass and herbaceous vegetation. This territorial pipit species forages on the ground for insects and seeds. Berthelot's pipit is territorial and usually seen singly or in pairs. The female Berthelot's pipit builds the ground-based nest, which is usually found under low shrubs or stones (Garcia-del-Rey and Cresswell, 2007; Avibirds European Birdguide, 2011; Spurgin et al., 2012). The trumpeter finch is a robust, seed-eating bird, widespread across warm arid regions around North Africa, the Middle East and the Canary Islands. Like the pipit, it inhabits stony desert regions, nesting in rocky crevices or underneath shrubs (Cramp and Perrins, 1994; Valera et al., 2003), but unlike the pipit, it is a gregarious, sociable species. The Spanish sparrow is a common inhabitant of farm and peri-urban regions around the Mediterranean including the Canary Islands, with the same gregarious behaviour as the house sparrow (*Passer domesticus*), which is also traditionally associated with human habitation, and persists as human population density increases (Shaw et al., 2008).

Over the non-breeding and breeding seasons for two years, birds were captured by baiting them with ground corn placed near the barn yards of dairy goat farms, with wide, spring-released nets that could be triggered remotely to trap five to 15 birds at a time, or with small individual spring-loaded traps baited with mealworms. Each captured bird was weighed and aged as a juvenile or adult since susceptibility to disease, regardless of species, is often different for young-of-the-year. The birds were examined closely for evidence of abnormalities, which consisted mainly of scaly, proliferative lesions on the legs, eyelids or face. If it was possible to collect a small sample of the abnormal tissue without harming the bird, a small portion was removed with a scalpel and fixed in formalin for future histopathologic evaluation. The number of prolific lesions on the face, legs and or feet was recorded, and a scale was created to rank the severity of the lesions on each individual as objectively as possible. Numerous birds had missing nails, partial or entire toes, which was recorded as well. Birds with missing digits had their own separate category because it was not possible to decisively rule out trauma or developmental etiologies.

A total of 893 birds were captured; Spanish sparrows (n = 128), trumpeter finches (n = 228), short-toed larks (n = 395) and Berthelot's pipits (n = 139). The relative number of birds with pox-like lesions differed dramatically among the four species, with the sparrows and finches that normally cohabit with humans and domestic animals, having no visible lesions during any collection period (Table 14.3).

Questions to consider when faced with this problem of an infectious disease that has a component of ecosystem health:

- Why were the short-toed larks and pipits, both normally selecting remote desert habitats and avoiding human environments, being trapped in the same nets as the sparrows and finches that are historically associated with humans and domestic animals?

Table 14.3 Prevalence of birds with pox-like lesions

Species	Total N	Breeding season*	Non-breeding season
Short-toed lark	395	49%	55%
Berthelot's pipit	139	22%	56%
Spanish sparrow	128	0%	0%
Trumpeter finch	228	0%	0%
		Juveniles	Adults
Short-toed lark	395	35%	57%
Berthelot's pipit	139	27%	33%

* 80–83% of birds from all four species were captured during the breeding season

- What factors may be contributing to developing clinical disease in these birds?
- What factors could influence the skewed distribution of the poxvirus infections among the four species?
- What investigative techniques could be carried out to confirm or refute your ideas?
- Who are the stakeholders that would be interested in/affected by this problem?
- With whom would you need to work to (1) determine the root of the problem, and (2) start crafting a solution?

Levels of poxvirus infection in native species in the Canary Islands (28 per cent of pipits, 50 per cent of larks) are even higher than those reported in native Hawaiian birds (17–35 per cent) that have been the most intensely studied populations regarding the epidemiology of avian poxvirus because of the concern that this virus is one factor responsible for the decline in populations of native birds in Hawaii. The pox problems in the Hawaiian species coincide closely with introductions of poultry and wild birds, as well as species of mosquitos that act as vectors for poxvirus (Tripathy et al., 2000; van Riper et al., 2002; Van der Werf, 2001). In the two susceptible species on the Canary Islands, a notable difference from the Hawaiian situation is that both affected and unaffected species are native to these islands.

This means that their susceptibility to developing clinical infection is related to other factors. Generally, young of the year, or juveniles of any species are more susceptible to infectious and parasitic diseases than adults are because their immune systems are not yet mature and maximally competent. That is not the case here. Something else is driving this dramatic, species-specific susceptibility. Severe degradation and denuding of the delicate but formerly productive desert habitat has coincided with the behavioural changes in the short-toed larks that finds them in farmyards, closely interacting with

other wild passerines and feeding with domestic species. Elsewhere in the world where these birds exist, they breed and forage exclusively in natural and semi-natural steppe habitats (Snow and Perrins, 1998, pp. 1034–1036; Suárez et al., 2002). Chronic stress is well-known to be immunosuppressive (Sapolsky et al., 2000), so the next logical step to better understand the extreme sensitivity to a common avian pathogen in these birds would entail measures of long term glucocorticoid levels in the affected populations along with studies of immunocompetence.

14.5 Summary and conclusions

Because the development of the Alberta oil sands is occurring at a fast pace, an active and continuous monitoring programme is needed to ensure the rate of development is balanced through maintaining a healthy ecosystem. By studying wild birds that use the boreal forest as breeding and nesting grounds, we present evidence of biological costs associated with exposure to air pollutants and the apparent capacity of the birds for compensating for such costs. It is important that these types of studies continue for several years to better assess long-term consequences of industrial development on native flora, fauna and the overall ecosystem.

As a final thought to consider, the two cases presented in this chapter, a transdisciplinary approach in which candid, well-informed, timely and efficient communication among researchers, government scientists and industry is of utmost importance if research findings are meant to be meaningful. Direct engagement of industrial partners in this type of research is especially valuable to increase the likelihood of research findings being incorporated into decisions by that industry. In addition, collaborative projects are needed to provide solid foundations for understanding complex effects of contaminants affecting biota, humans and the ecosystem. Such collaborations should include a variety of discipline experts including biologists, ecologists, veterinarians, toxicologists, environmental chemists, communication and public relations, environmental groups, sociologists, economics and other social sciences.

References

AB-SRD (2013). Alberta Greater Sage-grouse Recovery Plan 2013–2018. Alberta Environment and Sustainable Resource Development.

Aguirre, A.A. and Tabor, G.M. (2008). Global factors driving emerging infectious diseases. *Annals of the New York Academy of Sciences*, 1149, 1–3.

Avibirds European Birdguide (2011). *Berthelot's Pipit*, www.avibirds.com/euhtml/Berthelots_Pipit.html.

Basu, N., Scheuhammer, A.M., Bursian, S.J., Elliott, J., Rouvinen-Watt, K. and Chan, H.M. (2007). Mink as a sentinel species in environmental health. *Environmental Research*, 103, 130–144.

Bowerman, W., Best, D., Giesy, J., Kubiak, T. and Sikarskie, J. (1994). The influence of environmental contaminants on bald eagle (*Haliaeetus leucocephalus*) populations in the Laurentian Great Lakes, North America. In B.U. Meyburg and R.D. Chancellor (eds.), *Raptor Conservation Today*. London: Pica Press, pp. 703–791.

Brown, R.E., Brain, J.D. and Wang, N. (1997). The avian respiratory system: a unique model for studies of respiratory toxicosis and for monitoring air quality. *Environmental Health Perspectives*, 105, 188.

Burger, J. (2006). Bioindicators: types, development, and use in ecological assessment and research. *Environmental Bioindicators*, 1, 22–39.

Carrascal, L.M., Palomino, D., Seoane, J. and Alonso, C.L. (2008). Habitat use and population density of the houbara bustard *Chlamydotis undulata* in Fuerteventura (Canary Islands). *African Journal of Ecology*, 46, 291–302.

Charles, J., Sancey, B., Morin-Crini, N., Badot, P.-M., Degiorgi, F., Trunfio, G. and Crini, G. (2011). Evaluation of the phytotoxicity of polycontaminated industrial effluents using the lettuce plant (*Lactuca sativa*) as a bioindicator. *Ecotoxicology and Environmental Safety*, 74, 2057–2064.

Conti, M. and Cecchetti, G. (2001). Biological monitoring: lichens as bioindicators of air pollution assessment – a review. *Environmental Pollution*, 114, 471–492.

Cramp, S. and Perrins, C.M. (1994). *The Birds of the Western Paleartic*. Oxford: Oxford University Press.

Cruz-Martinez, L., Fernie, K.J., Soos, C., Harner, T., Getachew, F. and Smits, J.E. (2015). Detoxification, endocrine, and immune responses of tree swallow nestlings naturally exposed to air contaminants from the Alberta oil sands. *Science of the Total Environment*, 502, 8–15.

Cucu-Man, S.-M. and Steinnes, E. (2013). Analysis of selected biomonitors to evaluate the suitability for their complementary use in monitoring trace element atmospheric deposition. *Environmental Monitoring and Assessment*, 185, 7775–7791.

Czarnecki, J., Radoev, B., Schramm, L.L. and Slavchev, R. (2005). On the nature of Athabasca oil sands. *Advances in Colloid and Interface Science*, 114–115, 53–60.

Davis, D.K. (2005). Indigenous knowledge and the desertification debate: problematising expert knowledge in North Africa. *Geoforum*, 36, 509–524.

Dods, P.L., Birmingham, E.M., Williams, T.D., Ikonomou, M.G., Bennie, D.T. and Elliott, J.E. (2005). Reproductive success and contaminants in tree swallows (*Tachycineta bicolor*) breeding at a wastewater treatment plant. *Environmental Toxicology and Chemistry*, 24, 3106–3112.

Donázar, J.A., Negro, J.J., Palacios, C.J., Gangoso, L., Godoy, J.A., Ceballos, O., Hiraldo, F. and Capote, N. (2002). Description of a new subspecies of the egyptian vulture (*Accipitridae: Aeophron percjvofterus*) from the Canary Islands. *Journal of Raptor Research*, 36, 17–23.

Faber, D., and O'Connor, J. (1988). The struggle for nature: environmental crises and the crisis of environmentalism in the United States. *Capitalism Nature Socialism*, 1, 12–39.

Fairbrother, A., Smits, J. and Grasman, K. (2004). Avian immunotoxicology. *Journal of Toxicology and Environmental Health Part B: Critical Reviews*, 7, 105–137.

Garcia-del-Rey, E. and Cresswell, W. (2007). The breeding biology of the endemic Berthelot's pipit *Anthus berthelotii* in a harsh oceanic island environment (Tenerife, Canary Islands). *Ostrich-Journal of African Ornithology*, 78, 583–589.

Geist, H.J. and Lambin, E.F. (2004). Dynamic causal patterns of desertification. *Bioscience*, 54, 817–829.

Gentes, M.-L., Waldner, C., Papp, Z. and Smits, J.E. (2006). Effects of oil sands tailings compounds and harsh weather on mortality rates, growth and detoxification efforts in nestling tree swallows (*Tachycineta bicolor*). *Environmental Pollution*, 142, 24–33.

Giesy, J.P., Anderson, J.C. and Wiseman, S.B. (2010). Alberta oil sands development. *Proceedings of the National Academy of Sciences*, 107, 951.

Gosselin, P., Hrudey, S.E., Naeth, M.A., Plourde, A., Therrien, R., Van Der Kraak, G. and Xu, Z. (2010). Environmental and Health Impacts of Canada's Oil Sands Industry. Ontario: Royal Society of Canada Ottawa.

Government of Alberta (2013). *Alberta Oil Sands: About the Resource*, www.oilsands.alberta.ca/resource.html.

Hartman, C.A., Ackerman, J.T., Herring, G., Isanhart, J. and Herzog, M. (2013). Marsh wrens as bioindicators of mercury in wetlands of Great Salt Lake: do blood and feathers reflect site-specific exposure risk to bird reproduction? *Environmental Science and Technology*, 47, 6597–6605.

Henderson, K. and Coates, J.R. (2009). *Veterinary Pharmaceuticals in the Environment.* Paper presented at the American Chemical Society Symposium, Series 1018.

Hollamby, S., Afema-Azikuru, J., Waigo, S., Cameron, K., Gandolf, A.R., Norris, A. and Sikarskie, J.G. (2006). Suggested guidelines for use of avian species as biomonitors. *Environmental Monitoring and Assessment*, 118, 13–20.

Illera, J.C. (2001). Habitat selection by the Canary Islands stonechat (*Saxicola dacotiae*) (Meade-Waldo, 1989) in Fuerteventura Island, a two-tier habitat approach with implications for its conservation. *Biological Conservation*, 97, 339–345.

Medina, F.M., Ramírez, G.A. and Hernández, A. (2004). Avian pox in white-tailed laurel-pigeons from the Canary Islands. *Journal of Wildlife Diseases*, 40, 351–355.

Mo, L., Wu, J.P., Luo, X.J., Li, K.L., Peng, Y., Feng, A.H., Zhang, Q., Zou, F.S. and Mai, B.X. (2013). Using the kingfisher (*Alcedo atthis*) as a bioindicator of PCBs and PBDEs in the Dinghushan biosphere reserve, China. *Environmental Toxicology and Chemistry*, 32, 1655–1662.

Nain, S., Bour, A., Chalmers, C., and Smits, J.E. (2011). Immunotoxicity and disease resistance in Japanese quail (*Coturnix coturnix japonica*) exposed to malathion. *Ecotoxicology*, 20, 892–900.

National Research Council Committee on Animals as Monitors of Environmental Hazards (1991). *Animals as Sentinels of Environmental Health Hazards.* Washington, DC: National Academy Press.

Percy, K.E. (2013). Geoscience of climate and energy 11. Ambient air quality and linkage to ecosystems in the Athabasca oil sands, Alberta. *Geoscience Canada*, 40, 182–201.

Riemer, G. (2005). Land-use policy change and the ramifications for stewardship and waterfowl conservation in Saskatchewan. In T.A. Radenbaugh and G.C. Sutter (eds.), *Managing Changing Prairie Landscapes*. Regina: University of Regina Press, pp. 11–22.

Sapolsky, R.M., Romero, L.M. and Munck, A.U. (2000). How do glucocorticoids influence stress responses? Integrating permissive, suppressive, stimulatory, and preparative actions. *Endocrine Reviews*, 21, 55–89.

Schindler, D. (2010). Tar sands need solid science. *Nature*, 468, 499–501.

Shaw, L.M., Chamberlain, D. and Evans, M. (2008). The house sparrow *Passer domesticus* in urban areas: reviewing a possible link between post-decline distribution and human socioeconomic status. *Journal of Ornithology*, 149, 293–299.

Simpson, I.J., Blake, N.J., Barletta, B., Diskin, G.S., Fuelberg, H.E., Gorham, K., Huey, L.G., Meinardi, S., Rowland, F.S., Vay, S.A., Weinheimer, A.J., Yang, M. and Blake, D.R. (2010). Characterization of trace gases measured over Alberta oil sands mining operations: 76 speciated C2-C10 volatile organic compounds (VOCs), CO_2, CH_4, CO, NO, NO_2, NOy, O_3 and SO_2. *Atmospheric Chemistry & Physics Discussions*, 10, 18507–18560.

Smits, J.E. and Fernie, K.J. (2013). Avian wildlife as sentinels of ecosystem health. *Comparative Immunology, Microbiology and Infectious Diseases*, 36, 333–342.

Smits, J.E., Fernie, K., Bortolotti, G. and Marchant, T. (2002). Thyroid hormone suppression and cell-mediated immunomodulation in American kestrels (*Falco sparverius*) exposed to PCBs. *Archives of Environmental Contamination and Toxicology*, 43, 338–344.

Smits, J.E., Tella, J.L., Carrete, M., Serrano, D. and López, G. (2005a). An epizootic of avian pox in endemic short-toed larks (*Calandrella rufescens*) and Berthelot's pipits (*Anthus berthelotti*) in the Canary Islands, Spain. *Veterinary Pathology*, 42, 59–65.

Smits, J.E., Bortolotti, G.R., Sebastian, M., and Ciborowski, J.J. (2005b). Spatial, temporal, and dietary determinants of organic contaminants in nestling tree swallows in Point Pelee National Park, Ontario, Canada. *Environmental Toxicology and Chemistry* 24, 3159–3165.

Snow, D. and Perrins C.M. (1998). *The Birds of the Western Palearctic*, Vol. 2. Oxford: Oxford University Press.

Spurgin, L.G., Illera, J.C., Padilla, D.P. and Richardson, D.S. (2012). Biogeographical patterns and co-occurrence of pathogenic infection across island populations of Berthelot's pipit (*Anthus berthelotii*). *Oecologia*, 168, 691–701.

Stahl, R.G. (1997). Can mammalian and non-mammalian sentinel species data be used to evaluate the human health implications of environmental contaminants? *Human Ecological Risk Assessment*, 3, 329–335.

Suárez, F., Garza, V. and Morales, M.B. (2002). Habitat use of two sibling species, the short-toed *Calandrella brachydactyla* and the lesser short-toed *C. rufescens* larks, in mainland Spain. *Ardeola*, 49, 259–272.

Tripathy, D.N., Schnitzlein, W.M., Morris, P.J., Janssen, D.L., Zuba, J.K., Massey, G. and Atkinson, C.T. (2000). Characterization of poxviruses from forest birds in Hawaii. *Journal of Wildlife Diseases*, 36, 225–230.

Valera, F., Carrillo, C.M., Barbosa, A. and Moreno, E. (2003). Low prevalence of haematozoa in Trumpeter finches *Bucanetes githagineus* from southeastern Spain: additional support for a restricted distribution of blood parasites in arid lands. *Journal of Arid Environments*, 55, 209–213.

van Riper III, C., van Riper, S.G., Hansen, W.R. and Hackett, S. (2002). Epizootiology and effect of avian pox on Hawaiian forest birds. *The Auk*, 119, 929–942.

Van der Werf, E. (2001). Distribution and potential impacts of avian poxlike lesions in elepaio at Hakalau Forest National Wildlife Refuge. *Studies in Avian Biology*, 22, 247–253.

Viana, A. and Lucena Frédou, F. (2014). Ichthyofauna as bioindicator of environmental quality in an industrial district in the Amazon estuary, Brazil. *Brazilian Journal of Biology*, 74, 315–324.

Walker, B.L., Naugle, D.E. and Doherty, K.E. (2007). Greater sage-grouse population response to energy development and habitat loss. *The Journal of Wildlife Management*, 71, 2644–2654.

Wiener, J.G., Krabbenhoft, D.P., Heinz, G.H. and Scheuhammer, A.M. (2003). Ecotoxicology of Mercury. In D.J. Hoffman, B.A. Rattner, G.A. Burton and J. Cairns (eds.), *Handbook of Ecotoxicology*, 2nd edn. Boca Raton: Lewis Publishers, CRC Press, pp. 409–464.

Witter, M.S., Cuthill, I.C. and Bonser, R.H. (1994). Experimental investigations of mass-dependent predation risk in the European starling, *Sturnus vulgaris*. *Animal Behaviour*, 48, 201–222.

Wobeser, G.A. (1994). *Investigation and Management of Disease in Wild Animals*. New York: Plenum Press.

AGRICULTURAL SUSTAINABILITY (AND RESOURCES)

chapter 15

Integrated pest management (IPM): one of the earliest 'ecosystem approaches' to agricultural problem-solving

Tessa R. Grasswitz

Abstract

The concept of 'One Health' explicitly acknowledges that human health and wellbeing is intimately connected to the health of the rest of the environment. The need to safeguard human and environmental health while simultaneously reducing crop losses due to insects and other pests led directly to the development of integrated pest management (IPM) – an early example of this type of holistic thinking and a good example of an 'ecohealth' approach. In this chapter we will examine the importance of holistic crop management, giving some key examples of how this approach can be used to address pest problems in crops.

15.1 Introduction: development of the IPM concept

Tending crops played a key role in human evolution, and modern agriculture and horticulture continue to play an important role in our way of life. Crop losses due to insects, weeds and diseases were probably apparent early in the transition from natural to managed ecosystems as agriculture developed and evolved, with naturally diverse plant communities being gradually replaced by single-species stands. Even now, when humans have been farming for approximately 600 generations (Birch et al., 2011), such losses are still a feature of agricultural production: globally, estimates of annual losses due to pests range from 26 to 50 per cent for various arable crops and up to 80 per cent for some cotton crops (Oerke, 2006). In the US, it is estimated that insects destroy approximately 13 per cent of all potential crop yields, while diseases and weeds each account for an additional 12 per cent (Pimentel, 2005). Globally, the total amount of food currently lost to insects alone (both pre- and post-harvest) is reported to be sufficient to feed one billion people (Birch et al., 2011). Given the potential impact of pests, therefore, it is perhaps not surprising that deliberate attempts at crop protection are thought to date back to 2500 BCE (Oerke, 2006).

However, as new technologies have emerged to combat pest-related losses (particularly in the past 75 years), unforeseen effects have occurred that in some cases extend far beyond the point of application, adversely affecting both human and ecosystem health. Indeed, the whole concept of integrated pest management (IPM) was developed in response to various problems that became apparent with the introduction (and subsequent overuse) of the first synthetic organochlorine insecticides (e.g., DDT, aldrin and various others) in the 1940s and 1950s. DDT, for example, was widely used against such key pests as corn earworm (*Helicoverpa zea*), tobacco budworm (*Heliothis virescens*) and codling moth (*Cydia pomonella*) (among others). DDT and related compounds – initially hailed as 'silver bullets' for crop protection – heralded a new era of chemically based crop protection. However, the ready availability of these relatively cheap and (initially) very effective products led – particularly in the United States – to the widespread adoption of routine, fixed-schedule ('calendar') spraying of crops regardless of pest presence or population density. This eventually resulted in the development of insecticide resistance in target pests, as well as issues of primary pest resurgence and increases in so-called 'secondary' pests due to the destruction of their natural enemies (Stern et al., 1959). Control failures caused by problems such as these, together with concern regarding pesticide residues in food, stimulated the development of the IPM concept. At about the same time, the wider impact of these early synthetic pesticides on humans and other non-target species (including various fish, songbirds and raptors) was brought to the attention of a broader audience by the publication in 1962 of Rachel Carson's landmark book *Silent Spring* (Carson, 1962), resulting in widespread public concern.

The genesis of IPM is generally ascribed to Stern et al. (1959), who first articulated the concept of 'integrated control', which they defined as 'applied pest control which combines and integrates biological and chemical control' (Stern et al., 1959). Clearly, however, these authors had a broader vision in mind, as the following excerpt illustrates:

> To establish new, favorable balances [between crops and pests], it is first necessary to recognize the 'oneness' of any environment, natural or man-made. The populations of plants and animals (including man) and the non-living environment together make up an integrated unit, the ecosystem. If an attempt is made to reduce the population level of one kind of animal (for example, a pest insect) by chemical treatment, modification of cultural practices, or by other means, other parts of the ecosystem will be affected as well. For this reason, the production of a given food or fiber must be considered in its entirety. This includes simultaneous consideration of insects, diseases, plant nutrition, plant physiology, and plant resistance, as well as the economics of the crops.
>
> (Stern et al., 1959)

Given this holistic emphasis and the subsequent elaboration of the approach, IPM has been defined more comprehensively as follows:

> Integrated pest management (IPM) is an ecosystem-based strategy that focuses on long-term prevention of pests or their damage through a combination of techniques such as biological control, habitat manipulation, modification of cultural practices, and use of resistant varieties. Pesticides are used only after monitoring indicates they are needed according to established guidelines, and treatments are made with the goal of removing only the target organism. Pest control materials are selected and applied in a manner that minimizes risks to human health, beneficial and non-target organisms, and the environment.
>
> (University of California, 2014).

Ironically, as Kogan (1998) pointed out, prior to the development of synthetic pesticides, crop protection had traditionally incorporated a variety of complementary non-chemical tactics (one of the underpinnings of IPM as defined above), and some of these basic principles (e.g., cultural controls such as destruction of overwintering sites for pests and the importance of preserving natural predators) had been articulated in a number of publications prior to the paper by Stern et al. (1959) (e.g., Isley and Berg, 1924; Pickett et al., 1946). However, in the historical context in which it was developed, integrated control represented a radical departure from the prevailing paradigm of fixed-schedule spraying by emphasizing the importance of regular monitoring of pest densities and by introducing the use of economic injury levels and economic thresholds to guide spray decisions. The latter concepts were defined, respectively, as 'the lowest [pest] population density that will cause economic damage' and 'the density at which control measures should be [applied] to prevent an increasing pest population from reaching the economic injury level' (Stern et al., 1959). Although in practice it has often been difficult and research-intensive to develop robust economic (or 'action') thresholds, these concepts clearly emphasized the need to move away from fixed-schedule spray regimes to a more rational approach in which interventions with chemical or other control tactics were made only when absolutely necessary. The emphasis that Stern and his co-authors placed on developing an ecosystem approach to pest management also represented a major paradigm shift – one that has had a profound and lasting effect on both basic and applied entomological research. Today, more than 50 years after its publication, the article by Stern et al. has been acknowledged as the foundation of all modern IPM programmes (Naranjo and Ellsworth, 2009) and has been hailed as the 'most important pest control paper of 20th century' (Warnert, 2009).

15.2 Examples of successful IPM programmes in various agro-ecosystems

IPM in greenhouse production

Worldwide, production of food crops under protected cropping systems (either in traditional 'glasshouses' or in polythene-covered 'hoop-houses') is increasing, with the total global greenhouse vegetable area currently estimated at 411,262 hectares (Hickman, 2014), with an additional, largely unquantified, area devoted to glasshouse ornamentals. Protected crops are typically high-value commodities grown intensively on very limited acreage. The latter factor can restrict the range of insecticides available to growers, as the potential market may not be large enough to offset registration costs for pesticide manufacturers. A relative shortage of available products, combined with the reduced gene flow associated with an enclosed pest population, makes it likely that pests of protected crops will develop pesticide resistance more rapidly than pests of outdoor crops. However, the enclosed or semi-enclosed nature of protected cropping systems makes them much more amenable to the use of augmentative or innundative releases of mass-reared biological control agents than are outdoor crops. This approach was first used in the UK to control the greenhouse whitefly (*Trialeurodes vaporariorum*) on tomatoes more than 80 years ago (van Lenteren et al., 1996), and in some countries, such bio-intensive IPM programmes are now used on as much as 30 per cent of the total area of protected crops (Bale et al., 2008). Using biological control agents as the cornerstone of indoor pest management programmes has other benefits that are attractive to growers, including quicker application times compared to chemical spraying, improved worker health and safety, no mandatory re-entry interval (such as is required for most pesticides) and no risk of phytotoxicity (van Lenteren, 2009;

Graham, 2010). The latter is a particular concern to growers of ornamental plants, since only a small proportion of such species are tested during the product development process.

However, using purchased inputs of natural enemies as the foundation of indoor IPM programmes requires a rather different approach to that used in IPM programmes for field-grown crops, where the emphasis is on conserving naturally occurring (wild) beneficial insects and other potential control agents. Thus, while crop monitoring is important in both systems, it is particularly necessary in protected cropping, where pest populations can increase much more rapidly as a result of being isolated from their natural predators and because their host plants are produced under minimal abiotic stress in near-optimum environmental conditions (Pilkington et al, 2010). Consequently, purchased biological control agents must be introduced as soon as the pest is first detected if control is to be successful. Such meticulous monitoring and prompt action is particularly important given the inherent time-lags that occur between pest detection and effective biological control, which are due to (1) the time taken to order and ship mass-reared beneficials from suppliers, and (2) the fact that such organisms are often sold in life-stages other than that which actually exert control, such as eggs or adults of predaceous larvae (for example, green lacewings).

The need for rapid deployment of predators or parasitoids (parasitic wasps or flies that kill their hosts) has led to the development of so-called 'open rearing systems' or 'banker plants' (Plate 24) whereby natural enemies are introduced pre-emptively on a non-crop plant infested with a non-pest herbivore that supports the development and reproduction of the natural enemy. As such, these systems allow the natural enemy to persist for long periods in the absence of the target pest on the primary crop (Frank, 2010), while simultaneously ensuring that they are in place as soon as they are needed. In essence,

then, such systems constitute a preventative rather than a curative approach (Frank, 2010), which – although running counter to traditional IPM practices – may be much more cost-effective than repeated releases of larger numbers of beneficials (as in a traditional augmentative release programme). An additional benefit of banker plants is that they can be temporarily removed from a site should any pesticide applications be necessary, and returned once residues have declined to safe levels (Frank, 2010). At present, the best-known banker plant systems are targeted at aphid pests of broad-leaved crops, using cereal aphids such as *Rhopalosiphum padi* or *Sitobion avenae* on barley, wheat or oat plants to support populations of parasitoids (e.g., *Aphidius colemani*) or syrphid flies (Frank, 2010). Numerous attempts have been made to develop such systems for other species, with varying degrees of success (Frank, 2010; Parolin et al., 2013).

The success of these bio-intensive IPM systems is dependent not only on a high degree of knowledge and timely action on the part of growers, but also on the availability of competitively priced biological control agents for the key pests of individual crops, and/or selective pesticides for any pests for which no natural enemy is commercially available. In Europe, where greenhouse biological control is well-established, there are now more than 30 companies producing a total of more than 150 natural enemies (Bueno and van Lenteren, 2010). However, despite advances in mass-rearing processes and technology, expansion of greenhouse biological control into new regions may be limited – at least initially – by the availability of native natural enemies that can be successfully mass-produced. This factor also makes bio-intensive systems vulnerable to disruption by new invasive pests for which natural enemies are often unavailable, and that are becoming an increasing problem in most parts of the world (Bebber et al., 2014). Other potential disadvantages of biological control for protected crops – real or perceived – include cost (including the price of overnight shipping, which can be substantial), efficacy, and predictability (Frank, 2010).

There is general agreement that biological control is harder to implement for pests of glasshouse ornamentals than for those of vegetable crops, for a number of reasons. For example, producers of ornamentals often grow a much wider diversity of plant species (with a consequently broader range of potential pests), with a quicker turnover of individual crops and zero tolerance for pest damage on any part of the plant. Furthermore, a broader range of insecticides is often available for pests of ornamentals, since higher tolerances for pesticide residues (compared to edible crops) makes product registration easier (van Lenteren, 2009). Consequently, there is less incentive to switch to biologically based control programmes. As a result, it is estimated that, in Europe, more than 80 per cent of all biological control practised in protected cropping systems is for just three edible crops: tomato, cucumber and bell pepper (Bueno and van Lenteren, 2010). Consumer preferences and concerns regarding pesticide use have also had a major impact on the adoption of biological control on edible crops: in Europe in particular, some major supermarket chains have required growers to adopt such strategies as part of their own quality assurance schemes (Haynes et al., 2010).

In future, improvements in techniques for mass-rearing beneficials, coupled with advances in compatible greenhouse technologies, are likely to foster increased adoption of biologically based IPM in protected cropping systems. Examples of relevant innovations that are either currently available or near-market include the development of new biological controls for plant pathogens (van Lenteren, 2009), more effective materials for physically excluding pests such as thrips and aphids (Portorff and Panter, 2008), plastic coverings for hoop houses that selectively filter out UV light (decreasing certain insect and disease problems) (Díaz et al, 2006), and manipulation of greenhouse temperature, humidity and/or light intensity to selectively favour biological control agents over pests and diseases (Shipp et al., 2011). Such tactics could be readily integrated with biological control agents to form more broadly based programmes, making them more resilient and less prone to disruption by, for example, new invasive pests.

Cotton pest management in Arizona, USA

Historically, cotton has been one of the world's most heavily sprayed crops (Spurgeon, 2007) and has been classified as a 'pesticide dependent' commodity as a result (Dinham, 1993). It is currently grown in approximately 80 countries (Naranjo and Ellsworth, 2009) and occupies almost 2 per cent of the world's agricultural land area (calculated from data in Bruinsma, 2003, and Zhao and Tisdell, 2010). The pest complex associated with cotton varies in different parts of the world, and in Arizona some of the crop's most important pests originated elsewhere. The development of IPM in this region has therefore been driven by the need to manage key invasive species, and as such provides a pertinent case study for other crops.

The boll weevil (*Anthonomus grandis*), for example, is thought to have invaded Arizona from Central America, moving through Mexico and crossing into Texas in the late 1800s (Arizona Cotton Research and Protection Council, 2010). It subsequently spread within the state, and by the early 1960s had attained the status of an 'occasional pest', particularly in areas where so-called 'stub cotton' was produced (i.e., where the crop was grown as a short-term perennial, with the roots and main stem being allowed to persist from one season to the next). In 1965, in an effort to curtail the spread of the boll weevil, a state-wide ban on stub cotton was instituted along with a mandatory plough-down at the end of the growing season. The ban was lifted in 1978, and localized infestations of boll weevil were detected later that year (Spurgeon, 2007). By 1982, the problem had increased to the point where more than 44,000 acres of Arizona cotton had to be treated at least once for boll weevil (Arizona Cotton Research and Protection Council, 2010). The following year the ban on stub cotton was reintroduced and a boll weevil eradication programme was initiated (Arizona Cotton Research and Protection Council, 2010). The latter involved various tactics, including monitoring with pheromone traps to detect infestations, insecticide applications, and defoliation and destruction of plants as soon as possible after harvest to eliminate potential food and overwintering sites (USDA-APHIS, 2013; National Cotton Council of America, 2014). By 1991, no reproducing populations of boll weevil could be found in Arizona and it was considered eradicated from the state. Annual monitoring has continued ever since, but with only occasional interceptions (thought to be due to accidental transport of weevils on vehicles) (Arizona Cotton Research and Protection Council, 2010).

Eradication of key pests generally makes it correspondingly easier to develop integrated control programmes for remaining pests. In Arizona, real progress in cotton IPM was made following the elimination of a second exotic key pest, the pink bollworm (*Pectinophora gossypiella*). This pest, originally from India, has been an important pest of Arizona cotton since the 1960s (Naranjo and Ellsworth, 2010) and a variety of tactics have historically been used in its management. In addition to insecticides, these included sex-pheromone based mating disruption (Agnew, 1999) and cultural approaches such as shortening the cotton-growing season (Chu et al., 1996). The latter was achieved by delaying spring planting (to reduce the number of host plants available

for egg-laying by newly emerged females), early termination of irrigation (to reduce the number of late-season fruits for egg-laying and larval development) and prompt post-harvest crop destruction to reduce overwintering sites (Agnew, 1999). A major breakthrough occurred in 1996, when cotton cultivars became available in Arizona that had been genetically modified to produce insecticidal toxins from the bacterium *Bacillus thuringiensis* ('Bt'). The latter are selectively toxic to the larvae of Lepidoptera and were highly effective in controlling *P. gossypiella*. From 1997 onwards, the percentage of Arizona cotton acreage planted with 'Bt' cultivars increased steadily, reaching nearly 100 per cent by 2009 and effectively eliminating both damage due to the pink bollworm and the need to spray for it: since 2007, virtually no sprays have been applied for this pest in Arizona (Naranjo and Ellsworth, 2010).

Elimination of broad-spectrum insecticide sprays for *P. gossypiella* in turn made it possible to use more selective insecticides (e.g., insect growth regulators such as buprofezin and pyriproxyfen) for another important exotic pest, the sweet potato whitefly (*Bemisia tabaci*), and for native *Lygus* bugs (mainly *L. hesperus*). The use of these more selective insecticides helped conserve important natural enemies in the cotton ecosystem, which further reduced the need for intervention with insecticides. As a result, the average number of sprays applied for arthropod pests on Arizona cotton has fallen from 11.4 per hectare in 1990 to 1.7 in 2009, with concomitant economic and environmental benefits and 'unprecedented stability of ecosystem services' (Naranjo and Ellsworth, 2010).

Development of IPM in China

Agriculture has been practiced in China for more than 7,000 years (Liu et al., 2013) and, according to one report, China currently has a total of 1,648 agricultural pests (724 plant diseases, 838 insects and mites, 64 weeds and 22 rodents) (Zhang et al., 2011). Records of deliberate attempts at pest control first appeared in the Chinese literature in 240 BCE, and the first known attempt at applied biological control (i.e., the deliberate use of a tree ant (*Oecophylla smaragdina*) to control citrus pests in southern China) was recorded in 304 CE (Wang et al., 2003). Today more than 50 per cent of Chinese land is used for agriculture and a rich diversity of crops is grown under a variety of production systems, including both large- and small-scale organic production as well as conventional, high-input intensive systems, protected vegetable production under plastic or glass, and traditional integrated farming systems that combine crops with livestock and fish farming (Liu et al., 2013).

From the 1950s to the early 1970s, crop protection practices in China mirrored those in the US, with widespread use of broad-spectrum organochlorine insecticides such as BHC and DDT, and subsequent increases in public concern over pollution, insecticide resistance and residues in food (Wang et al., 2003). In 1975 the Chinese Ministry of Agriculture officially approved the concept of 'Integrated pest control with prevention first' as the national guiding principle for crop protection and from 1983 onwards, a successive series of national five-year plans was implemented to develop IPM techniques and programmes. By 2000, regionally appropriate IPM strategies for all principal cropping systems (rice, wheat, maize, cotton, soybean, vegetables and tree fruit) had been developed, tested and promoted on a large scale. Particular attention was paid to the development of action thresholds for major crop pests, which in some cases were sophisticated enough to take into account the likely impact of natural enemies and the ability of crops to compensate for pest damage. State support also resulted in a nationwide network for pest monitoring and forecasting that is particularly valuable for

predicting movements of major migratory pests (Wang et al., 2003). Furthermore, since 1998 the Chinese Ministry of Agriculture and the National Agro-technical Extension and Service Centre (NATESC) have partnered with the Food and Agriculture Organization of the United Nations (FAO) in conducting an annual national programme of Farmer Field Schools (FFS) aimed at promoting and training farmers in the use of IPM (Anon, 2014; Pontius et al., 2002).

The large-scale, state-supported approach to IPM in China has fostered the development and implementation of some highly innovative programmes that likely would not have been possible elsewhere. For example, approximately four million hectares of maize (the primary Chinese food crop in terms of planting area and total yield) are treated annually with innundative releases of mass-reared parasitic wasps (*Trichogramma* spp.) and other non-chemical control measures for Asian corn borer (*Ostrinia furnacalis*) and similar pests (Wang et al., 2014). This approach was first developed in the 1970s (Wang et al., 2003) and has been greatly refined and expanded since then. Currently, three species of *Trichogramma* are mass-reared on eggs of factitious hosts such as the Chinese oak silkworm (*Antheraea pernyi*) or stored product pests such as the rice moth (*Corcyra cephalonica*) and the Angoumis grain moth (*Sitotroga cerealella*). Mass production techniques are regionally optimized and highly mechanized, with some facilities having the capacity to produce more than 11 million wasps per day (Wang et al., 2014); typically, 150,000 to 300,000 wasps are released per hectare for each generation of corn borer (1–3 generations per year, depending on region). The timing of the first release is based on field monitoring of overwintered larvae, being made ten days after 15–20 per cent have pupated, followed by a second release six days later (Wang et al., 2014). In some areas, these releases have achieved up to 88 per cent parasitism of corn borer eggs and resultant reductions in crop damage in excess of

90 per cent (Wang et al., 2014). Furthermore, in areas where *Trichogramma* spp. have been released annually for many years, long-term reductions in corn borer and other lepidopteran pests have been observed, with concomitant ecological and economic benefits. For example, in one region the average number of corn borer egg masses decreased from approximately 100 per hundred plants in 1974 to 24 in 1981 (Wang et al., 2014). In addition, since corn fields treated with *Trichogramma* are not sprayed with insecticides, increases in the populations of other, endemic natural enemies have been observed, including parasitic wasps that attack the larval and pupal stages of the corn borer, and other species that contribute to the long-term, sustainable control of other corn pests (Wang et al., 2014).

In the context of IPM, however, it is important to realize that this is not a single-tactic approach: these large-scale innundative releases of biological control agents are integrated with other non-chemical control techniques, including the use of disease-resistant varieties and the replacement in crop rotations of spring maize by winter wheat, which reduces subsequent corn borer pressure on crops of summer maize (Wang et al., 2003). Where necessary, too, formulations of the lepidopteran-specific biopesticide *Bacillus thuringiensis* ('Bt') are applied via self-propelled, high-clearance sprayers (Wang et al., 2014). Other approaches are aimed at decreasing the survivorship of overwintered larvae and adults in corn stalk piles. These include treating infested piles with the entomopathogenic fungus *Beauveria bassiana*, and a trap-and-kill programme using light traps that attract adult moths as they emerge from overwintering. In 2010 this type of approach was officially endorsed by the Chinese Ministry of Agriculture as part of its 'Public Plant Protection, Green Plant Protection' programme, which serves as the current standard for crop protection in China (Wang et al., 2014).

15.3 Conclusions

Since the concept of IPM was first articulated more than 50 years ago, many successful IPM programmes have been developed and implemented around the world. Nevertheless, there are still notable barriers to wider adoption, including fluctuating commodity prices, new control products, new invasive pests and the perceived complexity of IPM. The latter has constrained not only the development of programmes targeted at single pests (or pest categories), but also the creation of truly interdisciplinary approaches to crop management that take into account all of the possible pests (including weeds, insects and diseases) that can affect a particular agroecosystem. A multiplicity of strategies developed for a number of individual pests on a particular crop decreases the likelihood of adoption by farmers and underlines the importance of including a sound understanding of the entire farming system (including farmer constraints) when developing IPM programmes.

Given this background, it is perhaps not surprising that in many cases it still requires a catastrophic control failure or other major crisis to force a change from single-tactic, chemical-intensive pest control to a more broadly based, ecologically sound approach. In some cases, one single-tactic approach is simply replaced by another, which can result in additional unforeseen problems. For example, in the Almería region of Spain (the primary area for the production of salad crops in the European Union), a highly chemically orientated approach to pest management was rapidly replaced by augmentative biological control following the detection in 2006 of residues of an illegal pesticide in peppers destined for export. In this case, a combination of effective pesticide residue monitoring, regional (EU) legislation, consumer concerns and consequent pressure from members of the supply chain combined to compel rapid change amongst the region's growers (Glass and González,

2012). IPM programmes based on mass releases of biological control agents were first adopted in pepper crops and subsequently in many others. In peppers alone the area estimated to be using biologically intensive IPM rose from 650ha in 2006/2007 to 7,500ha in 2008 (encompassing 100 per cent of the region's pepper-growing area). By 2009, a total of 23,500ha of Almería's pepper, tomato, cucumber, squash and eggplant crops (50 per cent of the area's total production) were reported to be using this approach (van der Blom et al., 2009), and this had increased to 26,372ha by 2014 (Sanchez et al., 2014). The resultant reduction in insecticide use permitted increased adoption of commercially produced bumblebees to improve fruit set (Glass and González, 2012), improved returns for growers (as compared to conventional chemical control programmes) (Sampson et al., 2009), and reduced the incidence of pepper samples with detectable pesticide residues (Glass and González, 2012). Nevertheless, the prophetic warning by Stern et al. (1959) that 'If an attempt is made to reduce the population level of one kind of animal (for example, a pest insect) by chemical treatment, modification of cultural practices, or by other means, other parts of the ecosystem will be affected as well' once again proved true: in this case, substitution of biological control for chemical control of the primary pests led to an increase in the pest status of species formerly kept in check by insecticides and hence considered to be of only minor importance (van der Blom et al., 2009).

There are other examples in which failing to adopt a holistic, ecosystem approach to pest management has had unintended consequences. Thus successful control of exotic *Opuntia* cacti in Australia by the deliberate introduction (in the early 1900s), of the South American moth *Cactoblastis cactorum*, subsequently led to other, more widespread, introductions of this species in other parts of the world. This eventually resulted in its accidental introduction into Florida, where it subsequently attacked various native cacti, including one extremely rare species (Cory and Myers, 2000); furthermore, it has now become a pest of a recently established exotic edible cactus, *Hylocerus* spp. (dragon fruit). In a similar vein, the widespread adoption of genetically modified crop varieties resistant to the herbicide glyphosate – and the consequent increased use of this material – have resulted in the development of glyphosate-resistant weeds (Duke, 2005; Powles, 2008), underlining importance of one of the fundamental tenets of IPM – that it is (or should be) a *multi-tactic* approach to managing pests.

The development of new tools and technologies for managing pests can be a mixed blessing: on the one hand – as shown by the example of cotton in Arizona – such tools can facilitate the development of pest management programmes that truly integrate a number of different approaches, with an overall reduction in pesticide use. On the other hand – as in the glyphosate example – they can merely result in the substitution of one tactic for another, with unfortunate consequences. At the time of writing, there is considerable interest in the pest management possibilities offered by RNA interference (RNAi) (a process whereby RNA molecules inhibit the expression of certain genes in target pests), which could be delivered either as topical sprays or via genetically modified plants (Lundgren and Duan, 2013). Technologies such as these pose new challenges for those charged with developing robust and appropriate risk assessment protocols, and for those seeking to properly integrate them into existing IPM programmes without adversely affecting non-target species. Mistakes have been made in the past by failing to adopt an ecosystem approach to pest management: let us hope that we are not condemned to repeat them.

References

Agnew, K. (ed.) (1999). *Crop Profile for Cotton in Arizona*, www.ipmcenters.org/cropprofiles/docs/Azcotton.pdf.

Anon (2014). *China National IPM Programme*, www.vegetableipmasia.org/Countries/China1.html.

Arizona Cotton Research and Protection Council (2010). Southwest Boll Weevil Eradication Program, www.azcotton.org/insect eradication/swbollweevil.html.

Bale, J.S., van Lenteren, J.C. and Bigler, F. (2008). Biological control and sustainable food production. *Philosophical Transactions of the Royal Society of London Series B: Biological Science*, 363, 761–776.

Bebber, D.P., Holmes, T. and Gurr, S.J. (2014). The global spread of crop pests and pathogens. *Global Ecology and Biogeography*, 23(12), 1398–1407.

Birch, A.N.E., Begg, G.S. and Squire, G.R. (2011). How agro-ecological research helps to address food security issues under new IPM and pesticide reduction policies for global crop production systems. *Journal of Experimental Botany*, 62, 3251–3261.

Bruinsma, J. (ed.) (2003). *World Agriculture: Towards 2015/2030. An FAO Perspective*. London: Earthscan.

Bueno, V.H.P. and van Lenteren, J.C. (2010). Biological control of pests in protected cultivation: implementation in Latin America and successes in Europe. In N. Barreto (ed.), *Memorias, XXXVII Congreso Sociedad Colombiana de Entomologia*, Bogota, Columbia, 30 June–2 July, pp. 261–269.

Carson, R. (1962). *Silent Spring*. Boston, MA: Houghton Mifflin.

Chu, C-C., Henneberry, T.J., Weddle, R.C., Natwick, E.T., Carson, J.R., Valenzuela, S.L., Birdsall, S.L. and Staten, R.T. (1996). Reduction of pink bollworm (Lepidoptera: Gelichiidae) populations in the Imperial Valley, California, following mandatory short-season cotton management systems. *Journal of Economic Entomology*, 89, 175–182.

Cory, J.S. and Myers, J. H. (2000). Direct and indirect ecological effects of biological control. *Trends in Ecology and Evolution*, 15, 137–139.

Díaz, B.M., Biurrún, R., Moreno, A., Nebreda, M. and Fereres, A. (2006). Impact of ultraviolet-blocking plastic films on insect vectors of virus diseases infesting crisp lettuce. *HortScience*, 41, 711–716.

Dinham, B. (1993). *The Pesticide Hazard: A Global Health and Environmental Audit*. London: Zed Books.

Duke, S.O. (2005). Taking stock of herbicide-resistant crops ten years after introduction. *Pest Management Science*, 61, 211–218.

Frank, S. D. (2010). Biological control of arthropod pests using banker plant systems: past progress and future directions. *Biological Control*, 52, 8–16.

Glass, R. and González, F.J.E. (2012). Biological control in the greenhouses of Almería and challenges for a sustainable intensive production. *Outlooks on Pest Management*, 23, 276–279.

Graham, S. (2010). Starting biocontrol programs in ornamental greenhouses. *Greenhouse Product News*, April, 26–29.

Haynes, I., Lamine, C., Wierzbicka, A., Szabo, Z., Lehota, J., Vandenberg, I., Buurma, J., Maraccini, E., Moonen, C., Williamson, S. and Paratte, R. (2010). Are supermarkets an appropriate tool for facilitating the transition to low input farming practices? In I. Darnhofer and M. Grötzer (eds.), *Building Sustainable Rural Futures: The Added Value of Systems Approaches in Times of Change and Uncertainty*. 9th European International Farming System Association Symposium, Vienna, Austria, 4–7 July, pp. 1855–1864.

Hickman, G.W. (2014). *International Greenhouse Vegetable Production – Statistics*. Mariposa, CA: Cuesta Roble Greenhouse Vegetable Consulting.

Isley, D. and Berg, W.J. (1924). *The Boll Weevil Problem in Arkansas*. University of Arkansas Agricultural Experiment Station Bulletin No. 190.

Kogan, M. (1998). Integrated pest management: historical perspectives and contemporary developments. *Annual Review of Entomology*, 43, 243–270.

Liu, Y., Duan, M. and Yu, Z. (2013). Agricultural landscapes and biodiversity in China. *Agriculture, Ecosystems and Environment*, 166, 46–54.

Lundgren, J.G. and Duan, J.J. (2013). RNAi-based insecticidal crops: potential effects on nontarget species. *BioScience*, 63, 657–665.

Naranjo, S.E. and Ellsworth, P.C. (2009). Fifty years of the integrated control concept: moving the model and implementation forward in Arizona. *Pest Management Science*, 65, 1267–1286.

Naranjo, S.E. and Ellsworth, P.C. (2010). Fourteen years of *Bt* cotton advances IPM in Arizona. *Southwestern Entomologist*, 35, 437–444.

National Cotton Council of America (2014). Eradication Administration, Program Operations, and Components, www.cotton.org/tech/pest/bollweevil/eradication3.cfm.

Oerke, E-C. (2006). Crop losses to pests. *Journal of Agricultural Science*, 144, 31–45.

Parolin, P., Bresch, C., Ruiz, G., Desneu, N. and Poncet, C. (2013). Testing banker plants for biological control of mites on roses. *Phytoparasitica*, 41, 249–262.

Pickett, A.D., Patterson, N.A., Stulz, H.T. and Lord, F.T. (1946). The influence of spray programs on the fauna of apple orchards in Nova Scotia: I. An appraisal of the problem and a method of approach. *Scientific Agriculture*, 26, 590–600.

Pilkington, L.J., Messelink, G., van Lenteren, J.C. and le Motte, K. (2010). 'Protected biological control': biological pest management in the greenhouse industry. *Biological Control*, 52, 216–220.

Pimentel, D. (2005). Environmental and economic costs of the application of pesticides primarily in the United States. *Environment, Development and Sustainability*, 7, 229–252.

Pontius, J., Dilts, R. and Bartlett, A. (ed.) (2002). *From Farmer Field School to Community IPM: Ten Years of IPM Training in Asia*. Rome: FAO, www.fao.org/docrep/005/ac834e /ac834e00.htm#Contents.

Portorff, L.P. and Panter, K.L. (2008). Integrated pest management and biological control in high tunnel production. *HortTechnology*, 19, 61–65.

Powles, S.B. (2008). Evolved glyphosate-resistant weeds around the world: lessons to be learnt. *Pest Management Science*, 64, 360–365.

Sampson, C., Eekhoff, D., Hernandez-Parra, R. and Lewis, J. (2009). The economic benefits of adopting integrated pest management in protected pepper, chrysanthemum and strawberry crops. *IOBC/WPRS Bulletin*, 49, 15–20.

Sanchez, C., Gallego, J.R., Gamez, M. and Cabello, T. (2014). Intensive biological control in Spanish greenhouses: problems of the success. *International Journal of Biological, Veterinary, Agricultural and Food Engineering*, 8, http://internationalscienceindex.org/publications/9999557/intensive-biological-control-in-spanish-greenhouses-problems-of-the-success.

Shipp, L., Johansen, N., Vänninen, I. and Jacobson, R. (2011). Greenhouse climate: an important consideration when developing pest management programs for greenhouse crops. *Acta Horticulturae*, 893, 133–143.

Spurgeon, D.W. (2007). Ecologically based pest management in cotton. In O. Koul and G.W. Cuperus (ed.) *Ecologically Based Integrated Pest Management*. Wallingford: CABI International, pp. 367–405.

Stern, V.M., Smith, R.F., van den Bosch, R. and Hagen, K.S. (1959). The integration of chemical and biological control of the spotted alfalfa aphid: the integrated control concept. *Hilgardia*, 29, 81–101.

University of California (2014). Definition of Integrated Pest Management, www.ipm.ucdavis.edu/ GENERAL/ipmdefinition.html.

USDA-APHIS (2013). *Questions and Answers: Boll Weevil Eradication Factsheet*, www.aphis.usda.gov/publications/plant_health/2013/faq_boll_weevil_erad.pdf.

van der Blom, J., Robledo, A., Torres, S. and Sanchéz, J.A. (2009). Consequences of the wide-scale implementation of biological control in greenhouse horticulture in Almería, Spain. *IOBC/WPRS Bulletin*, 49, 9–13.

van Lenteren, J.C. (2009). IPM in greenhouse vegetables and ornamentals. In E.B. Radcliffe, W.D. Hutchison and R.E. Cancelado (ed.), *Integrated Pest Management*. Cambridge: Cambridge University Press, pp. 354–365.

van Lenteren, J.C., van Roermund, H.J.W. and Sütterlin, S. (1996). Biological control of greenhouse whitefly (*Trialeurodes vaporariorum*) with the parasitoid *Encarsia formosa*: how does it work? *Biological Control*, 6, 1–10.

Wang, Z-Y., He, K-L., Zhao, J-Z. and Zhou, D-R. (2003). Integrated pest management in China. In K.M. Maredia, D. Dakouo and D. Mota-Sanchez (ed.), *Integrated Pest Management in the Global Arena*. Wallingford: CABI Publishing, pp. 197–207.

Wang, Z-Y., He, K-L., Zhang, F., Lu, X. and Babandreier, D. (2014). Mass rearing and release of *Trichogramma* for biological control of insect pests of corn in China. *Biological Control*, 68, 136–144.

Warnert, J. (2009). The 50th anniversary of a great idea. *California Agriculture*, 63, 160–161.

Zhang, W-J., Jiang, F-B. and Ou, J-F. (2011). Global pesticide consumption and pollution: with China as a focus. *Proceedings of the International Academy of Ecology and Environmental Sciences*, 1, 125–144.

Zhao, X. and Tisdell, C. (2010). A comparative economic study of China's and Australia's cotton production: differences, trends and analysis. In T.H. Lee (ed.), *Agricultural Economics: New Research*. Hauppauge: Nova Science Publishers, pp. 37–65.

chapter 16

Colony collapse disorder and other threats to honey bees

Ernesto Guzman-Novoa

Abstract

Honey bees have played an important role in human history. Not only are they valuable pollinators of horticultural crops but they are also important for the sustainability of many of the
wild and cultivated plants that we enjoy. Honey and other products produced by bees remain
popular in many parts of the world and it is estimated that, due to their role in crop pollination,
honey bees are responsible for the production of one-third of the food consumed in western
societies. In recent decades, many populations of wild and domesticated bees have been decimated as a result of changes to the environment and infectious disease. Due to the complex
ecology and important role of the honey bee in modern society, it has been necessary to apply
an interdisciplinary approach to conserve remaining bee populations and to better understand
the reasons for the current worldwide population decline.

16.1 Introduction

Currently, managed and natural ecosystems
are threatened by large-scale declines in honey
bee (*Apis mellifera* L.) populations, mainly in
countries of the northern hemisphere. Between
2006 and 2014, American, Canadian and
European beekeepers lost about one-third of
their bee colonies each year (Currie et al., 2010;
Guzman-Novoa et al., 2010; CAPA, 2014; van
Engelsdorp et al., 2008; Stankus, 2014). These
substantial losses of colonies are unprecedented
and have endangered the continuous supply of
honey bees as pollinators of flowering plants,

which has strong economic and ecological
implications.

The term 'colony collapse disorder' (CCD)
has been coined to characterize the massive loss
of honey bee colonies (van Engelsdorp et al.,
2009) and many suspects have been suggested as
potential culprits of CCD, but no clear explanation has yet been found. However, most scientists
agree that it is likely due to the interaction and
effect of a number of factors, ranging from parasites and viruses to colony transportation-related
stresses, single-source diets, inclement weather
and pesticides (Stankus, 2008, 2014). It seems
that a broad suite of stresses, acting in concert,

is taking its toll on honey bees. Stress in general increases human susceptibility to illness, and the same idea applies to honey bees. Stressed, their capacity to ward off primary infections of the well-known suite of larval and adult diseases is reduced. Moreover, stressed, their capacity to fight secondary infections is lessened.

Honey bees are valuable pollinators of horticultural crops; it is estimated that they are responsible for the production of one third of the food consumed in Western societies (Plate 25). Therefore it is important to establish multisectoral and interdisciplinary approaches to better understand the causes of CCD and to reduce the rate of colony losses. In this chapter, I discuss the antecedents, possible causes, implications and potential solutions of the massive die-offs of bees that have occurred in recent years worldwide.

16.2 Antecedents

CCD refers to a poorly understood syndrome characterized by an abrupt loss of worker bees in a honey bee colony, which leads to its collapse (van Engelsdorp et al., 2009). This disorder was first noticed in 2006 in eastern USA when beekeepers reported that their colonies were losing populations at an alarming rate (Stankus, 2008). Since then, massive colony losses have been reported not only from the USA, but also from Canada and European countries such as Spain, France, Italy, the UK and others, as well as from Asia (Stankus, 2014). Before CCD-like cases were first described, annual colony losses in the USA averaged less than 20 per cent for more than a decade, but since CCD was reported, more than 30 per cent of managed colonies in many countries collapse each year (van Engelsdorp et al., 2009). This death rate is at least two times the expected loss and has occurred every year for nine consecutive years. In extreme cases, a considerable number of beekeepers have reported

losing more than 90 per cent of their colonies (Stankus, 2014).

There have been events resembling CCD in the past. In those instances, other terms have been used to describe the syndrome, for example, 'disappearing disease', 'spring dwindle', 'May disease' and others whose causes have not yet been determined (Oldroyd, 2007). However, those cases of severe colony losses did not occur for nine years in a row as has been the case for CCD between 2006 and 2015.

16.3 Symptoms

CCD has been characterized as a multi-symptom syndrome (van Engelsdorp et al., 2009). Not all symptoms are observed in all cases, but those most frequently reported include a sudden disappearance of worker bees leading to weak, depopulated colonies, with little or no build-up of dead bees within or in front of the hives, presence of food stores not being consumed by bees, unattended brood and other less frequently observed symptoms. A collapsing colony shows too small a workforce for colony maintenance and that workforce is made up of young bees. Additionally, it has been reported that honey from CCD affected colonies does not seem to attract bees from other colonies, although it is not known why this occurs (Kevan et al., 2007; Stankus, 2008).

16.4 Impact and implications

The Western honey bee is a beneficial insect to humans and plants. Most people know about honey bees because they produce honey and because they sting. However, the importance of these insects lies more on their role as pollinators of flowering plants, which is necessary for their fertilization and ultimately their reproduction.

The availability of wild pollinators is already reduced due to modern agricultural practices and thus honey bees have become the major and most important managed pollinators. Not only do they pollinate flowers of agricultural crops but flowers of wild plants as well and, thus, play a critical role in the production of food and in sustaining biodiversity. They are responsible for pollination of approximately one third of the Western world's crop species, including almonds, peaches, soybeans, apples, pears, cherries, raspberries, cranberries, strawberries, watermelons, cantaloupes and cucumbers (McGregor, 1976). Many but not all of these plants can be pollinated by other insects, including other bee species. However, even though on a per-individual basis, many other insect species are actually more efficient at pollinating, on the crop types where honey bees are used, most native pollinators cannot be mass-produced and utilized (at a commercial scale) as easily or as effectively as honey bees. Numerous hives each containing thousands of bees can be moved from crop to crop, and they will visit many plants in large numbers, compensating via saturation for what they lack in efficiency. The commercial viability of these crops is therefore strongly tied to honey bees and to the beekeeping industry (McGregor, 1976).

The value of pollination by honey bees in agricultural crops ranges between US$9 billion and $18 billion a year, just in the United States (Stankus, 2008) and exceeds $120 billion globally (Gallai et al., 2009). Beyond the farm, if the central role of honey bees in sustaining plant life is considered, then it is easy to link these insects with maintenance of the planet's water, oxygen and carbon dioxide. The impact in biodiversity is huge because its ecological value is incalculable. Therefore, the role of honey bees as pollinators is central to life support systems on earth. It is then understandable that massive losses of honey bee colonies in consecutive years have strong economic and ecological implications.

16.5 Presumed causes

Many factors have been mentioned in the literature in association with CCD cases. However, when the information published on the potential culprits of this syndrome is analysed, the most frequently suspected causes of CCD include pathogens, pesticides, stress caused by transportation or malnutrition, deficient hive management, adverse climatic effects and other factors less frequently reported (Stankus, 2014). Currently, the consensus among scientists is that most CCD cases are caused by a combination of factors having additive or synergistic effects (Oldroyd, 2007; Van Der Sluijs et al., 2013; Williams et al., 2010). The combined effects of several factors may debilitate the bees' natural defences inhibiting their immune responses, which might make them more susceptible to diseases and parasites, with the end result of colony collapse.

Pathogens

Among pathogens, the most commonly found in CCD cases, are the ectoparasitic mite, *Varroa destructor*, and the microsporidian fungi *Nosema apis* and *Nosema ceranae* (Cox-Foster et al., 2007; Guzman-Novoa et al., 2010; Higes et al., 2008; Le Conte et al., 2010; van Engelsdorp et al., 2009). Viruses transmitted to bees by parasitic mites have also been found in CCD cases (Ball and Bailey, 1997; Berthoud et al., 2010; Carreck et al., 2010; Dainat et al., 2012; de Miranda et al., 2010).

Varroa destructor

V. destructor, an external parasite visible to the naked eye, is the most damaging single biotic agent affecting honey bees (Plate 26). Parasitism by this mite has killed millions of colonies worldwide, resulting in the loss of billions of dollars in agricultural crops (Sanford, 2001). *V. destructor* is a relatively new parasite of *A. mellifera* (less than 100 years of interaction), and therefore it is generally highly pathogenic to its host. *V. destructor* reproduces in bee brood, feeding on the haemolymph (blood) of larvae, pupae and, later, adult bees, thus shortening their life span (Schneider and Drescher, 1987). In addition, associated with varroa mite infestations is a complex of viral infections (Kevan et al., 2006) that have also been found in samples of bees taken from CCD affected colonies (Shen et al., 2005). Thus, *V. destructor* not only weakens their hosts by feeding on their blood, but also by transmitting viruses to them. Parasitism by *V. destructor* also can inhibit immune responses and favour viral infections in infested bees (Guzman-Novoa et al., 2013; Navajas et al., 2008; Yang and Cox-Foster, 2005). On the behavioural level, varroa mites hamper non-associative learning (Kralj et al., 2007), affect flight duration and orientation of foragers, and reduce the proportion of foragers that return to the hive (Kralj and Fuchs, 2006) with a consequent reduction in honey production (Emsen et al., 2014).

Researchers in Canada studied honey bee populations and collapse rates in more than 400 colonies, finding that *V. destructor* was associated with 85 per cent of the colony mortality cases. Additionally, varroa mite infestations significantly decreased spring and summer colony populations (Guzman-Novoa et al., 2010). The authors concluded that varroa mites alone or in combination with other factors could have a strong impact on the survivorship and populations of honey bee colonies.

Variability in susceptibility to *V. destructor* varies with host genotype. *Varroa* has been a major health problem for honey bees in most countries, but it does not appear to be a serious pest in southern Africa and in the South American tropics. The tropical climate and tropically adapted bees, such as the so-called Africanized honey bees (descendants of *A. m. scutellata*),

both play a role in maintaining reduced levels of mite infestation (Guzman-Novoa et al., 1999; Medina-Flores et al., 2014). Known mechanisms of resistance against *V. destructor* in honey bees include high levels of expression of hygienic and grooming behaviour (Arechavaleta-Velasco and Guzman-Novoa, 2001; Boecking and Spivak, 1999; Guzman-Novoa, 2011; Guzman-Novoa et al., 2012; Page and Guzman-Novoa, 1997), as well as reduced susceptibility to mite infestation and reproduction (Emsen et al., 2012; Guzman-Novoa, 2011). Since some of the above mechanisms have a genetic component, it should be possible to breed for resistance against varroa mites in honey bee populations to reduce the dependency on synthetic miticides to control the parasite.

Honey bee viruses

Recent studies suggest that *V. destructor* may be so harmful to honey bees not only because of its feeding on the insect's haemolymph, but also because it transmits and favours the multiplication of honey bee viruses. As evidence accumulates, it is clearer that viruses play an important role in deteriorating bees' health. Increases in the incidence and levels of several honey bee viruses have been observed with *V. destructor* as an inducer or vector of several of them (Genersch and Aubert, 2010). The viruses most commonly found in surveys of honey bee colonies worldwide, are deformed wing virus (DWV), acute bee paralysis virus (ABPV), sac brood virus (SBV), black queen cell virus (BQCV), Kashmir bee virus (KBV) and Israeli acute paralysis virus (IAPV) (Ball and Bailey, 1997; Genersch and Aubert, 2010). DWV, ABPV and KBV have been associated with cases of bee mortality (Ball and Bailey, 1997; Berthoud et al., 2010; Carreck et al., 2010; de Miranda et al., 2010; Francis et al., 2013; Martin et al., 2012), and IAPV has been related to CCD (Cox-Foster et al., 2007).

In particular, DWV has been frequently found in samples of bees taken from collapsed or weakly populated colonies that are heavily infested with *V. destructor* (Francis et al., 2013; Martin et al., 2012). DWV is a RNA virus that produces several symptoms on affected bees, such as impaired behaviour, deformed appendages, like wings and legs (Plate 27), and reduced overwintering colony survival (Dainat et al., 2012; Highfield et al., 2009). Indeed, DWV replication is triggered by *V. destructor* feeding on the bees (Martin et al., 2012).

Studies have shown some evidence indicating resistance to viruses in certain honey bee strains (Emsen et al., 2015; Hamiduzzaman et al., 2015; Locke et al., 2014). If the variability in susceptibility to viruses is at least partially genetic in origin, it would be possible to select bees for virus resistance in addition to controlling varroa mite infestations to reduce virus transmission in honey bee colonies.

Nosema apis and Nosema ceranae

Nosema disease or nosemosis is one of the most prevalent diseases of Western honey bees (Matheson, 1993). This disease is caused by the fungi *Nosema apis* and the newly detected *N. ceranae*, spore-forming microsporidians that are obligate intracellular parasites which infect epithelial cells of the honey bee midgut or ventriculus (Fries, 1997). Newly emerged bees become infected by ingesting *Nosema* spores (Plate 28) when cleaning combs soiled with faeces from affected bees or during feeding or grooming (Fries, 1997). Spores germinate quickly after entering the ventriculus, and the epithelial cells of this organ are infected when the vegetative stage of the parasite is introduced by way of the hollow polar filament. The vegetative stage multiplies and in 6–10 days the infected epithelial cells become filled with new spores. Maturation of spores occurs and epithelial cells burst, releasing infective spores into the midgut lumen to be excreted with the faeces and the cycle is repeated (Bailey and Ball, 1991). The disease impairs the digestion of pollen, thereby shortening the life of the bee. *Nosema* induced mortality is most noticeable in spring, as bees are restricted from cleansing flights by cold weather (Fries, 1997). The necessary winter confinement of honey bees in cold climates puts beekeeping operations especially at risk of *nosema* infection in Northern countries. Additionally, nosema infections decrease honey production and increase queen supersedure (Bailey and Ball, 1991).

N. apis was thought to be the only *Nosema* species to infect Western honey bees and to cause nosema disease in these insects until just a few years ago. It was recently found that *N. ceranae*, a parasite of the Asian honey bee, *Apis cerana*, also infects *A. mellifera* in different continents (Higes et al., 2006; Klee et al., 2007). This 'new' *Nosema* species has been associated with the collapse of thousands of colonies in parts of Europe (Higes et al., 2006, 2008; Martín-Hernández et al., 2007; Paxton, 2010) and thus could be a likely suspect of colony losses in the USA and Canada. However, because studies conducted so far have shown inconsistent results, the relative weight of nosema disease in the mortality of colonies is still a controversial matter (Cox-Foster et al., 2007; Fries, 2010; Guzman-Novoa et al., 2010; Stankus, 2014; van Engelsdorp et al., 2008). It is possible, however, that the same *nosema* species may cause varying degrees of damage to honey bees in different geographical locations due to differences in pathogenicity and virulence, and/or differences in environmental effects (Martín-Hernández et al., 2007; Fries, 2010).

The control of nosemosis in *A. mellifera* has been almost exclusively done using the antibiotic bicyclohexylammonium fumagillin (fumagillin), which is isolated from the fungus *Aspergillus fumigatus* (Huang et al., 2013). This antibiotic has been used for more than 60 years and, in most of the world, is the only antibiotic approved for use in controlling *N. apis* and *N. cer-anae* in honey bees. Fumagillin has been shown to be effective in reducing infection levels of *N. apis* (Webster, 1994) as well as *N. ceranae* (Higes et al., 2011; Williams et al., 2008). However, Huang et al. (2013) showed that decreasing levels of fumagillin lead to *N. ceranae* resistance and infection levels greater than those in untreated, infected hives. It is because of this resistance and the ever-present risk of antibiotic contamination of honey that research into natural, alternative treatments for *N. ceranae* is so greatly needed.

Pesticides

Some pesticides are highly toxic to bees and have been found to be involved in multiple incidents of acute poisoning of these insects (Plate 29). It is, however, not possible to estimate what proportion of CCD cases can be solely attributed to pesticides. Neonicotinoid insecticides in particular, have been frequently mentioned as a possible cause of CCD in recent years. However, the magnitude of the damage caused by these pesticides is controversial; while some reports conclude that neonicotinoids harm bees in the amounts typically used in crops, others claim that the evidence is not conclusive (Van Der Sluijs et al., 2013).

Neonicotinoids, pesticides that have a chemical structure similar to that of nicotine, were developed during the last decades of the twentieth century and are today the most widely used insecticides, accounting for 25 per cent of the world's pesticide market (Jeschke et al., 2011). Neonicotinoids act on the nicotinic nAChRs receptors of insects and by binding to the target site mediate the excitatory synaptic transmission in the central nervous system causing a neurotoxic effect; as a consequence, the insects experiment an accumulation of acetylcholine that leads to paralysis and death (Jeschke et al., 2011).

Neonicotinoids can be sprayed on crops but they are mostly used as seed dressings and act systemically by spreading through the tissues of plants as they grow, protecting them from many insects. They can also be found in the pollen and nectar of plants, which may impact the health of non-target insects such as the honey bee. Clothianidin, the neonicotinoid insecticide most commonly used to coat corn and soybean seeds, is highly toxic to bees. The estimated oral LD50 of clothianidin is 4 ng/bee, about 10,000 lower than that of DDT (Goulson, 2013). Besides potential exposure by nectar and pollen consumption, bees can also be exposed to this insecticide by visiting contaminated non-target vegetation growing near crops, such as dandelions. Exposure of honey bees to high levels of clothianidin has been documented through contact with dust drifting from seeding machines during sowing (Krupke et al., 2012). This talc, released into the air, is carried out by the wind and may contaminate vegetation visited by bees. This seems to have been the source of contamination in the cases of high bee mortality reported in the provinces of Ontario and Quebec, Canada, in 2012 and 2013. During the spring of 2012, Health Canada's Pest Management Regulatory Agency (PMRA) received an unusually high number of reports of honey bee mortalities from corn-growing areas. These reports coincided with the planting of clothianidin-treated corn seed. From their investigation, PMRA concluded that the neonicotinoid insecticide used to coat corn seeds contributed to the majority of these cases of bee mortality. In the spring and summer of 2013, PMRA continued to receive reports of honey bee mortality from locations where clothianidin-treated corn and soybean seeds were being used (Health Canada, 2013).

The above evidence and other reports in the literature (Blacquière et al., 2012; Goulson, 2013) clearly show that clothianidin and other neonicotinoid insecticides can cause acute toxicity and mortality in honey bees under certain conditions in field settings, such as when dust containing the insecticide is released into the air during sowing. Thus, the exposure of honey bees to neonicotinoid insecticides is likely unavoidable during planting if apiaries are located in corn and soybean growing areas. The other means of neonicotinoid exposure is through the collection of pollen and nectar of seed-treated plants by forager bees (Blacquière et al., 2012). Therefore, an important question is whether the typical levels of exposure encountered by bees in the pollen or nectar of neonicotinoid-treated corn and soybean are likely to significantly impact honey bees at the individual and colony levels. The literature indicates that concentrations of neonicotinoids applied as seed dressings may reach 9 ppb in nectar and 51 ppb in pollen based on the mean maximum levels obtained from several studies (Goulson, 2013). Considering these values and the amount of nectar and pollen that larvae and adults of honey bees can consume, it seems unlikely that they will be exposed to LD50 concentrations of neonicotinoids (4–5 ng/insect; Suchail et al., 2000) in the short term, but the persistence of neonicotinoids means that the pesticides could accumulate over time in the honey bee body, resulting in negative impacts on bee health.

Although some studies using field-realistic doses in pollen and nectar showed no significant lethal effects on bees (Cresswell, 2011; Cutler and Scott-Dupree, 2007; Schmuck et al., 2001), there is evidence of significant neonicotinoid sublethal effects on honey bee foragers. It has been found, for example, that exposure to sublethal doses of neonicotinoids may result in reduced olfaction (Yang et al., 2012; Williamson and Wright, 2013), learning and foraging ability (Decourtye et al., 2004; Henry et al., 2012), which may lead to disruption of foraging activity, possibly preventing them from finding their way back to the hive (Bortolotti et al., 2003). Neonicotinoids also impair the bees' memory, which again may result in failure to return to

the hive and may affect other behaviours that in turn negatively impact the whole colony. Moreover, neonicotinoids can reduce longevity and affect immune responses, reproduction, metabolism and other physiological mechanisms (Desneux et al., 2007). When sublethal doses of neonicotinoids suppress the bees' immune system, debilitated bees show an increase of viral infections (Di Prisco et al., 2011). Therefore, long-term effects of neonicotinoids may affect population dynamics and colony survival. A recent study showed that 60 per cent of queens heading neonicotinoid-exposed colonies were superseded within one year post-exposure, but not control colonies (Sandrock et al., 2014).

Thus far, studies have primarily examined potential causative factors of CCD in isolation. However, in real-world conditions, honey bees are likely exposed to multiple stresses in any given year, such as sublethal neonicotinoid exposure, *V. destructor* parasitism and DWV infection that together may cause CCD-like symptoms. However, not much evidence has been generated on the interactive effects of neonicotinoids and pathogens. Only two studies have examined the interaction of neonicotinoids with honey bee parasites, such as *Nosema* (Alaux et al., 2010; Pettis et al., 2013), and there has been no study examining the synergistic effects of neonicotinoids and *V. destructor* on honey bee health, two of the main suspects of colony mortality. Therefore, more research on the effect of multiple factors is warranted, as well as more field studies involving neonicotinoids and other factors.

Miticides used in hives

The current approach for controlling parasitic mites is the use of synthetic acaricides. However, these products have significant disadvantages; they can leave residues and accumulate in beeswax and thus comb cells may contain them at levels that could be harmful to larvae and to adult bees. Residues of these chemicals could also contaminate honey, making it unsafe for human consumption (Rosenkranz et al., 2010). Laboratory experiments have shown that miticides can shorten the length of life of bees, impair their learning ability, affect the queen's egg laying rate and suppress the expression of immune-related genes (Boncristiani et al., 2012). Therefore, miticides may also play a role in cases of CCD. Additionally, if mites become resistant to the active ingredients in miticides, populations of *Varroa* will increase, which may result in colony collapse.

Migratory beekeeping-related stress

Most CCD cases in the USA have been reported from operations that practice migratory beekeeping. Beekeepers rent hives to growers to pollinate different crops and thus, they are transported on trucks, sometimes thousands of kilometres and several times a year. For example, close to 1.5 million hives are brought to California from all over USA to pollinate almonds. The management of hives involved in this activity, including confining bees inside hives by closing their entrances, moving hives on trucks, subjecting them to extreme temperatures and placing them in field with monocultures, is stressful to the bees. When entrances are removed, it is usual to find numerous cadavers of bees at the bottom board of hives. Transportation may also inhibit the immune system of bees, increasing their susceptibility to pathogens and insecticides (Stankus, 2014).

Nutritional stress

Bees that are transported and used for pollination services on large monocultures are placed in environments where little or no food choice is available to them; they are basically forced to feed upon a single source of pollen, that of the crop being pollinated. A single source of pollen may not contain all the nutrients required to sustain bee health. Conversely, bees of hives that are not rented for pollination have access to a variety of pollen sources that theoretically would provide a more balanced diet to rear their larvae. It is known that a diverse diet of a mixture of pollens from different plant sources is beneficial to bees (Schmidt et al., 1987, 1995). For example, bees fed with a blend of pollen sources show higher expression levels of immune-related genes making them more resistant to pesticides (Schmehl et al., 2014). Thus, nutritional imbalance could explain, at least in part, some of the observed symptoms in CCD cases. Moreover, the pollen and nectar of some crops such as almonds may be toxic to bees when exposed to them for long periods (Kevan and Ebert, 2005).

Deficient hive management

Sometimes honey bee colonies do not receive proper management because beekeepers split them late in the season or because they are not sufficiently fed in periods of scarcity. Similarly, if colonies are not adequately treated against parasites and diseases or are not re-queened when required, hives could contain weakly populated colonies at the end of the season, right before winter. Thus, deficient management may contribute to increase the probability of colony collapse. Guzman-Novoa et al. (2010) found that weak colonies, likely resulting from deficient hive management, was the second cause of colony mortality in their study.

Other factors

In addition to the above, many other factors have been mentioned as possible culprits of CCD, some of them with little or no scientific support. For example, it has been suggested that electromagnetic radiation from cellular phones, genetically modified crops, global warming, reduced genetic variability of bees and micro-organisms not yet discovered, could be potential causes of CCD. However, thus far, none of these claims have been supported with consistent research data.

16.6 Potential solutions

Efforts to mitigate losses of honey bee colonies require the collaboration of beekeepers, scientists and regulatory agencies. Considerable efforts and resources are being invested by governments across the globe to halt the deterioration of honey bee health. Scientists continue testing hypotheses related to bee declines to provide further insights into the problem and strategies to improve hive management. In fact, CCD-related research has already yielded some promising results in our understanding of this complex syndrome. Also, *Varroa*-resistant bee stocks are being bred, and experiments with new soft chemicals to control parasitism by *Varroa* and *Nosema* are being conducted, as well as others aimed at reducing pathogen levels in combs. Additionally, researchers are working on the development of balanced diets to supplement colonies used for pollination, and protocols of best management practices that will provide beekeepers with guidelines to improve the health of their bees are under development.

Current best management practices (BMP) include recommendations on hive equipment, pesticide protection, bee health, nutrition and honey harvest. Beekeepers should follow practices that help reduce the impact of CCD-related factors on honey bee health such as old comb replacement in brood chambers, disinfection or sterilization of beekeeping equipment, use of screened bottom boards in hives, wrapping hives to increase overwinter survival, monitor-

ing hives for varroa levels, inspecting colonies for signs of diseases, re-queening colonies with stock selected for disease resistance or hygienic behaviour, treating colonies against diseases using registered medicaments and following label instructions, supplementing feed to colonies before winter, uniting weak colonies with populated colonies during fall, having colonies inspected and certified by animal health authorities when trading bees or equipment, etc. Plant growers could also contribute to decrease the rate of colony losses by implementing BMP such as planting with seeders adapted to minimize drift of toxic material, avoiding spraying insecticides when crops are blooming and during the day. Growers could also implement IPM practices to use pesticides only when needed. Moreover, they could also advise beekeepers to move colonies before applying a pesticide.

Programmes and initiatives to encourage the resurgence and conservation of wild pollinators and to protect managed pollinators have been implemented in several European countries, as well as in the USA and Canada, although with modest results so far. These initiatives involve the revision of conservation practices to provide sustainable habitat for pollinators, the provision of pollinator-friendly vegetation, and outreach campaigns to increase the awareness about the importance of pollinators. Ideally, agricultural ecosystems should be managed in ways that provide a friendly environment to pollinators without sacrificing yields and profit; for example, by leaving portions of uncultivated land. Other practices such as planting several crops instead of monocultures and decreasing the use of pesticides would extend the number and diversity of wild pollinators. Economic incentives should be provided through ecosystem services so that bee pollination becomes ecologically based rather than management based. Therefore, strategies aimed at combining economic prosperity with environmental sustainability should be further developed and supported.

Despite the above efforts made to control some of the factors associated with CCD and to increase wild pollinators, not much has been done to significantly decrease the impact of pesticides on bee populations. Regulatory policies are currently considered and implemented in different countries. The European Union, for example, invoked the precautionary principle to support their decision of banning the use of three neonicotinoid pesticides, despite the fact that the scientific evidence is still incomplete and inconclusive. They argued that there was sufficient circumstantial and laboratory evidence to infer that neonicotinoids might have a significant impact on pollinators' survival. In Canada, specifically in Ontario, the provincial government has passed regulations that will restrict the use of neonicotinoid insecticides based on proven need by the growers. Meanwhile, the USA government continues debating about whether or not restrictive policies on the use of neonicotinoids should be implemented in that country.

16.7 Conclusion

Overall, it seems that a number of factors acting alone or in combination, are stressing out honey bees, affecting their health and survivorship. More research is needed to establish the relative contribution of multiple factors on CCD cases, as well as to find solutions to ameliorate honey bee health and to diminish the impact of the suspected causes of CCD on honey bee colonies. Additionally, policies and practices that promote friendly environments to pollinators are required, while maintaining productivity in agricultural ecosystems, something not easy to achieve, but hopefully possible in the future.

References

Alaux, J.L., Brunet, C., Dussaubat, F., Mondet, S., Tchamitchan, M., Cousin, J., Brillard, A., Baldy, L.P., Belzunces, Y. and Le Conte, Y. (2010). Interactions between *Nosema* microspores and a neonicotinoid weaken honeybees (*Apis mellifera*). *Environmental Microbiology*, 12, 774–782.

Arechavaleta-Velasco, M.E. and Guzman-Novoa, E. (2001). Relative effect of four characteristics that restrain the population growth of the mite *Varroa destructor* in honey bee (*Apis mellifera*) colonies. *Apidologie*, 32, 157–174.

Bailey, L. and Ball, B.V. (1991). *Honey Bee Pathology*, 2nd edn. San Diego, CA: Academic Press.

Ball, B.V. and Bailey, L. (1997). Viruses. In R. Morse and K. Blottum (eds.), *Honey Bee Pests, Predators and Diseases*, 3rd edn. Medina, OH: A.I. Root Publishing Co., pp. 13-31.

Berthoud, H., Imdorf, A., Haueter, M., Radloff, S. and Neumann, P. (2010). Virus infections and winter losses of honey bee colonies (*Apis mellifera*). *Journal of Apicultural Research*, 49, 60–65.

Blacquière, T., Smagghe, G., van Gestel, A.M. and Mommaerts, V. (2012). Neonicotinoids in bees: a review on concentrations, side-effects and risk assessment. *Ecotoxicology*, 21, 973–992.

Boecking, O. and Spivak, M. (1999). Behavioral defenses of honey bees against *Varroa jacobsoni* Oud. *Apidologie*, 30, 141–158.

Boncristiani, H., Underwood, R., Schwarz, R., Evans, J.D., Pettis, J. and van Engelsdorp, D. (2012). Direct effect of acaricides on pathogen loads and gene expression levels in honey bees *Apis mellifera*. *Journal of Insect Physiology*, 58, 613–620.

Bortolotti, L., Monanari, R., Marcelino, J. and Porrini, P. (2003). Effects of sub-lethal imidacloprid doses on the homing rate and foraging activity of honey bees. *Bulletin of Insectology*, 56, 63–67.

CAPA (2014). *CAPA Statement on Honey Bee Wintering Losses in Canada*. Edmonton, AB: CAPA.

Carreck, N.L., Ball, B.V. and Martin, S.J. (2010). Honey bee colony collapse and changes in viral prevalence associated with *Varroa destructor*. *Journal of Apicultural Research*, 49, 93–94.

Cox-Foster, D.L., Conlan, S., Holmes, E.C., Palacios, G., Evans, J.D., Moran, N.A., Quan, P.L., Briese, T., Hornig, M., Geiser, D.M., Martinson, V., vanEngelsdorp, D., Kalkstein, A.L., Drysdale, A., Hui, J., Zhai, J., Cui, L., Hutchison, S.K., Simons, J.F., Egholm, M., Pettis, J.S. and Lipkin, W.I. (2007).

A metagenomic survey of microbes in honey bee colony collapse disorder. *Science*, 318, 283–287.

Cresswell, J.E. (2011). A meta-analysis of experiments testing the effects of a neonicotinoid insecticide (imidacloprid) on honey bees. *Ecotoxicology*, 20, 149–157.

Currie, R.W., Pernal, S.F. and Guzman-Novoa, E. (2010). Honey bee colony losses in Canada. *Journal of Apicultural Research*, 49, 104–106.

Cutler, G.C. and Scott-Dupree, C.D. (2007). Exposure to clothianidin seed-treated canola has no long-term impact on honey bees. *Journal of Economic Entomology*, 100, 765–772.

Dainat, B., Evans, J.D., Chen, Y.P., Gauthier, L. and Neumann, P. (2012). Predictive markers of honey bee colony collapse. *PLOS One*, 7, e32151.

Decourtye, A., Devillers, J., Cluzeau, S., Charreton, M. and Pham-Delegue, M.H. (2004). Effects of imidacloprid and deltamethrin on associative learning in honeybees under semi-field and laboratory conditions. *Ecotoxicology and Environmental Safety*, 57, 410–419.

de Miranda, J.R., Cordoni, G. and Budge, G. (2010). The acute bee paralysis virus-Kashmir bee virus-Israeli acute paralysis complex. *Journal of Invertebrate Pathology*, 103, S30–S47.

Desneux, N., Decourtye, A. and Delpuech, J.M. (2007). The sublethal effects of pesticides on beneficial arthropods. *Annual Review of Entomology*, 52, 81–106.

Di Prisco, G., Zhang, X., Pennacchio, F., Caprio, E., Li, J., Evans, J.D., Degrandi-Hoffman, G., Hamilton, M. and Chen, Y.P. (2011). Dynamics of persistent and acute deformed wing virus infections in honey bees, *Apis mellifera*. *Viruses*, 3, 2425–2441.

Emsen, B., Petukhova, T. and Guzman-Novoa, E. (2012). Factors limiting the growth of *Varroa destructor* populations in selected honey bee (*Apis mellifera* L.) colonies. *Journal of Animal and Veterinary Advances*, 11, 4519–4525.

Emsen, B., Guzman-Novoa, E. and Kelly, P.G. (2014). Honey production of honey bee (Hymenoptera: Apidae) colonies with high and low *Varroa destructor* (Acari: Varroidae) infestation rates in eastern Canada. *Canadian Entomologist*, 146, 236–240.

Emsen, B., Hamiduzzaman, M.M., Goodwin, P.H. and Guzman-Novoa, E. (2015). Lower virus infections in *Varroa destructor*-infested and uninfested brood and adult honey bees (*Apis mellifera*) of a low mite population growth colony compared to a high mite population growth colony. *PLOS One*, 10, e0118885.

Francis, R.M., Nielsen, S.L. and Kryger, P. (2013).

Varroa-virus interaction in collapsing honey bee colonies. *PLOS One*, 8, e57540.

Fries, I. (1997). Protozoa. In R. Morse and K. Blottum (eds.), *Honey Bee Pests, Predators and Diseases*, 3rd edn. Medina, OH: A.I. Root Publishing Co., pp. 57–76.

Fries, I. (2010). *Nosema ceranae* in European honey bees (*Apis mellifera*). *Journal of Invertebrate Pathology*, 103, S73–S79.

Gallai, N., Salles, J.M., Settele, J. and Vaissiere, B.E. (2009). Economic valuation of the vulnerability of world agriculture confronted with pollinator decline. *Ecological Economics*, 68, 810–821.

Gensersch, E. and Aubert, M. (2010). Emerging and re-emerging viruses of the honey bee (*Apis mellifera* L.). *Veterinary Research*, 41, 54.

Goulson, D. (2013). An overview of the environmental risks posed by neonicotinoid insecticides. *Journal of Applied Ecology*, 50, 977–987.

Guzman-Novoa, E. (2011). Integration of biotechnologies/Genetic basis of disease resistance in the honey bee (*Apis mellifera* L.). In M. Moo-Young (ed.), *Comprehensive Biotechnology*, 2nd edn, Vol. 4. Amsterdam: Elsevier, pp. 763–767.

Guzman-Novoa, E., Vandame, R. and Arechavaleta-Velasco, M.E. (1999). Susceptibility of European and Africanized honey bees (*Apis mellifera* L.) to *Varroa jacobsoni* Oud. in Mexico. *Apidologie*, 30, 173–182.

Guzman-Novoa, E., Eccles, L., Calvete, Y., McGowan, J., Kelly, P.G. and Correa-Benítez, A. (2010). *Varroa destructor* is the main culprit for the death and reduced populations of overwintered honey bee (*Apis mellifera*) colonies in Ontario, Canada. *Apidologie*, 41, 443–450.

Guzman-Novoa, E., Emsen, B., Unger, P., Espinosa-Montaño, L.G. and Petukhova, P. (2012). Genotypic variability and relationships between mite infestation levels, mite damage, grooming intensity, and removal of *Varroa destructor* mites in selected strains of worker honey bees (*Apis mellifera* L.). *Journal of Invertebrate Pathology*, 110, 314–320.

Guzman-Novoa, E., Koleoglu, G. and Reyes-Quintana, M. (2013). Cellular immune response to varroa mite infestation in European and Africanized bees. *The Ontario Bee Journal*, 32, 19.

Hamiduzzaman, M.M., Guzman-Novoa, E., Goodwin, P.H., Reyes-Quintana, M., Koleoglu, G., Correa-Benítez, A. and Petukhova, T. (2015). Differential responses of Africanized and European honey bees (*Apis mellifera*) to viral replication following mechanical transmission or *Varroa destructor* parasitism. *Journal of Invertebrate Pathology*, 126, 12–20.

Health Canada (2013). *Evaluation of Canadian Bee Mortalities in 2013 Related to Neonicotinoid Pesticides.* Interim report as of 26 September. Ottawa: Canada.

Henry, M., Beguin, M., Requier, F., Rollin, O., Odoux, J.F., Aupinel, P., Aptel, J., Tchamitchian, S. and Decourtye, A. (2012). A common pesticide decreases foraging success and survival in honey bees. *Sciencexpress*, 336(6079), 1.

Higes, M., Martín-Hernández, R., and Meana, A. (2006). *Nosema ceranae*, a new microsporidian parasite in honeybees in Europe. *Journal of Invertebrate Pathology*, 92, 81–83.

Higes, M., Martín-Hernández, R., Botías, C., Bailón, E.G. González-Porto, A.V., Barrios, L., Del Nozal, M.J., Bernal, J.L., Jiménez, J.J., Palencia, P.G. and Meana, A. (2008). How natural infection by *Nosema ceranae* causes honeybee colony collapse. *Environmental Microbiology*, 10, 2659–2669.

Higes, M., Nozal, M.J., Alvaro, A., Barrios, L., Meana, A., Martín-Hernández, R., Bernal, J.L. and Bernal, J. (2011). The stability and effectiveness of fumagillin in controlling *Nosema ceranae* (Microsporidia) infection in honey bees (*Apis mellifera*) under laboratory and field conditions. *Apidologie*, 42, 364–377.

Highfield, A.C., El Nagar, A., Mackinder, L.C., Noël, L.M., Hall, M.J., Martin, S.J. and Schroeder, D.C. (2009). Deformed wing virus implicated in overwintering honeybee colony losses. *Applied and Environmental Microbiology*, 75, 7212–7220.

Huang, W.F., Solter, L.F., Yau, P.M. and Imai, B.S. (2013). *Nosema ceranae* escapes fumagillin control in honey bees. *PLOS Pathogens*, 9, e1003185.

Jeschke, P., Nauen, R., Schindler, M. and Elbert, A. (2011). Overview of the status and global strategy for neonicotinoids. *Journal of Agricultural and Food Chemistry*, 59, 2897–2908.

Kevan, P.G. and Ebert, T. (2005). Can almond nectar and pollen poison honey bees? *American Bee Journal*, 145, 507–509.

Kevan, P.G., Hannan, M.A., Ostiguy, N. and Guzman-Novoa, E. (2006). A summary of the Varroa-virus disease complex in honeybees. *American Bee Journal*, 146, 694–697.

Kevan, P.G., Guzman-Novoa, E., Skinner, A. and van Englesdorp, D. (2007). Colony collapse disorder in Canada: do we have a problem? *Hive Lights*, 20, 14–16.

Klee, J., Besana, A.M., Genersch, E., Gisder, S., Nanetti, A., Tam, D.Q., Chinh, T.X., Puerta, F., Ruz, J.M., Kryger, P., Message, D., Hatjina, F., Korpela, S., Fries, I. and Paxton, R.J. (2007). Widespread dispersal of the microsporidian *Nosema ceranae*, an emergent pathogen of the Western honey bee, *Apis mellifera*. *Journal of Invertebrate Pathology*, 96, 1–10.

Kralj, J. and Fuchs, S. (2006). Parasitic *Varroa destructor* mites influence flight duration and homing ability of infested *Apis mellifera* foragers. *Apidologie*, 37, 577–587.

Kralj, J., Brockmann, A. and Fuchs, S. (2007). The parasitic mite *Varroa destructor* affects non-associative learning in honey bee foragers, *Apis mellifera* L. *Journal of Comparative Physiology*, 193, 363–370.

Krupke, C.H., Hunt, G.J., Eitzer, B.D., Andino, G. and Given, K. (2012). Multiple routes of pesticide exposure for honey bees living near agricultural fields. *PLOS One*, 7, e29268.

Le Conte, Y., Ellis, M. and Ritter, W. (2010) *Varroa* mites and honey bee health: can *Varroa* explain part of the colony losses? *Apidologie*, 41, 353–363.

Locke, B., Forsgren, E. and de Miranda, J.R. (2014). Increased tolerance and resistance to virus infections: a possible factor in the survival of *Varroa destructor*-resistant honey bees (*Apis mellifera*). *PLOS One*, 9, e99998.

Martin, S.J., Highfield, A.C., Brettell, L., Villalobos, E.M., Budge, G.E., Powell, M., Nikaido, S. and Schroeder, D.C. (2012). Global honey bee viral landscape altered by a parasitic mite. *Science*, 336, 1304–1306.

Martín-Hernández, R., Meana, A., Prieto, L., Salvador, A.M., Garrido-Bailón, E. and Higes, M. (2007). Outcome of colonization of *Apis mellifera* by *Nosema ceranae*. *Applied and Environmental Microbiology*, 73, 6331–6338.

Matheson, A. (1993). World bee health report. *Bee World*, 74, 176–212.

McGregor, S.E. (1976). *Insect Pollination of Cultivated Crop Plants*. Washington, DC: USDA.

Medina-Flores, C.A., Guzman-Novoa, E., Hamiduzzaman, M.M., Aréchiga-Flores, C.F. and López-Carlos, M.A. (2014). Africanized honey bees (*Apis mellifera*) have low infestation levels of the mite *Varroa destructor* in different ecological regions in Mexico. *Genetics and Molecular Research*, 13, 7282–7293.

Navajas, M., Migeon, A, Alaux, C., Martin-Magniette, M., Robinson, G., Evans, J., Cros-Arteil, S., Crauser, D. and Le Conte, Y. (2008). Differential gene expression of honey bee *Apis mellifera* associated with *Varroa destructor* infection. *BMC Genomics*, 9, 301–310.

Oldroyd, B.P. (2007). What's killing American honey bees? *PLOS Biology*, 5, e168.

Page, R.E. and Guzman-Novoa, E. (1997). The genetic basis of disease resistance. In R. Morse and K. Blottum (eds.) *Honey Bee Pests, Predators and Diseases*, 3rd edn. Medina, OH: A.I. Root Publishing Co., pp. 469–492.

Paxton, R.J. (2010). Does infection by *Nosema ceranae* cause 'Colony Collapse Disorder' in honey bees (*Apis mellifera*)? *Journal of Apicultural Research*, 49, 80–84.

Pettis, J.S., Lichtenberg, E.M., Andree, M., Stitzinger, J., Rose, R. and van Engelsdorp, D. (2013). Crop pollination exposes honey bees to pesticides which alerts their susceptibility to the gut pathogen *Nosema ceranae*. *PLOS One*, 8, e70182.

Rosenkranz, P., Aumeier, P. and Ziegelmann, B. (2010). Biology and control of *Varroa destructor*. *Journal of Invertebrate Pathology*, 103, 96–119.

Sandrock, C., Tanadini, M., Tanadini, L.G., Fauser-Misslin, A., Potts, S.G. and Neumann, P. (2014). Impact of chronic neonicotinoid exposure on honeybee colony performance and queen supersedure. *PLOS One*, 9, e103592.

Sanford, M.T. (2001). Introduction, spread and economic impact of varroa mites in North America. In T.C. Webster and K.S. Delaplane (eds.), *Mites of the Honey Bee*. Mansfield, MA: Dadant and Sons, pp. 149–162.

Schmehl, D.R., Teal, P.E.A., Frazier, J.L. and Grozinger, C.M. (2014). Genomic analysis of the interaction between pesticide exposure and nutrition in honey bees (*Apis mellifera*). *Journal of Insect Physiology*, 71, 177–190.

Schmidt, J.O., Thoenes, S.C. and Levin, M.D. (1987). Survival of honey bees, *Apis mellifera* (Hymenoptera: Apidae), fed various pollen sources. *Annals of the Entomological Society of America*, 80, 176–183.

Schmidt, L.S., Schmidt, J.O., Rao, H., Wang, W. and Xu, L. (1995). Feeding preferences and survival of young worker honey bees (Hymenoptera: Apidae) fed rape, sesame, and sunflower pollen. *Journal of Economic Entomology*, 88, 1591–1595.

Schmuck, R., Shöning, R., Stork, A. and Schramel, O. (2001). Risk posed to honeybee (*Apis mellifera* L., Hymenoptera) by an imidacloprid seed dressing of sunflowers. *Pesticide Management Science*, 57, 225–238.

Schneider, P. and Drescher, W. (1987). The influence of *Varroa jacobsoni* on weight, development of hypopharyngeal glands, and longevity of *Apis mellifera*. *Apidologie*, 18, 101–109.

Shen, M.Q., Yang, X.L. and Cox-Foster, D. (2005). The role of varroa mites in infections of Kashmir bee virus (KVB) and deformed wing virus (DWV) in honey bees. *Virology*, 342, 141–149.

Stankus, T. (2008) A review and bibliography of the literature of honey bee Colony Collapse Disorder: a poorly understood epidemic that clearly threatens the successful pollination of billions of dollars of crops in America. *Journal of Agricultural and Food Information*, 9, 115–143.

Stankus, T. (2014). Reviews of science for science librarians: an update on honeybee colony collapse disorder. *Science and Technology Libraries*, 33, 228–260.

Suchail, S., Guez, D. and Belzunces, L.P. (2000) Characteristics of imidacloprid toxicity in two *Apis mellifera* subspecies. *Environmental Toxicology*, 19, 1901–1905.

Van Der Sluijs, J.P., Simon-Delso, N., Goulson, D., Maxim, L., Bonmatin, J.M. and Belzunces, L.P. (2013). Neonicotinoids, bee disorders and the sustainability of pollination services. *Current Opinion in Environmental Sustainability*, 5, 293–305.

van Engelsdorp, D., Hayes, J., Underwood, R.M. and Pettis, J. (2008). A survey of honey bee colony losses in the US, fall 2007 to spring 2008. *PLOS One*, 3, 1–6.

van Engelsdorp, D., Evans, J.D., Saegerman, C., Mullin, C., Haubruge, E., Nguyen, B.K., Frazier, M., Frazier. J., Cox-Foster, D., Chen, Y.P., Underwood, R., Tarpy, D.R. and Pettis, J.S. (2009). Colony Collapse Disorder: a descriptive study. *PLOS One*, 4, e6481.

Webster, T.C. (1994). Effects of fumagillin on *Nosema apis* and honey bees (Hymenoptera: Apidae). *Journal of Economic Entomology*, 87, 601–604.

Williams, G.R., Sampson, M.A., Shutler, D. and Rogers, R.E.L. (2008). Does fumagillin control the recently detected invasive parasite *Nosema ceranae* in Western honey bees (*Apis mellifera*)? *Journal of Invertebrate Pathology*, 99, 342–344.

Williams, G.R., Tarpy, D.R., van Engelsdorp, D., Chauzat, M.P., Cox-Foster, D.L., Delaplane, K.S., Neumann, P., Pettis, J.S., Rogers, R. E.L. and Shutler, D. (2010). Colony Collapse Disorder in context. *BioEssays*, 32, 845–846.

Williamson, S.M. and Wright, G.A. (2013). Exposure to multiple cholinergic pesticides impairs olfactory learning and memory in honeybees. *Journal of Experimental Biology*, 216, 1799–1807.

Yang, E.C., Chang, H.C., Wu, W.Y. and Chen, Y.W. (2012). Impaired olfactory associative behavior of honeybee workers due to contamination of imidacloprid in the larval stage. *PLOS One*, 7, e49472.

Yang, X. and Cox-Foster, D.L., (2005). Impact of an ectoparasite on the immunity and pathology of an invertebrate: evidence for host immunosuppression and viral amplification. *Proceedings of the National Academy of Sciences of the USA*, 102, 7470–7475.

chapter 17

Bovine spongiform encephalopathy – the mad cow crisis and its consequences for animal and human health

Sabine Gilch, Wilfreda (Billie) E. Thurston and Keri L. Williams

Abstract

Bovine spongiform encephalopathy (BSE) or mad cow disease belongs to the group of prion diseases that are transmissible and inevitably fatal neurodegenerative diseases of animals and humans. Prions are unconventional infectious particles that solely consist of a misfolded isoform of the host-encoded cellular prion protein. The outbreak of BSE in the late 1980s in the United Kingdom reached epidemic dimensions, and eventually the disease was transmitted to humans, giving rise to a new variant of Creutzfeldt-Jakob disease (vCJD). An outbreak in Canada in 2003 is discussed in terms of the impact on the farmers and ranchers. In this chapter, we discuss the health and social impact of the BSE crisis, and actions that were implemented to control the disease. We argue that a One Health approach to the disease would have included more attention to the families whose livelihoods were affected.

17.1 Prion diseases – overview

Prion diseases or transmissible spongiform encephalopathies (TSEs) are strictly fatal neurodegenerative disorders of humans and animals. They are characterized by spongiform lesions, astrocytosis and the accumulation of an aberrantly folded isoform (PrP^{Sc}) of the endogenously expressed cellular prion protein PrP^{C} in the brain. In humans, there are sporadic, genetic and infectiously acquired forms of prion diseases (Table 17.1; Prusiner, 1998; Weissmann et al., 1996). Examples in animals are scrapie of sheep and goats, chronic wasting disease (CWD) of deer, elk and moose and bovine spongiform encephalopathy (BSE) in cattle (Watts et al., 2006; Gilch et al., 2011). Definite diagnosis relies upon detection of abnormal prion protein deposition in the central nervous system (CNS) by ELISA, immunohistochemistry or immunoblot. All prion diseases are characterized by a long incubation period and a short clinical phase. Once the disease is recognized and intervention may be possible, the brain is already significantly damaged. In infectiously acquired prion diseases, post-exposure prophylaxis to prevent

Table 17.1 Etiologies of human prion diseases

Etiology	Disease and frequency	Mechanism
acquired	Kuru (pandemic in the 1950s, nowadays virtually extinct); iatrongenic Creutzfeldt-Jakob disease (CJD) (<5%), variant CJD (vCJD) (total so far 229)	Infection through environmental exposure to prions; exogenous
genetic	Familiar or genetic CJD (10–15%); Gerstmann-Sträussler-Scheinker syndrome (GSS); fatal familiar insomnia (FFI)	Mutation in the PRNP gene (more than 30 different types are known); endogenous
sporadic	Sporadic CJD (1 case per million per year worldwide, 85%)	Apparent spontaneous formation of PrP^{Sc}, endogenous

transport of prions to the brain is complicated because usually the time point of prion uptake is unknown. Therefore, to date, neither therapeutic nor prophylactic treatment is available (Gilch et al., 2008).

17.2 Prions – proteinaceous infectious particles

Prions are unique pathogens that represent a new biological principle. According to the protein-only hypothesis postulated by the later Nobel laureate S. Prusiner in the 1980s, prions consist solely of the misfolded and aggregated prion protein isoform PrP^{Sc}, and replicate auto-catalytically by recruiting PrP^{C} as a substrate for conformational transition into the pathological isoform without the necessity of genetic information encoded by nucleic acids (Prusiner, 1982). However, despite intensive research it took more than 20 years until considerable proof of evidence for the protein-only hypothesis was provided by the cell-free *in vitro* generation of prion infectivity from recombinant prion protein expressed in *E. coli*, without the addition of PrP^{Sc} as a template for conversion (Legname et al., 2004).

The exact molecular mechanism of prion conversion, however, is not yet completely understood. According to the most widely accepted seeded nucleation model (Lansbury and Caughey, 1995) the PrP^{Sc} isoform is in equilibrium with PrP^{C}, with the PrP^{C} conformation being strongly favoured. Under rare circumstances, PrP^{Sc} can assemble and form oligomeric seeds, which then act as a template for recruitment and conversion of PrP^{C} molecules. This converts the soluble, mainly α-helical PrP^{C} into the β-sheet rich, aggregated PrP^{Sc} isoform. Larger seeds or amyloids are formed, and can break up again into smaller oligomeric seeds. In case of prion infection, the rate-limiting step of seed formation is circumvented since these are introduced with the inoculum, and the entire process is accelerated (Plate 30).

Prions are highly resistant to inactivation measures that are applied for viruses or bacteria, such as UV light. In contrast, they can be destroyed by agents that denature proteins, such as urea or sodium hydroxide, by autoclaving at more stringent conditions at 134°C and 3 bars for extended time periods and by incineration (Alper et al., 1967).

Prions can be transmitted within and also between species, although limited by the phenomenon of the species barrier (Scott et al., 1993). One aspect governing species barrier is the similarity of the PrP primary structure between different species, with more likely transmissibility in case of the presence of less amino acid exchanges (Schatzl et al., 1995;

Wopfner et al., 1999). Prion diseases can even be zoonotic. Although a considerable species barrier was predicted for transmission of BSE to humans based on amino acid sequence comparisons of bovine and human PrP, BSE crossed this barrier and resulted in a new human prion disease, the variant CJD (vCJD). To date, BSE is the only example of a zoonotic prion disease.

17.3 Bovine spongiform encephalopathy

BSE or 'mad cow disease' was first described in the United Kingdom in 1987 (Wells et al., 1987) as a novel spongiform encephalopathy in cattle. Although some veterinarians reported an unusual neurological disorder in cattle already from April 1985, none of these animals were subjected to neuropathological analysis. It was in 1986 that an African nyala antelope (*Tragelaphus angasii*) at a British zoo was killed because of neurological signs, and in the brain of this animal, spongiform lesions were found (Jeffrey and Wells, 1988). When brains of cows demonstrating similar nervous signs were analysed, a spongiform encephalopathy was diagnosed. One year later it had been confirmed that BSE-infected cows harbour PK-resistant PrP and amyloid fibrils in the brain, similar to those found in scrapie-infected animals (Hope et al., 1988). Subsequently, the disease could be transmitted to mice (Fraser et al., 1992) and cattle (Dawson et al., 1990).

Epidemiological evidence suggests that at this time a significant number of British dairy cattle were already infected with BSE-causing prions (Bradley and Wilesmith, 1993). The clinical signs of BSE are related to a disease of the CNS, and are rather non-specific. Most common signs are ataxia, changes in temperament, such as nervousness or aggression and hyperesthesia to external stimuli, decreased milk production, or loss of body weight despite continued appetite.

As in all other prion diseases, there is no adaptive immune reaction, no inflammatory response and no disease markers are detectable in the cerebrospinal fluid (CSF). The mean incubation time is 4.5–5.5 years, and most animals are clinically affected at an age of 4–4.5 years. Currently, there are no tests available for diagnosis of BSE in living animals, although newly developed assays such as real-time quaking induced conversion assay (RT-QuIC; Wilham et al., 2010) – which enables the detection of minute amounts of PrP^{Sc}; for example, in the cerebrospinal fluid of CJD patients (Atarashi et al., 2011) – may be available for diagnosis of human and animal prion diseases in the future. Clinically suspect cows will be euthanized, and brain stem material is subject to diagnostic assays that are based on the detection of PK-resistant PrP^{Sc} by immunohistochemistry, immunoblot or enzyme-linked immunosorbent assay (ELISA). Along with PrP^{Sc} depositions, vacuolation is found in the brains of affected animals. In BSE, the appearance of so-called 'florid plaques' is characteristic, which are large amyloid PrP^{Sc} depositions, surrounded by vacuoles (Harman and Silva, 2009).

At that time in the mid-1980s, BSE was a new disease, and its origin was, and still is, enigmatic. However, in all cases, feed was used that contained meat and bone meal (MBM) as a protein source, which was produced from animal carcasses, pointing at MBM as a source of infection. Indeed, when feeding of MBM was banned in the UK in 1988, infection rates decreased by 80 per cent in the following year.

Despite the feed ban introduced in 1988 in the UK, new BSE cases were found in cattle born after the feed ban. Since maternal or horizontal spread is not a natural route of BSE transmission (Donnelly et al., 1997), geographical variation in incidence was analysed. It became obvious that the highest incidence of these cases was found in areas with high pig and/or poultry density. This led to the conclusion that cattle feed was cross-contaminated with pig and poultry feed containing ruminant protein, possibly during production in feed mills, during transport of feed, or at the farm (Hoinville et al., 1995; Stevenson et al., 2005). This explanation is reasonable, since BSE only requires low-dose exposure, and as little as 1mg of BSE-positive brain homogenate is enough to orally infect a cow (Wells et al., 2007). In order to further diminish the risk of BSE infection, it became illegal after 1996 to feed mammalian proteins to any farmed livestock, including pigs and poultry. These more stringent conditions were reinforced in all countries of the European Union in 2001. In addition, specified risk material (SRM) – which are bovine tissues containing BSE infectivity, including skull, spinal cord, eyes, tonsils, distal ileum and vertebrae column from cattle older than 30 months – have been banned for human consumption in the EU (Heim and Kihm, 2003).

These feed bans were highly efficient in reducing the case numbers in animals born after 1988. However, in the following years more than 40,000 animals born before the feed ban developed BSE, with a peak of more than 37,000 cows in 1993 and approximately 180,000 cases in total in the UK. After 1996, in the UK less than 200 cases were identified. Twenty other European countries were affected, with highest numbers in Portugal (1,082), France (1,023), Spain (785) and Switzerland (467). In North America, the first case was detected in Canada in 2003 (Stack et al., 2004), and in the same year in the USA, which was found in an animal imported from Canada. Overnight, the Canadian beef industry was devastated due to a shutdown of trade borders. In total, 18 cases were identified in Canada, and three cases in the USA. Outside Europe and North America, Japan reported 36 cases, and a few were identified in Brazil and Israel (www.oie.int/animal-health-in-the-world/ bse-specific-data/number-of-reported-cases-worldwide-excluding-the-united-kingdom). Most cases were not clinical, but identified by surveillance programmes. In 2001, an active surveillance programme for all slaughtered cattle for human consumption over an age of 30 months and for cattle over an age of 24 months that were subject to emergency slaughter, fallen stock or animals suspect or suffering from disease was implemented in the European Union. In Canada, a targeted surveillance programme is installed, and collected samples include cattle over 30 months that are dead, down, dying or diseased. In addition, all cattle exhibiting signs of BSE must be reported to the Canadian Food Inspection Agency (CFIA). Thereby, every year more than 30,000 samples are analysed, and the last positive sample was detected in 2015.

Despite all actions that were taken to limit new infections with BSE, the disease has already been transmitted not only among cattle, but also to other animals and to humans (Figure 17.1). These were mainly ruminants, such as kudu (*Tragelaphus strepsiceros*), eland (*Taurotragus oryx*), nyala (*Tragelaphus angasii*) or gemsbok (*Oryx gazella*) in zoological gardens in the UK or France (Kirkwood and Cunningham, 1994). Furthermore, both exotic – puma (*Puma concolor*), cheetah (*Acinonyx jubatus*) – and domestic cats were affected by BSE, whereas dogs appear to be resistant, although presumably they were equally exposed to BSE-contaminated food as were cats (Pearson et al., 1992). Natural cases of BSE in pigs were not reported; however, when introduced by an intracranial route, pigs can be infected, with an estimated incubation period of between 69 and 150 weeks (Wells et al., 2003). Experimentally, sheep and goat are also susceptible to BSE, both upon intracerebral and oral inoculation (Foster et al., 1994). BSE in small ruminants can be clearly distinguished from scrapie, and no naturally transmitted cases have been reported. Similarly, European red deer is susceptible to BSE only upon intracranial challenge (Dagleish et al., 2008).

Only minor numbers of new BSE cases are reported every year, demonstrating that the implemented regulations successfully prevented

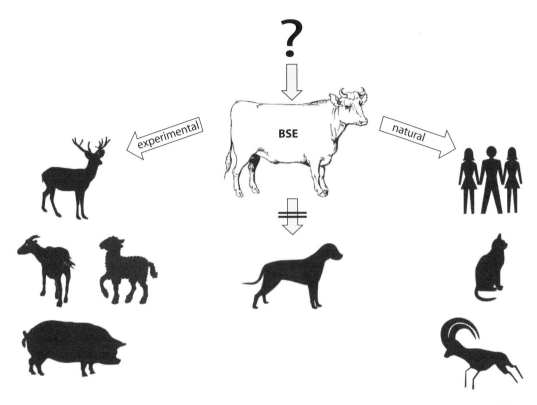

Figure 17.1 Interspecies transmission of BSE. The source of BSE remains enigmatic. Natural transmission of BSE occurred to humans, domestic and exotic cats, and exotic ungulates. Whereas dogs resist even intracranial inoculation, pigs and red deer are susceptible to experimental intracerebral inoculation. BSE was experimentally transmitted to sheep and goat intracerebrally and orally.

further spread of foodborne BSE. However, new concerns came up with the discovery of 'atypical' cases of BSE initially in France and Italy termed H-type and L-type BSE respectively, according to the biochemical signature of the associated PK-resistant PrP (Casalone et al., 2004), which allows us to distinguish these forms of BSE from the 'classical' foodborne BSE. Most of the affected animals were born before the reinforced feed ban in Europe. However, recently a case of H-type BSE in an animal born after the feed ban was reported (Guldimann et al., 2012). In contrast to classical BSE, all positive cows were older than eight years. L-type, but not H-type BSE is transmissible to transgenic mice expressing human PrP (Beringue et al., 2008; Kong

et al., 2008). The origin of atypical BSE is unclear, and both forms might represent sporadic BSE. However, one case of H-type BSE in the USA has been associated with a pathogenic mutation in the prion protein gene (Greenlee et al., 2012). To support the idea of sporadic BSE and assuming a similar incidence as known for sporadic prion disease in humans (1:1,000,000), controlled surveillance in large herds of older cows in a country free of BSE would be necessary, which is currently difficult to achieve. The finding of other BSE types now fuels concerns about re-emergence of BSE and the possibility of zoonotic transmission. It shows that it is important to run surveillance programmes for BSE, to thoroughly study the pathogenesis of atypical forms (Balkema-Buschmann et al., 2011), and to evaluate diagnostic rapid assays for their ability to detect atypical BSE prions in the currently used sample materials (Gray et al., 2012).

Overall, these data highlight the diversity of prion diseases. Whereas animal TSEs such as scrapie or CWD only have a narrow host range, BSE prions are less host-specific and able to convert PrP^C from an array of species and still retain their original molecular signature. This enabled to early determine a link between BSE and vCJD, a new human TSE that is strikingly different to all other human prion diseases.

17.4 Transmission of BSE to humans – variant Creutzfeldt-Jakob disease (vCJD)

In 1996, ten unusual cases of CJD (later termed vCJD) in younger individuals were reported in the UK (Will et al., 1996). Epidemiological investigation revealed that the new prion disease was only found in countries with BSE cases, mainly in the UK. There is evidence that all patients were residing in the UK or another country with confirmed BSE cases within a defined period (1980–1996) of high risk of exposure to BSE-contaminated products. Active surveillance did not reveal an increase in case numbers of CJD in younger patients in European countries other than the UK. This led to the conclusion that vCJD is causally linked to BSE, which is supported by several lines of experimental evidence. First, BSE was transmissible to cynomolgus macaques (*Macaca fascicularis*), a non-human primate model of human prion diseases. The molecular and clinical signatures were similar to vCJD, with florid plaques found in the brains and behavioural signs observed as an early indicator of disease (Lasmezas et al., 1996). Second, when brain homogenates from vCJD patients were injected into wildtype mice, the resulting disease could be clearly distinguished from

sporadic CJD (sCJD) by histopathological profiling of brain lesions and the recorded survival curves (Bruce et al., 1997). Third, the disease was transmissible to transgenic mice expressing bovine PrP, and in immunohistochemical and biochemical analysis vCJD behaved identical to BSE in these mice (Scott et al., 1999).

In humans, vCJD was mainly conspicuous because of the young age of affected individuals. Whereas the median age at death is 68 years in sCJD, it is 28 years in vCJD. Duration of the clinical phase in sCJD is around six months, in contrast to approximately 14 months in vCJD. Florid plaques are not found in sCJD, but are abundant in vCJD, and the clinical signs between the two forms of prion diseases are strikingly different, with psychiatric symptoms and ataxia being predominant in vCJD, and dementia in sCJD patients. In total, 229 cases of vCJD were reported, 177 of those were diagnosed in the UK.

In vCJD, a major involvement of the lymphoreticular system is evident, with prions found, for example, in tonsils, spleen and appendix, in contrast to BSE and sCJD, where prions are mainly contained in the brain (Ironside, 2012). This has led to further inter-human transmission of vCJD by blood or blood product transfusion. Currently, this is documented in three cases (Head et al., 2009; Hewitt et al., 2006; Wroe et al., 2006) where transmission resulted in clinical disease with an incubation period of 6.5–7.8 years. In addition, one asymptomatic case was discovered (Peden et al., 2004). This now raises the question how many individuals are 'silent' carriers of the infectious agent, and how many people might have become infected by blood transfusions.

Therefore, a large-scale survey on more than 30,000 archived appendices in the UK was performed. Out of these samples, 16 were positive for abnormal PrP deposits, indicating an overall prevalence of 493 per million population (Gill et al., 2013). Although co-factors that support infection with BSE prions and development of vCJD are mostly speculative, a single nucleotide polymorphism in the human *PRNP* gene encoding either methionine or valine at amino acid position 129 of the human PrP critically influences susceptibility to BSE infection and clinically apparent disease. To date, all cases of vCJD were found to be homozygous for methionine; however, heterozygosity or valine homozygosity may only prolong the incubation time rather than prevent the disease.

17.5 BSE and farmers and ranchers

The direct impact of prion diseases on humans has been small relative to other zoonotic diseases, such as avian influenza (H1N1). While vCJD is a deadly disease, it is also rare compared to other diseases and illnesses that are the concern of public health (e.g., depression, heart disease). The impact of BSE on the cattle industry and therefore on the health of farmers, ranchers[1] and their families was much greater, yet received minimal attention from health authorities. The impact was certainly linked to economics: the livelihoods of beef and dairy farmers and ranchers are vulnerable to weather, other diseases in their animals, other loss of animals (accident, predator), hay crop failures, feed prices, shipping costs and so on. Some of these (loss of one or two animals) have minimal impact, while others can have substantial impact economically. More importantly, none are under the control of the individual, except for the partial control exercised through vaccination and other health promotion efforts (including parasite control with anthelmintics) with the cattle. A lack of control in itself can threaten the mental health of people, but farming is also an occupation that differs from many in that the workplace and home are often not geographically different, family members including children are exposed, even temporary 'workers', and it can be a 365-day-a-year commitment (Thurston and Blundell-Gosselin, 2005) with emotional attachments to the geography, animals and broader community. The 2003 BSE event in Alberta, Canada was, in fact, preceded by a widespread drought in 2002 (Broadway, 2006), so it followed upon a previous threat to family wellbeing. Since the control of infectious diseases in animals and prevention of epidemics is contingent on the cooperation and good will of farmers and ranchers, it is imperative that health practitioners understand them and their context and work collaboratively in a One Health model.

Farming and ranching are dangerous occupations and the context in which the work occurs is unique (Fraser et al., 2005; Thurston et al., 2003b). Farms vary in size of the operation, age of the farmers and ranchers, and whether they are owned by the family or by a corporation. In fact, a large percentage of farmers and ranchers may also work off the farm; one study found that 31.7 per cent of male and 40.1 per cent of female respondents also worked off the farm (Thurston et al., 2003b). The vulnerability to injury is one of the stressors for farmers and ranchers (Thurston et al., 2003a) – if they don't work both on and off the farm they may lose the latter and their home. The fact that the workplace is also where home is situated also exposes other family members, especially children, to risk of injury or infection. High rates of stress among farmers and ranchers have been found in the United Kingdom (Simkin et al., 1998), although Thomas et al. (2003) found a lower percentage of psychiatric morbidity than in the general population of Britain. Although the sample was biased by a low response rate, Thomas et al. (2003) did find that farmers had a higher rate of thinking about suicide than non-farmers, especially when psychiatric morbidity was controlled. Dickens et al. (2014, p. 104) report that 'stress throughout the agricultural industry was nearly palpable' in a state of the United States when milk process dropped 'precipitously', suggesting that economic uncertainty is a major contributor to stress. Alston

(2012) reports that between 2002 and 2012, stress and depression increased among rural Australian men. Again, however, it is important to remember that sources of stress may vary and there may be differences between men and women on farms (Thurston et al., 2003a).

Individual farmers and ranchers are dependent on global markets to set the price they will receive for their product (Fraser et al., 2005). In 2002, nearly 100 per cent of Alberta's live cattle exports were to the US (Broadway, 2006). Almost immediately after the first case of BSE was identified in Canada in 2003, 40 countries, including the US, imposed a ban on the import of live ruminants, meat products and animal by-products from Canada. The US borders remained closed to cattle under 30 months until July 2005. The border was finally opened to all cattle in 2007. Serecon Management Consulting (2003, p. i., cited in Broadway, 2006) characterized this as the 'greatest threat and shock the Canadian agricultural industry has ever experienced' even before the consequences were fully understood. Jamaica, Canada's second largest beef importer in the Caribbean (C$4.5 million) did not open its borders until August 2014 (*The Cattle Site*, 2014), and Qatar and Honduras in October 2014 (*Meat and Poultry*, 2014).

When farmers and ranchers lose income the surrounding community and local economy are also affected. Members of parliament from across Canada reported on the broad economic impacts affecting truck drivers, car or farm equipment dealerships, restaurant owners and slaughterhouse owners, to name a few (Broadway, 2006). Broadway in his study of the impact of the BSE event on Barrhead, Alberta also reported that veterinarians who 'were straight beef were hit hard' (2006, p. 19) as farmers and ranchers were no longer able to afford their services. The economic impact was not equitable, however, and large producers, feedlots and meat packers made money after the BSE event. 'Barrhead's most prominent cattle feeder received a cheque for

$5.48 million, by contrast the cheque received by a family owned 300 head pure-bred operation . . . amounted to just $3,348.67.'[2] And later, 'little of the $2 billion spent by federal and provincial governments on BSE across Canada trickled down to average sized producers who are the heart of maintaining viable rural communities' (Broadway, 2006, pp. 17, 25). Farmers interviewed as a part of Mitra et al.'s (2009) study on the psychosocial and socioeconomic consequences of BSE reported feeling that they, rather than packing plants and feedlots who benefited from low cattle prices, shouldered the majority of the cost relating to the BSE crisis in Canada. This study also identified a ripple effect of BSE on the social fabric of agricultural communities as farmers perceived their communities to be shrinking as farm families were forced to move, resulting in school closures and a lack of attendance at important community events.

Canadian farmers and ranchers were surveyed about the impact of BSE on them, their families and communities in 2004. There were 273 respondents from 177 farms across Canada, although 42 per cent were from Alberta (Thurston, 2010a). More than half of the respondents (61 per cent) reported that their health had been impacted by the BSE outbreak. The majority were the fourth generation to have taken up farming or ranching and for more than 60 per cent of them, the farm had been in the family for two generations or more. 'About 45% of respondents were very stressed by not having enough time for entertainment and recreation and about 50% by having problems balancing work and family responsibilities. Not surprisingly, 30% were very stressed over conflicts with their spouse on spending priorities' (Thurston, 2010b). The study was originally planned to be longitudinal, but the funding was cut by PrionNet Canada one year into the work. The researchers concluded that in the management of BSE, 'Farmers and ranchers have not been heard nor represented' (Thurston and Brook, 2008).

Since interventions to protect other animals, farmers and ranchers, their families or the general public depend on the cooperation of producers, it is important to understand that they are personally affected by an outbreak. There were reports following the BSE outbreak in Alberta, for instance, that farmers were burying cattle that showed symptoms in order to avoid wholesale slaughter of their herds (Enevold, 2004). Thus, the risks to their and other people's health were being considered. Ricketts noted:

> The case of BSE represents a special challenge for [human] public health professionals because the initiative and the interventions necessary for the control of BSE lie within the animal health sector. As a direct result of this, it is to be expected that debate, disagreements, and occasionally dispute will populate the arena when animal health experts and public health experts talk about BSE.
>
> (Ricketts, 2006, pp. 212–213)

If a One Health model is employed, however, conflicts can be avoided as interdisciplinary collaboration becomes more normative, communication is enhanced and the intersections of animal and human wellbeing are more readily and more frequently acknowledged. Specialists in health promotion with humans have long recognized that risk communication, no matter how well done, is insufficient to ensure widespread uptake of public health recommendations (Russell et al., 2003).

17.6 Conclusion

We have shown in this chapter that TSEs are a group of infectious diseases that can potentially be passed from animals to humans. Since they are fatal diseases, the potential impact is very serious. The nature of the disease(s) and

their transmission warrants more investigation. Research with prions is challenged by the seriousness of the illness and the need for special biological containment in laboratories. Understanding more is a good investment in light of the spreading of CWD among wild living cervids, and its possible consequences for ecology, animal and human health, and also in the face of the seriousness of BSE and the impact that it has had on local and national economies, the health of rural communities and the threat of vCJD. There is so much variation in farm operations that a one-size-fits-all intervention is not likely to have uniform success (Thurston and Blundell-Gosselin, 2005), calling for a deep understanding of the issues from a multidisciplinary perspective. We have argued therefore that effective public health interventions in cases such as TSEs would benefit from a One Health model. This would require stakeholder engagement and involving both bench and social scientists who could translate research to the communities affected, and policymakers. In cases such as the TSEs where there remains much uncertainty with regard to risk, regulatory authorities need a very good plan to deal with public concerns that addresses the strategies of the Ottawa Charter for Health Promotion: build healthy public policy; create supportive environments; strengthen community action; develop personal skills; and reorient health services (World Health Organization, 1986). A One Health model of health promotion would not separate the animal and human health specialists and each would learn from the other. Veterinarians, prion researchers, farmers, farmers' association representatives, meat producers and human public health practitioners could develop a collaboration to undertake a One Health approach to BSE prevention. From this would come a multisectoral and multidisciplinary strategy; for instance, a region could develop a mental health promotion campaign that incorporated a role for veterinarians providing outreach to producers. Rural schools might be included to incorporate farm children and policies on farmer compensation might be analysed and changes recommended to government. The intersections of animal welfare and human wellbeing would therefore become better-known and the synergies of prevention efforts enhanced.

Endnotes

1 We use both farmers and ranchers, as producers tend to identify with one or the other label.
2 Conservatively, if farmers received C$1.27 per pound before BSE and an average weight was 650 pounds, the amount received would have been around $247,650 (Alberta Agriculture and Rural Development, 2014). It is not possible to be more precise without more knowledge of the actual population of cattle discussed.

References

Alberta Agriculture & Rural Development (2014). www1.agric.gov.ab.ca/general/progserv.nsf/all/pgmsrv187.

Alper, T., Cramp, W.A., Haig, D.A. and Clarke, M.C. (1967). Does the agent of scrapie replicate without nucleic acid? *Nature*, 214, 764–766.

Alston, M. (2012). Rural male suicide in Australia. *Social Science & Medicine*, 74, 515–522.

Atarashi, R., Satoh, K., Sano, K., Fuse, T., Yamaguchi, N., Ishibashi, D., Matsubara, T., Nakagaki, T., Yamanaka, H., Shirabe, S., Yamada, M., Mizusawa, H., Kitamoto, T., Klug, G., McGlade, A., Collins, S.J. and Nishida, N. (2011). Ultrasensitive human prion detection in cerebrospinal fluid by real-time quaking-induced conversion. *Nature Medicine*, 17, 175–178.

Balkema-Buschmann, A., Ziegler, U., McIntyre, L., Keller, M., Hoffmann, C., Rogers, R., Hills, B. and Groschup, M.H. (2011). Experimental challenge of cattle with German atypical bovine spongiform encephalopathy (BSE) isolates. *Journal of Toxicology and Environmental Health*, 74, 103–109.

Beringue, V., Herzog, L., Reine, F., Le, D.A., Casalone, C., Vilotte, J.L. and Laude, H. (2008). Transmission of atypical bovine prions to mice transgenic for human prion protein. *Emerging Infectious Diseases*, 14, 1898–1901.

Bradley, R. and Wilesmith, J.W. (1993). Epidemiology and control of bovine spongiform encephalopathy (BSE). *British Medical Bulletin*, 49, 932–959.

Broadway, M. (2006). *BSE's 'Devastating' Impact on Rural Alberta: A Preliminary Analysis*. University of Alberta, Department of Rural Economy, Edmonton, Canada.

Bruce, M.E., Will, R.G., Ironside, J.W., McConnell, I., Drummond, D., Suttie, A., McCardle, L., Chree, A., Hope, J., Birkett, C., Cousens, S., Fraser, H. and Bostock, C.J. (1997). Transmissions to mice indicate that 'new variant' CJD is caused by the BSE agent. *Nature*, 389, 498–501.

Casalone, C., Zanusso, G., Acutis, P., Ferrari, S., Capucci, L., Tagliavini, F., Monaco, S. and Caramelli, M. (2004). Identification of a second bovine amyloidotic spongiform encephalopathy: molecular similarities with sporadic Creutzfeldt-Jakob disease. *Proceedings of the National Academy of Sciences of the United States of America*, 101, 3065–3070.

The Cattle Site (2014). Jamaica opens borders to Canadian beef. *The Cattle Site*, www.thecattlesite.com/news/46417/jamaica-opens-borders-to-canadian-beef.

Dagleish, M.P., Martin, S., Steele, P., Finlayson, J., Siso, S., Hamilton, S., Chianini, F., Reid, H.W., Gonzalez, L. and Jeffrey, M. (2008). Experimental transmission of bovine spongiform encephalopathy to European red deer (*Cervus elaphus elaphus*). *BMC Veterinary Research*, 4, 17.

Dawson, M., Wells, G.A. and Parker, B.N. (1990). Preliminary evidence of the experimental transmissibility of bovine spongiform encephalopathy to cattle. *Veterinary Records*, 126, 112–113.

Dickens, S., Dotter, E., Handy, M. and Waterman, L. (2014). Reducing stress to minimize injury: the nation's first employee assistance program for dairy farmers and related photo documentary project. *Journal of Agromedicine*, 19, 103–106.

Donnelly, C.A., Ferguson, N.M., Ghani, A.C., Wilesmith, J.W. and Anderson, R.M. (1997). Analysis of dam-calf pairs of BSE cases: confirmation of a maternal risk enhancement. *Proceedings of the Royal Society B: Biological Sciences*, 264, 1647–1656.

Enevold, K. (2004). Ranchers taking advice to 'shoot, shovel & shut up'. *Calgary Sun*, 5 August.

Foster, J.D., Hope, J., McConnell, I., Bruce, M. and Fraser, H. (1994). Transmission of bovine spongiform encephalopathy to sheep, goats, and mice. *Annals of the New York Academy of Sciences*, 724, 300–303.

Fraser, C.E., Smith, K.B., Judd, F., Humphreys, J.S., Fragar, L.J. and Henderson, A. (2005). Farming and mental health problems and mental illness. *International Journal of Social Psychiatry*, 51, 340–349.

Fraser, H., Bruce, M.E., Chree, A., McConnell, I. and Wells, G.A. (1992). Transmission of bovine spongiform encephalopathy and scrapie to mice. *Journal of General Virology*, 73, 1891–1897.

Gilch, S., Krammer, C. and Schatzl, H.M. (2008). Targeting prion proteins in neurodegenerative disease. *Expert Opinion in Biological Therapy*, 8, 923–940.

Gilch, S., Chitoor, N., Taguchi, Y., Stuart, M., Jewell, J.E. and Schatzl, H.M. (2011). Chronic wasting disease. *Topics in Current Chemistry*, 305, 51–77.

Gill, O.N., Spencer, Y., Richard-Loendt, A., Kelly, C., Dabaghian, R., Boyes, L., Linehan, J., Simmons, M., Webb, P., Bellerby, P., Andrews, N., Hilton, D.A., Ironside, J.W., Beck, J., Poulter, M., Mead, S. and Brandner, S. (2013). Prevalent abnormal prion protein in human appendixes after bovine spongiform encephalopathy epizootic: large scale survey. *BMJ*, 347, f5675.

Gray, J.G., Dudas, S., Graham, C. and Czub, S. (2012). Performance analysis of rapid diagnostic tests on atypical bovine spongiform encephalopathy. *Journal of Veterinary Diagnostic Investigation*, 24, 976–980.

Greenlee, J.J., Smith, J.D., West Greenlee, M.H. and Nicholson, E.M. (2012). Clinical and pathologic features of H-type bovine spongiform encephalopathy associated with E211K prion protein polymorphism. *PLOS One*, 7, e38678.

Guldimann, C., Gsponer, M., Drogemuller, C., Oevermann, A. and Seuberlich, T. (2012). Atypical H-type bovine spongiform encephalopathy in a cow born after the reinforced feed ban on meat-and-bone meal in Europe. *Journal of Clinical Microbiology*, 50, 4171–4174.

Harman, J.L. and Silva, C.J. (2009). Bovine spongiform encephalopathy. *Journal of the American Veterinary Medicine Association*, 234, 59–72.

Head, M.W., Yull, H.M., Ritchie, D.L., Bishop, M.T. and Ironside, J.W. (2009). Pathological investigation of the first blood donor and recipient pair linked by transfusion-associated variant Creutzfeldt-Jakob disease transmission. *Neuropathology and Applied Neurobiology*, 35, 433–436.

Heim, D. and Kihm, U. (2003). Risk management of transmissible spongiform encephalopathies in Europe. *Revue scientifique et technique*, 22, 179–199.

Hewitt, P.E., Llewelyn, C.A., Mackenzie, J. and Will, R.G. (2006). Creutzfeldt-Jakob disease and blood transfusion: results of the UK Transfusion Medicine Epidemiological Review study. *Vox Sang*, 91, 221–230.

Hoinville, L.J., Wilesmith, J.W. and Richards, M.S. (1995). An investigation of risk factors for cases of bovine spongiform encephalopathy born after the introduction of the 'feed ban'. *Veterinary Records*, 136, 312–318.

Hope, J., Reekie, L.J., Hunter, N., Multhaup, G., Beyreuther, K., White, H., Scott, A.C., Stack, M.J., Dawson, M. and Wells, G.A. (1988). Fibrils from brains of cows with new cattle disease contain scrapie-associated protein. *Nature*, 336, 390–392.

Ironside, J.W. (2012). Variant Creutzfeldt-Jakob disease: an update. *Folia Neuropathologica*, 50, 50–56.

Jeffrey, M. and Wells, G.A. (1988). Spongiform encephalopathy in a nyala (*Tragelaphus angasi*). *Veterinary Pathology*, 25, 398–399.

Kirkwood, J.K. and Cunningham, A.A. (1994). Epidemiological observations on spongiform encephalopathies in captive wild animals in the British Isles. *Veterinary Records*, 135, 296–303.

Kong, Q., Zheng, M., Casalone, C., Qing, L., Huang, S., Chakraborty, B., Wang, P., Chen, F., Cali, I., Corona, C., Martucci, F., Iulini, B., Acutis, P., Wang, L., Liang, J., Wang, M., Li, X., Monaco, S., Zanusso, G., Zou, W.Q., Caramelli, M. and Gambetti, P. (2008). Evaluation of the human transmission risk of an atypical bovine spongiform encephalopathy prion strain. *Journal of Virology*, 82, 3697–3701.

Lansbury, P.T. and Caughey, B. (1995). The chemistry of scrapie infection: implications of the 'ice 9' metaphor. *Chemical Biology*, 2, 1–5.

Lasmezas, C.I., Deslys, J.P., Demaimay, R., Adjou, K.T., Lamoury, F., Dormont, D., Robain, O., Ironside, J. and Hauw, J.J. (1996). BSE transmission to macaques. *Nature*, 381, 743–744.

Legname, G., Baskakov, I.V., Nguyen, H.O., Riesner, D., Cohen, F.E., DeArmond, S.J. and Prusiner, S.B. (2004). Synthetic mammalian prions. *Science*, 305, 673–676.

Meat and Poultry (2014). Markets open for Canadian beef, cattle. *Meat and Poultry*, www.meatpoultry.com/articles/news_home/Global/2014/10/Markets_open_for_Canadian_beef.aspx?ID={2CB81B0E-571B-453A-BA9A-299057AA3877}&cck=1.

Mitra, D., Amaratunga, C., Sutherns, R., Pletsch, V., Corneil, W., Crowe, S., and Krewski, D. (2009). The psychosocial and socioeconomic consequences of bovine spongiform encephalopathy (BSE): a community impact study. *Journal of Toxicology and Environmental Health, Part A*, 72(17–18), 1106–1112.

Pearson, G.R., Wyatt, J.M., Gruffydd-Jones, T.J., Hope, J., Chong, A., Higgins, R.J., Scott, A.C. and Wells, G.A. (1992). Feline spongiform encephalopathy: fibril and PrP studies. *Veterinary Records*, 131, 307–310.

Peden, A.H., Head, M.W., Ritchie, D.L., Bell, J.E. and Ironside, J.W. (2004). Preclinical vCJD after blood transfusion in a PRNP codon 129 heterozygous patient. *Lancet*, 364, 527–529.

Prusiner, S.B. (1982). Novel proteinaceous infectious particles cause scrapie. *Science*, 216, 136–144.

Prusiner, S.B. (1998). The prion diseases. *Brain Pathology*, 8, 499–513.

Ricketts, M. (2006). BSE as a case study of public health and the public good. In J. Dwyer, C. Hedberg, T. Taylor and M. Wilson (ed.), *Institute of Medicine, National Academy of Sciences, Addressing Foodborne Threats to Health: Policies, Practices, and Global Coordination, Workshop Summary Forum on Microbial Threats*. Washington, DC: National Academies Press, pp.212–221. www.ncbi.nlm.nih.gov/books/NBK57091/pdf/TOC.pdf.

Russell, M. L., Thurston, W.E. and Henderson, E.A. (2003). Theory and models for planning and evaluating institutional influenza prevention and control programs. *American Journal of Infection Control*, 31, 336–341.

Schatzl, H.M., Da, C.M., Taylor, L., Cohen, F.E. and Prusiner, S.B. (1995). Prion protein gene variation among primates. *Journal of Molecular Biology*, 245, 362–374.

Scott, M., Groth, D., Foster, D., Torchia, M., Yang, S.L., DeArmond, S.J. and Prusiner, S.B. (1993). Propagation of prions with artificial properties in transgenic mice expressing chimeric PrP genes. *Cell*, 73, 979–988.

Scott, M.R., Will, R., Ironside, J., Nguyen, H.O., Tremblay, P., DeArmond, S.J. and Prusiner, S.B. (1999). Compelling transgenetic evidence for transmission of bovine spongiform encephalopathy prions to humans. *Proceedings of the National Academy of Sciences of the United States of America*, 96, 15137–15142.

Simkin, S., Hawton, K., Fagg, J. and Malberg, A. (1998). Stress in famers: a survey of farmers in England and Wales. *Occupational and Environmental Medicine*, 55, 729–734.

Stack, M.J., Balachandran, A., Chaplin, M., Davis, L., Czub, S. and Miller, B. (2004). The first Canadian indigenous case of bovine spongiform encephalopathy (BSE) has molecular characteristics for prion protein that are similar to those of BSE in the United Kingdom but differ from those of chronic wasting disease in captive elk and deer. *Canadian Veterinary Journal*, 45, 825–830.

Stevenson, M.A., Morris, R.S., Lawson, A.B., Wilesmith, J.W., Ryan, J.B. and Jackson, R. (2005). Area-level risks for BSE in British cattle before and after the July 1988 meat and bone meal feed ban. *Preventive Veterinary Medicine*, 69, 129–144.

Thomas, H.V., Lewis, G., Thomas, R.H., Salmon, R.L., Chalmers, R.M., Coleman, T.J., Kench, S.M., Morgan-Capner, P., Meadows, D., Sillis, M., and Softley, P. (2003). Mental health of British farmers. *Occupational and Environmental Medicine*, 60, 181–186.

Thurston, W.E. (2010a). *Farm and Ranch Family Health Survey – Information Sheet 1*. Department of Community Health Sciences, University of Calgary, Alberta, Canada.

Thurston, W.E. (2010b). *Farm and Ranch Family Health Survey – Information Sheet 2*. Department of Community Health Sciences, University of Calgary, Alberta, Canada.

Thurston, W.E. and Blundell-Gosselin, H.J. (2005). The farm as a setting for health promotion: results of a needs assessment in South Central Alberta. *Health & Place*, 11, 31–43.

Thurston, W.E. and Brook, R.K. (2008). *The Impact of Prion Diseases on Farm Family Health: Implications for Risk Management and Population Health. A Piece of the Puzzle is Missing*. Presentation to Sixth International Symposium, Public Health and the Agricultural Rural Ecosystem, Saskatoon, Saskatchewan, 19–23 October.

Thurston, W.E., Blundell-Gosselin, H.J., and Rose, S. (2003a). Stress in male and female farmers: an ecological rather than an individual problem. *Canadian Journal of Rural Medicine*, 8, 247–254.

Thurston, W.E., Blundell-Gosselin, H.J., and Vollman, A.R. (2003b). Health concerns of male and female farmers: implications for health promotion planning. *Canadian Journal of Rural Medicine*, 8, 239–246.

Watts, J.C., Balachandran, A. and Westaway, D. (2006). The expanding universe of prion diseases. *PLOS Pathogens*, 2, e26.

Weissmann, C., Fischer, M., Raeber, A., Bueler, H., Sailer, A., Shmerling, D., Rulicke, T., Brandner, S. and Aguzzi, A. (1996). The role of PrP in pathogenesis of experimental scrapie. *Cold Spring Harbour Symposia on Quantitative Biology*, 61, 511–522.

Wells, G.A., Scott, A.C., Johnson, C.T., Gunning, R.F., Hancock, R.D., Jeffrey, M., Dawson, M. and

Bradley, R. (1987). A novel progressive spongiform encephalopathy in cattle. *Veterinary Records*, 121, 419–420.

Wells, G.A., Hawkins, S.A., Austin, A.R., Ryder, S.J., Done, S.H., Green, R.B., Dexter, I., Dawson, M. and Kimberlin, R.H. (2003). Studies of the transmissibility of the agent of bovine spongiform encephalopathy to pigs. *Journal of General Virology*, 84, 1021–1031.

Wells, G.A., Konold, T., Arnold, M.E., Austin, A.R., Hawkins, S.A., Stack, M., Simmons, M.M., Lee, Y.H., Gavier-Widen, D., Dawson, M. and Wilesmith, J.W. (2007). Bovine spongiform encephalopathy: the effect of oral exposure dose on attack rate and incubation period in cattle. *Journal of General Virology*, 88, 1363–1373.

WHO (1986). www.who.int/healthpromotion/conferences/previous/ottawa/en.

Wilham, J.M., Orrú, C.D., Bessen, R.A., Atarashi, R., Sano, K., Race, B., Meade-White, K.D., Taubner, L.M., Timmes, A. and Caughey, B. (2010). Rapid end-point quantitation of prion seeding activity with sensitivity comparable to bioassays. *PLoS Pathogens*, 6, e1001217.

Will, R.G., Ironside, J.W., Zeidler, M., Cousens, S.N., Estibeiro, K., Alperovitch, A., Poser, S., Pocchiari, M., Hofman, A. and Smith, P.G. (1996). A new variant of Creutzfeldt-Jakob disease in the UK. *Lancet*, 347, 921–925.

Wopfner, F., Weidenhofer, G., Schneider, R., von, B.A., Gilch, S., Schwarz, T.F., Werner, T. and Schatzl, H.M. (1999). Analysis of 27 mammalian and 9 avian PrPs reveals high conservation of flexible regions of the prion protein. *Journal of Molecular Biology*, 289, 1163–1178.

Wroe, S.J., Pal, S., Siddique, D., Hyare, H., Macfarlane, R., Joiner, S., Linehan, J.M., Brandner, S., Wadsworth, J.D., Hewitt, P. and Collinge, J. (2006). Clinical presentation and pre-mortem diagnosis of variant Creutzfeldt-Jakob disease associated with blood transfusion: a case report. *Lancet*, 368, 2061–2067.

chapter 18

Global trends in food safety: One Health and trade

Susan C. Cork, Bonnie Buntain and Karen Liljebjelke

Abstract

The modern globalized economy of the twenty-first century has resulted in an increased level of social, political and economic interdependence as a result of the growing movement of people, produce and other commodities across national borders (Phillips, 2006; Vallat and Mallet, 2006). However, as a consequence of increased trade and travel there is a greater risk of transporting biological and other hazards, from country to country, on a large scale. With greater connectedness, new and emerging diseases have the potential to travel very fast to, and from, a large number of locations. As a consequence the development of an effective coordinated reporting can be difficult. Growing international trade in raw and processed plant and animal food commodities, and the development of a multinational market place, has resulted in an increased number of transboundary foodborne illnesses, many of which are zoonotic. Although some of the increased reporting is a result of better surveillance, it does highlight the need for international cooperation in disease reporting and for coordinated disease response and control initiatives (Kaferstein et al., 1997; King et al., 2004; Kobrin, 2008). Due to the volume of legal trade in live animals and animal commodities, and a recognition of the close link between food safety, food security, and human and animal health, there is also growing international awareness of the necessity of applying a One Health approach when developing and applying food safety regulations. At the formal trade level, this has largely occurred through the implementation of the internationally agreed standards outlined in the Sanitary and Phytosanitary (SPS) Agreement and the Codex Alimentarius (Vallat and Mallet, 2006). However, there is also a growing volume of illegal trade and a growth in 'bushmeat' markets in many parts of the world. These factors, along with cultural differences in food preferences have resulted in the need for a broader approach to the emerging food safety risks at the local, regional and global levels. The One Health approach to address food safety and other emerging animal, human and ecosystem concerns has been adopted in tripartite agreements among influential international organizations, such as the World Organisation for Animal Health (OIE), Food and Agriculture Organization of the United Nations (FAO) and World Health Organization (WHO) (FAO, 2013).

18.1 Disease and the food chain

Outbreaks of foodborne disease can have significant socioeconomic impacts on consumer food choices and other behaviour (Sockett, 1993; Knowles et al., 2007). Our understanding of the epidemiology of foodborne diseases has evolved in recent decades as a result of improvements in pathogen detection and better reporting systems. However, new pathogens have emerged to correspond with a changing food supply, a greater diversity of food preparation practices, changing food preferences and, in some parts of the world, an increase in the number of people with heightened susceptibility to foodborne diseases (i.e., immunocompromised and elderly people). This has posed a number of challenges for veterinary and public health agencies (Epp, 2008; BeVier, 2008). Alongside these changes, advanced technology and the growing global economy has facilitated the rapid transport of perishable foods, increasing the potential for human populations to be exposed to new or increased dosage of foodborne pathogens prevalent in distant parts of the world. Taking a One Health approach to food safety is an example of having to adapt to changing paradigms in which both the consumer as well as food producers and regulatory authorities need to work in partnership in order to ensure a safe and sustainable supply of food for communities across the globe (IOM, 2012) (see also Table 18.1).

Table 18.1 Applying the One Health approach to food safety. Adapted from King (2011), www.nap.edu/catalogue.php?record_id=13423.

Component	Previous approach	One Health approach
Problem-solving	Engaging technical experts to identify specific solutions to individual problems	Managing complex problems, broad interdisciplinary teams
Perspective	Fragmented approach, separate expertise (multidisciplinary but not integrated)	Systems approach, integrated expertise (interdisciplinary)
How work is done	Individuals working separately, lack of communication	Collaborative teams of multiple disciplines and perspectives
With whom work is done	Loose linkages, linear approach, duplication of efforts	Partnerships and strong linkages: government, academia, industry and the public/consumers engaged (transdisciplinary)
Where work is done	Focus on human illness	Closest to origin of problem/source of infection or contamination (root causes of determinants of health)
What is worked on	Single health domain	Human, animal and ecosystem/ environmental health domains
Surveillance and data	Limited to human health, disconnected from other domains	Interconnected systems, human and animal health, environmental health – shared data systems and collaborative interpretation
Timeframe	Reactive, emphasis on treating disease	Proactive, preventative and anticipatory

18.2 Foodborne disease control: a transnational challenge

The world has moved from a situation in which the majority of food was produced locally and sold in local markets to a system in which food is transported great distances and marketed through large chains of supermarkets. Despite international agreements providing a framework for import health and safety standards required for traded animal and plant-based products, the expansion of trade in fresh and processed primary produce has resulted in a number of significant biosecurity and resultant food safety breaches in recent years.

> Disease knows no boundaries and borders are porous to disease.
>
> (Kaferstein et al., 1997).

Processed products manufactured from raw ingredients imported from many different sources makes traceability difficult, and comprehensively tracking contaminated foodstuffs may be impossible – as illustrated by milk products and pet food contaminated with melamine initially produced in China but eventually disseminated in food supply chains around the world, resulting in illness and deaths in children and in pets (Brown et al., 2007; Ingelfinger, 2008).

The transnational transportation of animal and plant products contribute to the spread of infectious diseases, including those caused by foodborne bacteria, viruses and parasitic agents (Seimenis, 2008). International animal health and animal production food safety standards and guidelines have been developed by the OIE (see later section of this chapter) to encourage pre-processing food safety. These are used by the Codex Alimentarius in the development of food safety standards recognized by the World Trade Organization (WTO) to reduce the risk of

trading contaminated products, and by countries to develop their own food safety regulations. However, the degree of implementation of relevant regulations, and the extent of inspection and enforcement, varies from country to country, and sometimes within countries (Arambulo, 2008; Pires et al., 2009).

18.3 Factors affecting the changing pattern of foodborne diseases

Disease surveillance and pathogen detection

In industrialized countries, the systems for reporting foodborne disease outbreaks have become more sophisticated over the past few decades. This, along with better pathogen detection methods and the ability to trace the origin of infections to specific food products, has resulted in more awareness of food safety (Cooke, 1990; Hartung, 2008). Mild disease and sporadic cases of foodborne infection probably still go unreported, but better public education and greater media engagement in communicating potential food hazards and food recalls have contributed to enhanced reporting of many foodborne diseases.

Computer databases such as FoodNet in Canada, and PulseNet in the US, are used to identify individual foodborne bacterial strains, and are programmed to issue alerts when temporal or spacial clusters of disease are detected, or when a strain is associated with a particular food product or source (www.phac-aspc.gc.ca/foodnetcanada/index-eng.php, www.cdc.gov/pulsenet). In Europe, the European Food Safety Authority (EFSA) compiles and assesses data collected by individual member country food safety surveillance programmes, acting as an EU-wide food safety system assessing trends against historical data. The strain typing methods of the CDC PulseNet have been adopted by diagnostic laboratories on six continents, and the member country data has been compiled into an international foodborne pathogen database (www.pulsenetinternational.org). Because of the increasing importance of international trade of food, and the increasing mobility of the world population, international surveillance programmes are vital to identifying and controlling potential outbreaks of foodborne illness (www.efsa.europa.eu). These and other surveillance tools such as disease modelling, can be used to assist agencies to detect and prevent outbreaks of foodborne zoonoses earlier than in previous decades (Singer et al., 2007; Fosse et al., 2008a, 2008b; IOM, 2012).

Enhanced pathogen-detection methods, especially rapid molecular genetic techniques, have increased our ability to detect and trace pathogens associated with foodborne diseases. This has led to better reporting and a greater ability to implement food recalls and to issue alerts once a food source associated with a disease outbreak has been identified. Biosensors, immunoassays and PCR techniques are very sensitive and can be used to screen batches of commercial food products before sale as part of food-safety monitoring programmes. As new technologies have become available, current and emerging diseases have been more readily detected, thus allowing better reporting and more effective intervention in disease outbreaks. New molecular tools have also facilitated studies towards a better understanding of disease ecology (Chandra et al., 2008; Galligan and Kanara, 2008; Frank et al., 2011). Importantly these technologies have enabled regulatory agencies to develop policies and regulations that when adopted by industries and enforced by the government can result in prevention of food contamination at the regulated source.

Changes in food manufacturing and agricultural processes

With increasing knowledge of the ecology of foodborne pathogens, food safety guidelines must consider food production from the 'farm to the fork', i.e., from the farm setting, where the primary produce is grown, right through to the processing, shipping, storage, handling and preparation of food by the consumer (Beuchat and Ryu, 1997). Before food reaches the consumer, contamination can occur at any stage of the food production chain. In many parts of the world, modern food processing facilities are typically large and centralized compared with the traditional small family-run units where food was usually sold locally. In many countries there has been a drive, usually due to economic factors, to consolidate the food-producing sector (Howard, 2009). Technological changes in the food-manufacturing industry have enabled producers to maximize output but, although some risks have been minimized with modern processing methods, other risks have increased (Galligan and Kanara, 2008). Bulk food production has had a downside, for example, owing to the need to preserve food for wider distribution over long distances, appropriate conditions during transport and safe handling of food stuffs have become especially important to food safety (Siegford et al., 2008; Burton, 2009). A range of regulations have been developed and implemented in different countries to ensure that good handling practice is maintained by food producers and manufacturers, but compliance can vary from country to country and from company to company. Because of the rise of transnational food corporations and wide-scale distribution between and within countries, international agreements have been developed to ensure that minimum standards are set and enforced.

In reaction to consumer attitudes about large-scale agricultural production, an increase in the trade of fresh produce and the minimal treatment

Organic farming and foodborne pathogens

There remains a fair bit of controversy about the benefits and risks associated with organic food production, especially in relation to food quality and food safety. The accepted production methods for agricultural products to be considered organic vary from country to country. A well-managed organic farm can provide many environmental benefits and has socioeconomic value, especially when catering for small-scale niche markets (Hovi et al., 2003; Lund, 2006; Dangour et al., 2009). A recent study examining the prevalence of *Salmonella enterica* serotypes on processed chicken carcasses from large-scale commercial farms and small-scale free-range and organic farms demonstrated significant carriage of the pathogen on products from all farm types studied (Bailey and Cosby, 2005). Some studies have demonstrated a lower prevalence of antimicrobial resistance in bacteria isolated from animals on organic farms compared with those on conventional farms, although other studies have not seen differences (Schwaiger et al., 2008). Both large- and small-scale processing of organically produced products for international and national distribution has to comply with the same basic food safety standards as conventional products. Production standards, however, are usually set by national and international certification bodies that outline what management and intervention practices are required and/or allowed, as well as the production standards for growing, storage, processing, packaging and shipping of products considered organically produced.

processes required for some 'natural' and organic-based products has also occurred, leading to an increase in some foodborne diseases, especially in cases where the consumer fails to wash or prepare the product well. Raw fruits and vegetables have increasingly been identified as a source of foodborne infections (Beuchat, 2002; Noah, 2009). The increase in international trade in fruit and vegetables has increased exposure to foodborne pathogens on perishable products that are not easily disinfected, and intended to be consumed uncooked (www.cdc.gov/media/releases/2012/p0314_foodborne.html).

Emerging pathogens with improved survivability

In the past few decades, a number of new foodborne pathogens have been identified. Some of these represent the development of more virulent strains of pathogens including bacteria, such as *E. coli* O157:H7, and others have been discovered as a result of better detection methods. Newly recognized pathogenic strains of shiga-toxin producing *E. coli* (STEC) are now the target of food safety regulations in the US, with zero tolerance, having been declared food 'adulterants' in ground beef and trimmings (US Government Archives, 2012). It is widely argued that many of these new foodborne bacterial pathogen variants may have arisen as a result of selection pressure associated with livestock husbandry practices such as the use of antibiotics as growth promoters and the unique ecology of large-scale intensive agricultural production systems.

Antibiotic resistance has been reported in a wide range of enteric bacteria, including *E. coli*, *Salmonella enterica* and *Campylobacter* spp., but it is not known to what extent this is a result of natural selection versus a consequence of antibiotic use in both the human and animal population, and subsequent environmental contamination leading to selection pressure. It is also evident that many foodborne infections in industrialized nations, especially viral infections such as norovirus, reflect human-to-human transmission, with animals having a minor or insignificant role. However, other foodborne diseases such as listeriosis, *E. coli* O157:H7 and many outbreaks of campylobacteriosis have demonstrated links to livestock production and food preparation practices. Owing to the similarity of the clinical signs associated with a range of food- and waterborne diseases in the human population, the causative agent in many cases remains unconfirmed.

Other new and emerging diseases, such as severe acute respiratory syndrome (SARS), Nipah virus or new strains of Ebola virus, may be inadvertently spread across the world as a result of the increasing, and generally illegal, trade in bushmeat and animal parts intended for medicinal compounds, as well as being spread by humans as a result of international air travel (IOM, 2012). These isolated reports of emerging zoonotic pathogens that may occasionally be foodborne may reflect rare events, but they may also act as early indicators of diseases that may be exported around the world where biosecurity measures, and food safety and inspection standards are not enforced. As a result of the complex nature of the modern food supply it is important to engage interdisciplinary teams when developing guidelines for the safe production and handling of food.

18.4 Ensuring the safety of the food supply

Surveillance of foodborne disease outbreaks

Well-established surveillance systems play an important role in the early detection of foodborne

---

Illegal harvest and trade of bushmeat and emerging infectious disease

People around the world engage in the illegal harvest or poaching of wild animals in order to satisfy a growing population's need for dietary animal protein in the face of local food insecurity as well as the use wild meats and organs for cultural practices. The unregulated harvest of wildlife has consequences for the ecosystems impacted by the wholesale removal of animals; predator and prey species, pollinators and seed dispersers. In addition to causing direct harm to the environment, the hunters come in contact with the bodily fluids of animals, which may carry novel unrecognized viral and bacterial pathogens that may be zoonotic. An excellent example of an outbreak of a zoonotic disease originating from contact and consumption of wildlife occurred in China in 2002. A novel disease outbreak dubbed 'sudden acute respiratory syndrome' or SARS, was eventually traced back to the trapping and consumption of the Civet cat, considered a delicacy (Wang and Eaton, 2007). A new zoonotic Corona virus was described, and the Civet cat was identified as an intermediate carrier of the SARS virus, with local bat species found to be the definitive hosts. Human-to-human transmission of the virus occurred later in the outbreak, and it was eventually discovered that a genetic mutation in a single gene had enhanced the ability of the virus to infect a new host – human beings (Wang and Eaton, 2007).

Illegal movement of bushmeat across international borders may have serious consequences for both human and animal health, in addition to the negative effects on the ecosystems from which it is harvested.

diseases and their control. Early identification of the source of a disease outbreak is especially important where commodities are traded in high volumes internationally. Increased mass production means that disease outbreaks have the potential to affect hundreds or thousands of people in multiple countries. Examples of large foodborne disease outbreaks include more than 168,000 cases of salmonellosis in the UK in 1985, 224,000 cases of salmonellosis in the USA in 1993, >310,000 cases of hepatitis A in China in 1988, >3,050 cases of Norwalk-like virus in Australia in 1991 and >6,000 cases of *E. coli* O157 infection in Japan in 1996 (Kaferstein et al., 1997). Efficient surveillance and reporting can help to identify the source of a problem early and thereby prevent its spread; for example, a 1993 outbreak of listeriosis in France, caused by a potted pork product, involved 39 cases, including eight miscarriages and one death, the public health authorities traced it to its source within a week, quickly recalled the product, reducing further cases (Kaferstein et al., 1997). Early detection of disease outbreaks can also minimize direct and indirect costs, both in terms of human disease, economic burden and public health dollars.

Some food safety surveillance systems are hazard-focused and collate reports of non-compliance or problems in food safety audits (Marvin et al., 2009). As a complement to improved reporting of surveillance data, the principles of the hazard analysis and critical control point (HACCP) system adopted by the Codex Alimentarius (FAO, 1997) and the growing acceptance worldwide by industries and governments has resulted in a reduction in the number of foodborne disease outbreaks. In the US, the adoption of HACCP principles by food processors is associated with both a reduction in foodborne illness and economic burden of outbreaks (*Federal Register*, 61(144), 1996, pp. 38806–38989; Crutchfield et al. 1997). Application of HAACP programmes allow food

technologists and food inspectors to identify which critical food manufacturing processes are reasonably likely to reduce, control or prevent specific hazards likely to enter that process. These critical control points (CCPs) help ensure a scientific foundation for food safety preventive programmes when the HACCP principles are followed. Therefore, application of HACCP principles to food processing facilitates the identification of practices that may be potentially hazardous and allows manufacturers and food safety inspectors to suggest modifications which specifically address reduction of the pathogen or other food hazard (see box below).

Principles of the HACCP system

The HACCP system consists of the following seven principles:

PRINCIPLE 1: Conduct a hazard analysis.

PRINCIPLE 2: Determine the critical control coints (CCPs).

PRINCIPLE 3: Establish critical limit(s).

PRINCIPLE 4: Establish a system to monitor control of the CCP.

PRINCIPLE 5: Establish the corrective action to be taken when monitoring indicates that a particular CCP is not under control.

PRINCIPLE 6: Establish procedures for verification to confirm that the HACCP system is working effectively.

PRINCIPLE 7: Establish documentation concerning all procedures and records appropriate to these principles and their application.

(www.fao.org/docrep/005/Y1579E/y1579e03.htm; FAO, 1997)

Risk assessment and international food standards

Microbiological risk assessment can be used to provide an estimate of the probability of a specific pathogen or hazard being present in a given commodity as well as the likelihood of disease arising from the presence of a given amount of a specific pathogen or hazard in a specific population (Fosse et al., 2008a; Hallman, 2008). It can also be used to identify high-risk foods or processing methods (Swaminathan and Gerner-Smidt, 2007). However, although risk assessment is a useful tool, the conclusions derived from the risk assessment process must be viewed in context, as the assessment is usually qualitative. This is because there is often insufficient data available to produce a quantitative measure of the risks associated with a specific commodity. Essentially, risk assessment is a structured and objective process comprising four steps: hazard identification, hazard characterization, exposure assessment and risk characterization. Risk assessment, risk management and risk communication together constitute risk analysis. Risk analysis has a wide range of applications in food safety, ranging from informing national and international food safety policies to the implementation of specific sanitation measures to achieve pathogen reduction at certain points in the farm-to-fork (table) continuum. The process is well described in a number of publications (Murray, 2002; Mumford and Kihm, 2006; Ross, 2008; Wooldridge, 2008).

Risk assessment process steps

1. Hazard identification (i.e., the identification of biological, chemical and physical agents present in a particular food or group of foods that can cause illness).

2. Hazard characterization (i.e., the qualitative or quantitative evaluation of the nature of the illness associated with biological, chemical and physical agents that may be present in food).
3. Exposure assessment (i.e., the qualitative or quantitative evaluation of the likely intake of the hazard).
4. Risk characterization (i.e., the qualitative or quantitative estimation, including uncertainties, of the probability and severity of known impacts in a given population on the basis of hazard identification, characterization and exposure assessment).

(Murray, 2002; see also OIE, 2004)

Risk assessments are considered during the construction of science-based food safety regulation. In 2003, the US Department of Agriculture (USDA), in collaboration with the Food Safety Inspection Service (FSIS) of the USDA and the Centers for Disease Control and Prevention (CDC), released the results of a risk assessment predicting the risk of acquiring listeriosis from different food types (Swaminathan and Gerner-Smidt, 2007). As a result of risk assessments and the subsequent regulations implemented over the past decade to prevent *Listeria* in food commodities for sale to the public, the incidence of listeriosis in the USA declined, with reported cases reduced by 40 per cent between 1996 and 1998. However, despite these promising developments, outbreaks of listeriosis do still occur as illustrated in the *Listeria* contamination of cantaloupe melons in the USA in 2011, which resulted in 29 deaths and illness in 139 (mostly elderly) individuals. This outbreak was one of the few outbreaks of listeriosis attributed to fresh produce in the USA. The outbreak resulted in an in-depth investigation by the CDC and the voluntary recall of 300,000 cases of melons by the producer (IOM, 2012).

18.5 International agreements on food standards

The Codex Alimentarius Commission was created in 1963 by the FAO and WHO to develop food standards, guidelines and related texts such as codes of practice under the Joint FAO/WHO Food Standards Programme. The main purposes of this programme are protecting the health of consumers, ensuring fair trade practices in food trade and promoting coordination of all food standards work undertaken by international governmental and non-governmental organizations (Dawson, 1995; Droppers, 2006; Slorach, 2006). The Codex Alimentarius Commission adopts standards, codes of practices and other related texts that are prepared by specialized Codex Committees and ad hoc task forces. The WTO agreement on the Application of Sanitary and Phytosanitary Measures (SPS Agreement) considers that WTO members that apply the Codex Alimentarius Standards meet their obligations under this agreement. Scientifically based risk assessment plays an important role in the setting of Codex standards. Epidemiological data on foodborne diseases is important for the development of these risk assessments. A key example of this is the assessment of the risk of contracting listeriosis following the consumption of various products that may contain varying amounts of *L. monocytogenes*. In a joint study conducted by the USDA and the US Food and Drug Administration (FDA), foods were identified as being of high, medium and low risk with respect to harbouring *L. monocytogenes* (Swaminathan and Gerner-Smidt, 2007). High-risk foods included delicatessen meats, high-fat dairy products, soft unripened cheese and unpasteurized fluid milk. Medium-risk products included pasteurized milk, fresh soft cheeses, ready to eat (RTE) meals, salami, fruit and vegetables. To reduce the risk of products harbouring *L. monocytogenes*, good food production standards such as HACCP have been implemented but it is a challenge to reduce the risk to zero. In view of this, certain vulnerable sectors of society, including pregnant women, the elderly or immunocompromised are encouraged not to eat foods considered high to medium risk of containing listeria and other potential pathogens (www.cdc.gov/listeria/risk.html).

Increased trade opportunities following the Uruguay Round of multilateral trade negotiations in 1986–1994, and the increased liberalization of trade, caused concern between trading nations over the safety of imported food, and highlighted the need to develop transparent regulations to ensure that traded raw and processed products would be produced to the same standards as products in the country importing these products. This is relevant to biological, physical and chemical hazards with the potential to affect human health, as well as to chemical toxins, genetically modified agents and invasive microorganisms and pests that might have an effect on animal and plant health. The WTO emerged as an entity in 1995 (after the Uruguay Round) along with guidelines for the Application of Sanitary and Phytosanitary (SPS) measures designed to address concerns about the assessment and control of hazards in imported products. Along with the SPS measures, food safety issues are specifically addressed by the Codex Alimentarius Commission, which has standards, guidelines and recommendations to ensure food safety in traded products. The purpose of these standards is to facilitate trade among WTO members while ensuring that quality and safety standards are met.

In 2001, the WTO committee on Sanitary and Phytosanitary Measures clarified Article 4 of the SPS Agreement, outlining ways in which members could meet the concept of equivalence; that member countries may demonstrate that alternate methods and measures can meet the food safety and sanitation requirements of the importing country and provide the same level of health protection (www.wto.org/index.htm).

The increased volume of global food trade also highlights the need for consistent and effective surveillance and reporting to facilitate effective risk assessment of foodborne pathogens and hazards. In this regard, Article 5 of the SPS agreement explicitly requires WTO members to prepare, or refer to, scientific and consistent risk assessments. In addition, the World Health Organization (WHO) has recommended that the application of the HACCP system at every stage of the food chain represents an effective approach for governments to meet the terms outlined in the agreement.

The role of the World Organisation for Animal Health (OIE)

Human and animal health are interrelated in several key ways. The security of our food supply relies upon the health of our food animals. Increased international trade raises concerns not only about foodborne illness, but also about the possibility of movement of animal diseases across international borders. The need to fight animal diseases at global level led to the creation of the Office International des Epizooties (OIE) through an international agreement signed on 25 January 1924. In May 2003, the OIE became the World Organisation for Animal Health, but kept its historical acronym, OIE. The OIE is the intergovernmental organization responsible for improving animal health worldwide. It is recognized as a reference organization by the WTO and, as of April 2009, had a total of 174 member countries and territories. The OIE maintains permanent relations with 36 other international and regional organizations and has regional and sub-regional offices on every continent.

> ### The OIE mission
>
> - Guarantee the transparency of animal disease status worldwide.
> - Collect, analyse and disseminate veterinary scientific information.
> - Provide expertise and promote international solidarity for the control of animal disease.
> - Guarantee the sanitary safety of world trade by developing sanitary rules for international trade in animals and animal products.
>
> (See www.oie.int)

It is estimated that more than 60 per cent of known human infectious diseases have their source in animals (whether domestic or wild), as do 75 per cent of emerging human diseases and 80 per cent of the pathogens that could potentially be used in bioterrorism (ILRI, 2012). At the global level, the OIE has modernized its worldwide information system on animal diseases (including zoonoses) with the creation of World Animal Health Information Service (WAHIS), a mechanism whereby all countries are linked online to a central server that collects all the compulsory notifications sent to the OIE, covering 100 priority terrestrial and aquatic animal diseases. The WHO adopted the International Health Regulations in 1969, subsequently updating them several times and placing new obligations on its members with regard to disease reporting and surveillance in the human population (WHO, 2005). The OIE, WHO and FAO have since created the Global Early Warning System (GLEWS), a platform shared by the three organizations to improve early warning on animal diseases and zoonoses worldwide.

18.6 Foodborne disease and the globalized food supply – a case study

The globalization of legal and illegal trade in animals, animal parts and food has led to large-scale disease outbreaks that have been challenging to control, and have resulted in international trade disputes. In this section we present a recent case study illustrating the difficulties of investigating multinational outbreaks of foodborne disease.

Investigation of a multinational *E. coli* 014:H4 outbreak

In 2011, a novel strain of *Escherichia coli* 014:H4 bacteria caused a serious outbreak of foodborne illness initially focused in northern Germany in May and June (Frank et al., 2011). The illness was characterized by bloody diarrhoea, with a high frequency of serious complications, including haemolytic-uremic syndrome (HUS), a potentially fatal condition that requires urgent treatment (Borgatta et al., 2012). A handful of cases were reported in several other countries including Switzerland, Poland, the Netherlands, Sweden, Denmark, the UK, Canada and the US. All affected people had been in Germany or France shortly before becoming ill (EFSA, 2011).

The outbreak was originally thought to have been caused by an enterohaemorrhagic strain of *E. coli* (EHEC), but it was later shown to have been caused by an enteroaggregative strain of *E. coli* (EAEC) that had acquired the genes to produce Shiga toxins.

After a number of attempts to identify the original source of the bacteria it was eventually traced to fenugreek sprouts originating in Egypt (EFSA, 2011). In the interim, a number of other potentially contaminated products had been implicated in the outbreak, with significant financial impacts to the producers. The Robert Koch Institute advised against eating raw tomatoes, cucumbers and lettuces in Germany to prevent further cases. The media reaction to the outbreak and the uncertainty over the source of the contamination resulted in a significant public response with subsequent economic damage to many businesses growing salad vegetables (Beutin and Martin, 2012).

In May 2011, German health officials announced that cucumbers from Spain were identified as a source of the *E. coli* outbreak in Germany, issued an alert distributed to nearby countries, and withdrew them from the market. The European Commission said the two Spanish greenhouses suspected to be the sources had been closed, and soil and water samples were being analysed. Cucumber samples from the Andalusian greenhouses did not show *E. coli* contamination.

According to the head of the national *E. coli* lab at the German Federal Institute for Risk Assessment, the strain responsible for the outbreak had been circulating in Germany for ten years, and in humans, not in cattle. He said it is likely to have contaminated food via human faeces, and that the most probable source in the produce was cross-contamination.

In June 2011, a joint risk-assessment by the EFSA/ECDC made a connection between the German outbreak and a HUS outbreak in the Bordeaux area of France, in which infection with *E. coli* O104:H4 had been confirmed in several patients (ESFA, 2011). The assessment implicated fenugreek seeds imported from Egypt in 2009 and 2010 from which sprouts were grown as a common source of both outbreaks, but cautioned, 'there is still much uncertainty about whether this is truly the common cause of the infections', as tests on the seeds had not yet found any *E. coli* bacteria of the O104:H4 strain. The potentially contaminated seeds were widely distributed in Europe. Many countries took restrictive action. Egypt was the focus of the epidemiological investigation, but Egypt's Minister of Health Ashraf Hatem denied his nation had any patients infected with the new *E. coli* strain, due to the strict precautions brought in to test overseas tourists entering the country in June. The minister also told the Egyptian press the problem had nothing to do with Egypt and instead asserted, 'Israel is waging a commercial war against Egyptian exports'.

The EU's *E. coli* O104:H4 outbreak was estimated to have cost $2,840,000,000 due to expenses such as medical treatment and sick leave. It is estimated that more than 3,950 people were affected and 53 died, 51 of whom were in Germany. Consumers across Europe were shunning fruit and vegetables. EU farmers claimed to have losses up to $417,000,000 a week as ripe vegetables rotted in their fields and warehouses.

The definitive source of the outbreak was never identified.

Key resources

EFSA (European Food Safety Authority), www.efsa.europa.eu/en/press/news/120711.htm

European Union Press release, http://europa.eu/rapid/press-release_MEMO-11-366_en.htm

WHO, www.theguardian.com/world/2011/jun/02/e-coli-outbreak-who-bacterium-new-strain

European Union Presentations, http://ec.europa.eu/food/food/coli_outbreak_germany_presentations_en.htm

---

18.7 Conclusion

Many of the human diseases that have grown in importance in public health in recent decades are transmitted via the food supply. As the world has moved from a situation in which the majority of food was produced locally and sold in local markets to a system in which food is transported

great distances and marketed through large chains of supermarkets, the pathogen profile to which many human populations are exposed has expanded. Despite the international SPS agreement that provides a framework for the import health standards required for traded animal- and plant-based products the risk of transporting a pathogen from one country to another remains (Domenech et al., 2006). Current SPS requirements emphasize the importance of science-based risk assessment and hazard control programmes for the continued reduction of pathogens at relevant points of the 'farm-to-fork' food production chain. With the recognition of a need to take a broader interdisciplinary approach to monitor and respond to foodborne disease outbreaks the One Health concept has been applied effectively in the past decade. Since One Health encourages a multisectoral, transdisciplinary approach to food safety, it means that industry from farm to retail, multidisciplinary food safety experts all along the food chain, and consumers all share responsibility in preventing foodborne illnesses. Tools such as HACCP, risk analysis, and food safety surveillance programmes are critical for reducing risks to human health in the modern globalized society.

References

Arambulo, P. (2008). International programs and veterinary public health in the Americas – success, challenges, and possibilities. *Preventive Veterinary Medicine*, 86, 208–215.

Bailey, J.S. and Cosby, D.E. (2005). Salmonella prevalence in free-range and certified organic chickens. *Journal of Food Protection*, 68(11), 2451–2453.

Beuchat, L.R. (2002). Ecological factors influencing survival and growth of human pathogens on raw fruits and vegetables. *Microbes and Infection*, 4, 413–423.

Beuchat, L.R. and Ryu, J.H. (1997). Produce handling and processing practices. *Emerging Infectious Diseases*, 3, 459–465.

Beutin, L. and Martin, A. (2012). Outbreak of Shiga toxin-producing escherichia coli (STEC) O104:H4 in Germany causes a paradigm shift with regard to human pathogenicity of STEC strains. *Journal of Food Production*, 75(2), 408–418.

BeVier, G.W. (2008). What will the future bring, and how can we prepare for it? In G. Smith and A.M. Kelly (eds.), *Food Security in a Global Economy: Veterinary Medicine and Public Health*. Philadelphia: University of Pennsylvania Press, pp. 11–26.

Borgatta, B., Kmet-Lunacek, N. and Rello, J. (2012). E. coli O104: H4 outbreak and haemolytic-uraemic syndrome. *Med Intensiva*, 36(8), 576–583.

Brown, C.A., Jeong, K.S., Poppenga, R.H., Puschner, B., Miller, D.M., Ellis, A.E., Kang, K.I., Sum, S., Cistola, A.M. and Brown, S.A. (2007). Outbreaks of renal failure associated with melamine and cyanuric acid in dogs and cats in 2004 and 2007. *Journal of Veterinary Diagnostic Investigation*, 19, 525–531.

Burton, C.H. (2009). Reconciling the new demands for food protection with environmental needs in the management of livestock wastes. *Bioresource Technology*, 100, 5399–5405.

Chandra, V., Taneja, S., Kalia, M. and Jameel, S. (2008). Molecular biology and pathogenesis of hepatitis E virus. *Journal of Biosciences*, 33, 451–464.

Cooke, E.M. (1990). Epidemiology of foodborne illness: UK. *The Lancet*, 336, 790–793.

Cooper, J., Leifert, C. and Niggli, U. (eds.) (2007). *Handbook of Organic Food Safety and Quality*. Cambridge: Woodhead Publishing.

Crutchfield, S.R., Buzby, J.C., Roberts, T., Ollinger, M. and Lin. C.-T.J. (1997). *An Economic Assessment of Food Safety Regulations: The New Approach to Meat and Poultry Inspection*. Agricultural Economic Report No. 755, Economic Research Service, US Department of Agriculture, Washington, DC.

Dangour, A.D., Dodhia, S.K., Hayter, A., Allen, E., Lock, K. and Uauy, R. (2009). Nutritional quality of organic foods: a systematic review. *American Journal of Clinical Nutrition*, 90, 680–685.

Dawson, R.J. (1995). The role of the Codex Alimentarius Commission in setting food standards and the SPS agreement implementation. *Food Control*, 6, 261–265.

Domenech, J., Lubroth, J., Eddi, C., Martin, V. and Roger, F. (2006). Regional and international approaches on prevention and control of animal transboundary and emerging diseases. *Annals of the New York Academy of Sciences*, 1081, 90–107.

Droppers, W.F.G.L. (2006). OIE philosophy, policy and procedures for the development of food safety standards. *Revue Scientifique et Technique/Office International des Epizooties*, 25, 805–812.

EFSA (2011). Shiga toxin-producing *E. coli* (STEC) O104: H4 2011 outbreaks in Europe: taking stock. *European Food Safety Authority Journal*, 9(10), 2390.

Epp, T. (2008). Foodborne zoonoses: challenges for the veterinary profession. *Large Animal Veterinary Rounds*, 8(6), 1–6.

FAO (1997). www.fao.org/docrep/005/Y1579E/y1579e03.htm.

FAO (2013). www.fao.org/ag/againfo/home/en/news_archive/AGA_in_action/2013_Tripartite_partnership_at_the_human-animal-ecosystem_interface.html.

Fosse, J., Seegers, H. and Magras, C. (2008a). Prioritising the risk of foodborne zoonoses using a quantitative approach: application to foodborne bacterial hazards in pork and beef. *Review Scientifique et Technique – Office International des Epizooties*, 27, 643–655.

Fosse, J., Seegers, H. and Magras, C. (2008b). Foodborne zoonoses due to meat: a quantitative approach to a consequence risk assessment applied to pig slaughtering in Europe. *Veterinary Research*, 39, 1–16.

Frank, C., Werber, D., Cramer, J.P., Askar, M., Faber, M., an der Heiden, M., Bernanrd, H., Fruth, A., Prager, R., Spode, A., Wadl, M., Zoufaly, A., Jordan, S., Kemper, M.J., Follin, P., Muller, L., King, L.A., Rosner, B., Buchholz, U., Stark, K. and Kruase, G (2011). Epidemic profile of Shiga-Toxin-producing *Escherichia coli* O104: H4 outbreak in Germany. *The New England Journal of Medicine*, 365, 19.

Galligan, D.T. and Kanara, E. (2008). Technology, innovation, research, and development. In G. Smith and A.M. Kelly (eds.), *Food Security in a Global Economy: Veterinary Medicine and Public Health*. Philadelphia: University of Pennsylvania Press, pp. 43–50.

Hallman, W.K. (2008). Communicating about microbial risks in foods. In D.W. Schaffner (ed.), *Microbial Risk Analysis of Foods*. Washington, DC: American Society for Microbiology Press, pp. 205–262.

Hartung, M. (2008). Results of the zoonoses surveillance 2007 at foodstuffs in Germany. *Fleischwirtschaft*, 88, 114–122.

Hovi, M., Martini, A. and Padel, S. (eds.) (2003). *Socio-Economic Aspects of Animal Health and Food Safety in Organic Farming Systems*. Proceedings of the 1st SAFO Workshop, Florence, Italy, 5–7 September.

Howard, P.H. (2009). Consolidation in the North American food processing sector, 1997 to 2007. *International Journal of Sociology of Agriculture and Food*, 16, 13–30.

ILRI (2012). *Mapping of Poverty and Likely Zoonoses Hotspots*. Zoonoses Project 4. Report to Department for International Development, UK. Nairobi: International Livestock Research Institute.

Ingelfinger, J.R. (2008). Melamine and the global implications of food contamination. *New England Journal of Medicine*, 359, 2745–2748.

IOM (2012). *Improving Food Safety Through a One Health Approach*. Washington, DC: The National Academies Press.

Kaferstein, F.K., Motarjemi, Y. and Bettcher, D.W. (1997). Foodborne disease control: a transnational challenge. *Emerging Infectious Diseases*, 3, 503–510.

King, L. (2011). *What is One Health and Why is it Relevant to Food Safety?* Presentation given at the Public Workshop Improving Food Safety Through One Health, Forum on Microbial Threats, 13–14 December, Institute of Medicine, Washington, DC.

King, L., Marano, N. and Hughes, J.M. (2004). New partnerships between animal health services and public health agencies. *Revue Scientifique et Technique – Office International des Epizooties*, 23, 717–725.

Knowles, T., Moody, R. and McEachern, M.G. (2007). European food scares and their impact on EU food policy. *British Food Journal*, 109, 43–67.

Kobrin, S.J. (2008). Globalization: what caused it, and how will it end? In G. Smith and A.M. Kelly (eds.), *Food Security in a Global Economy: Veterinary Medicine and Public Health*. Philadelphia: University of Pennsylvania Press.

Lund, V. (2006). Animal welfare and ethics in organic agriculture. In P. Kristiansen, A. Taji and J. Reganold (eds.), *Organic Agriculture: A Global Perspective*. Wallingford: CAB International, pp. 187–199.

Marvin, H.J.P., Kleter, G.A., Prandini, A., Dekkers, S. and Bolton, D.J. (2009). Early identification systems for emerging foodborne hazards. *Food and Chemical Toxicology*, 47, 915–926.

Mort, M., Convery, I., Baxter, J. and Bailey, C. (2005). Psychosocial effects of the 2001 UK foot and mouth disease epidemic in a rural population: qualitative diary based study. *British Medical Journal*, 331.

Mumford, E.L. and Kihm, U. (2006). Integrated risk reduction along the food chain. *Annals of the New York Academy of Sciences*, 1081, 147–152.

Murray, N. (2002). *Import Risk Analysis: Animals and Animal Products*. Wellington: Ministry of Agriculture and Forestry.

Noah, N. (2009). Food poisoning from raw fruit and vegetables. *Epidemiology and Infection*, 137(3), 305–306.

OIE (2004). *Handbook on Import Risk Analysis for Animal and Animal products. Volume 1. Introduction and Qualitative Risk Analysis*. Paris: World Organisation for Animal Health.

Oloya, J., Doetkott, D. and Khaitsa, M.L. (2009). Antimicrobial drug resistance and molecular characterization of *Salmonella* isolated from domestic animals, humans, and meat products. *Foodborne Pathogens and Disease*, 6, 273–284.

Phillips, L. (2006). Food and globalization. *Annual Review of Anthropology*, 35, 37–57.

Pires, S.M., Evers, E.G., van Pelt, W., Ayers, T., Scallan, E., Angulo, F.J., Havelaar, A. and Hald, T. (2009). Attributing the human disease burden of food borne infections to specific sources. *Foodborne Pathogens and Disease*, 6, 417–424.

Ross, T. (2008). Microbial ecology in food safety risk assessment. In D.W. Schaffner (ed.), *Microbial Risk Analysis of Foods*. Washington, DC: American Society for Microbiology Press, pp. 51–98.

Schwaiger, K., Schmied, E.M.V. and Bauer, J. (2008). Comparative analysis of antibiotic resistance characteristics of Gram-negative bacteria isolated from laying hens and eggs in conventional and organic keeping systems in Bavaria, Germany. *Zoonoses Public Health*, 57(3), 171–180.

Seimenis, A.M. (2008). The spread of zoonoses and other infectious diseases through the international trade of animals and animal products. *Veterinaria Italiana* 44, 591–599.

Siegford, J.M., Powers, W. and Grimes-Casey, H.G. (2008). Environmental aspects of ethical animal production. *Poultry Science*, 87, 380–386.

Singer, R.S., Cox, L.A. Jr, Dickson, J.S., Hurd, H.S., Phillips, I. and Miller, G.Y. (2007). Modeling the relationships between food animal health and human foodborne illness. *Preventive Veterinary Medicine*, 79, 186–203.

Slorach, S.A. (2006). Assuring food safety: the complementary tasks and standards of the World Organisation for Animal health and the Codex Alimentarius Commission. *Revue Scientifique et Technique – Office International des Epizooties*, 25, 813–821.

Sockett, P. (1993). Social and economic aspects of food-borne disease. *Food Policy* 18, 110–119.

Swaminathan, B. and Gerner-Smidt, P. (2007). The epidemiology of human listeriosis. *Microbes and Infection*, 9, 1236–1243.

US Government Archives (2012). *Federal Register*, 77(105), 31975–31981, https://federalregister.gov/a/2012-13283.

Vallat, B. and Mallet, E. (2006). Ensuring good governance to address emerging and re-emerging animal disease threats: supporting the veterinary services of developing countries to meet OIE international standards on quality. *Revue Scientifique et Technique – Office International des Epizooties*, 25, 389–401.

Wang, L. and Eaton, B. (2007). Bats, civets and the emergence of SARS. Wildlife and emerging zoonotic diseases: the biology, circumstances and consequences of cross-species transmission. *Current Topics in Microbiology and Immunology*, 315, 325–344

WHO (2005). *International Health Regulations*, www.who.int/topics/international_health_regulations/en.

Wooldridge, M. (2008). Qualitative risk assessment. In: Schaffner, D.W. (ed.) *Microbial Risk Analysis of Foods*. American Society for Microbiology Press, Washington, DC, pp. 1–28.

chapter 19

Emerging markets and parasitic diseases

Brent Dixon

Abstract

Foodborne illnesses resulting from infections with protozoan parasites are an emerging problem in developed countries around the world, with numerous cases and outbreaks being reported in recent years. Fresh fruits and vegetables are of particular concern in this regard due, largely, to the demand for exotic or out-of-season fresh produce imported from developing countries where hygiene, sanitation and water quality may be poor, and where many potential sources of parasite contamination may exist. While there are many hurdles involved in testing foods, such as fresh produce, for the infectious stages of these parasites, and no standard methods currently exist, targeted surveillance studies for parasites on fresh produce have been done worldwide, and have generally demonstrated a high prevalence of contamination with protozoan parasites. A number of control measures at the pre- and post-harvest levels can be implemented to minimize the risk of contamination of fresh fruits and vegetables, or to physically remove the parasites or inactivate them following contamination. However, as these foods are often consumed raw with no further processing, there are few options at the consumer level for minimizing the risk of transmission and infection. Since many of these foodborne parasites can be transmitted from animals to humans and vice versa, either through direct contact with faeces containing infectious stages or indirectly through the consumption of contaminated water or foods, it is very important that a multidisciplinary One Health approach be adopted when investigating and managing foodborne parasitic diseases.

19.1 Introduction

The foodborne route of transmission of parasites is an important emerging issue in developed countries due to a variety of factors, including the globalization of the food trade, international travel, the increased number of immunocompromised and other susceptible individuals and changes in consumer habits. The foodborne protozoan parasites *Cryptosporidium* spp., *Giardia duodenalis*, *Cyclospora cayetanensis* and *Toxoplasma gondii* are of particular concern in this regard. All are commonly reported in humans worldwide and, with the exception of *C. cayetanensis*, are also highly prevalent in animals, and represent important zoonoses. *Cryptosporidium* spp., *G. duodenalis* and *C. cayetanensis* are all responsible for enteric illness in humans, while *T. gondii* infections are often asymptomatic, but may cause flu-like symptoms. Infections with *Cryptosporidium* spp. or *T. gondii* may result in severe and life-threatening illness in immuno-compromised individuals, and both are listed as AIDS-defining illnesses.

Numerous cases and outbreaks of foodborne illness due to infections with these parasites have been reported worldwide. Although the faecal-oral and waterborne routes of transmission are much more common for *Cryptosporidium* spp. and *G. duodenalis*, foodborne transmission is reported more frequently, and likely also accounts for more cases and outbreaks of infection with *C. cayetanensis* and *T. gondii*. For example, in the US, foodborne illnesses due to infection with *Cryptosporidium* spp., *G. duodenalis*, *C. cayetanensis* and *T. gondii* represent 8 per cent, 7 per cent, 99 per cent and 50 per cent, respectively, of the total number of illnesses reported annually (Scallan et al., 2011).

While some prepared foods have been implicated, most foodborne outbreaks have been associated with cyst- or oocyst-contaminated fresh fruits and vegetables, with the exception of *T. gondii*, which is more commonly associated with the consumption of raw or poorly cooked meats or organs, or with unpasteurized milk. Contamination of fresh produce with the infectious stages of protozoan parasites may occur through a number of different routes, involving either direct or indirect contact with the faeces of infected humans or animals. While the infectious stages of parasites have been commonly reported on fresh produce worldwide, there are many hurdles involved in testing foods for the presence of parasites, either in surveillance studies or as part of disease outbreak investigations.

Pre- and post-harvest control measures may be used to minimize the contamination of fresh produce with the infectious stages of parasites. These controls include, primarily, monitoring and enforcing the use of good-quality water for irrigation, washing and processing, as well as good hygienic practices by farm workers and food handlers. However, once contaminated, there are very few barriers to the transmission of parasitic infections associated with the consumption of fresh produce. For example, most of these parasites are highly resistant to common chemical disinfectants used in the food industry, and in routine water treatment. Even vigorous washing of the surface of contaminated produce is not fully effective in removing the infectious stages; nor is it even feasible in the case of more delicate fruits such as berries. Finally, fresh produce is very often consumed raw, with no further treatments such as freezing or cooking that would otherwise kill most contaminating parasites.

This chapter highlights the prevalence of protozoan parasites reported on fresh produce worldwide and the foodborne outbreaks that have been reported. It also discusses the possible sources of contamination and the challenges associated with the detection and control of these pathogens on fresh produce. Finally, a contemporary case study of *C. cayetanensis* on imported raspberries will be presented.

19.2 Prevalence of parasites on foods

Surveillance studies of foodborne parasites on a wide variety of fresh fruits and vegetables have been conducted in many countries around the world, with a wide range of prevalences reported. The variation is likely due to different levels of sanitation and hygiene, agricultural practices and methods used for detection (Dixon, 2015). Interestingly, the vast majority of these studies have been performed in developing countries in Africa, the Middle East and Central and South America, where the issue may be of greater public health concern and where contamination of produce may occur more frequently.

Although food is not as important in the transmission of *Cryptosporidium* spp. as water or person-to-person contact, numerous surveillance studies have nevertheless been done worldwide on *Cryptosporidium* spp. oocysts on fresh produce (Dixon, 2015). For example, cilantro and other fresh produce items collected from markets in Costa Rica were found to be contaminated with *Cryptosporidium* (Monge and Chinchilla, 1996; Calvo et al., 2004). Ortega et al. (1997) reported the presence of *Cryptosporidium* on a variety of green vegetables and herbs in a survey of vegetables collected from markets in Peru. Rzeżutka et al. (2010) reported the presence of *Cryptosporidium* on a variety of vegetables from areas of high livestock production in Poland. A very high prevalence (63.1 per cent) was reported on fresh produce samples irrigated with contaminated water in Spain (Amorós et al., 2010). Two studies done in Norway reported the presence of *Cryptosporidium* on lettuce and mung bean sprouts (Robertson and Gjerde, 2001; Robertson et al., 2002). Studies done in Canada reported the presence of *Cryptosporidium* in unpasteurized apple cider and on apples (Garcia et al., 2006), and spinach (Bohaychuk et al., 2009). More recently, Dixon et al. (2013) reported *Cryptosporidium* contamination in 5.9 per cent of retail leafy greens samples in Ontario.

As with *Cryptosporidium*, *Giardia* cysts have been detected on fresh produce in many countries around the world (Dixon, 2015). For example, 56 per cent of water spinach samples were found to be contaminated with *Giardia* in Cambodia (Anh et al., 2007). Several very recent studies have been done in Iran, including that by Ezatpour et al. (2013) who reported a distinct seasonality, with a higher prevalence in the spring than in the winter. Watercress and other leafy vegetables were found to be contaminated with this parasite in Egypt (Eraky et al., 2014). Abougrain et al. (2010) reported the presence of *Giardia* cysts on tomatoes, cucumbers, lettuce and cress in Libya. A number of surveillance studies were also done in Brazil. For example, da Silva et al. (1995) reported a 4.1 per cent prevalence of *Giardia* on vegetables sold at supermarkets in Rio de Janeiro. In Canada, Dixon et al. (2013) recently reported the presence of *Giardia* in 1.8 per cent of retail leafy greens samples.

A number of surveillance studies worldwide have reported the presence of *Cyclospora* on a variety of fruits and vegetables (Dixon, 2015). Tram et al. (2008) found *Cyclospora* spp. oocysts on all seven types of herbs, including lettuce, collected from farms and markets in Vietnam. These authors also detected oocysts in irrigation water on farms, and in 'sprinkling water' used to keep produce fresh in the markets. *Cyclospora*-like organisms have been found on green leafy vegetables and other fresh produce items in Nepal (Sherchand et al., 1999; Ghimire et al., 2005; Sherchand et al., 2010). In a survey of vegetables collected from markets in Peru, Ortega et al. (1997) reported the presence of *Cyclospora* on lettuce and two types of herbs. *Cyclospora* spp. was also reported on lettuce and other fresh produce items in Egypt (Abou el Naga, 1999; El Said Said, 2012) and Costa Rica (Calvo et al., 2004). Anh et al. (2007) reported *Cyclospora* spp. on water spinach collected in Cambodia. Recently, a Canadian study reported the presence of *Cyclospora* on 1.7 per cent of retail leafy greens (Dixon et al., 2013).

As there are few described methods for the detection of *Toxoplasma gondii* oocysts on produce, very little is known of the prevalence of this parasite. Al-Megrin (2010) reported a 1.1 per cent prevalence of *T. gondii* oocysts on leafy vegetables in Saudi Arabia. Another study reported the detection of *Toxoplasma* DNA by real-time PCR in 9.7 per cent of fruit and vegetable samples collected in Poland (Lass et al., 2012).

19.3 Sources of contamination

Contamination of fresh produce with the infectious stages of protozoan parasites may occur through a number of different routes, and at different stages, from farm-level to consumer-level. At the farm-level, contamination of fresh produce may occur during production, harvesting, packaging or transport. This contamination may occur directly from the hands of farm workers who are infected, or who are in close contact with infected individuals (e.g., baby in diapers), and may be associated with poor personal hygiene (Plate 31). Direct contamination of fresh produce may also occur through the application of animal faeces or human faeces ('night soil') as fertilizer to croplands. Finally, direct access to croplands by livestock and other animals represents another risk of contamination with protozoan parasites. Cats and other felines, for example, shed infectious *Toxoplasma gondii* oocysts into the environment, possibly resulting in the direct or indirect contamination of fresh produce. Farm practices may represent important risk factors in the contamination of produce due to the high prevalence of parasites, particularly *Giardia duodenalis* and *Cryptosporidium* spp. in animals (i.e., livestock, wildlife, companion animals) and in humans worldwide. Some genotypes of *G. duodenalis* (i.e., Assemblages A and B) and numerous species and genotypes of *Cryptosporidium* are zoonotic, most notably *C. parvum*, and may be transmitted between animals and humans, while others are thought to be host-specific and are of lesser concern in terms of public health. Furthermore, there is currently some evidence suggesting that the pathogenicity and virulence of these different species and genotypes may vary (Feng and Xiao, 2011; Bouzid et al., 2013).

Indirect contamination of produce with protozoan parasites at the farm-level may occur through the use of faecally contaminated water in irrigation, mixing of pesticides or washing of produce, hands or equipment, particularly in regions where water treatment and sanitation systems are poor. Parasites have, in fact, been detected in irrigation water in numerous studies (Thurston-Enriquez et al., 2002; Mota et al., 2009; Amorós et al., 2010). Wastewater irrigation, in particular, has been cited as an important source of contamination in a number of surveillance studies on fresh produce. *Giardia* and *Cryptosporidium*, for example, are commonly found in raw water sources which have been contaminated with human sewage or agricultural runoff. In endemic countries, *Cyclospora* oocysts are also frequently found in water sources used for these purposes. While *Toxoplasma* oocysts are shed exclusively by cats and other felines, waterborne disease outbreaks have been reported, and this remains a potential source of contamination of fresh produce. Even treated water, however, may represent a source of contamination, as the infectious stages of many parasites are much more resistant to chlorine than are bacterial pathogens.

At the consumer-level, direct contamination of fresh produce by infected food handlers, or those in close contact with infected individuals, is likely a major contributor, and in fact numerous foodborne outbreaks of parasitic illness have been epidemiologically associated with this source, as described in the following section. Another source of contamination may include the use of improperly treated water for washing the produce. Cross-contamination of fresh produce from other sources may also occur, for example *T. gondii* tissue cysts may be present in raw meats and could contaminate fresh produce if common knives or cutting boards are used without proper washing.

19.4 Disease outbreaks

Numerous disease outbreaks and cases associated with foodborne parasites have been reported worldwide, including a number of foodborne outbreaks of cryptosporidiosis associated with the consumption of fresh produce (Dixon et al., 2011). Uncooked green onions were epidemiologically associated with one such outbreak following a catered dinner in Washington State, US in 1997. In another outbreak in 1998, a large number of cases were associated with eating at a university cafeteria in Washington, DC. While no specific food item was implicated in this outbreak, an ill food handler with laboratory-confirmed cryptosporidiosis prepared raw produce used in meals served during the expected exposure period. More recently, an outbreak at a summer camp in North Carolina in 2009 was associated with sandwich-bar ingredients, including ham and lettuce, and possibly tomatoes and onions. There have also been several cryptosporidiosis outbreaks associated with drinking unpasteurized apple cider, all in the US (Mihajlovic et al., 2013). At least one of these outbreaks was attributed to the use of 'windfall' apples picked from an orchard floor contaminated with cattle faeces. Fresh produce has also been implicated in a number of recent cryptosporidiosis outbreaks reported in northern Europe (Robertson and Chalmers, 2013). For example, an outbreak in Sweden following a wedding reception resulted in gastroenteritis in both guests and restaurant employees. Fresh parsley was determined to be the most likely source of these illnesses. A large outbreak was associated with the consumption of peeled whole carrots, grated carrots or red peppers at a company cafeteria in Denmark. Again, the vegetables in this case were thought to have been contaminated by an infected food handler. Another outbreak reported in Finland in 2008 was thought to have been associated with the consumption of a contaminated lettuce mixture.

Several foodborne outbreaks of giardiasis have also been reported, particularly in the US. Some of these outbreaks have been associated with food handlers who were themselves infected, or who cared for infected individuals.

For example, an outbreak was reported following a party in New Jersey (Porter et al., 1990). The implicated food in this outbreak was fruit salad. The fruit salad was prepared by a woman who became ill nine days after the party. She had a young child in diapers who attended a day care and was subsequently found to be infected. Another outbreak was reported following a dinner for members of a church youth group in New Mexico (Grabowski et al., 1989). The most likely vehicles of transmission in this outbreak were taco ingredients including lettuce, tomatoes and onions. In an outbreak originating in the cafeteria of a corporate office in Connecticut, the probable vehicle was thought to be raw sliced vegetables served in the cafeteria and prepared by an infected, asymptomatic food handler (Mintz et al., 1993).

A very large number of foodborne outbreaks of diarrheal illness associated with infection with *Cyclospora cayetanensis* have been reported worldwide. In particular, outbreaks have occurred almost every year in North America since 1995, and have been largely associated with the consumption of fresh imported produce. These outbreaks, and the control measures put in place to minimize them, are further discussed later in this chapter.

Most foodborne outbreaks of toxoplasmosis have been associated with the consumption of raw or poorly cooked meats or organs, or raw goat's milk. There have been very few reported outbreaks of toxoplasmosis associated with fresh produce contaminated with *Toxoplasma gondii* oocysts. Recently however, Ekman et al. (2012) described an outbreak of acute toxoplasmosis in Brazil that was associated with the consumption of green vegetables. While toxoplasmosis is zoonotic, it was not determined whether the vegetables were contaminated with oocysts shed by cats or were cross-contaminated by *T. gondii*-infected raw meat.

Due to the many possible sources of contamination of these foods, and the often complex epidemiology, it is important that the One Health approach be adopted when investigating foodborne disease outbreaks such as these, and that experts from a variety of disciplines be involved, such as epidemiologists, parasitologists, medical and veterinary diagnostic experts, regulators, etc.

19.5 Food testing methodology

It is generally very difficult to make an association between the consumption of a certain food and human illness associated with a parasitic infection. This is due to a number of factors including the relatively long incubation period of these pathogens, and the problems in diagnosing and reporting human cases. The median incubation period for cyclosporiasis, for example, is about seven days (Ortega and Sanchez, 2010). Furthermore, the relatively short shelf-life of some foods, particularly fresh produce, adds to the problem. In many cases, the food(s) implicated following an epidemiological investigation are consumed, or disposed of, long before any testing could be initiated. As a result, foods are generally implicated in disease outbreaks based on epidemiological data rather than the actual detection of parasites. When portions of a suspected food item are still available, however, or during targeted food surveillance studies, rapid and sensitive methods for the detection of protozoan parasites are desired.

The number of parasites present in or on foods is generally much lower than that found in faecal material, and since protozoans will only multiply in the host, enrichment steps, such as those used in the detection of bacteria in foods, are not readily available. Furthermore, cysts and oocysts are often very difficult to wash off produce, making it very difficult to determine the level of contamination of raw foods in surveys, or to confirm the food source(s) involved in the event of an outbreak.

There are currently no standard methods for the detection of protozoan parasites in foods, and published methods are often inadequate, with low and variable recovery efficiencies. These methods are also limited in that they do not allow for determining the viability or infectivity of the parasites, which is of considerable importance in assigning a level of risk to consumers. Furthermore, microscopy-based detection methods often do not allow for speciation or genotyping of these parasites, and further molecular characterization is generally required.

The effective elution and concentration of protozoan parasites from foods is of considerable importance in their subsequent detection. Most published methods involve agitation of the fruits or vegetables in water or in buffer for elution, often in combination with detergents (Dixon et al., 2011). Elution of parasites, however, often results in the release of excessive debris particles, which can hamper microscopical analyses. When using molecular tools such as polymerase chain reaction (PCR), inhibiting compounds may be released, possibly resulting in false-negative results. To address these difficulties, concentration steps are often incorporated into the sample processing procedure. For example, the concentration of parasite cysts or oocysts generally involves centrifugation, sedimentation and/or flotation. Immunomagnetic separation has also been successfully used in concentrating *Giardia* cysts and *Cryptosporidium* oocysts from food debris, but the protocol can be technically difficult and the magnetic beads are relatively expensive.

Many of the same methods used in clinical diagnoses and environmental testing have been adapted and evaluated for foods. The majority of surveillance studies done worldwide, for example, have involved the use of microscopy for the detection of protozoan parasites on foods. A variety of microscopical techniques have been employed, including bright-field, differential interference contrast and immunofluorescence.

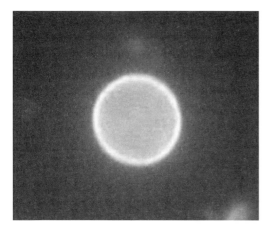 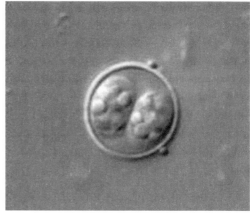

Figure 19.1 *Cyclospora cayetanensis* oocysts; (a) autofluorescing oocyst under UV light; (b) sporulated oocyst under differential interference contrast microscopy.

Immunofluorescence microscopy, using fluorochrome-labelled monoclonal antibodies has been used routinely for many years in water testing for the parasites *Giardia* and *Cryptosporidium,* and is now frequently used for their detection on foods as well. Although monoclonal antibodies are not commercially available against *Cyclospora cayetanensis*, the oocysts of this parasite are autofluorescent and can be readily identified on a microscope slide under ultraviolet (UV) light (Figure 19.1).

Polymerase chain reaction (PCR)-based methods have been used in detecting the presence of parasite DNA on foods. The amplification of a portion of the small subunit rRNA gene is probably the most commonly used PCR assay for the detection of *Cryptosporidium* spp., *G. duodenalis* and *C. cayetanensis* DNA on foods (Dixon et al., 2013). For example, Jinneman et al. (1998) used a nested 18S rRNA PCR method, in conjunction with a restriction fragment length polymorphism (RFLP) analysis, for the detection and identification of *Cyclospora* spp. from spiked raspberries. Very few methods have been described however, for the detection of *T. gondii* oocysts on foods. Lalonde and Gajadhar (2011) developed a real-time PCR and melting curve analysis for the detection and differentiation of *Cryptosporidium*

spp., *C. cayetanensis, T. gondii* and other coccidian oocysts in clinical and food samples. Lass et al. (2012) recently described a real-time PCR assay targeting the B1 gene for the detection of *T. gondii* DNA, and reported its presence on selected fruits and vegetables in Poland.

In addition to detection of cysts and oocysts on foods, molecular methods are also required to determine the species, genotypes and sub-genotypes of parasites on foods, which then allows for source tracking (i.e., determining possible sources of contamination of the food), as well as determining the risk to consumers. For example, PCR-positive food samples can be further characterized using restriction fragment length polymorphism (RFLP) analysis and/or DNA sequencing. In particular, small subunit rRNA-based molecular methods are often used for these purposes as they are particularly conducive to genotyping. Sequencing at the 60 kDa glycoprotein (gp60) locus is commonly used for sub-genotyping of some species of *Cryptosporidium* (Xiao, 2010), and provides for very high resolution molecular characterization.

The viability and/or infectivity of cysts and oocysts are also very important considerations in the risk management of foodborne protozoan parasites. Viability of cysts and oocysts may be determined using vital stains, evidence of sporulation (e.g., *C. cayetanensis* and *T. gondii*), and *in vitro* excystation, while infectivity assays are considerably more challenging and involve animal infectivity studies or, in the case of *Cryptosporidium*, cell culture. These analyses are, however, often subjective, time-consuming and/or expensive, and are not routinely done in surveillance studies or outbreak investigations.

19.6 Control measures

Since fresh produce is very often consumed raw, without any further processing, the development and implementation of effective control measures for minimizing the risk of contamination in the first place, or for physically removing the parasites or inactivating them following contamination are crucial in reducing the risk of illness in consumers.

At the pre-harvest stage, control measures may include the use of treated water for all activities, monitoring the health and hygiene of farm workers, improved on-farm sanitation, and restricted access of livestock and other animals to crop lands and to surface waters. Parasite contaminated water is thought to be an important source of contamination of fruits and vegetables at the farm level. As a result, it is imperative that only properly treated water be used for irrigation, washing fresh produce or washing hands and equipment. As chlorination, routinely used in water treatment, has little or no effect on the viability of protozoan parasites, filtration methods, and other technologies such as UV light and ozone should be used. Most of these technologies have been shown to be very effective in removing or inactivating parasites, but their added costs may be prohibitive to smaller communities or developing regions. Finally, it is very important that water used on-farm be regularly tested for the presence of organisms that act as indicators of faecal contamination, or for specific pathogens such as *Cryptosporidium* and *Giardia*.

Good hygienic practices by farm workers involved in the cultivation, harvesting, processing or packaging of fresh produce is another very important means of reducing the likelihood of contamination at the farm-level. In endemic regions in particular, the health of farm workers should be monitored and ill employees should be restricted from all food handling activities. The availability of toilets and hand-washing facilities for farm workers is an important part of this control measure, as are on-farm educational programmes on hygiene and public health.

Fresh produce may become faecally contaminated in the field through direct access by livestock, wildlife and companion animals, many of which are infected with the same species and genotypes of parasites as humans, and serve as reservoirs of parasitic infection (Plate 32). It is imperative, therefore, that these animals be physically restricted from crop lands or vegetable gardens wherever possible. As livestock are also important sources of water contamination, these animals should not have access to surface water subsequently used for drinking or agricultural purposes, and agricultural runoff should be minimized. While composted animal and human faeces are widely used in the fertilization of crops, the effectiveness of composting in destroying parasites is not yet clear. Olson et al. (1999) concluded that the application of cattle manure onto crop fields should be done in warmer weather and only following at least 12 weeks of storage to inactivate *Cryptosporidium* oocysts and *Giardia* cysts. However, Van Herk et al. (2004) demonstrated that composting manure was effective in inactivating both of these parasites when temperatures exceeded 55°C for just 15 days.

The environmental resistance of infectious stages of protozoan parasites should also be taken into consideration with respect to the control of parasites at the farm-level. Considerable data is available on the survival of *Cryptosporidium* spp. and *Toxoplasma gondii* oocysts under different environmental conditions, and the infectious stages of most parasites are quite resistant to adverse environmental conditions such as high and low temperatures. While desiccation readily kills or inactivates most protozoan parasites, some fruits and vegetables have moist, irregular surfaces that may protect the contaminating parasites from drying out.

As with the pre-harvest control measures already discussed, post-harvest controls include primarily the use of treated water for washing and processing produce and for cleaning hands and equipment, as well as the monitoring and enforcement of good personal hygiene in food handlers. The use of chemical and physical disinfectants, directly on foods, or on working surfaces and equipment, should also be considered as potential barriers to foodborne transmission of protozoan parasites. While most protozoan parasites are thought to be very resistant to the chemical disinfectants commonly used in the food industry (Dixon et al., 2011), some disinfectant gases have been shown to be quite effective. For example, Ortega et al. (2008) demonstrated that gaseous chlorine dioxide was effective as a sanitizer against *Cryptosporidium parvum*, and a microsporidian species, on basil and lettuce leaves, while *C. cayetanensis* oocysts were not affected.

In terms of physical disinfection, a variety of technologies have been shown to be effective against parasites on fresh produce or in juices. Pasteurization, for example, has been demonstrated to be effective in inactivating *Cryptosporidium parvum* oocysts in apple cider (Deng and Cliver, 2001). Irradiation has also been suggested as a possible means of decontaminating fresh fruits and vegetables. Appropriate irradiation doses to eliminate the infectivity of *T. gondii* oocysts have been published, and it was suggested that similar irradiation procedures would kill *C. cayetanensis* oocysts attached to fresh raspberries or other fruits and vegetables (Dubey et al., 1998). High hydrostatic

pressure, or high pressure processing, has also shown promise in the inactivation of protozoan parasites in juices and on fresh produce (Slifko et al., 2000; Lindsay et al., 2008). While some parasites demonstrate resistance to short-term household freezing, commercial freezing appears to be effective in destroying the infectious stages of protozoan parasites on berries and other produce items as no outbreaks have been associated with frozen products.

There are also some important control points at the food handler or consumer-level. As with all enteric pathogens, good personal hygiene, particularly frequent hand-washing, is of considerable importance in reducing the risk of transmission. In light of the numerous foodborne outbreaks associated with food handlers who are themselves ill, or who are caring for children or others with diarrheal illness, these individuals should not be involved in the preparation of food. Since this measure may be difficult to enforce, the use of disposable gloves should be considered for workers in the food industry.

While rinsing of fresh fruits and vegetables with water is recommended for reducing the risk of transmission of pathogens, it is unlikely that this practice will remove all parasite cysts or oocysts from the foods. Furthermore, delicate fruits such as raspberries will not tolerate anything more than a gentle rinse. In terms of freezing, since parasites have shown variable resistance to household freezing, this treatment should not be recommended as the sole means of inactivation in foods. For example, recent studies suggest that *C. cayetanensis* oocysts are relatively resistant to short exposures to household freezing (Ortega and Sanchez, 2010). While there is little data available on the effectiveness of cooking temperatures against protozoan parasites, cooking or baking likely serve as final barriers against transmission. It is important to note, however, that most of the produce items implicated in disease outbreaks are typically consumed raw.

19.7 Case study: *Cyclospora* on imported fresh berries

The organism responsible for cyclosporiasis was first recognized as a cause of human illness in the late 1970s. The causative agent, however, was not identified as a coccidian protozoan parasite until 1993, when it was named *Cyclospora cayetanensis* (Ortega et al., 1993). The sexual stage of the lifecycle of *C. cayetanensis* results in the development of oocysts, which are shed in the host's faeces. Ingestion of sporulated oocysts by human hosts may result in an infection causing profuse and prolonged diarrhoea and a variety of other symptoms including abdominal pain, nausea, vomiting, fatigue, fever and loss of appetite (Ortega and Sanchez, 2010). *C. cayetanensis* has, in fact, been identified as a cause of diarrhoeal illness in humans in North, Central and South America, the Caribbean, Southeast Asia, Eastern Europe, the UK, India and Africa (Ortega and Sanchez, 2010). Most of the prevalence data, however, comes from studies done in endemic regions including Nepal, Haiti, Peru and Guatemala.

Many of the earlier outbreaks of cyclosporiasis were thought to have resulted from the consumption of faecally contaminated drinking water, and the waterborne route continues to be an important mode of transmission in some countries. Person-to-person transmission (i.e., the faecal–oral route) is considered to be unlikely due to a relatively long sporulation period of seven to 15 days (Ortega and Sanchez, 2010), which must occur before oocysts become infectious. Zoonotic transmission has also been suggested, and *Cyclospora*-like organisms, and/or PCR positives for *Cyclospora*, have been observed in the faeces of chickens, ducks, dogs, monkeys, chimpanzees and baboons (Ortega and Sanchez, 2010; Chacín-Bonilla, 2010). However, to date, there is little more than anecdotal evidence for this method of transmission to humans. So, unlike *Giardia* and *Cryptosporidium*, *C. cayetanensis* is not considered to be a zoonotic parasite, and direct or indirect contamination of fresh produce with the faeces of livestock or other animals is not likely a factor in its transmission.

Since 1995, numerous foodborne outbreaks and cases of cyclosporiasis have been reported in the US and Canada. While two small outbreaks associated with fresh produce occurred in the US during the spring and summer of 1995, the first large foodborne outbreak of cyclosporiasis in North America occurred in 1996. As summarized by Herwaldt et al. (1997), a total of 1,465 cases of diarrheal illness due to *Cyclospora* infection were reported in the US and Canada during May and June of 1996. The only exposure that was consistently epidemiologically linked to *Cyclospora* infection was the consumption of fresh raspberries imported from Guatemala. In the spring of 1997, another outbreak of diarrheal illness due to cyclosporiasis was reported in the US and Canada, and involved 1,012 cases (Herwaldt et al., 1999). Fresh Guatemalan raspberries were again the only food common to all events. In subsequent years, fresh berries and a variety of other fresh produce items (e.g., mesclun, coriander, snow peas and basil) were epidemiologically linked to cyclosporiasis outbreaks in North America (Ortega and Sanchez, 2010; Dixon et al., 2011). When a country of origin was identified, most of the fresh produce items linked to illnesses were found to be imported from a variety of Latin American countries. Although the reasons are not entirely clear, a distinct seasonality has also been noted in these outbreaks, with the vast majority occurring in the spring and early summer (Chacín-Bonilla, 2010). Most recently, there were large multistate outbreaks in the US in the late spring and summer of 2013, which were associated with the consumption of imported leafy greens and fresh coriander (Centers for Disease Control and Prevention, 2013). Canada also reported an outbreak that summer that was associated with fresh leafy greens. Foodborne outbreaks of cyclosporiasis were, again, investigated in the US and Canada during the summer of 2014.

As discussed previously in this chapter, worker hygiene and water quality on farms, particularly in endemic regions, are important factors in the risk of contamination of produce with *C. cayetanensis* oocysts. These sources of contamination, and others, were thoroughly investigated following the large foodborne outbreaks of cyclosporiasis in North America in the late 1990s in an effort to minimize the contamination of fresh berries and to reduce the numbers of foodborne infections. The result of these investigations was the application of a hazard analysis critical control point (HACCP)-based approach at exporting raspberry farms and packaging plants in Guatemala. This plan involved stringent control measures, especially with respect to worker hygiene and water quality. Despite these control measures, however, further outbreaks associated with Guatemalan berries were reported in North America, suggesting that there may have been compliance problems, or that the control measures were ineffective or not directed against the actual sources of contamination (Herwaldt, 2000).

In the case of fresh berries, once contaminated, there are few or no control measures available to remove or to inactivate contaminating *C. cayetanensis* oocysts. The surface of raspberries is uneven, with many hairs and crevices that may prevent the oocysts from being easily washed off, and since raspberries are very delicate fruits, vigorous washing is not possible. The surface of raspberries also likely provides the oocysts some protection from desiccation in the field and during storage. As with other protozoan parasites, *C. cayetanensis* are likely resistant to most chemical disinfectants used in the food industry (Dixon et al., 2011). Furthermore, raspberries are generally consumed fresh, without any cooking or freezing. In light of these considerations, and in response to the continuing outbreaks of cyclosporiasis, the US and Canada drafted import policies which allowed importation of fresh Guatemalan raspberries during the fall season only, as there had not been any disease outbreaks during that time of year. While numerous other types of fresh produce have been implicated in subsequent years, cyclosporiasis outbreaks linked to fresh berries have only been reported rarely since 2000, and none of these have been specifically linked to Guatemalan berries. This suggests that in the absence of effective pre- and post-harvest control measures to minimize contamination of fresh produce in the country of origin, and with the very limited control measures available at the consumer-level, import restrictions are necessary and effective in protecting consumers. Although there are few effective control measures available to the consumer with respect to *Cyclospora*, and other parasites, on fresh produce, food safety education is also important.

19.8 Conclusions

Transmission of parasites through the consumption of fresh produce is an emerging public health issue in developed countries due to a number of different factors, the most important of which is the increasingly global food trade and the demand for exotic and out-of-season fruits and vegetables. Numerous cases and outbreaks of foodborne disease associated with the consumption of contaminated fresh produce have been reported worldwide. *Cyclospora cayetanensis*, in particular, has been responsible for annual foodborne disease outbreaks in North America since 1995, with a total of more than 900 cases being associated with the consumption of fresh produce in 2013 and 2014 alone. While a very large number of surveillance studies on fresh produce have been done in developing regions, there is relatively little prevalence data available from developed countries. Furthermore, there are numerous hurdles in testing foods for the presence of parasites in surveillance studies or in outbreak investigations and, as a result, the incidence of foodborne illness due to infection with protozoan parasites is likely underestimated. Contamination of fresh produce with the infectious stages of protozoan parasites may occur through a number of different routes, involving either direct or indirect contact with the faeces of infected humans or animals. Once contaminated, however, there are few barriers available to inactivate, destroy or remove parasites from fresh produce before consumption.

Further research and surveillance work is needed, therefore, to advance our knowledge on this emerging issue and to feed into risk assessments and guidelines or policies aimed at minimizing the risk of infection to consumers. Specifically, work is needed to determine the baseline prevalence of foodborne protozoan parasites on a variety of fresh fruits and vegetables, both imported and domestic. The use of molecular methods for determining the species, genotypes and sub-genotypes of parasites isolated from fresh produce will provide valuable information regarding the potential source(s) of contamination and the risk of infection to humans. Furthermore, the development of methods for the accurate determination of parasite viability and/or infectivity will be of great value. Studies on potential control measures and disinfectants to minimize contamination and to remove or inactivate parasites on fresh produce will also be very important. Finally, due to the many possible sources of contamination of these foods, and the often complex epidemiology, it is also important that a multidisciplinary One Health approach be adopted when investigating and managing foodborne parasitic diseases.

References

Abou el Naga, I.F. (1999). Studies on a newly emerging protozoal pathogen: *Cyclospora cayetanensis*. *Journal of the Egyptian Society of Parasitology*, 29, 575–586.

Abougrain, A.K., Nahaisi, M.H., Madi, N.S., Saied, M.M. and Ghenghesh, K.S. (2010). Parasitological contamination in salad vegetables in Tripoli-Libya. *Food Control*, 21, 760–762.

Al-Megrin, W.A.I. (2010). Prevalence of intestinal parasites in leafy vegetables in Riyadh, Saudi Arabia. *International Journal of Tropical Medicine*, 5, 20–23.

Amorós, I., Alonso, J.L. and Cuesta, G. (2010). *Cryptosporidium* oocysts and *Giardia* cysts on salad products irrigated with contaminated water. *Journal of Food Protection*, 73, 1138–1140.

Anh, V.T., Tram, N.T., Klank, L.T., Cam, P.D. and Dalsgaard, A. (2007). Faecal and protozoan parasite contamination of water spinach (*Ipomoea aquatica*) cultivated in urban wastewater in Phnom Penh, Cambodia. *Tropical Medicine and International Health*, 12(S2), 73–81.

Bohaychuk, V.M., Bradbury, R.W., Dimock, R., Fehr, M., Gensler, G.E., King, R.K., Rieve, R. and Romero Barrios, P. (2009). A microbiological survey of selected Alberta-grown fresh produce from farmers' markets in Alberta, Canada. *Journal of Food Protection*, 72, 415–420.

Bouzid, M., Hunter, P.R., Chalmers, R.M. and Tyler, K.M. (2013). *Cryptosporidium* pathogenicity and virulence. *Clinical Microbiology Reviews*, 26, 115–134.

Calvo, M., Carazo, M., Arias, M.L., Chaves, C., Monge, R. and Chinchilla, M. (2004). Prevalence of *Cyclospora* sp., *Cryptosporidium* sp., microsporidia and fecal coliform determination in fresh fruit and vegetables consumed in Costa Rica. *Archivos Latinoamericanos de Nutrición*, 54, 428–432.

Centers for Disease Control and Prevention (2013). *Cyclosporiasis Outbreak Investigations – United States, 2013 (Final Update)*, www.cdc.gov/parasites/cyclosporiasis/outbreaks/investigation-2013.html.

Chacín-Bonilla, L. (2010). Epidemiology of *Cyclospora cayetanensis*: a review focusing in endemic areas. *Acta Tropica*, 115, 181–193.

da Silva, J.P., Marzochi, M.C.A., Camillo-Coura, L., Messias, A.A. and Marques, S. (1995). Estudo da contaminação por enteroparasitas em hortaliças comercializadas nos supermercados da cidade do Rio de Janeiro. *Revista da Sociedade Brasileira de Medicina Tropical*, 28, 237–241.

Deng, M.Q. and Cliver, D.O. (2001). Inactivation of *Cryptosporidium parvum* oocysts in cider by flash pasteurization. *Journal of Food Protection*, 64, 523–527.

Dixon, B.R. (2015). Transmission dynamics of foodborne parasites on fresh produce. In A. Gajadhar (ed.), *Foodborne Parasites in the Food Supply Web: Occurrence and Control*. Cambridge: Woodhead Publishing Ltd.

Dixon, B.R., Fayer, R., Santin M., Hill, D.E and Dubey, J.P. (2011). Protozoan parasites: *Cryptosporidium, Giardia, Cyclospora*, and *Toxoplasma*. In J. Hoorfar (ed.), *Rapid Detection, Characterization and Enumeration of Food-Borne Pathogens*. Washington, DC: ASM Press, pp. 349–370.

Dixon, B.R., Parrington, L., Cook, A., Pollari, F. and Farber, J. (2013). Detection of *Cyclospora, Cryptosporidium* and *Giardia* in ready-to-eat packaged leafy greens in Ontario, Canada. *Journal of Food Protection*, 76, 307–313.

Dubey, J.P., Thayer, D.W., Speer, C.A. and Shen, S.K. (1998). Effect of gamma irradiation on unsporulated and sporulated *Toxoplasma gondii* oocysts. *International Journal of Parasitology*, 28, 369–375.

Ekman, C.C.J., Chiossi, M.F. do V., Meireles, L.R., de Andrade Junior, H.F., Figueiredo, W.M., Marciano, M.A.M. and Luna, E.J.A. (2012). Case-control study of an outbreak of acute toxoplasmosis in an industrial plant in the state of São Paulo, Brazil. *Revista do Instituto de Medicina Tropical de São Paulo*, 54, 239–244.

El Said Said, D. (2012). Detection of parasites in commonly consumed raw vegetables. *Alexandria Journal of Medicine*, 48, 345–352.

Eraky, M.A., Rashed, S.M., El-Sayed Nasr, M., El-Hamshary, A.M.S. and El-Ghannam, A.S. (2014). Parasitic contamination of commonly consumed fresh leafy vegetables in Benha, Egypt. *Journal of Parasitology Research*, www.hindawi.com/journals/jpr/2014/613960.

Ezatpour, B., Chegeni, A.S., Abdollahpour, F., Aazami, M. and Alirezaei, M. (2013). Prevalence of parasitic contamination of raw vegetables in Khorramabad, Iran. *Food Control*, 34, 92–95.

Feng, Y. and Xiao, L. (2011). Zoonotic potential and molecular epidemiology of *Giardia* species and giardiasis. *Clinical Microbiology Reviews*, 24, 110–140.

Garcia, L., Henderson, J., Fabri, M. and Oke, M. (2006). Potential sources of microbial contamination in unpasteurized apple cider. *Journal of Food Protection*, 69, 137–144.

Ghimire, T.R., Mishra, P.N. and Sherchand, J.B. (2005). The seasonal outbreaks of *Cyclospora* and *Cryptosporidium* in Kathmandu, Nepal. *Journal of Nepal Health Research Council*, 3, 39–48.

Grabowski, D.J., Tiggs, K.J., Hall, J.D., Senke, H.W., Salas, A.J., Powers, C.M., Knott, J.A., Nims, L.J. and Sewell, C.M. (1989). Epidemiologic notes and reports common-source outbreak of giardiasis. *Morbidity and Mortality Weekly Report*, 38, 405–407.

Herwaldt, B.L. (2000). *Cyclospora cayetanensis*: a review, focusing on the outbreaks of cyclosporiasis in the 1990s. *Clinical Infectious Diseases*, 31, 1040–1057.

Herwaldt, B.L., Ackers, M.-L. and the *Cyclospora* Working Group (1997). An outbreak in 1996 of cyclosporiasis associated with imported raspberries. *New England Journal of Medicine*, 336, 1548–1556.

Herwaldt, B.L., Beach, M.J. and the *Cyclospora* Working Group (1999). The return of *Cyclospora* in 1997: another outbreak of cyclosporiasis in North America associated with imported raspberries. *Annals of Internal Medicine*, 130, 210–220.

Jinneman, K.C., Wetherington, J.H., Hill, W.E., Adams, A.M., Johnson, J.M., Tenge, B.J., Dang, N.-L., Manger, R.L. and Wekell, M.M. (1998). Template preparation for PCR and RFLP of amplification products for the detection and identification of *Cyclospora* sp. and *Eimeria* spp. oocysts directly from raspberries. *Journal of Food Protection*, 61, 1497–1503.

Lalonde, L.F. and Gajadhar, A.A. (2011). Detection and differentiation of coccidian oocysts by real-time PCR and melting curve analysis. *Journal of Parasitology*, 97, 725–730.

Lass, A., Pietkiewicz, H., Szostakowska, B. and Myjak, P. (2012). The first detection of *Toxoplasma gondii* DNA in environmental fruits and vegetables samples. *European Journal of Clinical Microbiology and Infectious Diseases*, 31, 1101–1108.

Lindsay, D.S., Holliman, D., Flick, G.J., Goodwin, D.G., Mitchell, S.M. and Dubey, J.P. (2008). Effects of high pressure processing on *Toxoplasma gondii* oocysts on raspberries. *Journal of Parasitology*, 94, 757–758.

Mihajlovic, B., Dixon, B., Couture, H. and Farber, J. (2013). Qualitative microbiological risk assessment of unpasteurized fruit juice and cider. *International Food Risk Analysis Journal*, 3, 1–19.

Mintz, E.D., Hudson-Wragg, M., Mshar, P., Cartter, M.L. and Hadler J.L. (1993). Foodborne giardiosis in a corporate office setting. *Journal of Infectious Diseases*, 167, 250–253.

Monge, R. and Chinchilla, M. (1996). Presence of *Cryptosporidium* oocysts in fresh vegetables. *Journal of Food Protection*, 59, 202–203.

Mota, A., Mena, K.D., Soto-Beltran, M., Tarwater, P.M. and Cháidez, C. (2009). Risk assessment of *Cryptosporidium* and *Giardia* in water irrigating fresh produce in Mexico. *Journal of Food Protection*, 72, 2184–2188.

Olson, M.E., Goh, J., Phillips, M., Guselle, N. and McAllister, T.A. (1999). *Giardia* cyst and

Cryptosporidium oocyst survival in water, soil, and cattle feces. *Journal of Environmental Quality*, 28, 1991–1996.

Ortega, Y.R. and Sanchez, R. (2010). Update on *Cyclospora cayetanensis*, a food-borne and water-borne parasite. *Clinical Microbiology Reviews*, 23, 218–234.

Ortega, Y.R., Sterling, C.R., Gilman, R.H. Cama, V.A. and Díaz, F. (1993). *Cyclospora* species – a new protozoan pathogen of humans. *New England Journal of Medicine*, 328, 1308–1312.

Ortega, Y.R., Roxas, C.R., Gilman, R.H., Miller, N.J., Cabrera, L., Taquiri, C. and Sterling, C.R. (1997). Isolation of *Cryptosporidium parvum* and *Cyclospora cayetanensis* from vegetables collected in markets of an endemic region in Peru. *American Journal of Tropical Medicine and Hygiene*, 57, 683–686.

Ortega, Y.R., Mann, A., Torres, M.P. and Cama, V. (2008). Efficacy of gaseous chlorine dioxide as a sanitizer against *Cryptosporidium parvum*, *Cyclospora cayetanensis*, and *Encephalitozoon intestinalis* on produce. *Journal of Food Protection*, 71, 2410–2414.

Porter, J.D.H., Gaffney, C., Heymann, D. and Parkin, W. (1990). Food-borne outbreak of *Giardia lamblia*. *American Journal of Public Health*, 80, 1259–1260.

Robertson, L.J. and Chalmers, R.M. (2013). Foodborne cryptosporidiosis: is there really more in Nordic countries? *Trends in Parasitology*, 29, 3–9.

Robertson, L.J. and Gjerde, B. (2001) Occurrence of parasites on fruits and vegetables in Norway. *Journal of Food Protection*, 64, 1793–1798.

Robertson, L.J., Johannessen, G.S., Gjerde, B.K. and Loncarevic, S. (2002). Microbiological analysis of seed sprouts in Norway. *International Journal of Food Microbiology*, 75, 119–126.

Rzeżutka, A., Nichols, R.A., Connelly, L., Kaupke, A., Kozyra, I., Cook, N., Birrell, S. and Smith, H.V. (2010). *Cryptosporidium* oocysts on fresh produce from areas of high livestock production in Poland.

International Journal of Food Microbiology, 139, 96–101.

Scallan E., Hoekstra, R.M., Angulo, F.J., Tauxe, R.V., Widdowson, M.A., Roy, S.L., Jones, J.L. and Griffin P.M. (2011). Foodborne illness acquired in the United States – major pathogens. *Emerging Infectious Diseases*, 17, 7–15.

Sherchan, J.B., Cross, J., Jimba, M., Sherchand, S. and Shrestha, M.P. (1999). Study of *Cyclospora cayetanensis* in health care facilities, sewage water and green leafy vegetables in Nepal. *Southeast Asian Journal of Tropical Medicine and Public Health*, 30, 58–63.

Sherchand, J.B., Sherpa, K., Tandukar, S., Cross, J.H., Gajadhar, A. and Sherchand, J.B. (2010). Infection of *Cyclospora cayetanensis* in diarrhoeal children of Nepal. *Journal of Nepal Paediatric Society*, 30, 23–30.

Slifko, T., Raghubeer, E. and Rose, J. (2000). Effect of high hydrostatic pressure on *Cryptosporidium parvum* infectivity. *Journal of Food Protection*, 63, 1262–1267.

Thurston-Enriquez, J.A., Watt, P., Dowd, S.E., Enriquez, R., Pepper, I.L. and Gerba, C.P. (2002). Detection of protozoan parasites and microsporidia in irrigation waters used for crop production. *Journal of Food Protection*, 65, 378–382.

Tram, N.T., Hoang, L.M.N., Cam, P.D., Chung, P.T., Fyfe, M.W., Isaac-Renton, J.L. and Ong, C.S.L. (2008). *Cyclospora* spp. in herbs and water samples collected from markets and farms in Hanoi, Vietnam. *Tropical Medicine and International Health*, 13, 1415–1420.

Van Herk, F.H., McAllister, T.A., Cockwill, C.L., Guselle, N., Larney, F.J., Miller, J.J. and Olson, M.E. (2004). Inactivation of *Giardia* cysts and *Cryptosporidium* oocysts in beef feedlot manure by thermophilic windrow composting. *Compost Science and Utilization*, 12, 235–241.

Xiao, L. (2010). Molecular epidemiology of cryptosporidiosis: an update. *Experimental Parasitology*, 124, 80–89.

chapter 20

Antimicrobial resistance and food safety

Karen A. Liljebjelke

Abstract

Antimicrobial resistance is a clear example of a One Health problem. The global nature of the problem necessitates a global response. The stakeholders include physicians, veterinarians, food producers and processors, and every person on earth who may need antibiotic therapy in the future. Global food security is at risk. In order for this One Health problem to be addressed, all stakeholders worldwide must participate in the discussion of the problem and proposed solutions. The uses of antimicrobials in modern agricultural systems by veterinarians and food producers has been identified as one factor contributing to the increasing prevalence of antimicrobial resistance in foodborne pathogens and environmental bacteria. In particular, the non-therapeutic use of antibiotics with analogs to those in human medicine, as growth promoting substances in animal feeds, has been identified as a risk for selection and dissemination of antimicrobial resistance against antibiotics of critical importance to medicine. The complex ecology of bacterial genetics adds significant complexity to assessment of risk and formulation of effective counter measures. The World Health Organization (WHO), World Organisation for Animal Health (OIE) and Food and Agriculture Organization of the United Nations (FAO) are spearheading the global response, promoting education of physicians, veterinarians and the general public, and championing elimination of non-therapeutic use of antibiotics in food animal production for the purpose of growth promotion.

20.1 Antimicrobial resistance: a global One Health crisis

Antibiotic resistance used to be a concern only for clinicians treating individual human or animal patients with bacterial diseases. Almost as soon as antibiotics had begun to be used as a regular part of medicine, doctors began to notice that there were infections that were resistant to treatment.

In the past 30 years, resistance to the antimicrobial compounds used in human and veterinary medicine has increased greatly. Now, there are bacterial infections that are resistant to almost every antibiotic available. Once it was realized that antimicrobial resistance (AMR)

The campaign to preserve antibiotic effectiveness for human health

Despite decades of surveillance data documenting the steady increase in antimicrobial resistance among both pathogenic and environmental bacteria, governments have been slow to act on creating legislation controlling how antibiotics are used in human medicine, veterinary medicine and agriculture. The reasons for this inaction are numerous, including conflicting scientific opinion, political influence from medical and agricultural lobbying groups, lack of critical information on antimicrobial usage and lack of buy-in for the idea of antibiotic stewardship.

Thirty years ago Dr Stewart Levy of Tufts University School of Medicine formed the Alliance for the Prudent Use of Antibiotics (APUA), a non-profit group with the purpose of increasing the general public's awareness of the problem of antimicrobial resistance. Their campaign 'Keep antibiotics working', seeks to reduce the use of antibiotics in animal agriculture, particularly those used as feed additives for the promotion of growth that are also used in human medicine, and those of the same antibiotic classes used in human medicine. APUA has been urging the US Food and Drug Administration (FDA) to create regulation that would remove approval for use of antibiotics in animals for non-therapeutic purposes (www.tufts.edu/med/apua/index.shtml).

---

was beginning to cause serious problems, the human medical profession and the veterinary medical profession were at odds as to whether medical or veterinary use (or misuse) of antibiotics was the major cause of the problem (Bailar and Travers, 2002). A growing awareness of the complex ecology of infectious diseases, as illustrated by the influenza viruses flowing between wildlife, livestock and people in the environment, has promoted the value of adopting a One Health approach in addressing issues of human, animal and environmental health, including antimicrobial resistance.

As the concept of 'One Health' has developed, antimicrobials are now being considered as belonging to the global society as a whole, and not to one particular profession or nation. This gestalt shift has changed the way epidemiologists and infectious disease experts analyze the vast amount of data that has been collected on AMR, and has changed the way national and international regulatory bodies assess risk and recommend regulation of antimicrobial use in medicine and agriculture (WHO, 2014). The One Health approach to thinking about the

problem of AMR has also given rise to the concept of stewardship in use of antimicrobials. Applying the idea of stewardship to antibiotic use relies on the basic principle that these medically important drugs belong to everyone, not just to the person prescribing or the person using them, and that their effectiveness must be maintained for the good of humanity, now, and for the future.

20.2 Modern agricultural systems

The human population of the earth, currently estimated at 7.3 billion people, continues to grow, and with this growth, there are more mouths to feed (www.census.gov/popclock). In the developed and developing nations, populations continue to urbanize, moving out of the countryside and into cities and small family farms are being replaced by larger and larger farms due to the economy of scale (www.who.int/gho/urban_health/situation_trends/urban_population_growth_text/en). The World Health Organization (WHO) estimates that 54 per cent of the world population lives in urban centres. These socioeconomic factors have changed the way animals are raised for food. Critics use the term 'factory farming', but the terms 'intensive animal production' and 'industrial livestock production' are equally as descriptive of modern agriculture. The growing demand for food and dietary animal protein, at prices affordable to the average person, has driven the changes in livestock-rearing methods that have in turn increased the use of antimicrobials in agriculture. Regardless of what terms are used to describe livestock production in the modern age, changes in agricultural practice worldwide have had a significant impact on the use of antimicrobials and on the development of antimicrobial resistance.

20.3 Global food security and One Health

The Food and Agriculture Organization (FAO) convened the World Food Summit in Rome, Italy in 1996 (www.fao.org/wfs). The FAO defined food security as existing 'when all people at all times have access to sufficient, safe, nutritious food to maintain a healthy and active life' (www. who.int/trade/glossary/story028/en). As the world population grows, food security is a real concern for people of many nations. However, in order to be sustainable, global food security must be achieved while minimizing the effects of intensive agriculture on the global ecosystem. Ecologically sustainable agriculture has to address land and water use, fertilizer runoff, CO_2 emissions, climate change, genetically modified organisms, animal waste, infectious disease, food safety and antimicrobial resistance.

20.4 Antimicrobial use in livestock production

The term 'antimicrobial' encompasses a large group of natural and synthetic chemical compounds that kill or inhibit the growth of microbes: bacteria, protozoa, viruses and fungi. Antibiotics are antimicrobial compounds that kill or inhibit the growth of bacteria. Sanitizing and disinfecting agents are also considered antimicrobials, and resistance against these compounds has also been observed. When contemplating the complex issues surrounding antimicrobial resistance (AMR), these distinctions must be taken into account.

Antibiotics are used in livestock production for three purposes: (1) treatment of disease; (2) prophylaxis for disease prevention; (3) promotion of growth or increased feed efficiency. In livestock production, antibiotics are delivered to animals by a variety of methods depending on the reason for use, the type of livestock, and the production system: (1) treatment of individual animals via injection, or delivery in food or water; (2) delivery of antimicrobial to the entire herd or flock via food or water (Bailar and Travers, 2002; Cromwell, 2002).

Treatment of an individual animal with antibiotics by any delivery method can result in the selection of antibiotic resistance among the bacterial populations residing on the skin or in the respiratory or gastrointestinal tract. Treatment of an individual animal does lessen the chance of resistance occurring because the administration and dosing of a single animal will be more accurate, ensuring that the antibiotic chosen will reach the site of infection in a dose high enough to be therapeutic, and lethal for the bacteria causing disease.

Individual treatment is the norm in companion animal and zoo medicine. The mass medication delivery method via food or water is the norm in production animal medicine, due to the difficulty and cost of handling individual animals, the need for segregating treated animals, and risk factors for disease spread among closely confined groups of livestock animals. The use of mass medication delivery methods can increase the risk of selection of antimicrobial resistance because although the effective dosage is calculated on the basis of average food and water consumption per animal, the actual amount of antibiotic consumed per animal may vary greatly. When bacteria are exposed to sub-therapeutic amounts of antimicrobial (below the established minimum inhibitory concentration) the bacteria in the population may not be killed or inhibited in growth. Exposure to sub-lethal concentrations of antibiotics induces complex and varied stress responses in the exposed bacteria, which have been shown to induce genetic mutation, resulting in antibiotic resistance (Kohanski et al., 2010), and to induce the exchange of mobile genetic elements carrying resistance genes, resulting in the selection of resistant populations (Beaber et al., 2004; Davies et al., 2006).

20.5 The use of antibiotics to promote growth

The growing demand for food and dietary animal protein, at prices affordable to the average person, has driven the changes in livestock rearing methods that have in turn increased the use of antimicrobials in agriculture. Sixty years ago it was discovered that adding certain antibiotic compounds to poultry feed formulations improved both the feed efficiency (weight gained per weight of food consumed) of flocks and their overall health (Diarra and Malouin, 2014; Dibner and Richards, 2005). The practice was subsequently adopted by the swine and cattle industries with similar results. In the US, growth promoting antibiotics (AGP) are estimated to be currently used in 90 per cent of swine production and 60 per cent of poultry production

(Chapman and Johnson, 2002; Cromwell, 2002; Diarra and Malouin, 2014; Dewey et al., 1999). The use of AGP in animal production has led to considerable economic gains through the improvement of performance of poultry, swine and cattle. Many studies have shown that inclusion of AGP in swine feed improves growth by an average of 16.4 per cent and feed efficiency by 6.9 per cent (Cromwell, 2002).

The mechanisms by which the addition of sub-therapeutic amounts of antibiotics to animal feed produce these effects is still largely the subject of scientific conjecture (Dibner and Richards, 2005). The most plausible explanation of the biological mechanism is that long-term exposure of the gastrointestinal microbiome to sub-therapeutic levels of antibiotics leads to microbial population changes that reduce the presence and effects of bacterial pathogens, thereby producing the observed effects of increased herd health and feed efficiency (Dibner and Richards, 2005).

It is this use of antibiotics in animal production that has generated the most criticism and concern regarding the development and dissemination of antimicrobial resistance (O'Brien, 2010). The positive effects on animal production efficiency and animal welfare have been overshadowed by growing evidence that this practice has made a considerable contribution to the problem of AMR on a global scale, and specifically to increasing antimicrobial resistance in some foodborne pathogens of animal origin (Bengtsson and Wierup, 2006; Borza, 2002; McEwen and Fedorka-Cray, 2002; Swartz, 2002). The economic improvements achieved by improved animal health, weight gain and feed efficiency have come at the cost of antibiotic resistance and consumer confidence. The new realities of consumer pressure, trade restriction and regulation will result in the decreased use of antibiotics for the purpose of growth promotion in food animals.

20.6 The development of antimicrobial resistance

Antibiotics, compounds that inhibit the growth of bacteria, are naturally occurring substances produced by bacteria to compete, it is believed, for nutrients with other microbes living in the same ecosystem. Antibiotics have probably existed for as long as there has been bacteria and, likewise, the means to resist killing by antibiotics, antibiotic resistance, has also likely always existed, this survival advantage conferred by antibiotic-resistance genes.

The year 1945 marked the start of the large-scale use of the beta-lactam antibiotic penicillin in medicine. The cephalosporins, an antibiotic molecule that also has a beta-lactam ring structure, were discovered during the 1950s, the so-called golden age of antibiotics. Over time we have made modifications to the chemical structure of the basic cephalosporin molecule in order to improve its ability to kill both gram positive and gram negative bacteria, increasing its spectrum. Even today, the beta-lactam antibiotics, which include the penicillins, cephalosporins and carbepenams, are the drugs of choice for treating infections due to their broad spectrum and low toxicity for both human and veterinary patients (Bush and Macielag, 2010).

What has changed in recent history is the scale of the natural microbial ecology of antibiotic versus antibiotic resistance. The use of many tons of the beta-lactams in animal production, therapeutically and for growth promotion, has exposed vast and varied microbial ecosystems to intense selection pressure for the acquisition and dissemination of resistance against the beta-lactam class of antibiotics (Aminov, 2009; Garriss et al., 2009). As we continue to modify the cephalosporin beta-lactams in the laboratory, we drive evolution of the beta-lactamase enzymes that are produced by bacteria to resist the action of these antibiotics. As we discovered or created the first, second, third and fourth generation cephalosporins, the bacterial beta-lactamase enzymes evolved to inactivate each successive generation of antibiotic. It is an arms race that we cannot win.

20.7 The dissemination of resistance genes

Is selfish DNA responsible?

Could the environment provide a broader playground for the mobile antibiotic resistance encoding elements to promote their own diversity?

(Garriss et al., 2009)

The unique genetic mechanisms of bacteria and their ability to acquire and 'trade' extrachromosomal DNA on mobile genetic elements is another reason why we must abandon the arms race and implement One Health strategies in order to reduce the prevalence of antimicrobial resistance and maintain the usefulness of antibiotics in medicine.

On the bacterial chromosome are the genes for proteins essential to existence and reproduction. Bacteria are unique in possessing extrachromosomal DNA, in the form of a closed circular loop called a plasmid. These plasmids carry genes that are not essential for existence but enhance survival, the accessory genome. Among the genes commonly found on plasmids are antimicrobial resistance genes. Bacteria can transfer resistance genes to another bacterium via plasmids, and through a large and varied group of genetic structures called mobile genetic elements (MGE). These pieces of DNA can be mobilized separately or along with plasmids (horizontal transmission), as well as be transferred to the next generation through cell division (vertical transmission).

One of the major concerns in regard to AMR is the co-selection of resistance genes resulting in multiple-drug-resistance (MDR). Both plasmids and MGEs can possess multiple resistance genes, and when selection pressure is applied to a bacterial population, the selection for resistance against one antimicrobial will cause the increase in resistance against other antibiotics as well, because the resistance genes are physically linked on the plasmid or MGE, and are passed from one bacterium to another as a package (Chowdhury et al., 2014; Garriss et al., 2009). Co-selection of AMR may explain the increased prevalence of resistance against antibiotics that are no longer used in animal production, or that have never been used in animal production (Chowdhury et al., 2014). Co-selection of resistance genes may also explain why the 'background' prevalence of resistance has been gradually increasing in the resistome (Chowdhury et al., 2014; Wright, 2010).

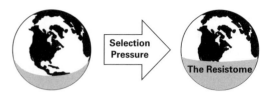

Figure 20.1 Illustration of the effect of antimicrobial selection pressure on the resistome, the absolute number of antimicrobial resistance genes in existence on earth.

'baseline' prevalence of resistance against antibiotics no longer in use that has been observed in surveillance data (Wright, 2010). This concept is illustrated in Figure 20.1. How long it might take for this baseline prevalence to subside after global reduction in antibiotic use is unknown, and may be confounded by the issue of co-selection of resistance mediated by MGEs (Garriss et al., 2009).

20.8 The resistome – environmental reservoir of resistance genes

If antibiotic compounds are natural and have always existed, and antibiotic resistance genes are natural and have always existed, it follows that there is a huge 'library' of resistance genes present in the microbes that inhabit the ecosystems of the earth (Martínez, 2008). Antimicrobial resistance is inevitable because resistance genes exist to counter all of the antimicrobials that exist. This is the concept of the resistome (Wright, 2010).

Now consider this line of thinking in light of the pollution of the environment with antimicrobial compounds that is occurring. The greatly increased prevalence of AMR genes that has been observed in both pathogens and in environmental bacteria may be the result of large-scale selection pressure. It suggests that the sheer number of antimicrobial resistance genes on earth has increased, increasing the

20.9 Transfer of resistance and food safety

The issue of antibiotic use in animal production and the development and dissemination of antibiotic resistance is often discussed in the context of food safety (Bailar and Travers, 2002; Borza, 2002). There are two means by which an antibiotic-resistant bacterium originating from a livestock production facility could be responsible for an antibiotic-resistant infection in a human or animal consumer of animal derived food:

- **Direct transfer:** The major bacterial food safety pathogens are *Salmonella*, *E. coli*, listeria and campylobacter. Any of these organisms can acquire antibiotic resistance, and will cause foodborne disease if ingested in a quantity equal to or greater than their infectious dose.
- **Indirect transfer:** Bacteroides and *Enterococcus* species are bacteria found in the digestive tract

flora of humans and animals. Different animal species have their own species of bacteroides and *Enterococcus*. These bacteria are commonly found on meats, occurring as a result of faecal contamination during slaughter and processing. When ingested, these bacteria generally do not cause foodborne illness. If the livestock are given antibiotics, their gastrointestinal bacteria will be exposed to the selection pressure to acquire antibiotic resistance genes from other bacteria in the gut microbiome (Borgeois et al., 2003; Shoemaker et al., 2001). When antibiotic-resistant bacteria are consumed on food, there is the potential for the bacteria to transfer their resistance genes to the bacteria in the gut microbiome of the consumer (Borgeois et al., 2003; Shoemaker et al., 2001). If the person (or animal) then gets a bladder infection from exposure to their own gastrointestinal bacteria, and, if that bacterium is resistant, the infection may be difficult to treat.

Figure 20.2 is an example of how antibiotic resistance genes will flow between different bacterial species, and between microbial ecosystems.

There is scientific evidence to support that both of these types of resistance gene transfers do occur in the context of antibiotic use in animal production and the development of antibiotic resistance in foodborne pathogens (Bailar and Travers, 2002). However, studies finding associations between the use of an antibiotic and the presence of antibiotic resistance do not demonstrate a causal link between use and resistance for all foodborne bacteria. This is most likely due to the complex nature of resistance gene ecology.

20.10 Effects of removing antibiotic growth promoters on antimicrobial resistance

Although the evidence linking the use of antibiotics as growth promoters in animal production and the rise of antibiotic resistance in foodborne pathogens is convincing for only some combinations of AGP use and AMR in particular bacterial species, the European Union decided to invoke the precautionary principle, and enact regulation to phase out the use of AGP in animal

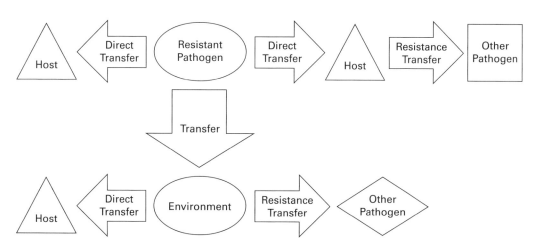

Figure 20.2 Diagram illustrating the direct and indirect transfer of antimicrobial resistance from foodborne bacterial pathogens to other bacteria.

production (http://eur-lex.europa.eu/LexUriServ. do?uri=OJ:L:2003:268:0029:0043:EN:PDF).

The most compelling evidence incriminating the use of AGP in the development of AMR of human health significance are studies examining the decline in vancomycin-resistant *Enterococcus* species isolated from swine production subsequent to the ban on use of avoparcin as an AGP in swine (Aarestrup et al., 2001).

Due to the complex nature of bacterial genetic exchange, and the role of co-selection of packages of genes transferred by mobile genetic elements, the effect of withdrawing AGP antibiotics on the prevalence of the corresponding AMR may vary considerably from one AGP/AMR/bacteria combination to another.

20.11 Antimicrobial resistance in foodborne pathogens and public health

Although there is some hyperbole and finger-pointing regarding the causes of increasing antimicrobial resistance, the threat to human and animal health is real, and concrete measures must be taken to prevent the development and dissemination of resistance.

We are already seeing infections with common bacteria such as *E. coli* and *Salmonella* that are considered multiple-drug-resistant (MDR), having resistance against three or more classes of antibiotics. It has been shown that antibiotic-resistant bacteria are more virulent and cause

---

Are we entering a post-antibiotic era?

In their 2014 publication, *Antimicrobial Resistance: Global Report on Surveillance*, the World Health Organization (WHO) made the following statement summarizing the current state of antibiotic resistance in common bacterial pathogens around the world:

> Increasingly, governments around the world are beginning to pay attention to a problem so serious that it threatens the achievements of modern medicine. A post-antibiotic era – in which common infections and minor injuries can kill – far from being an apocalyptic fantasy, is instead a very real possibility for the 21st century.
>
> (WHO, 2014)

Among the bacteria commonly causing both nosocomial and community-acquired infections, they analysed national surveillance data for some that can cause foodborne illness; *E. coli*, *Staphylococcus aureus*, *Shigella* sp. and *Salmonella enterica* serotypes. Analysis of surveillance data from 86 member states revealed that the frequency of resistance against third-generation cephalosporins and fluoroquinolones in *E. coli* is greater than 50 per cent. The frequency of resistance against fluoroquinolones in *Salmonella* serotypes and *Shigella* sp. associated with foodborne illness is greater than 25 per cent.

Antimicrobial resistance trends like these are a serious concern for human health. The third-generation cephalosporins are the treatment of choice for invasive infections with *E. coli*, *Salmonella* and *Shigella* due to the broad spectrum and safety profile for these antibiotics. The fluoroquinolones are the second tier choice of treatment for these infections due to their cost and concerns over side-effects. High prevalence of resistance against these two classes of antibiotics will have real consequences for treatment of foodborne illness (WHO, 2014).

worse disease, even if the bacteria are not resistant to all antibiotics and should be treatable (Travers and Barza, 2002). The association between AMR and worse patient outcome is thought to be due to co-selection of virulence factor genes along with antimicrobial resistance genes present on mobile genetic elements that are transferred between bacteria.

20.12 The social licence to operate

The public concerns about food safety, stewardship of antimicrobials, and environmental protection are central to the concept of the social licence to operate. The social licence granted to those involved in animal agriculture is based on trust and the assurance that they share the same ethical principles as the people who consume the food products that come from those animals.

As science comes to understand the complex ecology of antimicrobial resistance, and as public attitudes and values change, the social licence to operate for those involved in intensive animal production industries will be challenged, and the industries will have no choice but to adjust their antimicrobial use practices.

20.13 Drivers of change

The Center for Science in the Public Interest (CSPI) is a non-profit consumer advocacy organization that provides information to the public and policymakers on food, health and the environment. Their stated mission is to represent the interest of the citizen before regulatory, judicial and legislative bodies. In October 2014, the organization resubmitted a petition on behalf of the citizens of the US to the US Department of Agriculture Food Safety and Inspection Service (USDA-FSIS) asking that antibiotic-resistant *Salmonella enterica* serotypes Heidelberg, Hadar, Newport and Typhimurium, those most com-

monly associated with foodborne illness from the consumption of meat, poultry and eggs, be declared adulterants. In the petition, the CSPI based its request on the assumption that resistant *Salmonella* are created by exposure to antibiotics during poultry production. The same petition submitted in May 2015, was denied by the USDA-FSIS in August, 2015, citing the need for more data. In their rejection, the USDA-FSIS responded that antimicrobial resistant microbes can be present in food animals even if they haven't been exposed to antibiotics during food animal production. In addition, they claim that *Salmonella* are usually killed during the normal cooking processes for meat, poultry and eggs, and therefore do not present an unavoidable hazard.

The USDA-FSIS defines food to be considered adulterated when 'it bears or contains any poisonous or deleterious substance which may render it injurious to health; but in case the substance is not an added substance, such article shall not be considered adulterated under this clause if the quantity of such substance does not ordinarily render it injurious to health' (USDA-FSIS, 2011, Part 1, 601 (m)(1)).

The CSPI petition is relying on the precedent set by the FSIS declaration of two other foodborne bacterial pathogens as adulterants in meat products. The bacterium *Listeria monocytogenes* was declared to be an adulterant of ready to eat (RTE) products because it is introduced to the food during processing and handling, and because these products are intended to be eaten without further cooking, they present a risk to health. The toxigenic *E. coli* strain O157:H7 was declared to be an added substance because it too contaminates the meat products during processing, and that it is a risk to health because of the consumer preference for undercooked or 'rare' beef, which may still contain live bacteria not killed during cooking. As new toxigenic strains of *E. coli* are being characterized and associated with foodborne illness, these too are being declared adulterants (USDA-FSIS, 2011).

Substances declared adulterants evoke a zero-tolerance response from the USDA-FSIS. This means that if food inspection surveillance samples test positive for the substance, the animal carcasses, meat or products will be condemned and must either be reprocessed or destroyed, and cannot be used in human food.

Declaring specific bacteria as adulterants is feasible because individual HAACP programmes can be developed to keep the bacteria from contaminating food products during slaughter and processing.

The 'baseline' of antimicrobial resistance has been increasing for decades, perhaps due to the co-selection of AMR genes on mobile genetic elements that are transferred as a package, or as a result of antibiotic selection pressure on the global 'resistome', the AMR genes available in the environment. Can a HAACP programme be devised to keep resistant bacteria from contaminating animal carcasses during processing? Imagine the repercussions of declaring the presence of AMR in foodborne bacteria as food adulterants.

In North America and Europe the consumers of food products are driving change to agricultural practices affecting animal welfare, food safety and antimicrobial resistance. The general public, the consumers of food, are ultimately the 'customers' of agricultural industries, and as such, their opinions and buying power will inevitably shape agricultural practices and the use of antibiotics in animal production.

20.14 Current actions to reduce risk

There are many factors contributing to the worldwide emergence and dissemination of antibiotic resistance, and a multipronged approach is required for success in reducing the prevalence of AMR.

In 2014, the World Health Organization issued a report titled *Antimicrobial Resistance:* *Global Report on Surveillance*, calling for increased surveillance of resistance, harmonized between countries as the basis for informing global strategies, monitoring the effectiveness of public health interventions and detecting new trends and threats. In May 2014, the 67th World Health Assembly requested the director-general to develop a draft global action plan to combat antimicrobial resistance, which was adopted at the 68th Health Assembly in May 2015. The plan includes global standards for medical and veterinary education on AMR, stewardship and prudent use principles.

The Centers for Disease Control and Prevention (CDC) has developed guidelines and recommendations for antimicrobial stewardship for physicians and hospitals to reduce inappropriate antibiotic usage (July 2012 Update Antibiotic Stewardship Drivers and Change Package, Prepared by the Institute for Healthcare Improvement). In Canada, a consortium of healthcare agencies from Alberta and British Columbia have created a public health awareness campaign called 'Do bugs need drugs?' aimed at educating healthcare providers and the general public about the proper use of antibiotics.

The US Food and Drug Administration (FDA) uses the 'principle of proof' as its guideline for gathering scientific evidence for risk assessment when taking action and creating new regulations regarding use of antimicrobials as growth promoters in food animals. In May 2015, the FDA published a proposed rule that includes additional reporting requirements for sponsors of antibiotics approved for use in food-producing animals to obtain estimates of sales to producers of major food-producing species (cattle, swine, chickens and turkeys). The aim is to collect additional data that would improve understanding about how antimicrobials are sold, distributed and used in the major food-producing species, to help the FDA further target its efforts to ensure judicious use of medically important antimicrobials. In 2014, the FDA announced the

Veterinary Feed Directive (VFD) rule. This regulation is part of the FDA's strategy promoting the judicious use of medically important antibiotics in food-producing animals, as it brings the use of antibiotics in animal feed directly under the oversight of licensed food supply veterinarians.

20.15 Conclusions

In an increasingly connected and increasingly populated world, there are no borders for antibiotic-resistant bacteria. An international coordinated effort directed at responsible use of antimicrobials will be required for any positive effect on the prevalence of AMR in the global ecosystem. The One Health approach must include global buy-in of the concepts of stewardship and prudent use principles. Medical education must improve understanding of AMR, AMU and prudent use principles for students. Coordinated collection of AMR and AMU data will aid in our understanding of the relationships between AMU and AMR in human and veterinary pathogens and environmental bacteria. Further regulation and restriction of the use of AGP antibiotics may be deemed necessary, but these may come at a cost to agricultural production and animal welfare until effective alternatives can be found. Because of the complex ecology of resistance gene transfer, the effects of these efforts on the prevalence of resistance genes in the global resistome are difficult to predict.

References

Aarestrup, F., Seyfarth, A., Emborg, H., Pedersen, K., Hendriksen, R. and Bager, F. (2001). Effect of abolishment of the use of antimicrobial agents for growth promotion on occurrence of antimicrobial resistance in fecal enterococci from food animals in Denmark. *Antimicrobial Agents and Chemotherapy*, 45, 2054–2059.

Aminov, R. (2009). The role of antibiotics and antibiotic resistance in nature. *Environmental Microbiology*, 11, 2970–2988.

Bailar, J. and Travers, K. (2002). Review of assessments of the human health risk associated with the use of antimicrobial agents in agriculture. *Clinical Infectious Diseases*, 34(S3), S135–S143.

Beaber, J., Hochhut, B. and Waldor, M. (2004). SOS response promotes horizontal dissemination of antibiotic resistance genes. *Nature*, 427, 72–74.

Bengtsson, B. and Wierup, M. (2006). Antimicrobial resistance in Scandinavia after ban of antimicrobial growth promoters. *Animal Biotechnology*, 17, 147–156.

Borgeois, N., Savard, B., Moubareck, C., et al. (2003). Interspecies transfer of vancomycin resistance from poultry *Enterococcus faecium* to human *Enterococcus faecalis* in digestive tract of human flora associated mice. In *Abstracts of the Forty-third Interscience Conference on Antimicrobial Agents and Chemotherapy*, Chicago, IL. Washington, DC: American Society for Microbiology.

Borza, M. (2002). Potential mechanisms of increased disease in humans from antimicrobial resistance in food animals. *Clinical Infectious Diseases*, 34(S3), S123–S130.

Bush, K. and Macielag, M. (2010). New β-lactam antibiotics and β-lactamase inhibitors. *Expert Opinion on Therapeutic Patents*, 20, 1277–1293.

Chapman, H. and Johnson, Z. (2002). Use of antibiotics and roxarsone in broiler chickens in the USA: analysis for the years 1995 to 2000. *Poultry Science*, 81, 356–364.

Chowdhury, P., McKinnon, J., Wyrsch, E., Hammond, J. and Charles, I. (2014). Genomic interplay in bacterial communities: implications for growth promoting practices in animal husbandry. *Frontiers in Microbiology*, 5(394), 1–11.

Cromwell, G. (2002). Why and how antibiotics are used in swine production. *Animal Biotechnology*, 13(1), 7–27.

Davies, J., Spiegelman, G. and Yim, G. (2006). The world of subinhibitory antibiotic concentrations. *Current Opinion in Microbiology*, 9, 445–453.

Dewey, C., Cox, B., Straw, B., Bush, E. and Hurd, S. (1999). Use of antimicrobials in swine feeds in the United States. *Journal of Swine Health and Production*, 7, 19–25.

Diarra, M. and Malouin, F. (2014). Antibiotics in Canadian poultry productions and anticipated alternatives. *Frontiers in Microbiology*, 5(282), 1–15.

Dibner, J. and Richards, J. (2005). Antibiotic growth promoters in agriculture: history and mode of action. *Poultry Science*, 84, 634–643.

Food and Drug Administration (2014). *2009 Summary Report on Antimicrobials Sold or Distributed for Use in Food-Producing Animals*. Washington, DC: Center for Veterinary Medicine, Department of Health and Human Services.

Garriss, G., Waldor, M. and Burrus, V. (2009). Mobile antibiotic resistance encoding elements promote their own diversity. *PLOS Genetics*, 5, e1000775.

Kohanski, M., DePristo, M. and Collins, J. (2010). Sublethal antibiotic treatment leads to multi-drug resistance via radical-induced mutagenesis. *Molecular Cell*, 37, 311–320.

Martínez, J. (2008). Antibiotics and antibiotic resistance genes in natural environments. *Science*, 321, 365–367.

McEwen, S. and Fedorka-Cray, P. (2002). Antimicrobial use and resistance in animals. *Clinical Infectious Diseases*, 34(S3), S93–S105.

O'Brien, T. (2010). *Policy Brief and Recommendations #1: Misuse of Antibiotics in Food Animal Production: Preserve Antibiotics for the Future*. Alliance for the Prudent Use of Antibiotics, www.tufts.edu/med/apua.

Shoemaker, N.B., Vlamakis, H., Hayes, K. and Salyers, A.A. (2001). Evidence for extensive resistance gene transfer among Bacteroides spp. and among Bacteroides and other genera in the human colon. *Applied and Environmental Microbiology*, 67(2), 561–568.

Swartz, M. (2002). Human diseases caused by food-borne pathogens of animal origin. *Clinical Infectious Diseases*, 34(S3), S111–S122.

Travers, K. and Barza, M. (2002). Morbidity of infections caused by antimicrobial-resistant bacteria. *Clinical Infectious Diseases*, 34(S3), S131–S135.

USDA-FSIS (2011), *Federal Register*, 76(182), 58157–58158, www.fsis.usda.gov/OPPDE/rdad/FRPubs/2010-0023.pdf.

WHO (2001). *WHO Global Strategy for Containment of Antimicrobial Resistance*. Geneva: World Health Organization.

WHO (2014). *Antimicrobial Resistance: Global Report on Surveillance*. Geneva: World Health Organization.

Wright, G. (2010). Antibiotic resistance in the environment: a link to the clinic? *Current Opinion in Microbiology*, 13, 589–594.

chapter 21

Shrimp farming in Sri Lanka: a case study at the interface of human, shrimp and environmental health

Jessica Wu, Sylvia Checkley, Trisha Westers,
Theresa Burns, Carl Ribble and Craig Stephen

Abstract

Aquaculture is the fastest growing animal production sector in the world. Global demand for fish and other seafood has increased significantly with world per capita consumption increasing from 9.9kg in the 1960s to 19.2kg in 2012. The Democratic Socialist Republic of Sri Lanka is an island country in the Indian Ocean located off the south-east coast of India. Shrimp farming in Sri Lanka started in the late 1970s and has grown significantly as a primary industry. However, in addition to difficulties with disease outbreaks, shrimp farmers in Sri Lanka have also faced social and environmental constraints as well as questions about environmental sustainability. Conflict over changes in land use, such as converting traditional paddy and coconut fields to shrimp farms, has led to a loss of traditional livelihoods for some people. This case study investigates how shrimp farming can be a sustainable option for household food security in post-war Sri Lanka. The benefits of taking a holistic ecohealth approach to establishing an aquaculture initiative, such as shrimp farming, are also examined.

21.1 Introduction

Aquaculture, the cultivation of aquatic organisms, is the fastest growing animal production sector in the world (FAO, 2012). Global demand for fish and other seafood, including molluscs, has increased significantly with world per capita consumption in the 1960s of 9.9kg increasing to 19.2kg in 2012 (FAO, 2014). Fish constitutes approximately 17 per cent of animal protein consumption in the global population, with some coastal countries such as Sri Lanka exceeding 50 per cent of their intake of protein from fish (FAO, 2014).

With a growing global population, agricultural growth will be the key to reducing malnutrition and hunger (FAO et al., 2013). Smallholder farming, including aquaculture, is considered to be a key pathway for alleviating extreme poverty (Godfray et al., 2010; HLPE, 2013). Aquaculture can contribute to poverty alleviation and enhance food security directly through production of fish and aquatic products as well as increased employment and income generation. In many countries, aquaculture has been shown to improve the status of women by encouraging direct participation (Ahmed and Lorica, 2002; Kawarazuka and Béné, 2010).

The Democratic Socialist Republic of Sri Lanka is an island country in the Indian Ocean. It is located just off the southeast coast of India. The country has a total land area of 65,610km², 1,340km of coastline and 7,490km² of inland and aquaculture-appropriate area (such as lagoons, man-made lakes and freshwater bodies) (Agriculture and Environmental Statistics Division, 2005). The population of Sri Lanka, as of 2013, was estimated to be 20.5 million people, with 77 per cent in rural areas, 18 per cent in urban areas and 5 per cent in estates (Sri Lanka Department of Census and Statistics, 2012). There were reported to be more women than men (10.6 million women) and life expectancy at birth for women was 76.7 years and 71.7 years for men (Sri Lanka Department of Census and Statistics, 2001). The country is ethnically and religiously diverse with 75 per cent Sinhalese, 11 per cent Sri Lankan Tamil, 4 per cent Indian Tamil, 9 per cent Sri Lanka Moor, 0.2 per cent Burgher and 0.2 per cent Malay (remaining percentage made up of other minor ethnic groups), and 70 per cent Buddhist, 13 per cent Hindu, 10 per cent Muslim, 6 per cent Roman Catholic and 1 per cent other Christian (Sri Lanka Department of Census and Statistics, 2012). The two national languages are Sinhala and Tamil.

In 1983, ethnic conflict in the north and east part of the country erupted between the Sinhalese and Tamils. The civil war continued until May 2009, with significant impacts on the population, environment and the economy (Arunatilake et al., 2001). The 26 December 2004 Indian Ocean tsunami also had significant impact, affecting two-thirds of the Sri Lankan coastline (eastern to the south-western coast). The death toll from this disaster reached 31,000, with nearly half a million people displaced (Yamada et al., 2006). The decades-long civil war, compounded by environmental destruction from the tsunami, resulted in significant challenges for the country with increased poverty, food insecurity, displaced persons and a lack of livelihood options. With significant aquatic resources, the government of Sri Lanka considered aquaculture development as an important opportunity to diversify livelihoods and to increase household income (Harris, 2007).

In the case study presented below, we examine the establishment and success of shrimp farming in Sri Lanka. Information is provided on the current status of the industry and we present some important considerations for the expansion of the industry. The value of taking a One Health approach is also considered.

The specific issues examined in the case study are:

- Who is involved in shrimp farming?
- How are women involved in the industry?
- How sustainable is shrimp farming currently?
- Does shrimp farming contribute to poverty alleviation through ensuring food security?
- How do farmers obtain information about best farming practices?

21.2 Case study background

Shrimp farming in Sri Lanka started in the late 1970s in the Batticaloa district of the Eastern Province (EP). The farms in this region were largely abandoned in the 1980s due to civil unrest and the industry spread to the Puttalam district in the North-Western Province (NWP). The industry boomed in the NWP in the 1980s and 1990s, with a number of multinational companies and medium-scale entrepreneurs owning a large proportion of farms (Drengstig, 2013). In the 1990s, disease became a significant problem in cultivated shrimp with the introduction of *Penaeus monodon* nucleopolyhedrovirus virus, white spot syndrome virus and yellow head disease (Munasinghe et al., 2010, 2012). This led to the abandonment of many farms and, starting in the late 2000s, the industry was maintained by smallholder farmers with semi-intensive practices in both the NWP and EP. The NWP and the EP have a number of differences including socio-demographics (e.g., religion and ethnicity in the regions), as well as their shrimp farming activities. For example, while the NWP has struggled with shrimp disease on shrimp farms, there were no reports of disease on shrimp farms in the EP.

In addition to difficulties with disease outbreaks, shrimp farmers in Sri Lanka have also faced social and environmental constraints. Conflict over land use, such as converting traditional paddy and coconut fields, has led to a loss of traditional livelihoods for some people (Siriwardena, 1999). Once the land is abandoned, it is often unsuitable for conversion back into usable agricultural land (Primavera, 1997). Conflicts between shrimp farmers and with community members have also arisen. As the industry was initially unregulated and unplanned, ponds were constructed with the water outlet canal adjoining to the water inlet canal of another farmer (Corea et al., 1995). This has had negative consequences for water quality as well as causing increased disease transmission between ponds. Spillover salinization of ground water has also led to conflict as domestic water wells and agricultural water sources have been affected (Bergquist, 2007; Siriwardena, 1999). Environmental constraints have included water pollution and destruction of mangroves. The Dutch Canal connects lagoons along the coast of the NWP and this canal supplies brackish water to more than 70 per cent of the shrimp farms in the area (Corea et al., 1995). This canal also receives effluent from farms and therefore water quality has greatly deteriorated. Mangrove forests are ecologically and economically important areas that protect against erosion, provide shelter for breeding and growth of aquatic organisms and birds, and are a source of wood (Alongi, 2002). The development of shrimp farming has been considered to be a primary cause for the loss of mangroves in Sri Lanka (Corea et al., 1998; Dahdouh-Guebas et al., 2002; Senarath and Visvanathan, 2001). These are all issues that present challenges that will need to be addressed in a holistic way by interdisciplinary teams working with community members and policymakers.

Smallholder shrimp farming still holds promise as a way to alleviate poverty in Sri Lanka. Historically, the country had a successful shrimp export market and, given the right support, there is a real potential to revive the industry (Landesman et al., 2009). Shrimp farming expansion is particularly attractive due to high export demand for shrimp and the potential for significant profit when production is successfully executed (FAO, 2012). While the costs and benefits must be weighed carefully, there is the belief that establishing extensive or semi-intensive shrimp farming, which is more environmentally and socially sustainable, can benefit the rural poor (Burns et al., 2013; Galappaththi, 2013; Landesman et al., 2009). However, measuring sustainability is challenging because numerous definitions of sustainability exist. One of the most widely recognized definitions of sustainability comes from the Brundtland Report (see box), which states that 'sustainable development should meet the needs of the present without compromising the ability of future generations to meet their own needs' (World Commission on Environment and Development, 1987). The focus of this report was on environmental protection, but in low-income countries, productivity and social issues are also important. In agricultural sustainability, the three main pillars of sustainability should be included. These include the economic, social and environmental pillars (Gómez-Limón and Sanchez-Fernandez, 2010; Pope et al., 2004; Pretty, 2008; Van Cauwenbergh et al., 2007). Sustainability is key to the successful application of an ecohealth approach.

The *Brundtland Report*

The *Brundtland Report* was released by the Brundtland Commission in October 1987. This is a document that coined and defined the meaning of the term 'sustainable development'. The Brundtland Commission's mission was to provide impetus for the international community to work towards sustainable development together. It was officially dissolved in December 1987 after releasing the *Brundtland Report,* which was also known by the title *Our Common Future* (World Commission on Environment and Development, 1987).

An understanding of the gender dimension in development issues is important and must be addressed in order to move towards gender equality and gender equity. Gender equality is 'a state in which people enjoy equal rights, opportunities, and rewards, regardless of whether they were born female or male', and gender equity refers to 'fairness and impartiality in the treatment of women and men, according to their respective needs' (FAO, 2009a). Equity does not mean identical treatment, but recognizes that equal treatment is dependent on meeting different needs. Rural women make up a large proportion of the world's poor, and are often marginalized with regard to their access to education, land and other resources. It has been found that there can be an overall economic advantage to communities that ensure increased employment opportunities for women.

In contrast, unequal access to, and control of, resources negatively affects community productivity. Opportunities for income generation and control over household resources by women also positively influences individual household food security and children's health and education, because women generally spend more money on food and on children's needs (World Bank and IFAD, 2009; World Bank, 2011).

Poverty and a lack of food are closely related. Food security is defined as 'when all people, at all times, have physical and economic access to sufficient, safe, and nutritious food to meet their dietary needs and food preferences for an active and healthy life' (World Food Summit, 1996). Food security is a complex concept with multiple dimensions. It is composed of four key components: availability, accessibility, utilization and, more recently, stability (FAO, 2009b). The consequences of food insecurity have been associated with negative physical and psychological outcomes including being underweight, poor growth, chronic disease, poor social skills and depression (Cook and Frank, 2008; Cook et al., 2004; Hadley and Patil, 2006; Jyoti et al., 2005; Seligman et al., 2007), which has downstream economic consequences in terms of decreased productivity, lower GDP and an increased cost for healthcare (Arcand, 2001; FAO, 2001; Stein and Qaim, 2007; Wang and Taniguchi, 2003). In Sri Lanka, a reported 22.8 per cent of the population were considered undernourished between 2011 and 2013. However, this is an improvement of 32 per cent since 1990.

To feed a growing population, increased productivity is a priority in agriculture and aquaculture (FAO, 2009c). Achieving this increased productivity includes not only ensuring increased access to resources but also access to relevant information and knowledge to help farmers do their job well. Community-based 'social learning' is an important avenue for learning and information, particularly in rural, lower-income countries where technical information and formal extension services may be limited (Bandiera and Rasul, 2006; Conley and Udry, 2001; Hartwich and Scheidegger, 2010; Thuo et al., 2013). Social learning is often defined as the process of interactions between people through shared experiences, roles and environments that involve the generation of knowledge but also refers to subsequent changes in behaviour reflected in farming practices (Blackmore, 2007; Milbrath, 1989; Muro and Jeffrey, 2008).

Case study population

Inclusion criteria for participation in the case study were smallholder shrimp farmers in Sri Lanka, defined as a farm containing five or fewer ponds, where the farmer was actively working on the farm and no delegation of decision-making was given to a manager or any other person. A total of 165 farms were surveyed in the North-Western Province (NWP) and 60 farms in the Eastern Province (EP). The shrimp farming industry in the NWP is more established than the EP.

Data collection

A cross-sectional study of smallholder shrimp farmers was completed from June to August 2011. Teams of two interviewers able to speak the local language were hired and trained to administer a structured questionnaire. The questionnaire was developed to obtain self-reported information on (1) demographic and socioeconomic status, (2) household food insecurity, (3) gender roles, (4) sustainable shrimp farming practices and (5) social networks of information exchange. Basic demographic information (age, sex, ethnicity, religion, education) was also collected for each member of the household, as well as household characteristics (type of housing, ownership, etc.), household assets

and farming assets (production animals owned). The Household Food Insecurity Access Scale (HFIAS) was used to measure food security (Ballard, 2011; Coates et al., 2007). The HFIAS is an experiential questionnaire that consists of nine questions that assess anxiety, quantity and quality of food intake that may be decreased due to a lack of economic access (Coates et al., 2007). The basis for this method is that people experience food insecurity in predictable ways and these can be captured by responses to specific questions.

Scientific literature and consultation with local experts guided development of sustainability indices specific to the shrimp farming industry in Sri Lanka. The framework was adapted from the Sustainability Assessment of Farming and Environment (SAFE) model (Van Cauwenbergh et al., 2007) that utilizes the concept of the three pillars of sustainability: social, economic and ecological factors. These pillars, along with the industry specific shrimp health factors, form four sub-indices. The social pillar included variables related to interactions with other farmers and workers. The economic pillar referred to variables such as the costs of farming and sales. The ecological pillar related to environmental factors such as water use and use of chemicals. Shrimp health referred to disease in shrimp, farm biosecurity and health monitoring. Higher values for the indices indicate greater sustainability.

The study of the network of information exchange was based on social network methods (Scott, 2013), where the network refers to connections that farmers use to exchange information about shrimp farming, hereafter referred to as the information network (IN). To obtain information on this network, farmers were asked to name contacts that farmers may use or have used for the purpose of information-seeking regarding shrimp farming practices. Contacts were enumerated from questions in the structured survey and included community members and farmers as well as government, industry and academic experts. The total number of contacts is termed *degree* and the overall information network degree (IND) is the total count of unique individuals identified by farmers.

Results

Demographic information between each province showed differences. The median age was higher in the EP (46 years) compared to the NWP (39 years). Shrimp farming households in the NWP were mostly Sinhalese and Catholic, while in the EP shrimp farmers were primarily Moors and Muslim. For education, 62 per cent of shrimp farmers in the NWP had a high school or greater education while 49 per cent of shrimp farmers in the EP had the equivalent. There was a larger proportion of shrimp farmers and spouses that had no education in the EP compared to the NWP; however, there was also a larger proportion of shrimp farmers and spouses in the EP that had completed the graduate certificate of education (GCE) advanced level of education.

Men were involved in all aspects of shrimp farming. This included daily feeding, harvesting shrimp, cleaning the ponds, monitoring for disease and guarding the ponds overnight. A large proportion of women in the EP (71 per cent) were not involved in shrimp farming at all, in comparison to women in the NWP (20 per cent) that reported they were not involved in shrimp farming. Women in the EP were involved in cleaning, while women in the NWP reported daily feeding, cleaning the pond and guarding the ponds as tasks they performed on the farm.

Household food security was high among shrimp farmers in both provinces (Table 21.1). Only a small proportion of shrimp produced on farms was consumed within the household with 1 per cent and 1.3 per cent of total shrimp yield retained for household consumption in the NWP and EP, respectively.

Farms in the NWP had higher overall sustainability scores than farms in the EP despite the presence of disease. In the NWP, the mean sustainability score was 59.7 (95 per cent CI: 58.5–60.9). In the EP, the mean sustainability score was 54.3 (95 per cent CI: 52.3–56.4). Mean index scores for the social, ecological, and health pillars were significantly higher in the NWP compared to the EP.

The median IND for farmers was two in both the NWP and the EP (NWP quartile 1 (Q1) = 1, quartile 3 (Q3) = 4; EP Q1 = 1, Q3 = 3). The range of INDs in the two provinces was similar (NWP 0–8, EP 0–9). A large proportion of people that farmers sought information from were other farmers. Of the 49 individuals identified by farmers in the EP, there were nine people also named in the NWP.

In the NWP, farmer INDs differed by ethnicity. For the Sinhalese, median network degree was 1 (Q1 = 1, Q3 = 2), while the median network degree for Tamils was 4 (Q1 = 1, Q3 = 5), and for the Moors median network degree was 5 (Q1 = 4, Q3 = 5). These differences were

Table 21.1 Household food insecurity based on the HFIAS, by province

Food insecurity of the household	North-Western Province (n = 157)	Eastern Province (n = 59)
Severely food insecure	3.8%	1.7%
Moderately food insecure	1.9%	3.4%
Mildly food insecure	5.1%	8.5%
Food secure	89.2%	86.4%

statistically significant. Networks for the three ethnicities in the NWP appeared quite different visually, with the Sinhalese network more highly connected to experts at NAQDA (National Aquaculture Development Authority), while the Moor and Tamil networks were more highly connected to other farmers.

21.3 Conclusions

In Sri Lanka, the shrimp farming industry is male-dominated. There are differences in ethnicity and religion of farmers in the two provinces. This may indicate a preference for some groups of people to work in the industry. The differences in women's involvement in shrimp farming may have important implications for promoting increased participation of women. While having a separate income may be empowering, the extra work of activities on the household farm may be more of a burden. The increased time required in maintaining a farm may only be an additional encumbrance to women who are already responsible for maintaining the household and for childrearing activities (Felsing et al., 2000). It should also be recognized that there may be sociocultural challenges to overcome with regard to increasing women's participation in aquaculture and shrimp farming. While some women may need to work outside of the home out of economic necessity, households that can afford to keep women restricted to household work may consider themselves as having a better status (Williams et al., 2002). Similarly, women who are faced with economic difficulties may go against culturally imposed restrictions and become involved in a greater range of activities in order to earn any form of income (Felsing et al., 2000).

The majority of shrimp farmers were found to be food secure. The closest comparable data for the NWP is based on the National Household Income and Expenditure Surveys (HIES) from the Department of Census and Statistics in Sri Lanka. From the 2009–2010 data, the Puttalam district (the district with shrimp farms in the NWP) had a range of 29–47 per cent of the population considered to be food insecure (Mayadunne and Romeshun, 2013). For the EP, due to serious concerns of food insecurity post-war, the United Nations World Food Programme has taken a targeted interest in ongoing food insecurity assessment. Data from 2011 for the Batticaloa district (the district with shrimp farms located in the EP) indicate approximately 51 per cent food secure with 32 per cent moderately food insecure and 17 per cent severely food insecure based on Food Consumption Scores (WFP et al., 2012). From this research, shrimp farming households in these same districts are more food secure compared to the general population in the same area. This may indicate that either shrimp farming can lead to food security or that more food secure households are part of the shrimp farming industry. The measures of food insecurity from these studies utilized different methods; therefore, direct comparisons between these studies must be interpreted with caution as different dimensions of food security are assessed.

Shrimp farms in the NWP appeared to be more sustainable than the EP, despite more problems with shrimp health. Disease has historically been a limiting factor in the short-term survival of farms and therefore the government and farmers have made changes to regulations and practices to improve farm sustainability (Weerakoon, 2007). Therefore, disease in the farms in the NWP may have stimulated adoption of more sustainable practices in comparison to the EP, which has yet to experience disease. Farmers in the EP may consider adopting more sustainable practices sooner than later as a pre-emptive measure if disease becomes a problem for these farms. Farms in the NWP also have room for improvement in sustainability and this study provides useful baseline sustainability measures.

The network data indicates that farmers rely on other farmers for information. The low connectivity between farmers may reflect a choice in keeping information to themselves, a lack of availability of time to cultivate multiple relationships, and a matter of convenience in proximity of other farmers, all factors seen in other farming communities (Bodin and Crona, 2009; Mostert et al., 2007; Rist et al., 2007). These factors may hinder social learning; however, this cannot be fully validated from this study. Bandiera and Rasul (2006) demonstrated that adoption of technology among sunflower farmers in northern Mozambique was positive with fewer connections but negative when the network was larger. Similarly in Ghana, information is still able to flow through limited pathways and sources among pineapple farmers (Conley and Udry, 2001). A low number of connections for information exchange may not affect farmers negatively.

Networks appear to be separated by language. Sinhalese farmers had greater connections to the NAQDA and this may indicate a gap in extension for non-Sinhala-speaking shrimp farmers. Tamil and Moor farmers were also more highly connected to other farmers. If information on more sustainable practices or awareness of a disease outbreak were desired, it would be most efficient to access highly connected individuals to spread this information. Feed input suppliers may be more important in the Sinhala-speaking network, while influential farmers may be more important to inform in the Tamil-speaking network.

Overall, the smallholder shrimp farming industry is male-dominated, with differing ethnic and religious makeup in the EP versus the NWP. Methods to involve women in the industry would need to consider cultural and social norms and preferences in each region, The development of shrimp farming has also been considered to be a primary cause for environmental damage, including water pollution, salinization and the loss of mangroves in Sri Lanka. However, the majority of shrimp farmers are food secure. These are all complex issues that present challenges that will need to be addressed by interdisciplinary teams working with community members and policy makers in Sri Lanka.

References

Agriculture and Environmental Statistics Division (2005). *Fisheries and Aquatic Resources of Sri Lanka.* Colombo: Government of Sri Lanka.

Ahmed, M. and Lorica, M.H. (2002). Improving developing country food security through aquaculture development – lessons from Asia. *Food Policy, 27,* 125–141.

Alongi, D.M. (2002). Present state and future of the world's mangrove forests. *Environmental Conservation,* 29, 331–349.

Amlaku, A., Sölkner, J., Puskur, R. and Wurzinger, M. (2012). The impact of social networks on dairy technology adoption: evidence from Northwest Ethiopia. *International Journal of AgriScience, 2,* 1062–1083.

Arcand, J.L. (2001). *Undernourishment and Economic Growth: The Efficiency Cost of Hunger.* Rome: FAO.

Arunatilake, N., Jayasuriya, S. and Kelegama, S. (2001). The economic cost of the war in Sri Lanka. *World Development, 29,* 1483–1500.

Ballard, T., Coates, J., Swindale, A. and Deitchler, M. (2011). *Household Hunger Scale: Indicator Definition and Measurement Guide.* FANTA-2 Bridge, FHI 360, Washington, DC.

Bandiera, O. and Rasul, I. (2006). Social networks and technology adoption in northern mozambique. *The Economic Journal,* 116, 869–902.

Bergquist, D.A. (2007). Sustainability and local people's participation in coastal aquaculture: regional differences and historical experiences in Sri Lanka and the Philippines. *Environmental Management,* 40, 787–802.

Blackmore, C. (2007). What kinds of knowledge, knowing and learning are required for addressing resource dilemmas? A theoretical overview. *Environmental Science & Policy,* 10, 512–525.

Bodin, Ö. and Crona, B.I. (2009). The role of social networks in natural resource governance: what relational patterns make a difference? *Global Environmental Change,* 19, 366–374.

Burns, T.E., Wade, J., Stephen, C. and Toews, L. (2013). A scoping analysis of peer-reviewed literature about linkages between aquaculture and determinants of human health. *EcoHealth*, 11(2), 227–240.

Coates, J., Swindale, A. and Bilinsky, P. (2007). *Household Food Insecurity Access Scale (HFIAS) for Measurement of Food Access: Indicator Guide (v.3)*. Washington, DC: Food and Nutrition Technical Assistance Project, Academy for Educational Development.

Conley, T. and Udry, C. (2001). Social learning through networks: the adoption of new agricultural technologies in Ghana. *American Journal of Agricultural Economics*, 83(3), 668–673.

Cook, J.T. and Frank, D.A. (2008). Food security, poverty, and human development in the United States. *Annals of the New York Academy of Sciences*, 1136, 193–209.

Cook, J.T., Frank, D.A., Berkowitz, C., Black, M.M., Casey, P.H., Cutts, D.B., Meyers, A.F., Zaldivar, N., Skalicky, A. and Levenson, S. (2004). Food insecurity is associated with adverse health outcomes among human infants and toddlers. *The Journal of Nutrition*, 134, 1432–1438.

Corea, A., Jayasinghe, J., Ekaratne, S., Johnstone, R. (1995). Environmental impact of prawn farming on Dutch Canal: the main water source for the prawn culture industry in Sri Lanka. *Ambio*, 24, 423–427.

Corea, A., Johnstone, R., Jayasinghe, J., Ekaratne, S., Jayawardene, K. (1998). Self-pollution: a major threat to the prawn farming industry in Sri Lanka. *Ambio*, 27(8), 662–668.

Dahdouh-Guebas, F., Zetterstrom, T., Ronnback, P., Troell, M., Wickramasinghe, A. and Koedam, N. (2002). Recent change in land-use in the Pambala-Chilaw Lagoon complex Sri Lanka. *Environment, Development and Sustainability*, 4, 185–200.

Drengstig, A. (2013). *Aquaculture in Sri Lanka: History, Current Status, and Future Potential*. Trondheim: AquaNor Exhibition.

Emirbayer, M. (1997). Manifesto for a relational sociology 1. *American Journal of Sociology*, 103, 281–317.

FAO (2001). *The State of Food and Agriculture*. Rome: Food and Agriculture Organization.

FAO (2009a). *Gender Equity in Agriculture and Rural Development*. Rome: Food and Agriculture Organization.

FAO (2009b). *Declaration of the 2009 World Summit on Food Security*. Rome: Food and Agriculture Organization.

FAO (2009c). *How to Feed the World in 2050*. Rome: Food and Agriculture Organization.

FAO (2012). *The State of World Fisheries and Aquaculture 2012*. Rome: Food and Agriculture Organization.

FAO (2014). *The State of World Fisheries and Aquaculture 2014*. Rome: Food and Agriculture Organization.

FAO, IFAD and WFP (2013). *The State of Food Insecurity in the World 2013: The Multiple Dimensions of Food Security*. Rome: Food and Agriculture Organization.

Felsing, M., Brugere, C., Kusakabe, K. and Kelkar, G. (2000). *Women for Aquaculture or Aquaculture for Women?* Geneva: INFOFISH International.

Galappaththi, E.K. (2013). *Community-Based Shrimp Aquaculture in Northwestern Sri Lanka*. Master of Natural Resources Management, University of Manitoba.

Godfray, H.C.J., Beddington, J.R., Crute, I.R., Haddad, L., Lawrence, D., Muir, J.F., Pretty, J., Robinson, S., Thomas, S.M. and Toulmin, C. (2010). Food security: the challenge of feeding 9 billion people. *Science*, 327, 812–818.

Gómez-Limón, J.A. and Sanchez-Fernandez, G. (2010). Empirical evaluation of agricultural sustainability using composite indicators. *Ecological Economics*, 69, 1062–1075.

Hadley, C. and Patil, C.L. (2006). Food insecurity in rural Tanzania is associated with maternal anxiety and depression. *American Journal of Human Biology*, 18, 359–368.

Harris, C. (2007). Towards Sustainable Development in Aquaculture, www.thefishsite.com/articles/372/towards-sustainable-development-in-aquaculture.

Hartwich, F. and Scheidegger, U. (2010). Fostering innovation networks: the missing piece in rural development. *Rural Development News*, 1, 70–75.

HLPE (2013). *Investing in Smallholder Agriculture for Food Security*. A report by the High Level Panel of Experts on Food Security and Nutrition of the Committee on World Food Security, Rome.

Hoang, L.A., Castella, J.-C. and Novosad, P. (2006). Social networks and information access: implications for agricultural extension in a rice farming community in northern Vietnam. *Agriculture and Human Values*, 23, 513–527.

Jyoti, D.F., Frongillo, E.A. and Jones, S.J. (2005). Food insecurity affects school children's academic performance, weight gain, and social skills. *The Journal of Nutrition*, 135, 2831–2839.

Kawarazuka, N. and Béné, C. (2010). Linking small-scale fisheries and aquaculture to household nutritional security: an overview. *Food Security*, 2, 343–357.

Landesman, L., Amandakoon, H.P. and Varley, J.W. (2009). *Sri Lanka Connecting Regional Economies*

(USAID/CORE): Assessment of Aquaculture and Inland Fisheries in Eastern Sri Lanka. Washington, DC: USAID.

Mayadunne, G. and Romeshun, K. (2013). Estimation of prevalence of food insecurity in Sri Lanka. *Sri Lankan Journal of Applied Statistics*, 14, 27–40.

Milbrath, L.W. (1989). *Envisioning a Sustainable Society: Learning Our Way Out*. Albany, NY: State University of New York Press.

Mostert, E., Pahl-Wostl, C., Rees, Y., Searle, B., Tàbara, D. and Tippett, J. (2007). Social learning in European river-basin management: barriers and fostering mechanisms from 10 river basins. *Ecology & Society*, 12(1), 19.

Munasinghe, M.N., Stephen, C., Abeynayake, P. and Abeygunawardena, I.S. (2010). Shrimp farming practices in the Puttallam District of Sri Lanka: implications for disease control, industry sustainability, and rural development. *Veterinary Medicine International*, 2010.

Munasinghe, M.N., Stephen, C., Robertson, C. and Abeynayake, P. (2012). Farm Level and Geographic Predictors of Antibiotic Use in Sri Lankan Shrimp Farms. *Journal of aquatic animal health*, 24, 22-29.

Muro, M. and Jeffrey, P. (2008). A critical review of the theory and application of social learning in participatory natural resource management processes. *Journal of Environmental Planning and Management*, 51, 325–344.

Pope, J., Annandale, D. and Morrison-Saunders, A. (2004). Conceptualising sustainability assessment. *Environmental Impact Assessment Review*, 24, 595–616.

Pretty, J. (2008). Agricultural sustainability: concepts, principles and evidence. *Philosophical Transactions of the Royal Society B: Biological Sciences*, 363, 447–465.

Primavera, J.H. (1997). Socio-economic impacts of shrimp culture. *Aquaculture Research*, 28, 815–827.

Rist, S., Chidambaranathan, M., Escobar, C., Wiesmann, U. and Zimmermann, A. (2007). Moving from sustainable management to sustainable governance of natural resources: the role of social learning processes in rural India, Bolivia and Mali. *Journal of Rural Studies*, 23, 23–37.

Scott, J. (2013). *Social Network Analysis*. Thousand Oaks, CA: SAFE Publications Inc.

Seligman, H.K., Bindman, A.B., Kanaya, A.M. and Kushel, M.B. (2007). Food insecurity is associated with diabetes mellitus: results from the National Health Examination and Nutrition Examination Survey (NHANES) 1999–2002. *Journal of General Internal Medicine*, 22, 1018–1023.

Senarath, U. and Visvanathan, C. (2001). Environmental issues in brackish water shrimp aquaculture in Sri Lanka. *Environmental Management*, 27, 335–348.

Siriwardena, P.P.G.S.N. (1999). *National Aquaculture Sector Overview – Sri Lanka*, www.fao.org/fishery/countrysector/naso_sri-lanka/en.

Sri Lanka Department of Census and Statistics (2001). *Population and Housing Characteristics*. Colombo: Government of Sri Lanka.

Sri Lanka Department of Census and Statistics (2012). *Census of Population and Housing*. Colombo: Government of Sri Lanka.

Stein, A.J. and Qaim, M. (2007). The human and economic cost of hidden hunger. *Food & Nutrition Bulletin*, 28, 125–134.

Thuo, M., Bell, A.A., Bravo-Ureta, B.E., Lachaud, M.A., Okello, D.K., Okoko, E.N., Kidula, N.L., Deom, C.M. and Puppala, N. (2013). Effects of social network factors on information acquisition and adoption of improved groundnut varieties: the case of Uganda and Kenya. *Agriculture and Human Values*, 31(3), 339–353.

Van Cauwenbergh, N., Biala, K., Bielders, C., Brouckaert, V., Franchois, L., Garcia Cidad, V., Hermy, M., Mathijs, E., Muys, B., Reijnders, J., Sauvenier, X., Valckx, J., Vanclooster, M., Van der Veken, B., Wauters, E. and Peeters, A. (2007). SAFE: a hierarchical framework for assessing the sustainability of agricultural systems. *Agriculture, Ecosystems & Environment*, 120, 229–242.

Wang, X. and Taniguchi, K. (2003). *Does Better Nutrition Enhance Economic Growth? The Economic Cost of Hunger*. Geneva: Food and Agriculture Organization.

Weerakoon, D. (2007). Towards sustainability of black tiger shrimp Penaeus monodon farming in Sri Lanka. *Aquaculture Asia*, 12, 3.

WFP, Ministry of Economic Development and Hector Kobbekaduwa Agrarian Research and Training Institute (2012). *Food Security in the Northern and Eastern Provinces of Sri Lanka*. Rome: World Food Programme.

Williams, M.J.C., Choo, P.S., Matics, K., Nandeesha, M.C., Shariff, M., Siason, I., Tech, E. and Wong, J.M.C. (eds.) (2002). *Global Symposium on Women in Fisheries*. In, Penang, Malaysia, http://pubs.iclarm.net/resource_centre/WF_328.pdf.

World Bank (2011). *Gender Equality and Development*. Washington, DC: World Bank.

World Bank and IFAD (2009). *Gender and Agriculture Sourcebook*. Washington, DC: World Bank.

World Commission on Environment and Development

(1987). *Our Common Future*. Oxford: Oxford University Press.

World Food Summit (1996). *Rome Declaration on World Food Security and World Food Summit Plan of Action*. Rome: World Food Summit.

Yamada, S., Gunatilake, R.P., Roytman, T.M., Gunatilake, S., Fernando, T. and Fernando, L. (2006). The Sri Lanka tsunami experience. *Disaster Management & Response*, 4, 38–48.

chapter 22

Waterborne disease and public health in Vietnam and Bangladesh

David C. Hall and Quynh Ba Le

Abstract

The impact of waterborne diseases such as cholera has been devastating in Bangladesh during periods of extreme flooding and colibacillosis is known to be a problem for communities in Vietnam, particularly where raw fish are consumed. The two case studies presented in this chapter examine waterborne disease on small-scale integrated (SSI) farms in two different situations. In Vietnam, SSI farms were found to have unacceptably high levels of *E. coli* in drinking water sources; associated factors included poultry on farm and perceived skills in livestock management. In Bangladesh, improving dairy production contributed to financial stability necessary for coping with cyclone and flood damage, but it also brought the opportunity to adjust management of livestock waste to reduce risk of waterborne contamination during flooding. In both cases, farmers expressed keen interest in further knowledge of the interactions of humans, animals and their environment and how a One Health approach could benefit their communities.

22.1 Introduction

Water has a profound influence on the health of animals, humans and their environment. It is essential for all forms of life and is often a critical element in improving the wellbeing of individuals and communities, whether through quality or access to supply. Access is often a constraint in low-income communities due to poor coverage, inadequate volume or excessive costs for filtration and purification. Undetected naturally occurring inorganic contaminants such as arsenic are known to occur in large areas of some countries, while microbiological contaminants may compromise the quality of water in any geographic region resulting in severe disease epidemics.

This chapter presents two case studies relating to mitigation of waterborne disease. The first examines specifically the level of coliforms in the drinking and household water on small-scale farms in Vietnam and the potential role that perceptions of health hazards can play in mitigation strategies. The second case study is a broader examination of the recurring threat of waterborne disease in Bangladesh during flooding with specific reference to an intervention strategy and the impact it had on agricultural productivity for communities.

22.2 Drinking water contamination on small-scale integrated (SSI) farms in Vietnam

Introduction

Vietnam's economic growth relies primarily on agricultural production and industrialization associated with rapid urban development. However, the majority of farmers who practice small-scale integrated (SSI) farming benefit the least from national social economic policies and economic growth (Morley, 2010). About ten million rural inhabitants still live without adequate sanitation in Vietnam and 9.3 million lack safe drinking water (VPMO, 2010). Although farmers consider water the most important agricultural input, more than 70 per cent of SSI farmers use contaminated water for drinking and on-farm purposes. While awareness of water supply and environmental sanitation is a limiting factor (MoC, 2000; MoC and MARD, 2000), a number of other risk factors for transmission of water-related zoonotic diseases are related to SSI farming including proximity of poultry flocks to water sources, increased density of ponds and streams, and temporal flooding (Gilbert et al., 2008; Pfeiffer et al., 2009).

Understanding the uses of water on-farm is particularly important to understanding attitudes to water quality as well as SSI farmers' perceptions of risk of microbial contamination (Dinh et al., 2004; Nguyen et al., 2008; Tran et al., 2010). The value of incorporating a One Health approach including attention to the role of perceptions will be discussed in this case study, which summarizes research investigating

how to influence current SSI farming management practices and improve drinking water quality on SSI farms. This case study will be useful for SSI farmers, health workers, veterinarians, researchers and policymakers in promoting a One Health approach to improving rural water quality and reduce risk factors for transmission of waterborne zoonotic diseases.

Integrated agriculture on small-scale farms in Vietnam

More than 80 per cent of Vietnamese farmers own some form of livestock and are dependent on agriculture for their livelihoods (Pica-Ciarmarra et al., 2011) and nearly 90 per cent raise poultry (Hall et al., 2006). Integrated aquaculture/agriculture farming in Vietnam, known as the VAC model, is a popular form of small-scale integrated farming in which farmers combine livestock, crop and fish production in an integrated manner using livestock waste as both a source of food for fish and a source of nutrients for soils (Vu et al., 2007). Unfortunately, livestock waste can also be a source of contamination of on-farm water on any farm if not managed appropriately. In some communities, consumption of raw fish from SSI farms is also known to cause illness including colibacillosis due to *E. coli* found in the water in which fish are raised (Chi et al., 2009).

In general, the level of awareness among SSI farmers of health risk factors associated with emerging infectious diseases (EIDs) is low (Keraita et al., 2010). For example, a common way to deal with sick animals is sell or eat them, potentially exposing consumers to EIDs. Lack of awareness as a risk factor can be compounded by limited access to veterinary and other health services in rural areas. This makes it more important for SSI farmers to understand the proper management of animal waste and the useful role it can play on SSI farms as a fertilizer or food for fish. In the past decade, improper management of livestock including poultry and their waste on SSI farms has been implicated in disease transmission including colibacillosis and avian influenza (MoH and MARD, 2011).

Integrated agriculture is an important part of the rural culture and livelihoods of Vietnam. Assessing sources, uses and quality of water in the context of SSI farming can help provide better under-standing of potential health risk factors that could bring about undesirable health consequences for farmers, animals and their environment.

Rural drinking water

This case study summarizes research conducted by Le and Hall (2015) on 600 SSI farms in North and South Vietnam (Thai Binh and An Giang provinces respectively) to investigate sources of water, frequencies of use, basic indicators of drinking water quality and perceptions of the risks of EIDs due to microbial contamination of water. The farms were selected based on low income of residents, small farm size (typically less than 1ha), presence of livestock and, in most cases, fish. SSI farmers in both provinces depended on multiple sources of water for drinking (see Table 22.1). Water from drilled wells and rivers/canals were used by most of the farmers in Thai Binh and An Giang respectively. A high proportion of the farmers in An Giang (73 per cent) reported that they rarely or almost never used dug wells and drilled well water as one of their sources of water for drinking. In Thai Binh,

Table 22.1 Mean and median frequency of use of on-farm water used for drinking in Thai Binh and An Giang Provinces, Vietnam

Province/water Sources	Mean and median frequency of use for drinking[a]			
	Obs	Mean[b]	Std. Dev.	Median
Thai Binh				
Rain	196	3.4*	1.3	4
Drilled well	231	3.2*	1.3	4
Bottled	169	2.4	1.1	2
Pipe	61	2.4	1.4	2
Dug well	40	1.6*	1.0	1
Pond	143	1.0*	0.2	1
River/canal	143	1.0*	0.2	1
An Giang				
River/canal	297	3.0*	1.3	4
Pipe	243	2.6	1.7	2
Bottled	280	2.5	1.2	3
Rain	277	2.4*	1.0	2
Pond	271	1.3*	0.6	1
Drilled well	219	1.0*	0.2	1
Dug well	217	1.0*	0.1	1

a. based on 300 farms in each province. 1 = Never, 2 = Rarely, 3 = Sometimes, 4 = Often, 5 = Very often
b. * indicating values are significantly different between two provinces at p<0.01

Table 22.2 Comparison of mean pH, turbidity and *E. coli* colony forming units (cfu) of on-farm water used for drinking in Thai Binh and An Giang Provinces, Vietnam

Variable Province	Rainwater	Pipe water	Well water[e]	Bottled water	River water (fl.)
pH[a]					
Thai Binh	6.4**	6.4**	6.5**	—	—
An Giang	7.9**	7.5**	16.8**	9.4	7.0
Turbidity (Nephelometric Turbidity Unit)[b]					
Thai Binh	0.8**	0.9*	3.6	—	—
An Giang	1.3**	2.0*	3.9	0.8	7.6
E. coli (cfu/100 ml)[c]					
Thai Binh	61.8**	19.5**	27.0**	—	—
An Giang	11.1**	7.1**	107.1**	8.0	12.8
Frequency of use[d]					
Thai Binh	3.4	2.4	2.4	2.4	1.0
An Giang	2.4	2.7	1.0	2.5	3.0

a. mean pH of all sources of water was not smaller than 6.5 nor significantly greater than 8.5 at p<0.1
b. mean turbidity of well and river water was significantly greater than 2 at p<0.01
c. mean E. coli in all sources of water was significantly greater than 0 at p<0.01
d. frequency of use of the source water for drinking using (1 = Never, 2 = Rarely, 3 = Sometimes, 4 = Often, to 5 = Very often)
e. both drilled and dug wells
** indicating values that are significantly different between two provinces at p<0.05
* indicating values that are significantly different between two provinces at P<0.01

48 per cent of farmers indicated that pond water or river/canal water was never or rarely used as a source of drinking water. Farmers in both provinces used combinations of different sources of water for domestic purposes. Among these sources of water for domestic purposes, drilled wells and rivers/canals were used frequently by 84 per cent of the farmers in Thai Binh and 97 per cent of the farmers in An Giang. In both provinces, farmers rarely or never used water from bottles, pipes, and dug wells for domestic purposes.

With reference to basic indicators of drinking water quality set by the World Health Organization (WHO) and the Vietnam Ministry of Health (i.e., pH, turbidity and level of *E. coli*), the quality of water on the participating farms was low. Bottled water, rainwater and pipe water had turbidity levels (see Table 22.2) that met the national standards level of turbidity for drinking water (i.e., maximum turbidity of 2 NTUs). However, well water and flocculated river water exceeded the maximum turbidity level for drinking water (3.7 and 7.6 NTUs respectively). Mean turbidity in rain and pipe water in An Giang farms was almost double that found in Thai Binh; however, mean levels of *E. coli* in An Giang in those same two water sources were much lower than that in Thai Binh. Conversely, mean *E. coli* levels in well water used for drinking in An Giang farms was about four times higher than that in Thai Binh farms. Another study of pipe water in rural areas of the Mekong Delta also found that *E. coli* was commonly detected in pipe water (Wilbers et al., 2014). The levels[1] of *E. coli* in rainwater, well water and river water used by the farmers in our study can clearly be classified/scored as unacceptably high risk.

On-farm water management

Farmers relied on various sources of water for drinking including pond/lake, river/stream/canal, rainwater collection, piped water, hand-dug wells, drilled wells and bottled water (MoC and MARD, 2000; MoH, 2009). The percentages of SSI farmers that had access to improved sources[2] of water for drinking were slightly greater than the Vietnam national average for rural areas (i.e., 95 per cent) published by World Bank. Although farmers used multiple sources of water for drinking, the frequencies of use were varied among sources of water. This variation needs to be considered when developing rural water interventions in the study areas. In Thai Binh, observations of farm settings and in-depth interviews showed that rainwater was considered a valuable high-quality source of water, and farmers used it most for drinking compared to other sources. In Thai Binh, the majority of farms reported using drilled well water for drinking compared to other sources. However, drilled well water was second to rainwater in terms of the frequency of use. Rural water interventions should prioritize rainwater and drilled well water as these sources were used frequently by most of Thai Binh farmers. They did not use dug wells very often, noting that it had become increasingly harder to dig water wells.

The other reason farmers did not favour dug wells was the low quality of water in dug wells; an unpleasant odour in the water of shallow dug wells was perceived as indicating low-quality water, possibly contaminated by livestock waste and pesticides. In An Giang, on the other hand, the most frequently used source for drinking was river/canal water. This reflects the more comprehensive network of river branches and canals in the Mekong River Delta in An Giang compared to that of the Red River Delta in Thai Binh (Nguyen, 2007). The number of SSI farmers in An Giang who had water from pipes for drinking was four times greater than in Thai

Binh. However, these SSI farmers rarely used water services due to the economic barriers (i.e., they were not able to pay to connect to piped water networks or monthly fees) as well as the availability of other sources of on-farm water for drinking. Wilbers et al. (2014) reported limited use of pipe water by rural household in the Mekong Delta due to similar reasons.

Dug wells and drilled wells were common in An Giang with more than two-thirds of farmers reporting access to and use of dug wells and drilled wells for drinking. However, the corresponding mean frequencies of use for drinking indicated rare use for both dug wells and drilled wells. Water interventions in An Giang may need to focus on solutions for using river/canal water for drinking in the short and medium term. More research is needed to explore how to improve accessibility and affordability of piped water supply networks for rural farmers.

Attributes of farmers linked to mitigation strategies

The Health Beliefs Model and the Theory of Planned Behaviour (Janz and Becker, 1984; Becker, 2012) suggest that perceptions of a personal threat together with belief in benefits and barriers of an action will predict the likelihood of their behaviours. In other words, it is reasonable to assume that people make decisions related to their health based on their belief that these decisions will somehow mitigate undesirable outcomes. Examination of the association between SSI farmers' perceptions of risk factors for transmission of water-related zoonotic diseases and their corresponding engagement in mitigating strategies should shed light on possible policy interventions directed at reducing the risk of waterborne disease.

With the use of questionnaires and one-on-one interviews, data were collected from the SSI farmers addressing personal demographics, farm descriptors, perceptions and attitudes relating to risk and mitigation, and preferences relating to drinking water storage and use. Drinking water samples submitted by the farmers were analysed for levels of *E. coli* in a high quality government laboratory. Using probit regression analysis, we investigated the relation between presence of *E. coli* in drinking water and demographics, perceptions and mitigation of waterborne disease (Table 22.3). In numerous model specifications, we consistently found several significant predictors of the presence of *E. coli* in drinking water including gender of decision-makers, whether or not chickens were continuously raised on the farm and stated perceptions of the farmer relating to effectiveness in managing livestock and in managing water sources and storage. It is interesting to note there were differences in positive or negative association of some variables depending on water source (e.g., presence of chickens had a negative association with *E. coli* presence in rainwater; farmers generally did not prevent chickens from accessing rainwater collection points whereas well water collection and storage was covered, preventing access by chickens). Farmers' perception of their ability to manage livestock seemed to be consistent with reduced likelihood of *E. coli* presence (farmers who were better able to manage livestock had lower levels of well water *E. coli*). Level of education, years of farming and income were frequently significant in most models, although not as consistently as the other variables described. Perceptions of susceptibility to avian influenza and various barriers to action (e.g., lack of animal health services in the community) were also significant predictors for many models.

The model illustrated in Table 22.3 had moderately good predictive value in terms of correctly classifying outcomes and has promise for identifying farm and farmer characteristics that one might want to address when developing supportive policy options for improving rural water quality. For example, targeting only farmers with the lowest levels of income or education would not be as effective as consideration for continuous presence of poultry on farm. We also found that the presence of other livestock were significant predictors of *E. coli*, but not fish, suggesting livestock raising has more to do with explaining contamination of *E. coli* in drinking water than does growing fish. We do not report here the differences between provinces that should be a further consideration for policy development.

While the quality of on-farm water for drinking was low (most of the water samples were contaminated with *E. coli* and failed to meet the quality standards for drinking and domestic water set by WHO and the government of Vietnam), testing of water for coliforms alone can be intermittent. In addition to making uncomplicated affordable presence/absence tests for *E. coli* in drinking water available for farmers and communes, it is equally important to build capacity for inspecting and improvement of household water sanitation, and on-farm water public health management. Farmers indicated willingness to pay for affordable tests but they also expressed strong interest in improving their knowledge of water management, as well as access to water filtration and purification equipment.[3]

22.3 Waterborne disease, flooding and small-scale farmers in Bangladesh

The second case study in this chapter describes the problem of waterborne disease in Bangladesh associated with annual flooding, and reports on specific findings from interventions in the Districts of Bogra, Jamalpur and Sirajganj. Bangladesh is one of the most densely populated countries as well as one of the poorest, with a population of 160 million (UNDP, 2015; World Bank, 2015). More than 75 per cent of

Table 22.3 Association of presence of *E. coli* in drinking water with demographics, perception and mitigation in Thai Binh and An Giang Provinces, Vietnam

Variable	RAINWATER				WELLWATER			
	Coef.	SD	z	P>|z|	Coef.	SD	z	P>|z|
Years farming	0.0439*	0.0248	1.7700	0.0760	–0.0231	0.0157	–1.4700	0.1430
Education (years)	0.0434	0.0733	0.5900	0.5540	0.0225	0.0531	0.4200	0.6720
Gender (dummy vars)								
– Male (hhld decisions)	0.2954	0.4584	0.6400	0.5190	–0.6649**	0.3186	–2.0900	0.0370
– Female (lvstck mgmt)	1.0007*	0.5617	1.7800	0.0750	–0.2363	0.3447	–0.6900	0.4930
Chickens raised (dummy)	0.9681**	0.4370	2.2200	0.0270	–0.9968*	0.5334	–1.8700	0.0620
Fish raised (n)	0.3256	0.4740	0.6900	0.4920	0.4286	0.6318	0.6800	0.4970
Susc to AI (domstc wtr)	–0.9139*	0.4877	–1.8700	0.0610	–0.4342	0.2725	–1.5900	0.1110
Susc to AI (pond wtr)	0.7412	0.5226	1.4200	0.1560	n/a			
Barriers: not knowing	1.0759**	0.4921	2.1900	0.0290	0.0833	0.2963	0.2800	0.7790
Barriers: peer pressure	–0.7924	0.5123	–1.5500	0.1220	n/a			
Livestock management	–1.3004**	0.5423	–2.4000	0.0160	–0.8941***	0.3617	–2.4700	0.0130
Water management	1.1422**	0.5793	1.9700	0.0490	0.8071**	0.3753	2.1500	0.0320
Mitigation: lost income	–0.7204	0.4536	–1.5900	0.1120	–0.3617	0.2898	–1.2500	0.2120
Mitigation: peers	–0.5092	0.4065	–1.2500	0.2100	0.9157*	0.5194	1.7600	0.0780
Mitigation: disease	0.6563	0.4405	1.4900	0.1360	–0.2656	0.3849	–0.6900	0.4900
On–farm income	–0.4451	0.5612	–0.7900	0.4280	0.1118	0.1368	0.8200	0.4140
Satisf w/ drinking wtr	1.1051	0.9457	1.1700	0.2430	–0.2568	0.5586	–0.4600	0.6460
(constant)	–2.6090	1.4312	–1.8200	0.0680	1.9459	1.0307	1.8900	0.0590

n = 121
LR chi2(17) = 40.88 Prob > chi2 = 0.0010
Log likelihood = –48.4151 Pseudo R2 = 0.2968
Correctly classified = 76.86%

n = 146
LR chi2(15) = 24.27 Prob > chi2 =0.0607
Log likelihood = –73.5927 Pseudo R2 = 0.1415
Correctly classified = 76.03%

Bangladeshis live in rural village areas where the poverty rate is greater than 63 per cent. As for Vietnam, livestock is relied on by the majority of poor rural Bangladeshis as a main source of income as well as nutrition and for soil nutrients. One of the most challenging factors to sustaining livelihoods, particularly in poor rural areas, is the annual flooding and destruction of homesteads that occurs from cyclones (Cash et al., 2013; Sarker et al., 2013) and natural runoff from melting snows in the Himalayas. During these annual events, rivers are overburdened and flood waters breach embankments, surround flatlands, engulf homes and wash away property including livestock. Char dwellers, individuals who live in villages built on small islands (i.e., chars) in rivers, often are most vulnerable to loss of homes and livelihoods during the annual flooding. Waterborne disease is a particular concern during and after flooding events because of the rapid widespread distribution in the water of faecal matter from humans and animals, resulting in cholera and other life-threatening gastroenteritic diseases. These events can be so widespread that up to two-thirds of the entire country can be submerged in water for weeks, as occurred in 1998.

Bangladesh has learned to prepare for and respond to such disasters, relying particularly on the role of community mobilization of prevention and response services as well as science-based policy support to predict areas most vulnerable and to effect rapid deployment of life-sustaining resources (government of Bangladesh, 2008; Chowdhury et al., 2013). This approach requires transdisciplinary cooperation among many fields of expertise including hydrologists, health professionals and community leaders, illustrating the value of a One Health approach to disaster management.

A number of non-governmental organizations and international development agencies have been working with chars areas to minimize the damage to communities caused by annual flooding, emphasizing prevention through homestead restructuring but also mitigation of the impact of consequences through preparedness and response coordination. A particularly successful joint project between the Governments of Bangladesh, the UK (UKaid), and Australia (AusAID) is the Chars Livelihoods Programme[4] (CLP). The CLP has benefitted more than 900,000 villagers through broad One Health-oriented projects and activities that address human and animal health, livestock development, market access and growth, gender equity, education and local community empowerment and participation in implementing solutions. A key element of the CLP programme has been redesign of homes in at least two ways: (1) homes were elevated above potential flood water level with the use of a plinth base, and (2) water hygiene at all times has improved by installing latrines in villages to manage human waste more appropriately.

Bangladesh Agricultural University (BAU) has also partnered with local NGOs in the Chars regions of Sariakandi Upazila of Bogra District, Islampur Upazila of Jamalpur District, and Belkuchi Upazila of Sirajganj District to address integrated agricultural systems with particular focus on fish, dairy, and vegetable farming (Hall et al., 2012). The study area includes more than one million people in roughly 175,000 households earning less than $400 per annum. With the assistance of local NGOs, interventions to mitigate the effects of flooding included many of the elements also addressed by CLP including access to basic healthcare, latrine installation and education. Beginning in November 2009, the BAU study identified a sample size of 1,500 villagers for the study reported here covering 300 households. Participants chose development options that included improved dairy cow management and other forms of improved integrated agriculture. Comparisons were made between productivity and economic impact in villages where both indigenous and crossbred dairy cattle were used.

Compared to indigenous cattle, the crossbred cattle were more productive, had healthier reproductive cycles and longer lactation lengths, and produced heavier calves. However, indigenous cattle are more difficult to access are somewhat more demanding in terms of management skills. For those reasons, the study also reported economic impact of interventions for indigenous dairy cattle (very brief results are reported in this chapter and in Table 22.4; further details can be found in peer-reviewed literature, PhD dissertations and NGO reports).

Table 22.4 Economic variables for Bangladeshi dairy cattle in livelihoods study

Variable	District		
	Bogra[1]	Jamalpur	Sirajganj
Number of dairy cattle	109	115	153
Cow purchase price (Taka)[2]	13,560.73 (1386.40)	13,800.13 (1414.38)	14,079.22 (1709.04)
Feed costs (Taka/cow)	4535.26[a] (1903.03)	3799.52[d] (2496.61)	5079.96[a,d] (5403.63)
Veterinary costs (Taka/cow)[3]	340.00 (297.97)	309.17 (304.20)	348.04 (341.89)
Milk revenue (Taka/cow)	6543.03[a] (4750.07)	7462.09[a] (6469.00)	6942.28[a] (7361.07)
Manure revenue (Taka/cow)	726.61[c] (371.61)	450.21[a,c] (348.60)	664.28[a] (591.29)
Dairy profit (Taka/cow)[4]	2319.52[a] (4982.62)	3581.78[a] (6388.75)	2076.24[a] (4974.55)
Milk revenue to feed costs ratio	1.76[a] (1.43)	2.83[a] (3.39)	1.60[a] (1.68)
Returns on investment[5,6]	1.06[b] (0.74)	0.92[c] (0.60)	1.07[b,c] (1.10)

1 Data are reported as means followed by standard deviation.
2 All financial figures are in Bangladesh Taka. One $US = 70.5 Bangladeshi Taka, 1 January 2011.
3 Veterinary costs include deworming, vaccines and cost of para-veterinary services.
4 Profit = [(milk revenue + manure revenue) – (purchase price + feed costs + veterinary costs)].
5 Returns on investment = [(value of milk revenue + manure revenue + cow value + calf value) – (purchase price + feed costs + veterinary costs)]/purchase price.
6 For ROI cow and calf values at the end of the study were included whether or not producers sold their cow or calf at the end of the lactation.
a, d: Significant difference of means within row ($p < 0.01$); b: Significant difference of means within row ($p < 0.1$) and c: Significant difference of means within row ($p < 0.05$).

Some significant differences existed in economic impact for indigenous dairy cattle owners between districts (e.g., milk revenue, feed costs). In all districts, the ratio of milk revenue to feed costs was positive, although the return-on-investment in Jamalpur was slightly below a minimally acceptable 1.0. Cash flow was reportedly a problem during dry seasons when local dairy market middlemen were much less willing to transport milk to processing centres. The latter is one indicator of the need for consideration of dairy market development in conjunction with interventions in dairy production and health. More recent work in the region has shown continued progress in expanding profitability and integration with mixed agricultural systems (Ahmed, 2015).

An important element of the project was helping dairy farmers understand the importance of proper manure management, cow udder hygiene, livestock housing and the role animals play in both human health and, when not properly managed, emerging infectious disease. One of the most significant changes with respect to waterborne disease has been movement of cattle out from small homes and into corralled or barn-shed areas. This has reduced human exposure to livestock waste and has allowed farmers to manage livestock waste as a resource more effectively, reducing the spread of microbiological hazards during times of flooding.

This study showed that modest interventions in dairy production as part of a larger livelihoods programme can contribute the financial and economic security needed in order to build coping strategies for surviving the devastating effects of cyclones and flooding in Bangladesh, including the health impact of poorly managed livestock waste. It also emphasizes the need for economic and social equity in communities facing the same challenges as millions of other Bangladeshis during severe flooding. This has been noted as an important component of coping strategies and community resilience (Pelling, 2003).

22.4 Conclusions

The complexity of small-scale integrated farming is easy to overlook. These two case studies illustrate some of the public health risks and challenges when working with systems in which multiple species and water are in a close proximity. They also serve as reminders of the importance of community participation when studying SSI farming and in developing solutions to environmental challenges, particularly where waterborne disease is a threat in poorly managed systems. The case study from Vietnam suggests understanding perceptions and attitudes to risk management is critical when formulating policy support for interventions. If farmers do not perceive E. coli originating from livestock and tracked from fish ponds into their drinking water as a credible threat to their families' health, then there will be weak adoption of suggested changes.

In both Vietnam and Bangladesh, study participants expressed keen interest in learning more about the source of waterborne hazards and how to manage the risks of waterborne disease effectively. In particular, participants requested better understanding of the relation between health of animals, humans and their environment, and how interventions could be part of their on farm mitigation strategies for reducing the risk of waterborne diseases.

The two case studies examined in this chapter vary substantially in the circumstances that led to need for intervention. Both cases, however, bear similarity in that they illustrate the significance of vulnerability when examining risk of waterborne disease due to the same hazard (E. coli in this case). Poverty, lack of access to markets, weak delivery of health services for humans and animals, and limited formal education can all worsen vulnerability of communities, worsening the impact of hazards. The benefit of a One Health approach in each case was recognition of the need to address the multiple elements of each complex problem.

Endnotes

1. While the presence of *E. coli* in drinking water does not conclusively indicate water is unsafe for drinking (presence of faecal coliforms would be more conclusive but also considerably more costly), presence of *E. coli* is recommended by WHO as an indicator organism for assessing microbial safety of drinking water (WHO and OECD, 2003).
2. 'Improved sources of water' refers to pipe water into dwelling, pipe water to yard/plot, public pipe or standpipe, tube well or borehole, protected dug well and rainwater.
3. An industrial partner worked with the participants during the study to ensure they were aware of affordable filtration and purification options.
4. Details of CLP activities can be found online at several sites including www.clp-bangladesh.org, www.gbs-bd.org/chars-livelihoods-programme-clp, www.facebook.com/CLPBangladesh *and* www.linkedin.com/company/chars-livelihoods-programme-clp-?trkInfo=tas%3Achars%2Cidx%3A1-1-1.

References

Ahmed, J.U. (2015). Unpublished PhD dissertation results and personal communication. Bangladesh Agricultural University, Department of Agribusiness and Marketing, Mymensingh, Bangladesh.

Becker, M.H. (2012). *The Health Belief Model and Personal Health Behavior*. Health Education Monographs.

Cash, R.A., Halder, S.R., Husain, M., Islam, M.S., Mallick, F.H., May, M.M., Rahman, M. and Rahman, M.A. (2013). Reducing the health effect of natural hazards in Bangladesh. *The Lancet*, 382, 2094–2103.

Chi, T.T.K., Murrell, K.D., Madsen, H., Khue, N.V. and Dalsgaard, A. (2009). Fishborne zoonotic trematodes in raw fish dishes served in restaurants in Nam Dinh Province and Hanoi, Vietnam. *Journal of Food Protection*, 11, 2236–2435.

Chowdhury, A.M.R., Bhuiya, A., Chowdhury, M.E., Rasheed, S., Hussain, Z. and Chen, L.C. (2013). The Bangladesh paradox: exceptional health achievement despite economic poverty. *The Lancet*, 382(9906), 1734–1745.

Dinh, N.P., Long, H.P., Tien, N.T.K., Hien, N.T. and Phong, L.H. (2004). Risk factors for human infection with avian influenza A H5N1, Vietnam. *Emerging Infectious Diseases*, 12, 1841–1847.

Gilbert, M., Xiao, X., Pfeiffer, D.U., Epprecht, M., Boles, S., Czarnecki, C. et al. (2008). Mapping H5N1 highly pathogenic avian influenza risk in Southeast Asia. *Proceedings of the National Academy of Sciences*, 105, 4769–4774.

Government of Bangladesh (2008). *National Plan for Disaster Management 2008–2015*. Dhaka: Disaster Management Bureau, Ministry of Food and Disaster Management.

Hall, D.C., Thao, T.D., Minh, D.V. and Lien, L.V. (2006). *Competitiveness of the Livestock Sector in Vietnam*. World Bank research document, WB-EASRD and FAO-TCIP.

Hall, D.C., Alam, M.G.S, and Raha, S.K. (2012). Improving dairy production in Bangladesh: Application of integrated agriculture and ecohealth concepts. *International Journal of Livestock Production*, 3(3), 29–35.

Janz, N.K. and Becker, M.H. (1984). The Health Belief Model: a decade later. *Health Education and Behavior*, 11, 1–47.

Keraita, B., Drechsel, P., Seidu, R., Amerasinghe, P., Cofie, O. and Konradsen, F. (2010). Harnessing farmers' knowledge and perceptions for health-risk reduction in wastewater-irrigated agriculture. In P. Drechsel, C.A. Scott, L. Raschid-Sally, M. Redwood and A. Bahri (eds.), *Wastewater Irrigation and Health: Assessing and Mitigating Risk in Low-Income Countries*. London: Earthscan, pp. 337–353.

Le, Q.B. and Hall, D.C. (2015). *Risky Practices and Water Related Disease Transmission on Vietnamese Small-Scale Integrated Farms*. Invited paper presented at the Society for Risk Analysis annual meeting, Washington, DC, 6–10 December.

MoC (2000). *Vietnam National Rural Clean Water Supply and Sanitation Strategy up to 2020*. Ministry of Agriculture and Rural Development. Hanoi: Ministry of Construction.

MoC and MARD (2000). *National Rural Clean Water Supply and Sanitation Strategy Up to the Year 2020*. Hanoi: Ministry of Construction and Ministry of Agriculture and Rural Development.

MoH (2009). National Technical Regulation on Domestic Water Quality (QCVN 02: 2009/BYT). Hanoi: Department of Preventive Medicine and Environment, Ministry of Health.

MoH and MARD (2011). *The Vietnam Integrated National Operational Program on Avian Influenza, Pandemic Preparedness and Emerging Infectious Diseases (APEID) 2010–2015: Strengthening Responses and Improving Prevention through a One Health Approach*. Hanoi: Vietnam Ministry of Agriculture and Rural Development and Ministry of Health.

Morley, C. (2010). *Bio-Security Stakeholder Analysis, Vietnam (Rep. No. OSRO/RAS/604/USA B6)*. Rome: Emergency Centre for Transboundary Animal Diseases, Food and Agriculture Organization of the United Nations.

Nguyen, H.N. (2007). *Flooding in Mekong River Delta, Vietnam*. Hanoi: UNDP.

Nguyen, T.V., Kitajima, M., Nguyen, M.H., Matsubara, K., Takizawa, S., Katayama, H., Oguma, K. and Ohgaki, S. (2008). Bacterial contamination of raw vegetables, vegetable-related water and river water in Ho Chi Minh City, Vietnam. *Water Science and Technology*. 58, 2403–2411.

Pelling, M. (2003). *The Vulnerability of Cities*. London: Earthscan.

Pfeiffer, J., Pantin, J.M., To, T.L., Nguyen, T. and Suarez, D.L. (2009). Phylogenetic and biological characterization of highly pathogenic H5N1 avian influenza viruses (Vietnam 2005) in chickens and ducks. *Virus Research*, 142, 108–120.

Pica-Ciarmarra, U., Tasciotti, L., Otte, J. and Zezza, A. (2011). *Livestock Assets, Livestock Income and Rural Households: Cross-Country Evidence from Household Surveys (Rep. No. ESA Working Paper No. 11-17)*. Rome: World Bank, FAO, AU-IBAR, ILRI.

Sarker, M.H., Huque, I., and Alam, M. (2013). Rivers, chars, and char dwellers of Bangladesh. *International Journal of River Basin Management*, 1, 61–80.

Tran, H.P., Adams, J., Jeffery, J.A.L., Nguyen, Y.T., Vu, N.S. and Kutcher, S.C. (2010). Householder perspectives and preferences on water storage and use, with reference to dengue, in the Mekong Delta, southern Vietnam. *International Health*, 2, 136–142.

UNDP (2015) http://data.un.org/CountryProfile.aspx?crName=Bangladesh.

VPMO (2010). *Organisation of the National Poverty Survey to Prepare for the Implementation of the Social Security Program and Policy in the Period of 2011–2015*. Report No. 1752/ CT-TTg). Vice-Prime Minister's Office (VPMO), government of Vietnam.

Vu, T.K.V., Tran, M.T. and Dang, T.T.S. (2007). A survey of manure management on pig farms in Northern Vietnam. *Livestock Science*, 112, 288–297.

WHO and OECD (2003). *Assessing Microbial Safety of Drinking Water: Improving Approaches and Methods.* London: IWA Publishing.

Wilbers, G.J., Sebesvari, Z. and Renaud, F.G. (2014). Piped-water supplies in rural areas of the Mekong Delta, Vietnam: water quality and household perceptions. *Water*, 6, 2175–2194.

World Bank (2015). *Bangladesh's Chars Livelihoods Programme (CLP)*, http://data.worldbank.org/country/bangladesh.

chapter 23

One Health and community-based human and animal healthcare: a case study from Afghanistan

John Woodford, Joanna McKenzie, Peter Jolly and Ron Jackson

Abstract

In Afghanistan, the European Union (EU) and World Bank have supported the Directorate of Animal Health, Ministry of Agriculture, Irrigation and Livestock (MAIL) through the Animal Health Development Programme (AHDP) and the National Horticulture and Livestock project (NHLP) to develop and expand an animal disease surveillance system that engages private-sector, community-based veterinary practitioners to detect, report and investigate suspected occurrences of notifiable animal diseases on behalf of the state veterinary service. Concurrently, the United States Agency for International Development (USAid) has been funding a similar approach towards creating a disease early warning system (DEWS) in the human health sector through the network of non-government primary health organizations that are distributed throughout Afghanistan. In this chapter we examine the history of the One Health concept and describe a case study in Afghanistan in which the application of this concept has been highly successful.

23.1 Background: transition of 'One Medicine' to 'One Health' approaches in human and veterinary public health

The concept of 'One Medicine' is not new. As long ago as 200 BCE, the earliest surviving texts suggest that the Greek and Egyptian priest-healers of that period gained much of their knowledge of treating both humans and animals as a result of their involvement in making animal

sacrifices, learning anatomy from the dissection of the animal carcasses this involved (Schwabe, 1978). Between the second and fifth centuries CE, several of the works that comprise the Hippocratic corpus suggest that animal dissections were often used as a means of developing treatments for human medical conditions. What is perhaps more surprising is that around the fourth century CE, some of the Egyptian-Greek physicians were the first to become specialized in either human or animal medicine, thus creating the beginnings of professional elitism that is the bane of the One Health philosophy in modern times. These early medical practitioners (*iatros*), many of whose clients came from the wealthy upper class, chose to distance themselves from veterinary practitioners (*hippiatros*), fearing that their clients might consider it degrading to be treated by a physician who also treated horses. Some of these physicians, however, also specialized in treating horses as they became valuable status symbols amongst the same wealthy upper classes (Schwabe, 1978).

Although Calvin Schwabe has been widely credited with coining the phrase 'One Medicine' in his book *Veterinary Medicine and Human Health* (Kaplan and Scott, 2011), a search of the literature by Cassidy (forthcoming) finds earlier references to its use (e.g., Schmidt, 1962; Allam, 1966; Cass, 1973). Schwabe used the term to describe the collaborative relationships between the medical and veterinary professions that began to emerge after the end of the Second World War, when the US Public Health Service (USPHS) and the World Health Organization (WHO) began to recruit veterinary practitioners to work alongside medical doctors in order to create a new professional cadre with a broad base of expertise going beyond the traditional boundaries of food safety and zoonotic disease control to include: veterinary and medical education, biomedical research and environmental protection (Schwabe, 1991). Those early interdisciplinary collaborative initiatives between the veterinary and medical professions resulted in a clearer understanding of the complex interrelationships between man, domestic pets, livestock, wildlife and the environment, the growth of 'veterinary public health' as a distinct discipline and led to the beginnings of the science of analytical epidemiology as we know it today.

Perhaps one of the most significant milestones in the history of 'One Medicine' was the discovery that infection of milkmaids with the cowpox virus conferred protection against small-

pox, made by a humble Dorset (England) farmer, Benjamin Jesty, in 1774. However, it was Edward Jenner who, 22 years later, became world famous for his work in developing and field-testing the first vaccine against smallpox using the cowpox virus, replacing the common, but less safe, practice of variolation, which had been discovered two centuries earlier in China (Needham, 1999, p. 134). Jenner has been credited with saving more human lives than any other single person in the modern history of human medicine, and the term 'vaccination', derived from the name of the cowpox virus (*Vaccinia*), came into common medical usage. The true importance of these events from the perspective of the title of this chapter is that this is an excellent early example of how giving credence to a community-based observation made such an important contribution to the prevention and cure of human and animal diseases.

The 'One Medicine' concept has gradually evolved from those institutional settings involving the veterinary and medical professions in Europe and America during the post-war period, into a global 'One Health' multidisciplinary movement with seemingly endless boundaries. The trigger for the 'One Health' movement in recent years undoubtedly has its origins in the 1997 outbreak of highly pathogenic avian influenza (HPAI) caused by the H5N1 avian influenza virus, amid fears that this virus would mutate into a virus capable of spreading from human to human and resulting in a human influenza pandemic similar in scale to the catastrophic Spanish flu pandemic at the end of the First World War, when between 50 and 100 million people died (Taubenberger and Morens, 2006). The HPAI epidemic that spread rapidly from Southeast Asia to Africa, Asia and Europe through a combination of trade and migratory birds followed closely on the heels of a series of other dramatic zoonotic (and other) disease outbreaks including the West Nile virus outbreak starting in New York in 1990, the UK foot and mouth disease outbreak of 2001, the severe acute respiratory syndrome (SARS) outbreak in 2003, monkey pox in the US in 2003 and BSE in the US in 2003, each of which attracted a frenzy of media attention and the recognition that emerging diseases in animals can cross intercontinental boundaries very rapidly and have far-reaching human health consequences as well as serious socioeconomic impacts. The combination of these events led to unprecedented political support and a call for much closer international collaboration for disease surveillance and control. Thus in January 2006, at the International Ministerial and Pledging Conference in Beijing, co-hosted and jointly organized by the Chinese government, the EU and the World Bank, a Global Response to Avian Influenza (GRAI) trust fund was launched with the immediate pledge of more than $US2 billion (Gibbs, 2005, 2014; Okello et al., 2011).

From 2006 onwards, the same consortium of donors and governments funded a series of further international ministerial conferences, attended by political leaders as well as human and animal disease control experts, and in 2010 the World Bank published a framework for the control of animal influenzas through the application of the One Health approach. The bank estimated that between 2005 and 2009 a total of US$4.3 billion was pledged for the international control of HPAI, a testament to the value of this approach (World Bank, 2010). During this same period, the major global agencies with an interest in human and animal health, in particular the WHO, the Food and Agriculture Organization of the United Nations (FAO), the World Organisation for Animal Health (OIE), UNICEF and the World Bank developed a framework for reducing the risks of infectious diseases at the human–animal–ecosystems interface (FAO, 2008). Although this framework focused more on emerging zoonotic diseases, it also recognized that the same approach would be appropriate to combat endemic 'neglected zoonoses' in developing countries. The report emphasized, however, that although the control of such diseases is in everyone's best interest, it would require long-term public and private investment (Gibbs, 2014). There are many examples where such an approach has worked in industrialized countries. For instance, while the US federal government funded research and other public activities, it was the owners of horses who paid for clinical treatment and vaccination of their animals against West Nile virus following the 1991 outbreak. Similarly in the UK, while both BSE and TB control programmes have been largely financed out of public funds, farmers have indirectly funded some of the costs (Okello et al., 2011).

Yet, although it would seem unrealistic to expect that this form of public–private partnership would work in developing countries, there are many examples of successful projects where livestock keepers have contributed to the cost of controlling zoonotic diseases for the sake of protecting human health (Okello et al., 2011). Novel public–private partnership approaches are now beginning to attract donor support. For example, in Uganda, the UK Department for International Development (DfID) is piloting a project that uses the sale of 'social impact bonds' to private investors to finance the initial costs of starting a tsetse fly/sleeping sickness control programme. Investors are repaid once defined outcomes are achieved (DfID, 2014). In Afghanistan, the EU and World Bank have supported the Directorate of Animal Health, Ministry of Agriculture, Irrigation and Livestock (MAIL) through the Animal Health Development Programme (AHDP) and the National Horticulture and Livestock Project (NHLP) to develop and expand an animal disease surveillance system that engages private-sector, community-based veterinary practitioners to detect, report and investigate suspected occurrences of notifiable animal diseases on behalf of the state veterinary service. Concurrently, the United States Agency for International Development (USAid) has been funding a similar approach towards creating a disease early warning system (DEWS) in the human health sector through the network of non-government primary health organizations that are distributed throughout Afghanistan.

The One Health programme for the surveillance, prevention and control of HPAI has been successful in establishing permanent inter-sectoral institutions coordinating the combined activities of human and animal health practitioners, especially in those countries where HPAI persisted or became endemic that have required longer-term support. However, in many other countries where the disease was brought under control relatively quickly, the funding has been reduced to the extent that these same institutions have no longer been seen to have any further relevance and in some cases have become dormant.

In South Asia, however, the One Health approach was revitalized in some countries in 2010 through the award of a grant from the European Commission Animal and Human Influenza Trust Fund, administered by the World Bank, to Massey University in New Zealand, to establish a 'Regional Training in Animal and Human Health Epidemiology in South Asia' programme. The project has created a 'One Health Network – South Asia', which is underpinned by a web-based communication and collaboration facility called Hubnet (www.hubnet.org.nz). The project has assisted in the conduct of a series of collaborative investigation projects (CIPs) in participating countries (Afghanistan, Bangladesh, Bhutan, India, Nepal, Pakistan and Sri Lanka), all of which have strengthened understanding and application of the One Health philosophy in these countries. A case study of the CIP that was undertaken in Afghanistan is used below to illustrate the very positive impact that the One Health approach has had in strengthening the linkages between the Ministry of Public Health (MoPH) and the MAIL at central, provincial, district and community levels, which in the future is hoped will help to combat several neglected zoonotic diseases.

23.2 Community-based human and animal healthcare systems and One Health initiatives for surveillance, prevention and control of zoonotic diseases in Afghanistan

Livestock play important roles in the livelihoods of almost 85 per cent of the rural population of Afghanistan, where farming systems can broadly be divided into two main categories. The majority of farmers are sedentary and practice a small-scale, largely subsistence level of mixed crop and livestock production. Within this production system, livestock generally plays a secondary role, providing the household with small quantities of eggs, milk and occasionally meat, but important by-products such as draught power for ploughing and transport, and dung that is used both as a fertilizer and as a fuel for cooking and heating during the long winters. At the other extreme, are pastoralists, who represent approximately 5–6 per cent of all livestock keepers but own close to 50 per cent of the small ruminants comprising the national flock. Pastoralism, or transhumance in Afghanistan, involves annual migration between the very extensive mountain pasture rangelands, which are grazed during the summer months, and the lower valleys during the winter. Due to a combination of rapid population increases and decades of internal conflict, resulting in changes in local power structures, the grazing patterns of many pastoralist groups are seriously threatened as former traditional lowland winter grazing lands have come under the plough and centuries-old grazing rights are often now being violated. Nevertheless, more than 70 per cent of the meat sold in the major city markets throughout Afghanistan is derived from the pastoralist production system. Both sedentary and pastoralist livestock production systems are low input and low output, making it challenging to establish an accessible and sustainable animal healthcare system, especially to the more remote rural communities. Similarly, it has been equally challenging for the state to provide even the most basic primary healthcare service in a country that has been ravaged by internal conflict for more than 50 years.

By the end of the Russian occupation of Afghanistan (1979–1989), government medical, veterinary and other agriculture services had all but collapsed as more than five million people, including most of the trained professionals, escaped the conflict, fleeing to the refugee camps in Iran and Pakistan or going into exile in Europe and America.

Since 1989, a continuous, long-term programme of donor investment using non-governmental organizations (NGOs) as their implementation partners, has helped to rebuild both public and private sector institutions involved in human and animal healthcare and agriculture. Much of this investment has resulted in services at the community and district levels being operated by private sector para-professionals due to the lack of suitable government infrastructures and very poor public sector staffing levels. Today, in the human health sector there are now 43 regional and provincial hospitals, of which 35 are operated by the MoPH, 62 district hospitals and more than 2,200 comprehensive and basic health centres, approximately 95 per cent of which are operated by private doctors and paramedics supervised and supported by more than 35 different NGOs.

Although the state veterinary service has established six well-staffed regional offices in the provincial capitals of Kandahar, Jalalabad, Ghazni, Kunduz, Mazar-e-Sharif and Herat, many of the remaining 28 provincial veterinary offices do not yet have a complete professional cadre of staff and cannot therefore effectively carry out many of the core functions of a state

veterinary service. However, there are currently estimated to be in the region of 1,200–1,500 veterinary field units (VFUs), which have been established at the district and village levels. VFU distribution more or less corresponds to human and animal population densities, but is heavily influenced by security, leaving the southern half of Afghanistan less well covered. Almost all of the VFUs are operated by a veterinary para-professional, 'paravet', with a minimum of six months' formal training, supported by approximately 15 different NGOs. In order to rationalize the delivery of largely private good animal health services, the government privatized 167 district level clinics in 2011/2012. These clinics now function as VFUs and although a very few are operated by a qualified veterinarian, most are managed by either health technicians (with a two-year diploma qualification) or paravets. Both the MAIL and the MoPH are developing disease surveillance systems through creating a public–private partnership with these privately operating community-based clinics and it is hoped that the One Health approach described below will lead to closer collaboration between the two disciplines.

23.3 Overview of human and animal disease surveillance systems and zoonotic disease prevalence in Afghanistan

There is a paucity of accurate data on the prevalence of both human and animal disease in Afghanistan. What little data that did exist up to the late 1970s, apart from that published in international journals, was mostly destroyed during the Taliban regime period of rule from 1998 to 2001. From that time onwards, both human and animal disease reporting has been very sporadic. Only recently are we beginning to see the picture change, as disease surveillance systems are becoming re-established. In the case of the human health sector, the disease early warning system (DEWS) was started in 2006 through funding provided mostly by the USAid and technical support provided by the WHO. The DEWS network is based upon establishing 'sentinel sites', which are either public or private health centres and include regional or provincial hospitals, district hospitals, and comprehensive and basic health centres at the community level. By 2013, the Afghanistan National Public Health Institute (ANPHI) had established 368 sentinel sites covering all 34 provinces and 88 per cent of districts in Afghanistan. Seventy per cent of the sentinel sites are either comprehensive or basic health centres, almost all of which are managed by paramedics with limited clinical diagnostic skills and almost no nearby access to diagnostic laboratory support. The selection of the sites is based on the geographic location, the estimated prevalence of communicable diseases in the area, availability of communication systems (internet/mobile phones) and population density (MoPH, 2013). For the time being, disease reporting is based upon a prioritised list (Table 23.1) of 15 clinical syndromes or specific disease entities each of which has been given a case definition based on clinical observation of signs and a description of symptoms reported by patients (DEWS Annual Report 2013, MoPH). The selection of these syndromes and disease entities

aims to not only provide the government with an early warning system to detect outbreaks of potential epidemic diseases, it is also designed to provide disease information which can be used to plan disease prevention and control interventions based on risk analysis. Traditional healers in both the human and animal health sector are known to be widespread but their numbers are not known and little is known about their relevance. However, it should be mentioned that almost 70 per cent of the rural population of Afghanistan is illiterate and not well informed of the benefits of modern medicine.

In the animal health sector, the establishment of a national animal disease surveillance network supported by central, regional and provincial veterinary diagnostic laboratory services has been given high priority through the EU-funded Animal Health Development Programme, which began in May 2006 (www.ahdp.net). The project has taken advantage of the existence of the VFU network, which was already well established. By the end of 2014, 168 VFUs were engaged under a 'sanitary mandate contracting (SMC) scheme', whereby private veterinarians, veterinary technicians and paravets are contracted to perform disease surveillance, reporting and outbreak investigations, and vaccination services (Hussain et al., 2011; AHDP, 2013). An additional 72 VFUs are planned to be added to the

Table 23.1 Prioritized list of diseases and clinical syndromes – DEWS.

S/N	Disease	S/N	Disease
1	Cough and cold	9	Pertussis
2	Pneumonia	10	Diphtheria
3	Acute watery diarrhoea (AWD)	11	Tetanus/neonatal tetanus
4	Acute bloody diarrhoea	12	Acute flaccid paralysis
5	AWD with dehydration	13	Malaria
6	Meningitis/severely ill child	14	Typhoid fever
7	Acute viral hepatitis	15	Haemorrhagic fever
8	Measles		

SMC scheme in 2015. The SMC scheme provides a useful contribution to the monthly earnings of the private service providers whose income from routine clinical service delivery is precarious. Thus the system helps to support the delivery of a much-needed animal health service and provides the government veterinary services with an early warning system to detect outbreaks of animal disease epidemics and useful animal disease information, which, as with the DEWS, can be used to plan animal disease prevention and control programmes based on risk analysis. The cost savings to government in terms of avoiding having to pay salaries to a district or village-based cadre of veterinary officers or animal health technicians to obtain animal disease information and provide vaccination services, which are only required on an ad hoc basis, are likely to be considerable.

The privatization programme mentioned above has reduced the cost of salaries for state-employed animal health service providers by an estimated $350,000/annum. Further research is needed to quantify both the costs and benefits of some of these innovative approaches towards disease surveillance, prevention and control in order to provide evidence for policymakers who, in many developing countries, remain unconvinced about the value of such private–public partnerships. A recent three-year longitudinal study comparing outcomes derived from the provision of animal health services by paravets compared with households that did not use paravets, conducted in three districts of Herat Province by the Dutch Committee for Afghanistan (DCA), has demonstrated a reduction in mortality of adult sheep and goats and lambs and kids of approximately 25 per cent and 26 per cent respectively and an increase in offtake of lambs and kids of 22 per cent (R. Briscoe and C. Bartels, pers. comm., 2015).

23.4 Case study: A survey of the sero-prevalence of brucellosis, Q fever and Crimean Congo haemorrhagic fever in humans and livestock in Herat Province, Afghanistan

Brucellosis is known to have been widespread in Afghanistan for many years, as is the case in all of its immediate neighbours. Only recently, however, has the disease attracted the attention of either the medical or veterinary professions, mostly due to a significant improvement in both human and animal disease surveillance and diagnostic capabilities but also because of the growth and institutionalization of the One Health programme.

Between August 2007 and June 2008 a total of 58 suspected human cases of brucellosis were detected in Bamyan Province through the DEWS reporting system. From these suspected cases, 19 samples were submitted for laboratory confirmation and 15 were found to be serologically positive. As a result of these findings, the Afghanistan National Public Health Institute (ANPHI), with technical support provided by the WHO and the FAO, launched a survey to investigate the outbreak more fully. A team including an epidemiologist, a medical doctor and a veterinarian were deployed to the area to determine the prevalence of antibodies to brucellosis and *Coxiella burnetii* in humans and animals and to investigate risk factors associated with brucellosis and *C. burnetii* infection. Blood samples were collected from 39 human patients selected from a list of 1,317 people who were suspected of being infected with brucellosis on the basis of a case definition from Punjab District Hospital. Of these 39 human samples, 23 (59 per cent) tested positive for brucellosis using the Rose Bengal Test (RBT). A further 16 samples were collected from the neighbouring district of Yakawlang, and 100 per cent of these were reported to be positive. From the same batch of 39 samples collected in Punjab District,

28 were tested by FAO at the Central Veterinary Diagnostic and Research Laboratory (CVDRL) and of these, 100 per cent were reported to be positive for brucellosis, and 96.4 per cent were reported as being positive for antibodies to *C. burnetii* using a PCR test (Saeed et al., 2013).

In Herat Province, between 2007 and 2012, a total of 39 confirmed human cases of Crimean-Congo haemorrhagic fever (CCHF) were recorded by the ANPHI. A serological survey conducted in Herat in 2008 revealed an overall sero-prevalence of antibodies to CCHF of 11.2 per cent in householders (sandwich/indirect ELISA VECTOR-BEST diagnostic kit (VECTOR-BEST, Novosibirsk, Russia)), 79.1 per cent in cattle and 75 per cent in sheep (in-house ELISA using the IbAr 10200 strain of CCHF as antigen) and anti-species IgG horseradish peroxidase–conjugated (Mustafa et al., 2011).

As a follow-up to all of these earlier studies, a CIP was developed jointly by MAIL and the MoPH with the assistance of the Massey University Institute of Veterinary, Animal and Biomedical Sciences under funding provided through the Regional Training in Animal and Human Health Epidemiology in South Asia programme referred to earlier in this chapter. The project was designed to examine the sero-prevalence of brucellosis, CCHF and Q fever in humans and livestock (adult female cattle, sheep and goats of breeding age), and to investigate risk factors associated with infection with these diseases in randomly selected villages in Herat Province. The study was conducted at the level of 204 randomly selected households from a total of 11 villages, six of which were pre-dominantly occupied by 'kuchi' (transhumant or semi-nomadic pastoralists) and five consisting of mainly sedentary households. Demographic and behavioural information was collected using a comprehensive questionnaire based on a knowledge, attitudes and practice (KAP) framework. The field study was conducted during the period 26 December 2012 to 17 January 2013.

The CIP was successfully implemented by an effective public–private partnership led by the ANPHI and MAIL working together with local Directorates of Agriculture, Irrigation, and Livestock (DAIL) and DEWS staff and Health Protection Research Organization (HPRO), a NGO supporting human health and the Dutch Committee for Afghanistan (DCA), a NGO supporting animal health. A key to success of this partnership was that all participants had a clear understanding of their role and the role of the other parties. This was achieved through a series of One Health workshops and meetings held at the central level in Kabul and then at the local level in Herat and in the districts where the study was to be conducted. At each of these workshops and meetings representatives from the MoPH and MAIL, as well as other key stakeholders with an interest in the prevention and control of zoonotic diseases were invited to participate. Prior to undertaking the fieldwork, training seminars were held at which private paravets and paramedics, selected as enumerators from the two local NGOs working in the field in Herat Province, DCA and HPRO, were trained in survey techniques. During the weeks before the launch of the field study, preparatory meetings were conducted with community elders and heads of households in the selected study villages by 'motivation teams' comprising the enumerators and their human and animal health supervisors, in order to explain the purpose of the study and what it would entail and to ensure their full cooperation.

A total of 1,143 blood samples was collected from sheep, 876 from goats, 344 from cattle and 1,017 from humans, and sera were separated at the provincial (regional) veterinary diagnostic laboratory in Herat. Only households with animals were selected for testing so the target population was 'households with animals'. The sample size of 200 animals per village was based on an expected prevalence of 4.5 per cent for brucellosis and an assumption that the epidemiology of brucellosis and Q fever (*Coxiella burnetii* infection) would be similar in sheep and goats.

Animal sera were screened for Brucella antibodies using the Rose Bengal Test (RBT – AHVLA Scientific) at the CVDRL Kabul. RBT positive samples were then tested using the AHVLA Scientific competition ELISA (c-ELISA) and the test results were interpreted in series. Difficulties were experienced at the Central Public Health Laboratory (CPHL) in Kabul, when a set of 300 human sera were initially tested using the RBT and all found to be negative. For that reason, it was decided to dispense with the RBT in the case of human sample testing and only use the c-ELISA. All sera from humans and animals were tested at the CVDRL for antibodies to Q fever using an indirect ELISA (LSI™ – LSIVET) for animal sera and a two phase ELISA (IBL international) for human sera. During the process of laboratory testing, technicians from the CPHL were given hands-on training in the ELISA techniques and interpretation of test results at the CVDRL.

The overall prevalence of antibodies to brucellosis in animals was 1.4 per cent (95 per cent, CI 0.7, 2.7) in sheep, 1.5 per cent (95 per cent, CI 0.7, 3.0) in goats and 0.3 per cent (95 per cent, CI 0.0, 3.2) for cattle, giving an overall sero-prevalence of 1.3 per cent (95 per cent, CI 0.7, 2.2) in all species. Brucella sero-positives were found in 25 (12.3 per cent) of the 204 households and ten out of 11 of the selected villages. These levels of sero-prevalence for brucellosis are lower than the national average which has since been determined by a national survey involving the collection and testing of 14,432 samples from cattle, sheep and goats in all 34 provinces of Afghanistan where the sero-prevalences for antibodies to brucellosis recorded were: 3.5 per cent (95 per cent, CI 3.1, 3.9) for sheep, 2.3 per cent (95 per cent, CI 2.3, 2.8) for goats and 2.6 per cent (95 per cent, CI 1.3, 3.0) for cattle (MAIL, Central Epidemiology Department, A. Hussain. and A.S. Maken Ali, pers. comm., 2015).

The overall sero-prevalence of brucellosis in humans in the 11 study villages was 5.21 per cent (95 per cent, CI = 1.8 – 14.3), and sero-positives were found in ten of the 11 villages selected for the study. Humans with evidence of previous exposure to brucellosis were found in 32 (15.7 per cent) of the 204 households and were strongly clustered in three (one sedentary and two *kuchi*) villages.

The results of sero-prevalence to *C. burnetii* were very surprising. In the case of animals, the sero-prevalence was 43.4 per cent (95 per cent, CI 34.7, 52.5) in sheep, 52.7 per cent (95 per cent, CI 43.8, 61.5) for goats and 5.2 per cent (95 per cent, CI 3.1, 8.6) for cattle, giving an overall prevalence of 41.3 per cent (95 per cent, CI 33.4, 49.6). For humans, the overall prevalence of antibodies to *C. burnetii* was 63.9 per cent (95 per cent, CI 57.0, 70.3) and sero-positives were found in 199 (97.5 per cent) of the 204 households surveyed and in all 11 villages. Of the 53 people found sero-positive for brucellosis, 47 were also positive for antibodies to *C. burnetii*. What was of particular interest was the high sero-prevalence (52.9 per cent (95 per cent, CI= 38.2, 67.1)) of antibodies to *C. burnetii* in the lowest age group, all 26 of whom were nine-year-olds. Unfortunately, partly due to a shortage of funds but also the lack of a validated serological test for CCHF in animals, no human or animal sera have as yet been tested for the presence of antibodies to CCHF.

Multivariate logistic regression analysis of this data to determine possible causality relationships between sero-positives and a number of putative risk factors related to demographics, health history, occupations and behavioural characteristics indicates a significantly higher sero-prevalence for brucellosis in all ruminant species in *kuchi* as opposed to sedentary villages (OR 2.6, 95 per cent, CI 1.1, 6.2). The high prevalence of antibodies to *C. burnetii* in children would suggest that risk factors for transmission of *C. burnetii* infection from animals to humans are not necessarily as closely related to high-risk occupational activities, which is certainly the case with brucellosis, since young children would be less likely to be involved in these types of activity than adult members of households. The high prevalence of antibodies to *C. burnetii* seen in children in this study is almost certainly due to the heavy contamination of the farm and household environment with a spore-like form of the organism, which survives readily under adverse climatic conditions (McCaughey, 2014). The KAP survey data found that almost all household members were engaged in several high risk activities, including slaughtering/butchering (19.8 per cent), assisting difficult births (42.3 per cent), shearing (58.2 per cent), removing ticks (61.1 per cent) and using unboiled milk (32.6 per cent). Aside from brucellosis and *C. burnetii* infection, the high prevalence of households (62 per cent) feeding raw offal to dogs would undoubtedly present a high risk for echinococcosis infection. The results from this analysis will be useful for developing appropriate extension and public awareness training materials (Akbarian et al., forthcoming).

This study has reinvigorated the One Health concept in Afghanistan and has helped to build a closer working relationship between the animal and human health sectors, especially at the provincial government level in Herat Province. A number of important One Health concepts are now being put into practice. To quote the principal investigator for the human health sector of this CIP: 'As a direct consequence of this CIP, a strong Zoonotic Disease Control Committee at the provincial level has been formed and strengthened by the CIP. The ZDCC is now considered as the official platform for implementation of One Health activities at the community level' (Z. Akbarian, pers. comm., 2014). The One Health activities will now include:

- Joint training programmes for community-level human and animal health workers in the use of standard operating procedures for safe sample collection, handling and transportation and the use of personal protective equipment (PPE).
- Preparation and use of training materials to improve the knowledge and understanding at the community level of the risk factors associated with zoonotic diseases, hygiene and sanitation, safe disposal of aborted foetuses and afterbirths.
- Joint training programme for control of CCHF (tick control) – awareness of the potential risk of hand-removal of ticks and other occupational hazards.
- Sharing of laboratory facilities for processing and testing of human and animal samples, joint training of human and animal laboratory technicians, especially at the provincial level.
- Planning and implementation of joint community awareness campaigns.

23.5 One Health and community-based human and animal care programmes

The One Health approach as a concept bringing together all of the disciplines in one way or another related to human and animal health and the environment has become widely adopted in the industrialized nations of the world and is well funded. In many developing countries, although the concept was initially adopted enthusiastically, the continued practical application of One Health activities has all but died away as the funding for HPAI surveillance and control programmes came to an end.

Nevertheless, the One Health approach is especially relevant for application in developing countries not the least because of the enormous benefits to be derived from the sharing of scarce human and financial resources for the surveillance, prevention and control of human and animal diseases. Whilst some human and animal diseases can be prevented, controlled or even eradicated through the use of vaccines and medicines, most illnesses affecting the rural poor and their livestock in developing countries occur largely as a consequence of a lack of access to clean water, poor standards of hygiene and a fundamental lack of understanding of disease causality. Solving each of these issues effectively requires an interdisciplinary and collaborative approach connecting human and animal health technicians, as well as other specialist service providers, with community members. Providing clean water, extension services and disease prevention and control interventions, however, are very costly. Almost all developing countries lack sufficient human and financial resources to bring about the desired state of physical, mental and socioeconomic wellbeing – in other words 'good health' – for all of their peoples. In spite of these challenges, in the case of food safety and the prevention and control of zoonotic diseases, in particular, professionally supervised community-based primary human and animal healthcare workers can play a crucial role in helping to resolve many of the issues through acting as extension agents to create better awareness as well as providing ready access to preventative and curative health services to communities in more remote or underserved areas.

23.6 Conclusions

The One Health approach to understanding, preventing and controlling human and animal disease and promoting stability within ecosystems provides senior policymakers in donor institutions as well as the governments of developing countries with a unique opportunity to develop strategies designed specifically to create closer working relationships between technical disciplines and to share the very limited resources available to them. Yet there still remain challenges. Decision-makers still lack sufficient quantitative evidence derived from cost–benefit or cost-effectiveness studies. Researchers implementing projects based on putting One Health concepts into practice are therefore strongly encouraged to incorporate systems for recording costs and evaluating benefits of the approaches being tested.

The case study described in this chapter illustrates the successful application of the One Health approach for disease investigation leading to a disease control programme based upon a more efficient and cost effective use of human and financial resources. Such an approach could be advocated as a useful starting point for many other developing countries where the benefits of the One Health approach have not yet been fully appreciated.

References

Akbarian, Z., Ziay,G., Schauwers, W., Noormal, B., Saeed, I., Qanee, A.H., Shahab, Z., Dennison, T., Dohoo, I., Jackson, R., (2015) Brucellosis and Coxiella burnetii infection in householders and their animals in secure villages in Herat province, Afghanistan: a cross sectional study. PLOS Neglected Tropical Diseases 9(10): thhp://dx.doi.org/10.1371/journal.pntd.0004112.

Allam, M.W. (1966). The MD and the VMD. *Pennsylvania Medicine*, 69(8), 57–60.

AHDP (2013). www.ahdp.net/reports/07%20AHDP II%20July%2013%20Report%20-final.pdf.

Cass, J. (1973). One Medicine – human and veterinary. *Perspectives in Biology and Medicine*, 16(3), 418–426.

Cassidy, A. (forthcoming). One Medicine? (Inter)disciplinary advocacy for animal and human health. In S. Frickel, M. Albert and B. Prainsack (eds.), *Critical Studies of Interdisciplinary Research*. Chapel Hill, NC: Rutgers University Press.

DfID (2014). *Social Impact Bond Pilot: Sleeping Sickness in Uganda*, http://devtracker.dfid.gov.uk/api/access/activities/GB-1-203604.

FAO (2008). *Influenza Coordination Contributing to One World, One Health: A Strategic Framework for Reducing the Risks of Infectious Diseases at the Human–Animal–Ecosystems Interface*. Consultation document at the international ministerial conference on avian and pandemic influenza at Sharm El-Sheikh, Egypt. Rome: FAO in collaboration with the OIE/WHO/UNICEF/World Bank and UN System.

Gibbs, E.P.J. (2005). Emerging zoonotic epidemics in the interconnected global community. *Veterinary Record*, 157, 673–679.

Gibbs, E.P.J. (2014). The evolution of One Health: a decade of progress and challenges for the future. *Veterinary Record*, 174, 85–91.

Halpin, B. (1981). *Vets, Barefoot and Otherwise*. Pastoral Network Paper No.11c. London: Overseas Development Institute.

Hussain, S.A., Rassoul, A.B., Shaghasy, M.N., Villon H., Tufan, M. and Woodford, J.D. (2011). An innovative means of establishing a national epidemio-surveillance network in Afghanistan. Épidémiologie et Santé Animale, 59/60, 425–427.

Kaplan, B. and Scott, C. (2011). *One Health History Question: Who Coined the Term 'One Medicine'?* www.vetmed.ucdavis.edu/onehealth/local-assets/pdfs/schwabe_coins_onemedicine#schwabe_coins_one-medicine.pdf.

McCaughey, C. (2014). Q fever: a tough zoonosis. *Veterinary Record*, 175, 15–16.

MoPH (2013). Disease Early Warning System (DEWS). Annual Report. Kabul: Ministry of Public Health.

Mustafa, M.L., Ayazi, E., Mohareb, E., Yingst, S., Zayed, A., Rossi, C.A., Schoepp, R.J., Mofleh, J., Fiekert, K., Akbarian, Z., Sadat, H. and Leslie, T. (2011). Crimean-Congo haemorrhagic fever, Afghanistan, 2009. *Emerging Infectious Diseases*, 17, 1940–1941.

Needham, J. (1999). Part 6: medicine. In *Science and Civilization in China: Volume 6, Biology and Biological Technology*. Cambridge: Cambridge University Press.

Okello, A., Gibbs, E.P.J., Vandersmissen, A. and Welburn, S.C. (2011). One Health and the neglected zoonoses: turning rhetoric into reality. *Veterinary Record*, 169, 281–285.

Saeed, K.M.I., Jamalludin, A., Ghiasi, A.F. and Ashgar, R.J. (2013). Concurrent brucellosis and Q fever infection: a case control study in Bamyan Province, Afghanistan. *Central Asian Journal of Global Health*, 2(2).

Schmidt, C.F. (1962). Editorial: One Medicine for more than one world. *Circulation Research*, 11(6), 901–903.

Schwabe, C.W. (1978). Cattle, priests and progress in medicine. In *Wesley W. Spink Lectures on Comparative Medicine*, Vol 4. Minneapolis: University of Minnesota Press.

Schwabe, C.W. (1984). *Veterinary Medicine and Human Health*, 3rd edn. Baltimore: Williams & Wilkins.

Schwabe, C.W. (1991). History of the scientific relationships of veterinary public health. *Scientific and Technical Review of the Office International des Epizooties (Paris)*, 10, 933–949.

Taubenberger, J.K. and Morens, D.M. (2006). 1918 influenza: the mother of all pandemics. *Emerging Infectious Diseases*, http://dx.doi.org/10.3201/eid1209.050979.

World Bank (2010). *Animal and Pandemic Influenza: A Framework for Sustaining Momentum: Synopsis of the Fifth Global Progress Report*, http://documents.worldbank.org/curated/en/2010/07/12915838/animal-pandemic-influenza-framework-sustaining-momentum-synopsis-fifth-global-progress-report.

Acknowledgements

The authors wish to acknowledge the role played by the principal actors involved in undertaking the One Health study on brucellosis, *Coxiella burnetii* infection and CCHF in Afghanistan. In particular we would like to thank Dr Zarif Akbarian (DEWS Regional Coordinator, MoPH, Herat), Dr Islam Saaed (Director of Surveillance, ANPHI, MoPH, Kabul), Dr Abul Hussain (head of Department of Epidemiology, MAIL, Kabul and MAIL central ZDCC representative), Dr Ghulam Ziay, Director, Central Veterinary, Diagnostic and Research Laboratory, Dr Maken Ali, W. Schauwers (Landell Mills Ltd. (UK), Technical Assistance to the Animal Health Development Programme – Phase II.), and the several human and veterinary para-professionals working with the NGO's DCA-VET & HPRO, Herat, Afghanistan.

We would also like to acknowledge the important contribution of Tania Dennison as a member of the CIP Team and Project Manager of the Animal Health & Development Programme Phase II.

chapter 24

Retinol status in mobile pastoralists in Chad: a case study

Lisa Crump, Mahamat Béchir, Bongo Naré
Richard Ngandolo and Jakob Zinsstag

Abstract

In this chapter we present a case study examining the important interaction between dietary nutrients and human and livestock health in pastoralists in Chad. Carotenoids are naturally occurring pigments found in plants and animals. They cannot be synthesized by animals and are only ingested through food. Certain carotenoids, in particular ß-carotene, can be converted into vitamin A. The latter is an important nutrient for the maintenance of health and plays an essential role in vision, particularly night vision, normal bone and tooth development, reproduction and the health of skin and mucous membranes. Retinol deficiency is a prevalent problem in mobile pastoralists in the Lake Chad area, with 30 per cent in the cold season, 25 per cent in the rainy season and 15 per cent in the dry season being found deficient. Vitamin A supplementation as part of an intervention of the Expanded Programme on Immunization (EPI) in children and women should be considered. In this case study we present the results of preliminary research performed by an interdisciplinary team including veterinary, medical, agricultural and geographic experts. Future work investigating ecosystem linkages should include mobile demographic surveillance of migratory routes and an agronomy component to facilitate adequate pasture sampling.

24.1 Introduction

In the Sahel, there are approximately 50 million mobile pastoralists, with estimates in Chad ranging up to two million (Rass, 2006). Pastoralists migrate in a seasonal cycle to manage livelihood risk through mobile lifestyles highly adapted to utilize limited resources to provide for the needs of their animals (Bille, 1997), but mobility and sociocultural factors limit their access to social services and effective interventions (Cohen, 2005; Münch, 2012). With the objective of improved access for mobile communities to social services, the Swiss Tropical and Public Health Institute has been active throughout the Sahel region with local partners for more than

15 years (Montavon et al., 2013). Initially, it was crucial to gain understanding of the local context and pastoralists' needs. The remote setting made it difficult, but not impossible, to conduct even basic research (Schelling et al., 2003). In order to maximally transform results into development actions, priorities were defined in a participatory manner using stakeholder workshops that included pastoralist representatives, local and national authorities and interdisciplinary researchers (Wyss et al., 2004; Münch, 2012). Because of the important role of animals for pastoralist livelihoods and the close contact between them and their livestock, a 'One Health' approach was adopted as the conceptual basis for the research. The defining feature of this collaboration between human and animal health, and their related outcomes, is an added value through closer cooperation in terms of improved wellbeing, financial savings or better service provision.

Work in Chad shows that the vast majority of pastoralists suffer from health problems but rarely visit health centres (Daugla et al., 2004; Schelling et al., 2005). Antenatal care is seldom sought (Münch, 2012), and women and children have very low vaccination coverage (Bechir et al., 2004). The pastoralist diet consists mainly of milk and cereals, and food security is periodically extremely difficult to ensure due to seasonality and market influence (Bechir et al., 2013). Globally, vitamin A deficiency (VAD) continues to be a significant public health issue and underlying cause of disease in developing countries (WHO, 2009). Even sub-clinical VAD increases mortality and severe morbidity from common diseases (Tanumihardjo et al., 1994). Vitamin A supplementation is associated with large reductions in mortality and morbidity in young children in a wide range of settings (Mayo-Wilson et al., 2011). Therefore, our research teams working in close partnership with the Chadian public health and livestock sectors included retinol status evaluation as part of health assessments investigated in the Lake Chad area.

24.2 Interdisciplinary field research: case study

The first study was a repeated cross-sectional design during the rainy and dry seasons in 1999 and 2000 (Zinsstag et al., 2002). Sixty per cent of the investigated Arab and Fulani mobile pastoralist women were retinol deficient (<0.7 µmol/L). The diet of the study population consisted nearly exclusively of millet, rice and maize along with milk and milk products. A 24-hour dietary recall study showed a significantly lower intake of cereal and milk in women with severe retinol deficiency (<0.35 µmol/L). Human serum retinol level was dependent on livestock milk retinol. A second study in 2008 in the same area investigated retinol status in mobile and sedentary women and children up to five years old at the end of the rainy season (Bechir et al., 2012). One in five semi-nomadic and sedentary women and one in 20 nomadic women were found to be retinol deficient (<0.7 µmol/L), with a similar trend in children. Children older than three years were significantly more likely to be retinol deficient than children less than one year of age. There was a positive correlation between both blood retinol level and mothers' milk retinol level and cow milk retinol level. A portable device for rapid retinol assessment (iCheck™, BioAnalyt GmbH) was found to be reliable under harsh field conditions.

In 2012–2013, we investigated environmental determinants of retinol status in mobile pastoralists in the same study area. Our hypothesis was that human vitamin A status fluctuates seasonally, and we postulated that data on the availability and quality of pastures could be good indicators of the nutritional and health status of Sahelian livestock and people. The research questions were:

- Do retinol levels in human blood, cattle milk and pasture grass vary according to season?
- Does the prevalence of retinol deficiency vary according to season and/or ethnic group?
- Are human blood and cattle milk retinol associated with pasture grass carotenoid levels or Normalized Difference Vegetation Index (NDVI) and Enhanced Vegetation Index (EVI)?
- Is portable photometry feasible for measuring carotenoids in pasture grass samples? Is it possible to record grazing patterns in pastoralist cattle?

Prior to beginning the study, the protocol was approved by the Ethics Commission of Basel (Switzerland) and the Ministry of Public Health (Chad). Stakeholder meetings were held in villages near the southern shore of Lake Chad to discuss the project with Chadian local authorities and pastoralist community leaders. A convenience sample of ten camps was selected, considering logistic constraints (travel and data collection time) and accessibility (projected camp locations based on known transhumance patterns), availability and history of previous cooperation. One camp subsequently declined participation due to change in migration route. There were three sampling intervals in the repeated cross-sectional study design. In each camp, seven men and seven women at least 15 years of age were selected from multiple households using ethical considerations first, in accordance with accepted local customs, and randomization criteria second. Each participant was interviewed to record demographic and seven-day dietary recall information. Whole blood was collected and analysed for retinol using portable devices (iCheck™). Pooled cow milk was collected from each household and similarly analysed. Two cows in the camp herds were fitted with logging collars, which recorded Global Positioning System (GPS) coordinates every two minutes during the daytime grazing period. Fodder samples were collected where the collared cows were grazing. The fodder samples were air-dried in the shade then stored in foil pouches for later processing. Analysis involved grinding, reconstituting and analysing the plant samples for carotene level using the iCheck™ device and high-performance liquid chromatography (HPLC). MODIS (Moderate Resolution Imaging Spectroradiometer) satellite data was accessed to record vegetation index values, with camp GPS coordinates used as the reference point. Due to satellite images pixel resolution (250m), there was one measurement per camp per sampling interval, which was used as the mean value.

A total of 327 human blood samples were analysed from nine camps, representing three ethnic groups (Fulani, Arab and Gorane), during three sampling intervals (September 2012 rainy season, January 2013 cold season and July 2013 dry season), as summarized in Table 24.1 (Crump et al., 2015). The mean human retinol levels by characteristic are listed in Table 24.2. Average values were highest in Gorane during the rainy season and highest in Fulani in the cold and the dry season. The lowest average values were seen in Arabs in all three seasons, as shown in Figure 24.1. Multivariable analysis, where season was included as a fixed study design effect and camp as a random effect, considered human retinol level as outcome. Lower retinol levels were associated with the cold and the dry season, with the cold season effect being larger. Arab ethnicity was associated with lower retinol levels. Consumption of >1L of milk per day was associated with higher retinol levels. The level of human retinol deficiency also varied according to season and ethnic group. During the rainy season, no Gorane participant was found to be retinol deficient (<0.7 μmol/L), while more than 20 per cent of Fulani and 50 per cent of Arab participants were affected. In the cold season, more than 10 per cent of Fulani, 40 per cent of Gorane and 50 per cent of Arabs were deficient. During the dry season, close to 10 per cent of Fuliani

Table 24.1 Sociodemographic characteristics of study participants

Participating camps (n)	Sep 2012 (rainy)	Jan 2013 (cold)	July 2013 (dry)	TOTAL
Fulani	4	4	4	
Arab	3	3	3	
Gorane	2	2	1	
Total camps/ interval	9	9	8	9
Human participants				
Fulani	56	57	42	155
Arab	29	42	33	104
Gorane	26	28	14	68
TOTAL humans	111	127	89	327
Male	52% (n = 58)	50% (n = 64)	44% (n =39)	49%
15–45 years	84% (n = 93)	84% (n = 107)	73% (n = 65)	81%

Table 24.2 Human blood retinol levels (µg/L)

			Rainy Sep 2012		Cold Jan 2013		Dry July 2013	
		n	mean	% deficient	mean	% deficient	mean	% deficient
Sex								
	Male	161	618	26	303	25	567	9
	Female	166	594	24	262	38	450	20
Age								
	15–45	265	600	28	282	35	538	14
	>45	62	637	11	287	15	402	17
Ethnicity								
	Fulani	155	597	23	349	12	583	7
	Gorane	68	984	0	264	43	545	7
	Arab	104	286	52	205	50	379	30
Milk consumption								
	≤1L/day	166	602	32	249	42	405	28
	>1L/day	161	613	14	325	18	541	9
Vegetable/fruit consumption								
	only in sauce	200	330	47	273	37	546	5
	1 or more/week	127	718	16	326	5	394	32

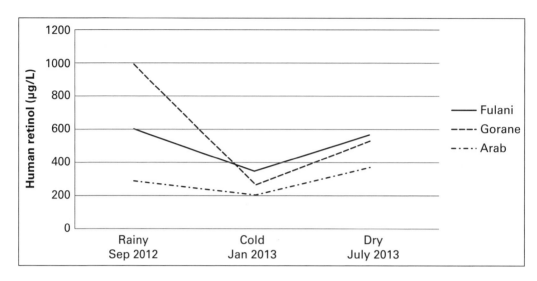

Figure 24.1 Human mean blood retinol by season: stratified by ethnic group.

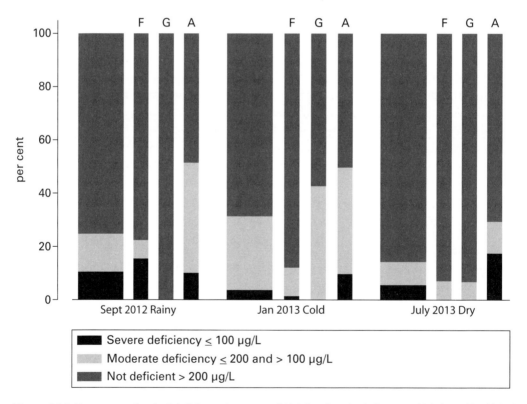

Figure 24.2 Frequency of retinol deficiency by season (thick bars) and ethnic group (thin bars: F = Fulani, G = Gorane, A = Arab).

and Gorane and 30 per cent of Arabs were deficient (Figure 24.2). Although the sample size was small when stratified by ethnic group, and we were unable to demonstrate a statistically significant difference, those of Arab ethnicity were three times as likely to be deficient and the odds of being deficient also increased in the cold season (OR 1.6). Those reported to drink more than 1L of milk per day had nearly three times lower odds of being deficient, and the difference was statistically significant, in line with previous work (Zinsstag et al., 2002). A total of 215 pooled cow milk samples were analysed, and milk retinol values were highest in the rainy season and lowest in the cold season. In multivariable models, mean milk retinol had a positive effect on human blood retinol level (Crump et al., 2015). The portable iCheck™ devices functioned well in ambient temperatures up to 45°C; however, when the air temperature was higher, they did not. The battery lifespan was acceptable (approximately 300 tests).

It proved feasible to use GPS loggers (M-241™, HOLUX, Taiwan) to record the grazing pattern of the cattle herds, although during the rainy season some herds were grazing in flooded pastures. In these cases, the collars were not utilized, and grazing sites were recorded as point coordinates using a handheld device (eTrex 10®, Garmin, USA). Fulani and Arab herders grazed the cows in or near the lake during the dry season, while the Gorane were away from the lake (defined as more than 4km). During the cold season, half of Fulani herders were at the lake and half were away, while the Arab and Gorane were away from the lake. During the rainy season, half of the Fulani remained on islands within the lake, while the other pastoralists migrated as far as 100km from the lakeshore. Even during the dry season when ambient temperatures were sometimes above 50°C, the loggers functioned for at least eight hours without battery replacement.

Analysis of the dried fodder samples proved to be problematic. We were unable to sufficiently optimize the process for extracting β-carotene using the portable iCheck™ device due to inability to grind the samples finely enough. A subset of the samples were analysed using HPLC, but there was a long time lag (one to six months) before processing and the number of samples analysed was small (n = 53). In these samples, grazed pasture carotene values were highest in the dry season and lowest in the cold season. The grass carotene values were not as expected; however, differences in husbandry and use of the pastoral ecosystem are a likely explanation (Jean-Richard et al., 2014). The dynamics of migratory patterns are likely to play an important role in determining the retinol status of mobile pastoralists and should be further investigated. Based on the variation in carotene content between duplicate HPLC analyses at different times on the same samples, it is also likely that in spite of the storage precautions taken the measured grass carotene values in this study were falsely low due to sample degradation between the time of collection and lab analysis.

Vegetation indices for the grazing sites were highest in the rainy season and lowest in the cold season. It was expected that the highest vegetation indices would be noted in the rainy season and the lowest in the dry season. Similarly to the pasture carotene values, differences in husbandry and ecosystem use are one likely explanation. Another contributing factor could be variation in the annual seasonal rain cycle. In this study, the dry season sampling interval was delayed from May until early July 2013 due to security restrictions in the study zone. At this time, the collected grazed grass samples were all green, whereas during a pilot test of the method, also carried out in the dry season but in May of 2012, the Fulani herds were grazing green grass continuously at the lakeshore, while the Arab herds moved to the vicinity of the lake for part of the day and the Gorane herds ate only standing hay. Although the vegetation indices were not statistically significantly different and the

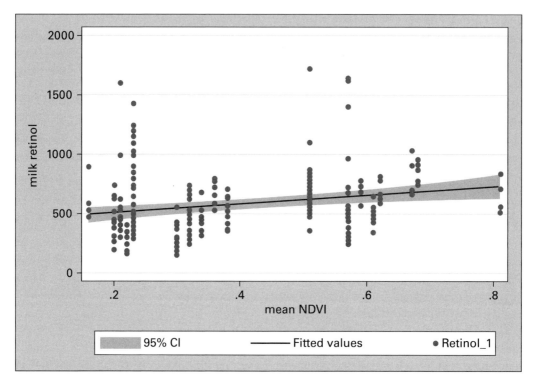

Figure 24.3 Individual milk retinol values against mean NDVI.

effect sizes were small, higher vegetation indices were associated with higher milk retinol levels (Figure 24.3).

This study considered a large amount of variation between season, ethnic group, sex and age with a relatively small sample size. This complex design is likely to have absorbed some of the differences that were present, possibly even obscuring some. It is difficult to demonstrate significant effects in clustered data, and the relatively small size of the clusters contributed to model instability. However, despite these limitations, we could establish that there are seasonal variations in human blood and cattle milk retinol levels and demonstrate a linkage from animals to humans through milk. We document seasonal variation in the grazed pasture grass and vegetation indices, but the linkages are less clear. A larger-scale study is necessary to investigate seasonal interethnic variation in human retinol levels and the vegetation linkage through cattle milk to human retinol. Future work investigating ecosystem linkages should include an agronomy component to facilitate adequate pasture sampling. The time from sampling to analysis of fodder should be decreased. In this study, there was only one sample collection interval per season, which provided an incomplete picture, given the dynamic nature of the growing season and long interval between sampling (four months and six months). It was impossible to consider the time period between fodder intake, rise in cow milk retinol concentration and blood retinol concentration in humans. Future work should utilize mobile phones to collect demographic surveillance data on the migration patterns of mobile pastoralists (Jean-Richard et al., 2014) in order to sample pasture sites grazed two weeks earlier and thus incorporate lag time.

Based on this study, stakeholders should be informed that retinol deficiency is a prevalent problem in mobile pastoralists in the Lake Chad area, with 30 per cent in the cold season, 25 per cent in the rainy season and 15 per cent in the dry season being found deficient. The Arab ethnic group may be disproportionally affected, at more than 50 per cent deficient during the rainy and cold seasons and 30 per cent deficient during the dry season. Vitamin A supplementation as part of an intervention of the Expanded Programme on Immunization (EPI) in children and women should be considered.

24.3 Conclusion

We can establish seasonal variations in human blood and cattle milk retinol levels. We demonstrate an ecological linkage from animals to humans, through milk. Rapid analysis using portable technology is feasible in remote populations. Retinol deficiency is a prevalent problem in mobile pastoralist adults in the Lake Chad area during certain time periods, and particularly in the Arab ethnic group. Options for improving retinol (and thus vitamin A) status include increasing milk consumption, food fortification and linking supplementation programmes to other interventions such as joint human and animal vaccination campaigns.

The added value to using a One Health approach to investigate this problem comes through improved accessibility and cost savings. The study area is remote and there is little access to health centres. Animal health and human health personnel share equipment and travel costs. Using a portable device for rapid diagnosis of vitamin A deficiency, perhaps even through screening of animal milk rather than human blood, is another way to increase accessibility, save costs and improve health outcomes.

References

Bechir, M., Schelling, E., Wyss, K., Daugla, D.M., Daoud, S., Tanner, M. and Zinsstag, J. (2004). An innovative approach combining human and animal vaccination campaigns in nomadic settings of Chad: experiences and costs. *Médecine tropicale: revue du Corps de santé colonial*, **64**(5), 497–502.

Bechir, M., Schelling, E., Kraemer, K., Schweigert, F., Bonfoh, B., Crump, L., Tanner, M. and Zinsstag, J. (2012). Retinol assessment among women and children in Sahelian mobile pastoralists. *EcoHealth*, **9**(2), 113–121.

Bechir, M., Zinsstag, J., Tidjani, A., Schelling, E., Ibrahim, A., Bonfoh, B. and Tanner, M. (2013). Food security and resilience among mobile pastoral and settled community around Lake Chad in Sahel. In Y. Srivastava (ed.), *Advances in Food Science and Nutrition*. Aurangabad: Queen's College of Food Technology & Research Foundation, pp. 90–106.

Bille, J. (1997). L'elevage pastoral doit renouer avec ses traditions d'equilibre. *Spore*, 68, 11.

Cohen, D. (2005). Providing nomadic people with health care. *BMJ*, 331(7519), 720.

Crump, L., Bechir, M, Mahamat, M.B., Ngandolo, B.N.R., Daugla, D.M., Hattendorf, J. and Zinsstag, J. (2015). Seasonal dynamics of human retinol status in mobile pastoralists in Chad. Acta Tropica, in Review.

Daugla, D.M., Daoud, S., Tanner, M., Zinsstag, J. and Schelling, E. (2004). Morbidity patterns in three nomadic communities in Chari-Baguirmi and Kanem, Chad. *Médecine tropicale: revue du Corps de santé colonial*, 64(5), 469–473.

Jean-Richard, V., Crump, L., Daugla, D., Hattendorf, J., Schelling, E. and Zinsstag, J. (2014). The use of mobile phones for demographic surveillance of mobile pastoralists and their animals in Chad: proof of principle. *Global Health Action*, 7, 23209.

Mayo-Wilson, E., Imdad, A., Herzer, K., Yakoob, M.Y. and Bhutta, Z.A. (2011). Vitamin A supplements for preventing mortality, illness, and blindness in children aged under 5: systematic review and meta-analysis. *BMJ*. 343, d5094.

Montavon, A., Jean-Richard, V., Bechir, M., Daugla, D.M., Abdoulaye, M., Bongo Naré, R.N., Diguimbaye-Djaibé, C., Alfarouk, I.O., Schelling, E., Wyss, K., Tanner, M., Zinsstag, J. (2013). Health of mobile pastoralists in the Sahel – assessment of 15 years of research and development. *Tropical Medicine & International Health*, 18(9), 1044–1052.

Münch, A. (2012). *Nomadic Women's Health Practice Islamic Belief and Medical Care among Kel Alhafra Tuareg in Mali*. Basel: Schwabe Verlag.

Rass, N. (2006). *Policies and Strategies to Address the Vulnerability of Pastoralists in Sub-Saharan Africa*, Rome: Food and Agriculture Organization.

Schelling, E., Diguimbaye, C., Daoud, S., Nicolet, J., Boerlin, P., Tanner, M. and Zinsstag, J. (2003). Brucellosis and Q-fever seroprevalences of nomadic pastoralists and their livestock in Chad. *Preventive Veterinary Medicine*, 61(4), 279–293.

Schelling, E., Daoud, S., Daugla, D., Diallo, P., Tanner, M. and Zinsstag, J. (2005). Morbidity and nutrition patterns of three nomadic pastoralist communities of Chad. *Acta Tropica*, 95(1), 16–25.

Tanumihardjo, S.A., Permaesih, D., Dahro, A.M., Rustan, E., Muhilal, Karyadi, D. and Olson, J.A. (1994). Comparison of Vitamin A status assessment techniques in children from two Indonesian villages. *The American Journal of Clinical Nutrition*, 60(1), 136–141.

WHO (2009). *Global Prevalence of Vitamin A Deficiency in Populations at Risk 1995–2005*. Geneva: World Health Organization.

Wyss, K., Bechir, M., Schelling, E., Daugla, D.M. and Zinsstag, J. (2004). Health care services for nomadic people: lessons learned from research and implementation activities in Chad. *Médecine tropicale: revue du Corps de santé colonial*, 64(5), 493–496.

Zinsstag, J., Schelling, E., Daoud, S., Schierle, J., Hofmann, P., Diguimbaye, C., Daugla, D.M., Ndoutamia, G., Knopf, L., Vounatsou, P. and Tanner, M. (2002). Serum retinol of Chadian nomadic pastoralist women in relation to their livestocks' milk retinol and beta-carotene content. *International Journal for Vitamin and Nutrition Research*, 72(4), 221–228.

CONCEPTS AND KNOWLEDGE TRANSFER

chapter 25

Human and animal health in a cultural context: Tanzania One Health field school

Frank van der Meer, Jennifer Hatfield and Karin Orsel

Abstract

In this chapter we provide context and examples of the integration of important concepts of One Health, global health, animal and human health and transdisciplinary collaborations during educational and research activities in the Ngorongoro region of Northern Tanzania. These activities are based on collaborations between researchers from different disciplines in partnership with local communities and stakeholders. Although the animal–human health challenges in this region of Tanzania are in many instances non-zoonotic in nature, we find value in using a One Health approach in which we draw knowledge and expertise from many disciplines and individuals, in order to mitigate the impact of diseases on the animal and human population. The added benefits of training human and animal health professionals side-by-side using this One Health approach, is illustrated in the example of our Tanzania field school. The principles, approaches and frameworks that inform our field school activities are also presented through the detailed articulation of a set of global health practice competencies. This field school is a joint initiative between the Faculties of Medicine (Cumming School of Medicine) and Veterinary Medicine (UCVM) of the University of Calgary (UofC) and the Catholic University of Health and Allied Sciences (CUHAS) in Mwanza Tanzania as well as community members and leaders in the Ngorongoro Conservation Area (NCA).

25.1 One Health and global health

One Health: developing an inclusive and comprehensive perspective

As stated by the American Veterinary Medical Association: 'One Health is the integrative effort of multiple disciplines working locally, nation- ally, and globally to attain optimal health for people, animals, and the environment' (AVMA, 2008). However, multiple challenges present themselves as we seek to implement a One Health approach to problem-solving. Integrating multiple disciplines in a practical way is complicated. Jacob Zinsstag and co-workers at the Swiss Tropical and Public Health Institute,

Basel[1] have reflected on the value of integrative conceptual and methodological developments of a One Health approach, but they identify that large portions of the thinking and actions pertaining to human and animal health still remain in separate disciplinary silos.

Expanding beyond perceived limitations of One Health notions to a broader understanding of the importance of ecological contexts has led to an inclusion of concepts such as 'human-environmental systems', also called 'social-ecological systems' (HSES) (Zinsstag et al., 2011). These frames of reference allow for the consideration of emerging properties and determinants of health that may arise from a systemic view, i.e., one that ranges from the level of molecules and microbes to the broader and applied ecological and sociocultural context, as well (Zinsstag et al., 2011). The ability to address health at the animal, human and environmental interface depends upon teams composed of many disciplines who collaborate and communicate effectively.

Recognizing these challenges we draw on a broad range of resources in order to create an experiential learning environment that seeks to prepare veterinary and health science trainees to engage in community capacity-building and research activities utilizing this more expansive and inclusive concept of One Health.

Global health competencies: developing a shared understanding of key concepts across disciplinary groups

The Cumming School of Medicine has adapted the Canadian Coalition for Global Health Research (CCGHR) conceptual frameworks and learning resources to frame a set of six core competencies for global health work applicable to clinical, educational or research-focused projects in resource constrained settings (Figure 25.1). All students, regardless of their educational or disciplinary background, receive training on

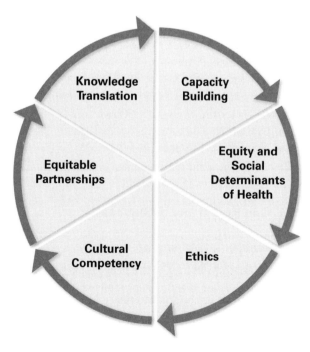

Figure 25.1 Core competencies of global health research.

global health competencies before and during participation in the Tanzania field school.

The broad foundational knowledge that is critical to engaging in global health activities is taught through semester-long or short intensive courses. These concepts are then carried forward as topics of discussion throughout the field school experience and form a set of commonly shared definitions, themes and competencies across disciplinary groups. The knowledge and skills needed to approach and analyse complex problems are reinforced so that trainees develop the ability to use these frames of reference to inform their approach to research and community engagement.

Regardless of disciplinary perspective we encourage an understanding and competence in the following concepts: As defined by the WHO, the determinants of health include: the social and economic environment, the physical environment and the person's individual characteristics and behaviours. Furthermore, income and social status, education, physical environment, social support networks, genetics, health services and gender are factors that influence the health of individuals. Health inequities are defined as the differences in health that are unnecessary, avoidable, unfair and unjust. The WHO has defined capacity-building as the development of knowledge, skills, commitment, structures, systems and leadership to enable effective health promotion. Developing community capacity is a foundation for good health promotion practice and assists in the ability of local communities to effectively uptake health interventions (Costello and Zumla, 2000; Simmons et al., 2011). We seek to mitigate the problems and limitations of the 'briefcase or parachute model' (Costello and Zumla, 2000), which is characterized by a 'top-down' approach to engagement where research or interventions are planned and implemented by outsiders with little community participation or negotiation. We foster and teach a 'partnership model' of research collaboration based

on *equitable partnerships*. This means that we demonstrate and model to the trainees how a research agenda or programme intervention is negotiated with researchers and community members from the host country to ensure that projects are jointly managed. The partnership assessment tool (PAT) (Afsana et al., 2009) developed by the Canadian Coalition for Global Health Research (CCGHR) is a valuable tool for developing and evaluating equitable mutually beneficial partnerships. We intentionally teach and actively discuss issues associated with *ethics* and ethical conduct of research in low and middle-income country settings. Much of this debate focuses on the controversies of internationally sponsored research (Bhutta, 2002). A nuanced understanding of the importance of ethical compliance and practice in LMICs is vital to reducing inequity. Furthermore, there is an important ethical debate on international guidelines for the conduct of research and the importance of adapting informed consent, improving community participation and the benefits and burdens of research on the local population (Bhutta, 2002). Regarding cultural competency, 'culture' implies the integrated pattern of human behaviour (including thoughts, communication, actions, customs, beliefs, values and institutions of a racial, ethnic, religious or social group). 'Competence' means that one has the ability to function effectively (Shiu-Thornton, 2003). We support our trainees in understanding the role of their own culture on their perceptions and seek to develop understanding of local history, cultural practices and an appreciation of differences and similarities between cultural groups. Finally we develop an understanding of the challenges and opportunities for knowledge translation (KT) within resourced constrained settings. KT was defined by Canadian Institutes of Health Research in 2006 as, 'the exchange, synthesis and ethically-sound application of knowledge – within a complex system of interactions among researchers and users – to accelerate the capture of the benefits of research for Canadians through improved health, more effective services and products, and a strengthened health care system'. This definition is adapted to apply to low and middle-income settings where resources and barriers to KT are significant and the need to integrate and plan KT from the inception of projects is critical.

Before, during and following participation in the Tanzania field school, these concepts and the associated competencies, developed through use and practice, are integrated in all aspects of the work undertaken, be it medical or veterinary of nature. This set of competencies complement programme-specific medical and veterinary clinical competencies (such as a knowledge of maternal child health, tropical (animal) diseases, epidemiology, education principles or basic research skills (see Plate 33).

25.2 Transdisciplinary approaches: respecting diverse perspectives

Drawing on the rich set of frameworks articulated above; how do we create an educational environment that fosters the understanding and application of these complex, integrated concepts while building on the competencies that we consider to be important?

To address these challenges we developed an experiential learning approach that draws on transdisciplinary scholarship. This is described well in the literature (Min et al., 2013). Transdisciplinary research performed in the Tanzania field school is based on an approach to understanding health issues that brings together disciplines and stakeholders in a setting where community representatives participate as co-researchers who provide knowledge based on their experiences. This transdisciplinary approach is used to enhance our understanding of the practical complexities of improving health at the animal–human–ecological interface.

Maasai pastoralists live a traditional lifestyle, closely linked to their livestock in the context of an ever-changing environment that they share with wildlife. Human and animal health problems cannot be considered in isolation. For example, due to the zoonotic nature of some diseases, such as brucellosis, the disease can impact humans, domestic ruminants and wildlife. Developing disease control recommendations warrants the development of an integrated approach that considers aspects as disparate as food safety, political forces, climate influences, cultural context, health services and disease transmission. We impress upon all our trainees, regardless of previous experience or knowledge, the complexity of the cultural and physical environment we are working in and the expertise required to understand and work toward solutions. The lenses afforded by social scientists, veterinarians, biomedical researchers, ecologists and local community members are all crucial.

The examples provided later in this chapter illustrate how we use a One Health approach to address common human and animal infectious diseases in our work with the NCA and we demonstrate how a single problem can be effectively tackled by using an interdisciplinary approach. We have found that this approach, when done well, leads to building trust and collaborative solutions.

A considerable amount of time and good will is needed to ensure the effective engagement of animal and human medical experts, government organizations, public health experts, diagnosticians, disease modellers, sociologists, anthropologists, education and economic experts among many others. Once 'experts' step over their discipline boundaries and share their knowledge in a logical and constructive way, effective and acceptable approaches to mitigating disease risks, and enhancing wellbeing, for both human and animal populations can develop (Figure 25.2). Central to the success of this

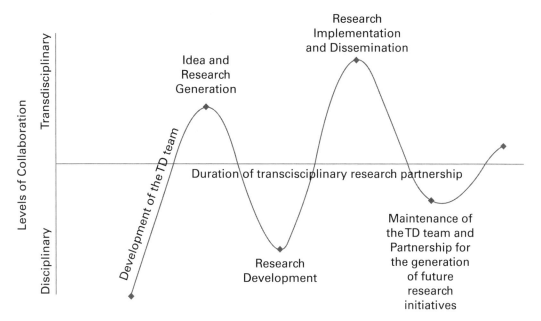

Figure 25.2 Development of collaboration during transdisciplinary research.

process is the building of local capacity and local adoption and implementations of recommendations to address issues and learning from the wisdom of our local partners to create appropriate interventions. We are constantly reminded of the value of community engagement and selecting health issues considered to be important by communities in the NCA.

25.3 In practice: the Tanzania field school

Over a period of nine years the Bachelor of Health Sciences/Cumming School of Medicine together with the Faculty of Veterinary Medicine and CUHAS has structured a field school near Endulen Hospital. The Endulen community is situated in the Ngorongoro Conservation Area (NCA) in Tanzania. The NCA was established as a shared resource for livestock keeping, tourism and wildlife. The NCA has been used by man for hunting and pastures for a long time. Maasai still use parts of the region for live-

stock rearing. Administrative authorities in the area are the Tanzania National Parks Authority (TANAPA) and Ngorongoro Conservation Area Authority (NCAA) (Thornton et al., 2007). The Ngorongoro district has only two hospitals, of which Endulen Hospital was established as a clinic for tuberculosis in the early 1970s by missionaries from Austria. Within 45 years, Endulen Hospital has grown into a health centre that provides care for approximately 80,000 individuals residing in the south-west of the Ngorongoro District. The majority of individuals within the Endulen Hospital's catchment area belong to the Maasai tribe. Currently the archdiocese of Arusha runs the hospital with support from the NCAA. As with many remote health facilities throughout Africa, Endulen Hospital faces many barriers to provide adequate care and treatment. Such barriers include shortages of human and material resources (Allen et al., 2011).

The field school consists of undergraduate and graduate students and is supervised by faculty members who are supported by postdoctoral fellows. This has created the unique opportunity for a One Health education and training environment. Inspired by the global health competencies already articulated we determined the key factors of success of the research training environment:

1. For long-term fruitful relationships of the academic partners with the local communities and governmental institutions, the field school must constantly strive to ensure mutual benefit.
2. The knowledge gained through research must serve the health needs of the NCA; this includes the agency that governs the conservation area and the Maasai population through increased knowledge to make informed decisions and increased quality of their livelihood.
3. Scholarly publications are generated with collaboration and capacity-building in mind.
4. High-quality educational opportunities are supported through robust research projects.
5. Funds obtained for research directly benefit education of students from both Tanzania and Canada.
6. Training of graduate students enables the creation of a learning environment that allows graduate students and postdoctoral fellows to develop leadership, mentoring and supervisory skills.
7. Local and indigenous knowledge must be sought out and acknowledged for its value.
8. Teams are assembled with a variety of disciplinary skills and perspectives.
9. Students are prepared through courses and mentoring in the core competencies of global health, Swahili and Maa language (general greetings and courtesy expressions), and the purpose and history of the research projects.
10. Team members should be selected for their solid individual disciplinary expertise and for their willingness to work in transdisciplinary teams.

25.4 Case studies illustrating One Health in the Tanzania field school: connecting with community

Case study 1: A modified photovoice method to assess the veterinary needs

As a component of a joint medicine–veterinary medicine One Health field school, we initiated an animal health needs assessment. We chose to use photovoice, as this research method has been used in a variety of public health programmes (Wang and Burris, 1994, 1997). It aims at giving voice to the disadvantaged, and documenting societal realities. In an extensive review (Catalani and Minkler, 2010) it was shown that among participatory projects, photovoice contributes to an enhanced understanding of community assets and needs, motivations and leads to empowerment of the participants. While the collaborative, capacity-building intent of the photovoice research approach has been clearly established; the method continues to evolve (Wang, 1999; Nykiforuk et al., 2011). The objective of this study was to explore the use of photovoice to build relationships with the NCA community and strengthen our understanding of their animal health needs.

The project took place in three different ecosystems in the NCA: highland plains, semi-arid savanna and savanna woodlands/forests (Homewood and Rodgers, 1991; Homewood et al., 2001). In each region, the community identified a woman, a *murran* (warrior, 15–35 years old), and an elder, representing the different gender and age groups, to participate in the study. In total, nine people were interviewed. A local translator of the *murran* age group facilitated all interviews. The Calgary Conjoint Health Research Ethics Board and the Tanzanian National Institute for Medical Research granted ethical approval. Participants gave informed consent for the pre-photovoice interview and debrief separately. They were informed that the photos and the stories accompanying them would be used to guide research within the NCA.

The photovoice methodology was adjusted to the NCA setting; participants used digital cameras and standard components of the photovoice approach; the photo display and group discussion sessions, were replaced with individual interviews using a laptop to display all the pictures taken by the participant for discussion. All interviews were recorded using a voice recorder. This approach allowed us to gather perspectives across the large geographic area of the NCA and acknowledge different priorities in ecosystems as well as positions in society. The outcomes of the study were used to inform future research and outreach projects based on the needs as expressed through this method.

This method has proven itself as useful to engage community members in the topic and empowered them to express their concerns related to animal and human health issues. Main topics discussed were: access to water for animal and human use, several diseases causing high mortality in especially young stock (East Coast fever, helminth infections) and the social cultural context of livestock keeping in the Maasai society. This unique method for gathering local perspectives arose from team members with a social science background and yielded excellent data on community perspectives and health priorities.

Using the knowledge obtained through photovoice, in combination with insights obtained through interviews with the hospital staff and community leaders a community-supported helminth infection study was initiated in both animals and humans exploring the parallels in helminth infection prevention and control (see Case Study 3).

Case study 2: Workshops on animal health

Responding to concerns raised by the community, and as a rapport and trust-building strategy, education programmes were developed. As research is a relatively slow process and results generated from our projects can take multiple years before they can be implemented in the field, we started with education programmes on the topics identified with the photovoice needs assessment. We designed multiple workshops with the core themes as identified: East Coast Fever treatment, use of Western drugs and anthelmintics in livestock, and prevention and treatment of bloat in cows in the early wet season.

The main questions we were confronted with were:

• How do we convey messages to a largely illiterate population that has a good practical knowledge on animal health?
• What can we learn from the community we work with?
• Where can we start building on existing knowledge?
• How do we adapt our Western veterinary knowledge to the local circumstances?
• How do we engage local stakeholders in the design and make the material locally relevant?

During the development phase of the research projects, our educational activities were focused on knowledge exchange. An exchange of material and ideas should ensure that our ideas were practical and applicable within the Maasai pastoralist system. Continuous tweaking of the messaging was needed to ensure that the workshops reached their goals (e.g., being culturally relevant and locally applicable): change of practice of animal treatment and in some cases husbandry. This learning process provided us with many insights of local perception of treatment practices of animals and ensured that our knowledge of the local constrains around livestock keeping was sufficient to make meaningful contributions in the discussions around these topics.

Lessons learned

The continuous feedback cycles with translators and the community were essential; development of materials and messages emerged over multiple iterations. The delivery of the workshop was the end of a consultation process that took many sessions. In this setting, information and nuances got lost in translation, especially when double translations (Maa–Swahili–English) needed to take place.

Visuals should be locally relevant, as relevance in an African context was not always sufficient. Therefore local adaptations were considered for the most effect; for example, being trustworthy and in retaining of knowledge. For example, a Maasai person that demonstrated the use of bed-nets was taken more seriously than a person from any other tribe who showed the same activity. Zebu cows were recognizable and community members preferred the picture that used this bovine breed to a figure with a Holstein cow. Even a demonstration of treatment on a healthy zebu cow could not easily convey the messages. Therefore pictures of animals showing clear signs of the disease, while any form of treatment takes place seemed essential. This obviously was more challenging to develop, but the message uptake seemed better.

An important aspect was that all take home materials needed to be sturdy and environment resistant; laminating handouts ensured a longer life for this material and better uptake through repetition.

Case study 3: One Health approach to a non-zoonotic disease; human and animal parasitism

The community identified parasitic infection as a priority in animals and the hospital identified parasitic infection in humans as a concern. This lead us to consider a research design that investigated gastrointestinal (GI) parasitism in animals and humans in the NCA Tanzania using a One Health approach that addresses both human and animal parasitism. There is a need to consider the importance of any particular disease constraint to the poor, estimate the potential impact achieved by controlling the infection, the probability of achieving that impact and the availability of resources to undertake the work through to completion. This led to our decision to work on GI parasitism in livestock and humans simultaneously as they are closely interlinked. GI parasitism in livestock, for example, results not just in mortalities but also in stunted growth, diarrhoea, etc. The current mitigation strategy for both human and livestock against the impact of parasites is to provide treatment options. Essential for the control of human parasitism is the application of mass drug administration programmes (MDA), increased hygiene, access to clean and potable water, housing standards for hygiene/sanitation and sustained socioeconomic development. MDA have been shown to be among the most cost effective control strategies (Turner et al., 2015). However, despite the donations by pharmaceutical companies of anthelmintics, there is currently no vision on the long-term sustainability of these programmes and the provision of long-lasting benefits (Parker and Allen, 2011). Drug administration in human and livestock populations have had undoubtedly a positive impact, helminth infections, however, persist and these parasites seemed to be resilient to the current intervention strategies. Understanding the social determinants as well as the biological and environmental characteristics of this persistence might prove to be crucial to reduce GI parasitism in the long term.

The project was led by a veterinary PhD student from Canada collaborating with the Tanzania partners (CUHAS Mwanza, Endulen Hospital, NCAA veterinary staff and local primary schools along with health officials from the area) and the team of the University of Calgary. We explored the diversity, ecology, transmission dynamics and socioeconomic impacts of parasites in humans and animals, with the goal of identifying risk factors for parasitism and developing mitigation strategies. We paralleled (or mirrored) the methodologies for human and animal parasitology research to (1) enhance education and engagement of stakeholders, (2) generate novel insights on parasite ecology and control by exploring these separate, but intricately linked, human and animal systems in a comparative framework, and (3) simultaneously and synergistically enhance health promotion in people and animals.

25.5 Conclusion

In this chapter we have discussed the conceptual frameworks that have informed our development of a One Health field school. We have sought to illustrate the value of creating an environment where transdisciplinary teams work with communities to design innovative research, new programme development and enhance engagement from all parties.

Endnotes

1 www.swisstph.ch/en.html.

References

Afsana, K., Habte, D., Hatfield, J., Murphy, J. and Neufeld, V. (2009). *Partnership Assessment Toolkit*. Canadian Coalition for Global Health Research, www.ccghr.ca/resources/partnerships-and-networking/partnership-assessment-tool.

Allen, L.K., Hatfield, J.M., Devetten, G., Ho, J.C. and Manyama, M. (2011). Reducing malaria misdiagnosis: the importance of correctly interpreting Paracheck Pf(R) 'faint test bands' in a low transmission area of Tanzania. *BMC Infectious Diseases*, 11, 308.

AVMA (2008). 'One Health Initiative Task Force', *One Health: A New Professional Imperative*. American Veterinary Medical Association, www.avma.org/KB/Resources/Reports/Documents/onehealth_final.pdf.

Bhutta, Z.A. (2002). Ethics in international health research: a perspective from the developing world. *Bulletin of the World Health Organization*, 80, 114–120.

Catalani, C. and Minkler, M. (2010). Photovoice: a review of the literature in health and public health. *Health Education and Behaviour*, 37, 424–451.

Costello, A. and Zumla, A. (2000). Moving to research partnerships in developing countries. *BMJ*, 321, 827–829.

Homewood, K. and Rodgers, W.A. (1991). *Maasailand Ecology: Pastoralist Development and Wildlife Conservation in Ngorongoro, Tanzania*. Cambridge: Cambridge University Press.

Homewood, K., Lambin, E.F., Coast, E., Kariuki, A., Kikula, I., Kivelia, J., Said, M., Serneels, S. and Thompson, M. (2001). Long-term changes in Serengeti-Mara wildebeest and land cover: pastoralism, population, or policies? *Proceedings of the National Academy of Sciences*, 98, 12544–12549.

Min, B., Allen-Scott, L.K., and Buntain, B. (2013). Transdisciplinary research for complex One Health issues: a scoping review of key concepts. *Preventive Veterinary Medicine*, 112, 222–229.

Nykiforuk, C.I.J., Vallianatos, H. and Nieuwendyk, L.M. (2011). Photovoice as a method for revealing community perceptions of the built and social environment. *International Journal of Qualitative Methods*, 10, 103–124.

Parker, M. and Allen, T. (2011). Does mass drug administration for the integrated treatment of neglected tropical diseases really work? Assessing evidence for the control of schistosomiasis and soil-transmitted helminths in Uganda. *Health Research Policy and Systems*, 9, 3.

Shiu-Thornton, S. (2003). Addressing cultural competency in research: integrating a community-based participatory research approach. *Alcoholism: Clinical and Experimental Research*, 27, 1361–1364.

Simmons, A., Reynolds, R.C. and Swinburn, B. (2011). Defining community capacity building: is it possible? *Preventive Medicine*, 52, 193–199.

Thornton, P., Boone, R., Galvin, K., Burnsilver, S., Waithaka, M., Kuyiah, J., Karanja, S., González-Estrada, E. and Herrero, M. (2007). Coping strategies in livestock-dependent households in East and Southern Africa: a synthesis of four case studies. *Human Ecology*, 35, 461–476.

Turner, H.C., Truscott, J.E., Hollingsworth, T.D., Bettis, A.A., Brooker, S.J., and Anderson, R.M. (2015). Cost and cost-effectiveness of soil-transmitted helminth treatment programmes: systematic review and research needs. *Parasites & Vectors*, 8, 355.

Wang, C. (1999). Photovoice: a participatory action research strategy applied to women's health. *Journal of Women's Health*, 8, 185–192.

Wang, C. and Burris, M.A. (1994). Empowerment through photo novella: portraits of participation. *Health Education Quarterly*, 21, 171–186.

Wang, C. and Burris, M.A. (1997). Photovoice: concept, methodology, and use for participatory needs assessment. *Health Education & Behavior*, 24, 369–387.

Zinsstag, J., Schelling, E., Waltner-Toews, D. and Tanner, M. (2011). From 'One Medicine' to 'One Health' and systemic approaches to health and well-being. *Preventive Veterinary Medicine*, 101, 148–156.

chapter 26

A One Health approach to disease investigation, prevention and control in Bhutan: anthrax case study

Nirmal K. Thapa, Tenzin Tenzin, Karma Wangdi, Tshering Dorji, Jambay Dorjee, Ratna B. Gurung, Kinzang Dukpa and Susan C. Cork

Abstract

During 2010, there was an outbreak of anthrax in which 43 domestic animals died in the Zhemgang district of central Bhutan. There were also eight cases of cutaneous anthrax in humans and one person died following systemic infection. All affected people had a history of contact with the carcasses of infected animals. The outbreak was contained by field staff from the Department of Livestock, Ministry of Agriculture and Forests, and the Department of Public Health, Ministry of Health, using a One Health approach. Concurrent treatment of affected people and sick animals, along with ring vaccination of neighbouring cattle, controlled the outbreak. Enhanced public awareness was created through meetings and a door-to-door advocacy campaign in the area impacted by the outbreak. Comprehensive disease preparedness and response guidelines were subsequently developed with the aim of ensuring an effective and coordinated approach to dealing with human and animal cases and to enhance regional awareness of anthrax in Bhutan. In the case study presented we illustrate how the Department of Livestock and the Department of Public Health in Bhutan have practiced a One Health approach to the control and prevention of zoonotic diseases such as anthrax.

26.1 The Himalayan Kingdom of Bhutan

Bhutan is a landlocked country (38,394km²) located in the Himalayas between India to the south, west and east, and the Tibetan autonomous region of China to the north. The country relies predominantly on primary agriculture and hydropower for its economic base (NAS, 2014). The terrain ranges from 180m above sea level at the Indian border to more than 7,500m above sea level in the high altitude mountain ranges, which remain home to migratory livestock, yak herders and wildlife. The majority of Bhutan's population (est. 673,000) continues to rely on agriculture that provides a livelihood for more than 55 per cent of the population (Labour Force Survey, 2013) and until a decade ago, agriculture was practiced on a subsistence basis (SYB, 2014). Farm crop production is supplemented by keeping different kinds of domestic animals such as cattle for draught work and milking, horses for transport, chickens for eggs and pigs for meat (in some parts of the country). At higher altitudes, herds of yaks and sheep are also kept for draught work and milking. The predominantly

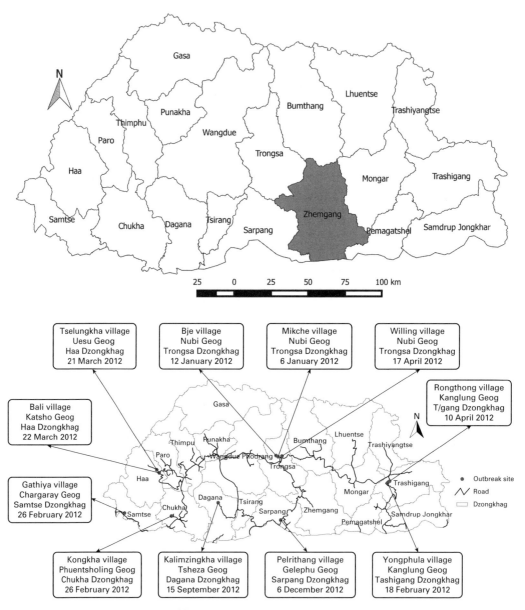

Figure 26.1 Administrative maps of Bhutan showing (above) the location of the anthrax outbreak in 2010 (Zhemgang) and (below) the locations of a number of outbreaks which occurred during 2012.

Buddhist population of Bhutan has great respect for the natural ecosystem and for the wild and domestic animals with whom they share their rural environment. Due to cultural concerns over commercial animal slaughter, much of the domestic meat supply continues to be imported from India.

Administratively, Bhutan is divided into 20 Dzongkhags or districts and each of these is further divided into smaller administrative units or Gewogs (see Figure 26.1). Each Gewog has a basic health unit (BHU) staffed by human health para-professionals and a livestock extension centre (LEC) or a renewal natural resources centre (RNRC) staffed by livestock extension personnel or veterinary para-professionals. These units provide a direct service to village communities. Additional support is provided by human health and veterinary professionals from the Dzongkhag headquarters and the regional level. Animal health services are overseen by the National Centre for Animal Health (NCAH) in Thimphu and are supplemented by livestock and veterinary staff based at Dzongkhag veterinary hospitals (DVH), satellite veterinary laboratories (SVLs) and regional livestock development centres (RLDCs). The latter offers a range of diagnostic services. Public health services at the Gewog and Dzongkhag level are supplemented by medical staff based in a network of regional hospitals. Advanced healthcare and diagnostic support is available in some of the main centres and in the capital city, Thimphu. The government of Bhutan has made a significant investment in staff training with 30 additional veterinarians added to the workforce since 2012 and a growing cadre of health professionals. In recent years, the road network in rural Bhutan has also been expanded but due largely to the terrain, travel in some remote regions continues to pose logistical challenges.

Bhutan is well known for its integrated approach to developing and using renewable natural resources as well as for promoting the concept of gross national happiness (Centre for Bhutan Studies, 2014). Government projects and new initiatives must align with priorities identified in the current (11th) five-year development plan and need to address national goals and objectives developed by Gross National Happiness Commission (GNHC, 2015). The agencies that oversee the operational work of the human health and animal extension services are the Department of Public Health (DoPH, Ministry of Health) and Department of Livestock (DoL, Ministry of Agriculture and Forests) respectively. These two government agencies have been working together to deal with key zoonotic diseases in Bhutan including anthrax, avian influenza, rabies and zoonotic parasites. In the following case study, we describe their collaborative response to an outbreak of anthrax which involved human and animal subjects in Zhemgang district, central Bhutan. Links to the webpages of the key agencies mentioned are provided in the reference section.

26.2 Anthrax, the disease

Anthrax is an acute infectious disease caused by the anaerobic bacterium, *Bacillus anthracis*. This organism is a relatively large, rod shaped, spore bearing bacterium measuring about one by nine micrometres in size. Anthrax derives its name from the Greek word for coal due to the black, coal-like scabs that *Bacillus anthracis* can cause on the skin of infected people (Spencer, 2003). The anthrax bacillus was initially shown to cause disease by the scientist Robert Koch in 1876 and since this time there have been many developments in the production of effective vaccines to protect humans and animals against the disease (Spencer, 2003). The ecology of the disease can be quite complex. In the environment, the bacterium rests as an endospore in the soil. Spores do not form in host tissues unless the infected body fluids are exposed to air. When nutrients are exhausted, resistant spores are formed that can survive in soils for decades. These spores then germinate when exposed to a nutrient-rich environment such as the tissues or blood of an animal or human host. Once ingested, inhaled or placed in an open wound, the bacterium can multiply rapidly and typically kills the animal host within a few days or weeks. There are some differences in species susceptibility to the disease with ruminants considered highly susceptible. This is thought to be partly the result of frequent traumatic injuries to the oral cavity of ruminants grazing pasture and forage plants and subsequent entry of the organism from the environment. The production of powerful exotoxins by the bacteria usually causes rapid death. Clinical cases of anthrax have been reported in many mammalian species including humans (Anon, 2008; WHO, 2015). Animals generally become infected through contact with soil-borne *B. anthracis* spores in areas where previous cases have occurred. Some outbreaks of the disease have also been traced back to contaminated food sources (Fasanella et al., 2013).

Humans usually become infected accidentally through contact with diseased animals or from handling the carcasses or by-products (such as skins and wool) of diseased animals. Infection typically occurs after introduction of the spore through a break in the skin (cutaneous anthrax) or entry through muscosa (gastrointestinal anthrax). Cutaneous anthrax is by far the most commonly reported (90 per cent of cases) form of the disease in humans (Spencer, 2003). After ingestion by macrophages at the site of entry, germination of the vegetative form occurs, followed by extracellular multiplication, together with the production of capsule and toxins. Consumption of meat from infected animals can pose a significant health risk to humans but human-to-human transmission is unlikely (Spencer, 2003; CDC, 2015). Inhalation anthrax can occur if spores (typically 1–2μm diameter) are inhaled and so precautions should be taken when han-

dling infected carcasses and animal products. Historically, human cases of inhalation anthrax (wool sorters' disease) have occurred where large-scale processing of infected hides and wool took place in an enclosed space (Spencer, 2003). Penicillin has long been considered to be the preferred treatment for human cases of the disease and, to date, very few cases of antibiotic resistance have been reported in naturally occurring strains. Post-exposure prophylaxis with antibiotics is generally reserved for cases considered at high risk of infection because of the long duration (60 days) of treatment required. Vaccination is available for humans but is not routinely recommended (Spencer, 2003).

Anthrax is globally widespread and sporadic cases and epizootics have been reported in livestock and wild animals in most parts of the world including North America, Asia and Europe. (Ahmed et al., 2010; Bales et al., 2002; Chakraborty et al., 2012a, 2012b; Harrison et al., 1989; Patra et al., 1998). In 2012, outbreaks of anthrax were reported in 67 countries and in all continents except Antarctica (WAHID, 2015). *Bacillus anthracis* is generally classified within the *B. cereus* group of bacteria along with *B. cereus, B. thuringiensis*, and *B. mycoides* by phenotype. It is the only obligate pathogen in this group. Although it is not possible to discriminate between species by 16S rRNA sequencing, multilocus variable number tandem repeat analysis and other molecular tools provide clear evidence that *B. anthracis* can be clearly differentiated from others of the *B. cereus* group. *B. anthracis* is generally considered to be one of the most molecular monomorphic bacteria characterized. All known strains have been classified into five separate categories (allowing for geographical identification) on the basis of variable numbers of tandem repeats in the variable region of the VrrA gene (Keim et al., 2000). Molecular characterization can be used to study the molecular epidemiology of outbreaks.

As mentioned above, the spores of anthrax are very resistant to environmental elements and can survive for decades in undisturbed earth. This can result in some areas of land being considered an ongoing source of infection. If the affected area is small it can be fenced off, but in most cases this is not feasible and routine vaccination is recommended especially where outbreaks have occurred on a regular basis. There are a wide range of vaccines available for use in livestock (Anon, 2008) and many countries produce their own vaccine products against the disease. Outbreaks have recently been reported in Australia, Africa and Asia (CFSPH, 2007) and often occur after heavy rainfall when anthrax spores get disturbed and brought to the surface (Anon, 2008). Anthrax is considered to be endemic in India and Bangladesh, and several outbreaks and sporadic cases have been reported in animals and humans (Ahmed et al., 2010; Chakraborty et al., 2012a, 2012b; Siddiqui et al., 2012). In Bhutan, sporadic outbreaks of anthrax occur annually among animals, especially ruminants, posing health risks to people who come into contact with the infected animals and their by-products (Tenzin et al., 2012).

Anthrax is a notifiable disease in Bhutan but routine vaccination of livestock is not recommended. However, in places where there have been outbreaks, vaccination is undertaken annually for three years. This is discontinued if no cases have been reported during that period. Sporadic cases have been reported from different parts of the country but historic cases may have gone unreported in both animals and humans due to the passive reporting system and the absence of clear prevention and control guidelines. As a result of this, it was felt necessary to develop comprehensive guidelines for dealing with anthrax on both the human and animal health side and for the departments of Livestock and Public Health to work together to develop a One Health approach (Ministry of Health, 2015).

The first edition of the anthrax guidelines (DoPH, 2013) was developed by the anthrax working group consisting of experts from the Department of Public Health and the Department of Livestock. This is one of several such documents being developed using the One Health approach. Similar guidelines have been developed for avian influenza and rabies and others will be developed for a priority list of zoonotic diseases of importance in Bhutan.

26.3 Zhemgang case study

In 2010 there was a major outbreak of anthrax in the Zhemgang district of central Bhutan (see Figure 26.1). The outbreak impacted 14 households in six different villages. Skin lesions were reported in eight people including a schoolchild. Livestock infected included 25 cattle (predominantly Jersey cross), eight horses, four pigs and six cats, which died over a six-week period (Thapa et al., 2014). The treatment for the human cases was the use of antibiotics (Procaine penicillin) and for animals it involved antibiotic treatment (penicillin) for sick animals and vaccination of healthy animals in the affected region using anthrax vaccines produced in-country at the Biological production unit at NCAH. A mass public awareness campaign was also implemented in the outbreak area.

Anthrax cases in cattle had previously been reported in Trongsa and Wangdue in 1989 and 1998 respectively. These cases had been linked to human deaths that were associated with the consumption of infected meat. In some districts of Bhutan, the local people have become familiar with the disease but in the 2010 outbreak it became apparent that many of the farmers in Zhemgang were not familiar with the characteristic clinical presentation of the disease nor were the communities aware of the zoonotic risk.

The 2010 anthrax outbreak began during July (summer) in cattle in a remote village. From July to September it spread to eight neighbouring villages, where humans also became infected. There had not been any previous cases reported in this region of Bhutan. The 2010 outbreak began after a period of heavy rainfall, which may have brought spores to the soil surface, where they could be ingested by ruminants grazing in the area (Thapa et al., 2014). As mentioned earlier in the chapter, ruminant livestock and some ruminant wildlife are highly susceptible to the disease (Anon, 2008). Due to the robust nature of anthrax spores, it is recommended that the carcasses of animals that have died from the disease are buried and not handled or butchered. In the case of wild or free-roaming animals, the carcasses are often predated by wild carnivores and spores can be widely distributed resulting in a disease risk to other animals in the area. With reports of several sudden deaths in cattle and skin lesions in humans who had handled these cattle (Plates 34 and 35), a multisectoral team from local and regional animal and public health offices in Bhutan visited the outbreak area to conduct an investigation and to establish a disease control programme.

A case of anthrax is suspected when an animal dies suddenly and becomes quickly bloated with a bloody discharge from the nose and other orifices; the disease is confirmed if rod-shaped bacilli are found by blood smear examination. Livestock extension staff in Bhutan are familiar with the clinical presentation of the disease and samples are usually collected to confirm the diagnosis of anthrax. This is because some other diseases can cause similar clinical signs. If livestock staff are called to a case early, they ensure that the carcasses of infected livestock are not opened and that dead animals are buried whole to avoid environmental contamination with the resistant anthrax spores and to minimize public health risk.

If anthrax is suspected, blood smears are taken from the ear vein of dead animals then fixed, stained and examined under the microscope in one of the Dzongkhag veterinary hospital laboratories. During the Zhemgang investigation, these samples were collected to confirm the

diagnosis and *B. anthracis* was later isolated from three samples (two ear tip and one nasal swab) collected from three cattle (from three separate villages). In this investigation, additional samples from animals with positive blood smears were also referred to the US Centers for Disease Control and Prevention (Atlanta, GA) for culture and strain characterization. Isolates were later characterized by molecular techniques (multilocus variable-number tandem repeat analysis) which detected the strain to be of B1 lineage (genotype 83) and canonical single-nucleotide polymorphism subgroup B.Br.001/002 unlike the A lineage of India and Bangladesh (Thapa et al., 2014).The significance of this finding is not yet clear, but anthrax bacteria may have entered the country through a variety of routes including imported products and then become established in some regions of the country.

In the index village, i.e., where the first cases were reported, a cow had died suddenly after a brief illness; the animal exhibited discharge of un-clotted blood from nostrils, and its carcass was bloated (Plate 34). The owner of the affected herd had opened the carcass and dressed the meat, which he shared or sold within the village for human consumption. Through tracing of subsequent cases it was revealed that transportation of infected meat to neighbouring villages resulted in the spread of disease with subsequent death among animal herds in eight other villages. In some instances, the horses that were used to carry contaminated meat also became infected and died of anthrax.

In the remote villages of Bhutan, meat from dead animals is often consumed because meat is in short supply and villagers often lack awareness of zoonotic diseases that might harm them. As in many other remote Bhutanese villages, the farmers in villages affected by this outbreak were unaware of the signs of anthrax in animals or of the public health implications of the disease. To address this, the investigation team held an education meeting involving the farmers and a teacher of the school to make villagers aware of the risks associated with anthrax and also door-to-door advocacy was conducted in the area. The villagers cooperated during the investigation and in the subsequent response to the disease, including the correct disposal of carcasses and recall and disposal of meat from the carcasses that had been kept for human consumption. Villagers were also actively engaged in the anthrax control measures such as the treatment of affected animals and ring vaccination of animals that had been in contact with infected animals.

During July–September, a total of 43 animals in nine villages died: 25 cattle, eight horses, four pigs and six cats (see Table 26.1). The infected cats were most likely exposed to B. anthracis through the ingestion of meat from infected carcasses because Bhutanese families often share their food with pet cats and dogs. Cases included predominantly adults with both males and females affected.

The collaborative interdisciplinary disease investigation engaged the local (Gewog) basic health unit (BHU) and LEC staff who found that, within one week of exposure to infected livestock, characteristic skin lesions developed on eight villagers who had handled and dressed the animal carcasses. Another person developed the systemic form of anthrax. The cutaneous lesions were the black eschars typical of anthrax (Taylor and Carslaw, 1967; Spencer, 2003), and occurred on the patients' necks, fingers, arms, feet, legs or cheeks (Plate 35). The person that died had developed abdominal cramps, vomiting and respiratory distress, which is suspected to be due to the gastrointestinal form of anthrax because it occurred at the same time as the cutaneous form in others was observed. This person had ingested contaminated meat, although due to the remote nature of the village, samples were not collected and the diagnosis could not be confirmed.

To stop the spread of disease, animal and public health authorities initiated various prevention and control measures including a campaign to create awareness among villagers and they also developed targeted education for students. BHU staff promptly treated clinically affected and exposed village people and also later referred cases to another BHU which had a resident doctor. The BHU staff also coordinated a farmers' meeting in the area involving schoolchildren and teachers. It is well-recognized that raising public awareness and effective knowledge translation are essential components for an effective One Health approach to dealing with zoonotic diseases.

LEC staff with assistance from the Dzongkhag and regional veterinary staff coordinated ring vaccination of cattle against anthrax (est. 445 animals in 11 villages) along with treatment of sick animals using antibiotics. This approach ensured that all potentially 'at risk' cattle within a defined radius of the area affected by the outbreak were protected against the disease. A programme to ensure the correct disposal of

Table 26.1 Cases reported during the Zhemgang outbreak (2014)

Species	Number at risk	Number of cases	Number of deaths
Bovine	350	27	25
Swine	70	4	4
Equine	100	8	8
Feline	60	6	6
Total	580	45	43

potentially infected carcasses in deep burial pits was also implemented along with recall, collection and disposal into burial pits of all potentially infected meat and hides from cattle that died of suspected or confirmed anthrax. These control measures, along with the education and care of exposed villagers eventually contained the outbreak.

Following this outbreak investigation in Zhemgang, the One Health team recommended the following measures:

- Development of comprehensive guidelines for anthrax surveillance among humans and animals.
- Recording of all notifiable disease outbreaks of the country in the transboundary animal diseases online information database (TAD Info). Hence, with the help of the information from TAD Info (National Centre for Animal Health, 2015), the establishment of surveillance for anthrax hot-spot areas could be initiated.
- Development of education programmes to teach persons at high risk (e.g., butchers, meat handlers working in the meat shop) about anthrax transmission.
- Ensure that the public are aware of the care of skin abrasions, and disease-prevention measures, including personal hygiene practices and encourage people not to eat meat from dead or sick animals.

26.4 Anthrax and public health – case discussion

In Bhutan, sporadic anthrax cases in animals are detected and reported every year; such cases pose health risks to humans (Tenzin et al., 2012). The emergence in 2010 of a significant anthrax outbreak in remote villages in central Bhutan was most likely linked to heavy rainfall, which can bring B. anthracis spores to the soil surface, where

they can be ingested by animals. The cutaneous anthrax cases described in this case study are similar to those reported at the human–animal interface in other countries. In 1979 and 1980, more than 6,000 human cases were associated with the slaughter of B. anthracis-infected cattle (Turner, 1980) and 25 cutaneous anthrax cases occurred in humans in Paraguay in 1987 after the slaughter of a single B. anthracis-infected cow (Harrison et al., 1989). Many cases of cutaneous anthrax have been reported in humans following the slaughter of sick or dead animals in India (Chakraborty et al., 2012a, 2012b), Bangladesh (Siddiqui et al., 2012) and China (Ting-Lu et al., 2012). For humans, the major risk factors for exposure to B. anthracis are direct or indirect contact with infected animals or contaminated animal products such as meat and animal skins. People at high risk for exposure, such as farm staff and butchers, should be made aware of those risks and of the public health implications of zoonotic diseases such as anthrax (WHO, 2015). Due to the close links between livestock and villagers in remote Bhutanese villages, any family member is potentially at risk if handling animals or animal products that are infected with anthrax. It is important that human and animal extension staff work closely together to ensure that clear and consistent messages are provided on the prevention and control of zoonotic diseases such as anthrax, rabies and avian influenza. These messages must also be clearly articulated at the department and ministry level. From the Zhemgang outbreak investigation and other cases in Bhutan, a number of recommendations have been developed and these have now been published as the 2013 guidelines for anthrax prevention and control in Bhutan.

26.5 One Health in Bhutan – summary

Globally, the emergence and re-emergence of infectious zoonotic diseases has been a major driver for the adoption of a One Health approach to disease management. In Bhutan, the emergence of highly pathogenic avian influenza (HPAI) caused by H5N1 virus in the region in 2003 provided an opportunity among the Department of Livestock (Ministry of Agriculture and Forests) and Department of Public Health (Ministry of Health) to work together to develop the National Influenza Pandemic Preparedness and Response Plan (NIPPRP) based on the One Health concept. The first outbreak of H5N1 in poultry in February 2010 brought human and animal health authorities together along with other relevant stakeholders to prevent and combat the disease in poultry and prevent its transmission to humans. This provided a solid collaborative base for the development of additional One Health initiatives. The relationships established during this time subsequently provided the foundations for the development and implementation of an effective rabies control programme and the development of the anthrax prevention and control guidelines. The anthrax investigation described in this chapter illustrates how the Department of Livestock and Department of Public Health worked together to control the outbreak using a One Health approach. The approach used was effective in controlling the outbreak and also raised public awareness in order to prevent future outbreaks of the disease in humans and animals. Knowledge translation and engagement of villagers in the control and prevention planning was also a key component of the approach.

References

Ahmed, B., Sultana, Y., Fatema, D.S.M., Ara, K., Begum, N., Mostanzid, S.M. and Jubayer, S. (2010). Anthrax: an emerging zoonotic disease in Bangladesh. *Bangladesh Journal of Medical Microbiology*, 4, 46–50.

Anon (2008). OIE, WHO & FAO: Anthrax in Humans and Animals, www.who.int/csr/resources/publications/anthrax_webs.pdf.

Bales, M.E., Dannenberg, A.L., Brachman, P.S., Kaufmann, A.F., Klatsky, P.C. and Ashford, D.A. (2002). Epidemiologic response to anthrax outbreaks: field investigations, 1950–2001. *Emerging Infectious Diseases*, 8, 1163–1174.

CDC (2015). *Anthrax Fact Sheet*, www.cdc.gov/anthrax.

Centre for Bhutan Studies (2014). www.bhutanstudies.org.bt.

CFSPH (2007). *Institute for International Cooperation in Animal Biologics & OIE: Animal Disease Information, Anthrax*. Center for Food Security & Public Health, www.cfsph.iastate.edu/Factsheets/pdfs/anthrax.pdf.

Chakraborty, A., Khan, S.U., Hasnat, M.A., Parveen, S., Islam, M.S., Mikolon, A., Chakraborty, R.K., Ahmed, B.N., Ara, K., Haider, N., Zaki, S.R., Hoffmaster, A.R., Rahman, M., Luby, S.P. and Hossain, M.J. (2012a). Anthrax outbreaks in Bangladesh, 2009–2010. *American Journal of Tropical Medicine & Hygiene*, 86, 703–710.

Chakraborty, P.P., Thakurt, S.G., Satpathi, P.S., Hansda, S., Sit, S., Achar A. and Banerjee, D. (2012b). Outbreak of cutaneous anthrax in a tribal village: a clinic-epidemiological study. *Journal of the Association of Physicians India*, 60, 89–93.

DoPH (2013). *Department of Public Health Guidelines for Preparedness, Surveillance and Control of Anthrax in Human and Animals in Bhutan*. Ministry of Health, Royal Government of Bhutan.

Fasanella, A., Garofolo, G., Hossain, M.J., Shamsuddin, M., Blackburn, J.K. and Hugh-Jones, M. (2013). Bangladesh anthrax outbreaks are probably caused by contaminated livestock feed. *Epidemiology & Infection*, 141, 1021.

GNHC (2015). *Gross National Happiness Commission*, www.gnhc.gov.bt/five-year-plan and www.gnhc.gov.bt/about-us.

Harrison, L.H., Ezzell, J.W., Abshire, T.G., Kidd, S. and Kaufmann, A.F. (1989). Evaluation of serologic tests for diagnosis of anthrax after an outbreak of cutaneous anthrax in Paraguay. *Journal of Infectious Diseases*, 160, 706–710.

Keim, P., Price, L.B., Klevytska, A.M., Smith, K.L., Schupp, J.M., Okinaka, R., Jackson, P.J. and Hugh-Jones, M.E. (2000). Multiple-locus variable-number tandem repeat analysis reveals genetic relationships within *Bacillus anthracis*. *Journal of Bacteriology*, 182, 2928–2936.

Labour Force Survey, Bhutan (2013). www.ilo.org/dyn/lfsurvey/lfsurvey.list?p_lang=en&p_country=BT.

Ministry of Agriculture and Forests (2015). www.moaf.gov.bt.

Ministry of Health (2015). www.health.gov.bt.

NAS (2014). *National Statistical Bureau of Bhutan*, www.nsb.gov.bt/main/main.php#&slider1=4 .

National Centre for Animal Health (2015). *Serbithang*, www.ncah.gov.bt.

Patra, G., Vassaire, J., Weber-Levy, M., Le Doujet, C. and Mock, M. (1998). Molecular characterization of *Bacillus* strains involved in outbreaks of anthrax in France in 1997. *Journal of Clinical Microbiology*, 36, 3412–3414.

Siddiqui, M.A., Khan, M.A.H., Ahmed, S.S., Anwar, K.S., Akhtaruzzaman, S.M. and Salam, M.A. (2012). Recent outbreak of cutaneous anthrax in Bangladesh: clinico-demographic profile and treatment outcome of cases attended at Rajshahi Medical College Hospital. *BMC Research Notes*, 5, 464.

Spencer, R.C. (2003). *Bacillus anthracis* (review). *Journal of Clinical Pathology*, 56, 182–187.

SYB (2014). *Statistical Year Book (Bhutan)*, www.nsb.gov.bt/publication/publications.php?id=3.

Taylor, L. and Carslaw, R.W. (1967) Cutaneous anthrax. *Lancet*, 1(7501), 1214–1216.

Tenzin, Dukpa, K., Tshering, Y. and Thapa, L. (2012). *Status of Notifiable Animal Diseases in Bhutan, 2011–2012*, www.ncah.gov.bt/reports.php?page=2.

Thapa, N.K., Tenzin, Wangdi, K., Dorji, T., Migma, Dorjee, J., Martson, C.K. and Hoffmaster, A.R. (2014). Investigation and control of anthrax outbreak at the human–animal interface, Bhutan, 2010. *Emerging Infectious Diseases*, 20(9), 1524–1526.

Ting-Lu, Z., Liang-Liang, C., Li, L., Ming-Lei, Z., Fang, Q., Liang, Y. and Chang-jun, B. (2012). Investigation of an outbreak of cutaneous anthrax in Banlu village, Lianyungang, China. *Western Pacific Surveillance Response Journal*, 3, 12–15.

Turner, M. (1980). Anthrax in humans in Zimbabwe. *Central African Journal of Medicine*, 26, 160–161.

WAHID (2015). World Animal Health Information Database: Detailed Country Disease Incidence (OIE). www.oie.int/wahis_2/public/wahid.php/diseaseinformation/statusdetail.

WHO (2015). *Anthrax*, www.who.int/csr/disease/Anthrax/en.

chapter 27

Development of One Health training programmes

David C. Hall and Stanley G. Fenwick

Abstract

One Health training has developed rapidly in the last five years from workshop-based teaching and learning to flexible modules addressing core One Health competencies to complete undergraduate and graduate degrees in One Health. Important elements of One Health training based on past and current programmes include: communication; cultural awareness; complexity and systems thinking; policy formulation; and some element of management and leadership training. An important consideration for instructors and designers of curriculum is the need to include opportunities to engage with transdisciplinary teams during training, whether in One Health research or application.

27.1 Introduction

Training in One Health is currently offered by a wide range of institutions ranging from purely academic programmes to informal training for professionals to components of regional projects supported by international development organizations. This chapter will briefly identify some of the characteristics of students claiming interest in One Health training, briefly identify several representative One Health training programmes currently on offer, and go into detail of two recently implemented programmes.

27.2 Characteristics of students of One Health

Students of One Health come from a variety of academic and professional backgrounds and express an assortment of One Health training needs and expected applications. Given the broadly defined nature of a One Health approach, this should not be surprising, but it does make it challenging for course developers to generate a One Health training programme that addresses the needs of the majority of individuals, rather than reflects the requirements of local health priorities. This requires some flexibility in how One Health modules are designed, which is an important point we address later in this chapter.

Based on questionnaire replies from more than 200 health professionals and students living in Canada,[1] Hall (2015) identified the characteristics of individuals claiming interest in taking some form of online training in One Health. Nearly two-thirds of respondents felt One Health training would be valuable to their career and to their profession (Plate 36), but fewer than 20 per cent reported they had engaged in some sort of formal One Health training such as taking courses outside their discipline. The most common reasons given were lack of awareness of training options, cost of training and time to complete training. More than 50 per cent of respondents reported they interacted more than once a month with a colleague outside their health discipline. The primary reason for engaging in One Health training was updating of knowledge; enhancing career options was a close second reason. Most participants also stated they would want certification following training, and would expect their employer to fund the costs of training.

Of those respondents who expressed interest in some form of continuing education (CE) in One Health, online or otherwise, the preference for top three preferred choices of CE environments for learning were self-paced with online modules (29.5 per cent), classroom interactive settings (20.5 per cent) and any media but self-paced on his/her own (20 per cent). Online interactive classrooms with a rigid schedule ranked least popular (10.5 per cent). Nearly half of respondents stated they could spend no more than one to three hours per week on CE.

These results reflect respondents surveyed in Canada. During One Health workshops in Asia from 2010 to 2012, similar questions were asked of about 100 Southeast Asian participants with similar backgrounds in health and related professions. More than 80 per cent of participants in these settings expressed strong preference for in-person workshop training with certification. Part of the difference may be due to the desire

expressed by the latter participants to attend workshops outside their office or country, meet new colleagues from other countries in their region and limited ability to access the internet for training during working hours.

Internet accessibility and bandwidth have been noted as constraints to online learning by other colleagues working in Southeast Asia with potential university participants,[2] although the rapid pace of low-cost access to the internet may make this a more reasonable option in the next few years. A co-taught university course in One Health between the Universities of Alberta and Calgary utilized the internet for live lectures between the two venues. Even in this setting where internet access and bandwidth is reliable and where technology is a low-level barrier for teaching, instructors found set-up and use of the internet could be a challenge to maintaining contact with both classrooms. More importantly, they found the lack of a personal connection with students in the classroom as opposed to visual and audio teleconferencing was intimidating and stifled a richer discussion among students. Nevertheless, options for improved online teaching are rapidly developing, with demand driven by students.

27.3 The Asia Partnership on Emerging Infectious Diseases Research (APEIR) and the BECA project

In 2006, the Asia Partnership on Emerging Infectious Diseases Research (APEIR)[3] was established as a research network linking One Health researchers, practitioners and government representatives from Cambodia, China, Lao PDR, Indonesia, Thailand and Vietnam. APEIR began largely in response to the spread of highly pathogenic avian influenza (HPAI) in the region and expanded its scope to all emerging infectious diseases in 2009. APEIR assists to facilitate communication and knowledge sharing among countries, aiming to mitigate the threat of emerging infectious diseases (EIDs) and their burden. Among the capacity-building objectives of APEIR are knowledge generation, coordination of research activities and enabling science-based policy formulation.

Expanding on and supportive of the network initiated by the APEIR partnership, the Building Capacity for Research and Practice in Ecosystem Approaches to Health in Southeast Asia' (hereafter 'BECA') project was active in Southeast Asia from early 2010 to March 2013. BECA was set up as a research and capacity-building project to investigate the processes involved in building the capacity for research and application of One Health approaches to health management among researchers, development practitioners and policymakers in Southeast Asia. The research also investigated the methodologies and tools that contribute to effective capacity-building in One Health approaches. The BECA project was funded by the International Development Research Centre (IDRC) and Australian Agency for International Development (AusAID), and implemented by several partners including the Universities of Calgary, Prince Edward Island, Guelph and VWB/VSF-Canada.[4]

Objectives and methods

The working hypothesis of the BECA project was that bringing actors together from different countries and institutions with an array of experience and expertise in the prevention of EIDs, public health, and health promotion will enable participants to investigate and respond more effectively to complex ecohealth issues, with a particular focus on EIDs. The BECA activities, linked with APEIR and other initiatives in the region, were designed to contribute in the longer term to an effective network of expertise in One Health approaches to managing health while

contributing to policy formulation. The target audiences of the project included academic researchers, government staff and extension personnel involved in promoting integration and application of One Health approaches in activities that directly benefit communities in need.

The BECA project used a number of methods and techniques to address objectives, including:

- Active participation of participants, particularly country level leaders (focal points).
- Knowledge-building through large group workshops and smaller focused meetings.
- Foundational knowledge training in specific ecohealth concepts.
- Sharing of lessons from application of ecohealth concepts (workshop settings, conference presentations, courses delivered elsewhere by BECA participants).
- Development of policy briefs.
- Participant contribution to workshop reports.
- Communication methods including dedicated internet site for sharing resources, online discussions, conference presentations and peer-reviewed (journal) articles.
- Linkages with other institutional initiatives.
- Monitoring and evaluation tools including questionnaires, elements of outcome mapping, one-on-one semi-structured interviews, structured telephone interviews, SWOT analysis, GAP analysis and performance indicator analysis.

A key to successful implementation of the BECA project was identification and active participation of country-level focal points who assisted in maintaining regular communication with project participants and guided activities of the workshops and meetings and application of ecohealth lessons in country-level projects. Focal points were particularly helpful in identifying potential participants and in-country collaborators, and often led discussions during workshops and meetings, encouraging participation of their fellow country participants. The project also relied heavily on recruitment of a skilled and diplomatic project manager, a position that was not easy to fill or maintain.

Workshops provided foundational knowledge training in specific One Health concepts, and sharing of lessons from application of One Health concepts identified by participants. The project participants found workshops useful for two key reasons: (1) participants appreciated guided and effective information transfer, and (2) workshops were an ideal method for engaging participants in learning and sharing of experiences. The workshop topics chosen were based on the following One Health themes[5] selected and agreed on by project leaders and, where possible, workshop participants:

- Fundamentals of ecohealth.
- Researchable issues in ecohealth.
- Using research to advise ecohealth policy formulation.
- Evaluation training in outcome mapping and other methods.
- Building on complexity.
- Policy briefs and project planning.
- Complexity frameworks and application.
- Implementing ecohealth in Southeast Asia.
- Project evaluation.
- Ecohealth application to rabies control in Bali, Indonesia.

While this list of topics is far from exhaustive, participants and project leaders felt it captured sufficiently the information needed for a participant to achieve moderate understanding of One Health concepts, and be able to apply these concepts in research project grant-writing and policy-reporting. These themes are similar to those of other One Health training projects that have since developed in the region and elsewhere.

Lessons shared, lessons learned

An important component of the BECA One Health training activities was sharing of participants' experiences. The BECA project design anticipated that participants would share One Health lessons from their various health projects and activities as well as apply lessons learned in a transdisciplinary context with their various project partners. Participants were generous in sharing One Health lessons from their various projects, and were enthusiastic to identify and discuss One Health opportunities they had not previously considered. This level of interaction was appreciated by all participants. However, although workshop participants were chosen in part based on self-identification of involvement in health research projects, participants reported that it was far more challenging to apply their new One Health knowledge, primarily for three reasons. First, many participants either lacked engagement with or were not part of the leadership structure of a health project, which they felt prevented them from applying new knowledge. Second, junior participants felt uneasy suggesting to more senior colleagues they had new ideas to approach management of health problems. Finally, participants expressed some frustration with the lack of a step-by-step application manual that might guide implementation of a One Health framework, such as might be used for risk assessment or benefit–cost analysis.

A further opportunity for sharing of lessons learned came with the training and subsequent exercise in writing a policy brief proposing a One Health approach to a health problem in participants' home countries. The BECA project observed a wide range of experiences and attitudes to engagement with policy formulation. For many participants, particularly those from countries with centrally planned economies, the notion that all stakeholders have a stake in input to policy formulation was a novel and sometimes worrying concept. For those participants, the important One Health lesson regarding knowledge to action was understood but implementation was considered the domain of government representatives and not scientists. A relatively uncomplicated solution was to rename 'policy briefs' as 'information bulletins' or 'advisory statements'. In summary, as a methodology for investigating researchable issues, developing skills in policy advocacy and communication, the BECA project learned that the policy brief is a valuable tool, but requires substantial leading and support writing to generate a final product.

Boundary partners and regional programmes

The BECA project made an effort to capitalize on initiatives already active in the region (e.g., APEIR) and to partner with institutions interested in developing new One Health training programmes. Key among the project boundary partners[6] and institutions were government agencies (Ministries of Health, Agriculture and Rural Development), academic institutions (e.g., Kunming Medical University, Chiang Mai University, Hanoi School of Public Health, Vietnam National Institute of Veterinary Research), local NGOs (e.g., CIVAS Indonesia), international government and research institutions (e.g., FAO-UN, ILRI) and provincial and district health officers. The BECA project was also acknowledged for its role, along with several other One Health capacity-building projects and partners, in contributing to development of several academic programmes (e.g., One Health programmes at the Hanoi School of Public Health, Chiang Mai University and Gadja Mada University, Indonesia) and two Ecohealth Resource Centres in Southeast Asia (EHRCs in Chiang Mai University, Thailand and Gadja Mada University, Indonesia). An important message is these initiatives were the result of multiple partners engaged in One Health training at application in Southeast Asia, often reflecting guidance from participants and project leaders who aimed to work towards common objectives.

27.4 The Southeast Asia One Health University Network

The Southeast Asia One Health University Network (SEAOHUN) was established with assistance from USAID[7] and the RESPOND project in 2011 as a consortium of research universities in Indonesia, Malaysia, Thailand and Vietnam with the objective of increasing transdisciplinary capacity of regional institutions to respond to outbreaks of emerging infectious diseases (EIDs) in Southeast Asia. SEAOHUN is achieving this objective by enabling collaboration between these universities in their efforts to build capacity and academic partnerships with government, national and regional stakeholders in responding to outbreaks of emerging infectious diseases in Southeast Asia (SEAOHUN, 2014).

Core competencies and technical modules

SEAOHUN began with and has maintained training in One Health core competencies and One Health technical modules as follows:

The seven One Health core competency modules are:

1. Collaboration and Partnership
2. Communication and Informatics
3. Culture, Beliefs, Values and Ethics
4. Leadership
5. Management
6. Policy, Advocacy and Regulation
7. Systems Thinking

The seven One Health technical modules are:

1. One Health Concepts and Knowledge
2. Fundamentals of Infectious Disease
3. Infectious Disease Management
4. Epidemiology and Risk Analysis
5. Fundamentals of Public Heath
6. Ecosystem Health
7. Behaviour Change

These competencies provide the skills, knowledge and technical training to apply expertise in a One Health context. The modules are considered interdependent in that an understanding of one competency (e.g., infectious disease management) would typically require understanding of concept and application of other competencies (e.g., behaviour change).

Competency training is adjusted to fit the needs and desired learning outcomes of individual institutions and countries. Table 27.1 shows the current approach used in Southeast Asia, illustrating slight modifications across countries. The One Health University Network is also upscaling activities in Africa, although we leave out discussion of those activities in this chapter for brevity and due to the early stage of development of the African dimension of the project.

The core competency modules are designed to be flexible enough that instructors can teach them as standalone modules or integrate them into the technical modules. For example, a SEAOHUN instructor aiming to deliver a session on how to change stakeholder behaviour might choose to teach culture and communication skills as separate units or choose to integrate those

Table 27.1 The RESPOND One Health competency framework applied by SEAOHUN in the region

RESPOND ONE HEALTH COMPETENCY FRAMEWORK					
Global Domains February 2014	SEAOHUN Regional Domains	Malaysia	Indonesia	Thailand	Vietnam
Management	Management	Management	Management	Planning and Management	Planning and Management
Communication	Communications and Informatics	Communication	Communication	Communications and Informatics	Communications and Informatics
Culture and Beliefs	Culture and Beliefs	Culture and Belief	Culture and Belief	Culture and Ethics	Culture and Beliefs
Leadership	Leadership	Leadership and Professionalism	Leadership and Professionalism	Leadership	Leadership
Collaboration and Partnership	Collaboration and Partnership	Collaboration and Partnership	Collaboration	Collaboration and Partnership	Collaboration and Partnership
Values and Ethics	Values and Ethics	Ethics	Values and Ethics		Values and Ethics
Systems Thinking	Systems Thinking	Systems Thinking	Systems Thinking	Systems Thinking	Systems Thinking
				One Health Knowledge	Policy, Regulation and Advocacy

concepts into teaching units addressing behaviour change. Similarly, part or all of a module(s) can be combined to form a new One Health course or inserted in existing courses. Course content can easily be adapted to fit local examples, content, and level of audience ability.

As well as course training, SEAOHUN participants are often engaged in research activities with universities, research institutes and national and international government organizations. Country level priorities will differ but the ability to adapt SEAOHUN teaching to fit the needs and priorities of country participants is an important element, making training more appropriate and outcomes more sustainable than they might be with an inflexible series of training modules.

The Vietnam One Health University Network (VOHUN)

We illustrate the application of the SEAOHUN training in One Health with reference to Vietnam where the programme has been active since November 2011. The project has brought together 17 universities in Vietnam specializing in teaching and research in medicine, veterinary science and public health. In order to facilitate implementation of activities in Vietnam, the Hanoi School of Public Health was identified as the Vietnam One Health University Network (VOHUN) National Coordinating Office. This has allowed for effective coordination between universities, research institutes, policy formulating agencies and IGOs.

The VOHUN programme expects to develop a One Health educational curricula leading to a Bachelor's degree as well as graduate degrees at both the MSc and PhD level. Both entry level and mid-career professionals will be eligible for training. VOHUN is also actively engaged in research activities, currently focusing on avian influenza, anthrax, rabies and waterborne as well as foodborne diseases.

For those members not actively taking course training or away from VOHUN centres, the VOHUN programme maintains collaboration and communication with the use of newsletters and an actively updated website (www.vohun. org). Numerous documents, modules and news can be found on the site, which is available in both Vietnamese and English. VOHUN members frequently participate in national and international meetings and conferences, as well as sharing their experiences and occasionally engaging in training with their counterpart university networks in Thailand (THOHUN), Malaysia (MyOHUN) and Indonesia (INDOHUN).

27.5 Additional One Health training projects

The activities of APEIR, the BECA project and the SEAOHUN training programme illustrate the rapidly growing interest and participation over the past five years in One Health training, both in terms of demand and development of training options. In an earlier report, Hall and Coghlan (2011) developed a bibliography of One Health projects and institutions engaged in One Health activities including training programmes, listing more than 100 entries. That listing is now well out of date, but a current listing is available on the website linked to this book, identifying training programmes ranging from short courses and online modules to university curricula and One Health degree programmes. A few of those programmes deserve mention here.

The Field Building Leadership Initiative (FBLI) (www.ecohealthasia.net) is a five-year initiative that focuses on One Health research, capacity-building and knowledge translation in order to solve human health problems associated with agricultural intensification and related challenges in China, Indonesia, Thailand and Vietnam. APEIR and the BECA project were two of many other initiatives and institutions including universities and research organizations active in the region that contributed lessons and input to development of the original FBLI framework. This is a good example of the development of One Health training, research, and application in the region that has benefitted from lessons of past programmes. Further details regarding the FBLI programme can be found on their website.

As One Health gains momentum, universities in at least five continents are offering One Health training in their curriculum. Typically these are optional courses or elements of other courses and programmes designed to develop core competency in transdisciplinarity, complexity and systems thinking, communication and cultural awareness. Many examples can be found in the United States including Tufts University, University of Minnesota and the University of Wisconsin-Madison, and in Canada at the Universities of Alberta, Calgary, Guelph, Saskatchewan and Prince Edward Island. A recent example of a baccalaureate programme is the One Health Undergraduate Degree Programme taught at Berry College in Georgia, US. The programme engages faculties and facilities from across campus, including the Berry One Health Center. Students typically enrol in a related life science major (e.g., animal science) while completing required and elective One Health coursework and undergraduate research projects.

In the EU, an interesting recent One Health training related development is the Network for Evaluation of One Health (neoh.onehealthglobal.net), a project supported by the EU COST (European Cooperation in Science and Technology) and coordinated by the Royal Veterinary College, University of London. The main objective of the NEOH network is not training but rather evaluation of One Health activities, which of course would reflect on training. The approach is currently quantitative and intended to guide policymakers in decisions regarding policy formulation embracing a wider One Health approach. NEOH exists as an open network bringing together expertise from a wide spectrum of disciplines.

27.6 Conclusions: common themes in One Health training

In terms of core competencies in One Health, some conclusions can be reached based on the material and curriculums of the BECA project, the SEAOHUN, and the various other academic and continuing education programmes noted in this chapter. Solid foundational knowledge in life sciences (which could be coincident with an undergraduate major in a complementary social science) seems necessary as a starting point, but not sufficient to address broader concepts such as complexity, communication and policy development. As well, lessons from past projects indicate opportunities to apply One Health training are an essential part of a successful One Health curriculum.

Beyond foundational knowledge in a life science, common elements of One Health training based on current offerings include the following: communication; cultural awareness; complexity and systems thinking; policy formulation; and some element of management and leadership training. Just as a practicing veterinarian or socioeconomist cannot be expected to develop high level competency without some degree of applied 'real world' experience, coursework alone will not generate One Health practitioners. In most One Health training programmes there is recognition that engagement with real-world problem-solving during training is essential. Typically this is achieved through participation in existing research.

What might be more important though is engagement in a real-world problem as a member of a transdisciplinary team, whether that team is researching problems or applying solutions. The importance of learning to work in a transdisciplinary group also highlights the need for One Health training programmes to consider learning platforms or formats. Research on demand for One Health training (Hall, 2015) and the experiences of One Health projects in Asia indicate that working in groups is not only desirable by trainees but also highly effective in building communication and transdisciplinary skills. As well, group work during training often solidifies the network building important to a One Health approach.

Finally, context matters. One of the reasons for the success of the SEAOHUN network is the flexibility it provides to country members to adapt lessons to suit their local One Health training needs and circumstances. Not only classroom materials and curricula but also field exercises should reflect health priorities at primarily the local level, but also country and regional level.

Endnotes

1   Respondents were selected from across Canada and identified themselves as either students or practitioners of: human or veterinary health including medicine, nursing, dentistry, chiropractic; animal science or biology; wildlife biology; and ecological sciences. Selection of respondents was equitably weighted for age, sex, location and income.
2   Pattamaporn Kittayapong, Mahidol University, Thailand, pers. comm., 2012, regarding options and barriers to setting up a co-taught One Health programme between universities in Thailand and Canada.
3   http://apeiresearch.net/new/main.php.

4   Veterinarians without Borders/Vétérinaires sans Frontières–Canada (VWB/VSF–Canada).
5   For the sake of maintaining the titles of the workshops and meetings, the term 'ecohealth' is preserved in this list.
6   Earle et al. (2001) define boundary partners as 'those individuals, groups, or organizations with whom the program interacts directly and with whom the program can anticipate opportunities for influence'. Even though the programme works with boundary partners to effect change, it does not control them. Thus, the power to influence development rests with them.
7   The United States Agency for International Development (USAid) funds the Emerging Pandemic Threats (EPT) programme that aims to strengthen capacity to prevent, detect and control infectious diseases in animals and people. The EPT has four main components/projects with the self-descriptive titles PREDICT, PREVENT, IDENTIFY and RESPOND. SEAOHUN is part of the RESPOND component.

References

Earle, S., Carden, F., and Smutylo, T. (2001). *Outcome Mapping: Building Learning and Reflection into Development Programs*. Ottawa: International Development Research Centre.

Hall, D.C. (2015). *Characteristics of Demand for On-line Training in One Health*. Working paper, University of Calgary.

Hall, D.C. and Coghlan, B. (2011). Implementation of the One Health Approach in Asia & Europe: How to Set Up a Common Basis for Action and Exchange of Experience. Brussels: EEAS-EU.

SEAOHUN (2014). *SEAOHUN One Health: An Introduction to the Southeast Asia One Health University Network*. Washington, DC: USAID.

chapter 28

Engagement of Indigenous peoples in One Health education and research

Stephanie Montesanti and Wilfreda (Billie) E. Thurston

Abstract

The term 'One Health' is increasingly being used in veterinary and human medicine to refer to the interdependence between the health of people, animals and entire ecosystems. The relationship between people, their environment and non-human entities is central to Indigenous understandings of health and wellbeing, which preceded the One Health concept. In this chapter we describe the Indigenous connection to land and its importance to the health and wellbeing of Indigenous populations in Canada and internationally, drawing mainly on Canada for specific examples. We applied the One Health approach to understand how government policies on natural resource management and First Nation governance continue to threaten Indigenous ways of life and ultimately impact their health and wellbeing. The One Health concept provides a useful framework in understanding current structural and systemic forces that have threatened the relationship that Indigenous people have to their land and animals.

28.1 Introduction

The Ottawa Charter for Health Promotion identified the importance of environments supportive to health, stating that the inextricable links between people and their environment are the basis for a socioecological approach to health (WHO, 1986). This WHO charter advocated for protection of natural and built environments, and conservation of natural resources as essential to the health of populations. The relationship between people, their environment and non-human entities, is central to Indigenous understandings of health and wellbeing. Indigenous peoples across the globe share a deep understanding of their land, and its spiritual connection with the people, a connection that plays a key role in providing safe and healthy environments (Burgess et al., 2009). The land is therefore a fundamental component of Indigenous culture and identity, having physical, spiritual, cultural and emotional bonds (Hudson-Rodd, 1998; Kirmayer et al., 2000; Brown, 2001; Scougall, 2002; Richmond et al., 2005).

Indigenous peoples have a long history of using a wide variety of natural resources as well as knowledge and traditional practices relating to the management of these resources. Colonization and treaty processes resulted in the loss of widespread access to traditional territories and relationships supporting the hunting, gathering, fishing and cultivation of traditional Indigenous foods (Morrison, 2011; Richmond et al., 2005). Structural processes (e.g., assimilative efforts of the Indian Act in Canada (1876), expansion of commercial agriculture, and environmental changes) have acted to significantly limit the ways in which Indigenous peoples can use and relate to environmental and non-human resources within their traditional territories (e.g., traditional, ceremonial and recreational activities) (Beckford et al., 2014; Wyatt, 2008). The processes through which Aboriginal people's access to the resources of their traditional environments is reduced has been referred to as 'environmental dispossession' (Richmond and Ross, 2009). The physical displacement of Indigenous peoples from their traditional lands and territories, in Canada and around the world, has negatively affected the collective wellbeing of Indigenous populations. Loss of land is argued to be among the most significant factors contributing to culture stress within Indigenous communities (Bartlett, 2003).

In this chapter we describe the Indigenous connection to land and its importance to the health and wellbeing of Indigenous populations in Canada and internationally. We provide an example of how Aboriginal farmers in Canada are in a different social context than their non-Aboriginal counterparts. This social context applies equally to fishers and hunters. We discuss colonial and treaty processes that have threatened Indigenous connections to the land and non-human entities. There is little academic literature on Indigenous farming in both historical and contemporary contexts. Consequently, there is limited knowledge of how government policies on agriculture and First Nations governance continue to threaten Indigenous ways of life on

reserves and ultimately impact their health and wellbeing. This is a symptom of the colonial past. Understanding how Indigenous agriculture, fishing and hunting have evolved is important for fields of veterinary and human public health that have much to offer in terms of a One Health approach to Indigenous communities. Effective participation and promotion of Indigenous rights is critical to the management and sustainability of Indigenous lands, the natural resources and the cultural identity of Indigenous peoples. Effective participation in research is now a requirement of many Indigenous peoples that requires a set of skills that veterinary and human public health researchers may not be taught. In this chapter, we will use the term 'Indigenous' to refer to Aboriginal peoples in an international context. However, we acknowledge that neither 'Aboriginal' nor 'Indigenous' has been used without controversy and no clear consensus exists on which label is most preferable. It is advisable when approaching a community to ask what term is preferred.

28.2 Background

Terminology

'Aboriginal peoples' is the term used to describe the original peoples who inhabited North America before European settlers arrived, and the descendants of those original peoples. Aboriginal peoples are First Nations (i.e., North American Indians), Métis and Inuit – each having unique heritages, languages, cultural practices and spiritual beliefs. Whereas the majority of First Nations and Métis live in the western provinces and Ontario, most Inuit live in Labrador and the Northwest Territories, Nunavut and the Yukon. 'Aboriginal' is the term commonly used in Canada. More recently scholars have pushed to replace the word 'Aboriginal' with the more uniting and less colonizing term

'Indigenous' (Institute for Aboriginal Peoples Health, 2013). 'Indigenous' is considered by some to be the most inclusive term, since it identifies Aboriginal communities in similar circumstances, while acknowledging their diverse histories (Asch, 2014).

Many Indigenous communities have experienced the full force of governmental assimilationist policies (e.g., the Indian Act (1876), residential schools, disenfranchisement). The Indigenous populations in Canada, the US, Australia and New Zealand share similar experiences of British colonization that have shaped Indigenous–settler relations in each country. First Nations (registered status and non-status Indians), Métis and Inuit in Canada, Australian Aboriginal and Torres Strait Islander peoples, New Zealand Maori, and American Indians and Alaska Native tribes in the US have each been subjected to oppression and marginalization through colonial policies (Wilson and Ellender, 2002).

Treaties and Indigenous land rights in Canada, US, Australia and New Zealand

There are differences with respect to Indigenous relations with central governments and to land rights in each country. Between 1871 and 1921, the Crown entered into treaties with various First Nations that enabled the Canadian government to actively pursue agriculture, settlement and resource development of the Canadian west and the north. Under these treaties, the First Nations who occupied these territories gave up large areas of land to the Crown. In exchange, the treaties provided for such things as reserve lands and other benefits such as farm equipment and animals, annual payments, ammunition, clothing and certain rights to hunt and fish (Asch, 2014). Eleven treaties were signed by the Crown with First Nations peoples in Canada.

Native title encompassed the interests of Indigenous people to benefit from activities on their ancestral lands, including the pursuit of subsistence. Recognition of native title and restoration of some land rights to Aboriginal Australians are very recent, while most American Indian nations have exercised at least some jurisdiction over reserved lands for decades and, in some cases, much longer, and some of those reserved lands are extensive. Many First Nations in Canada have some measure of control over reserved lands, but in nearly all such cases the lands are miniscule and First Nations do not have direct ownership (Cornell, 2004). Maori people, having suffered massive land losses over the years, have been engaged in a major effort in recent decades to regain significant lands and resources (Cornell, 2004).

In recent decades, there have also been changes in the relationships between Indigenous peoples and the federal state to promote Indigenous peoples rights. In Canada, Indigenous rights were included in the Canadian Constitution Act of 1982, and affirmed in the Royal Commission on Aboriginal Peoples, which examined the social, economic, legal and health status of Indigenous peoples (Aboriginal Affairs and Northern Development Canada, 1996). While there has been gradual movement towards increased recognition of Aboriginal and treaty rights since 1982, progress has been slow (Asch, 2014). Governments must consult Aboriginal communities when developments are proposed on their lands. However, consultation as currently practised is largely one-sided, with many communities feeling powerless in decisions about their lands (Asch, 2014). Current federal policy in the US recognizes tribal sovereignty.

In the US, tribes were granted new taxation powers in the 1980s, allowing them to better fund their own social programmes and, as in Canada, there has been devolution of control over health and social services to Indigenous communities since the mid-1980s (Cornell, 2004).

Self-governance is fundamentally designed to provide tribal governments with more control and decision-making authority over the federal financial resources provided to them. Federally recognized tribes in the US have a formal nation-to-nation relationship with the US government. However, federal regulations and laws that prevent tribal governments from equitable access to federal programmes on par with state and local governments have shaped the extent of tribal sovereignty (www.ncai.org).

In Australia, Indigenous peoples were granted rights to equal pay in 1965, and a 1967 referendum transferred some powers in respect to Indigenous peoples from the states to the federal government, leading to the establishment of an Indigenous representative body, the Aboriginal and Torres Strait Islander Commission (ATSIC). In New Zealand, the Treaty of Waitangi Act was amended in 1985 to strengthen the mandate of the Waitangi Claims Tribunal to hear claims of historical breaches of the treaty, and the 1993 Maori Land Law Act strengthened Maori land claims. New Zealand is the only one of the four countries in which there are a number of dedicated parliamentary seats for Indigenous people, and this number of Maori seats was increased in 1995 (Armitage, 1995).

Indigenous conceptualizations of health and wellbeing

In a majority of Indigenous communities with a close linkage to the land, the concept of health is holistic, involving physical, social, emotional, spiritual, cultural and environmental wellbeing (Committee on Indigenous Health, 1999; Lutschini, 2005; Boulton-Lewis et al., 2002) and is based on relationships with people and the land (Burgess et al., 2005). The land is described in Indigenous communities as 'a resource, which behaves as a living being and a life support system for humans' (Barrera-Bassols and Zinck,

2003, p. 232). International literature similarly identifies the centrality that land plays in Indigenous identity and health (Garnett et al., 2009; Hudson-Rodd, 1998; Kirmayer et al., 2000; Brown, 2001; Scougall, 2002; Richmond et al., 2005). Thus, the land is a fundamental component of Indigenous culture, and central to the health and wellness of Indigenous communities.

Indigenous peoples in Victoria, Australia, talk about 'caring for country' defined as having knowledge, sense of responsibility and inherent right to be involved in the management of traditional lands (Kingsley et al., 2009). For the Cree of Whapmagoostui in northern Quebec, health is about living a 'Cree way of life' that is imbued with robust connections to the physical and spiritual northern landscape (Adelson, 2000, p. 62). Health is 'inseparable from being able to hunt, pursue traditional activities, live well in the bush, eat the right foods, keep warm, and provide for oneself and others' (Adelson, 2000, p. 97). Anthropologist Naomi Adelson (2000) translates the Wemindji Cree term for 'health' as the subjective experience of 'being alive well'. This concern for 'being alive well' encompasses the wildlife and the land.

Bastein (2004) in her book *Blackfoot Ways of Knowing: The Worldview of the Siksikaitsitapi*, explains how that the Blackfoot Nations in the western prairies in Canada organize themselves according to their observations of the natural world and their understanding of the relationship with the environment (Bastein, 2004, p. 12). The belief system of the Blackfoot people includes a belief in the spiritual nature of the animals and their ability to communicate scared knowledge to humans (Bastein, 2004, p. 11). Some species often feature prominently in the language, ceremonies and narratives of Indigenous peoples and can be considered cultural icons. For instance, the bison has traditionally been considered a sacred animal in the Blackfoot culture and was part of ceremonies as well as a staple food source. However, with

European colonization, the relationship with the bison shifted from a ceremonial and survival relationship to one of commercial use (Bastein, 2004, p. 18). With the introduction of horses and guns, newly nomadic First Nations groups could shoot bison, speeding up the rate of the bison hunt (Isenberg, 2001). Commercialization and capitalism brought on by European contact resulted in the near-extinction of the bison (Isenberg, 2001).

Richmond and colleagues examined the perceptions of environment, economy and health among the 'Namgis First Nation community in Alert Bay, British Columbia, and found that their perceptions of health and wellbeing were intricately connected to economic choice and opportunity. The degree of autonomy over environmental resources allows Indigenous groups to have control and ownership in managing natural resources on their land that is accorded to them as a consequence of their land rights. Autonomy over environmental resources (i.e., land, water, wildlife, fish and minerals) allows First Nation communities the choice and opportunity to create economic development that empowers the community, thereby impacting their health and wellbeing (Richmond et al., 2005). The authors also argue that good health and wellbeing is dependent not only on economic development, but also on participation in the political decision-making that deeply undermines environmental resource development (Richmond et al., 2005).

28.3 One Health and Aboriginal epistemology and ontology

Public health for both humans and animals has traditionally been concerned with the prevention of disease and promotion of population health. However, public health researchers and practitioners continually grapple with complex problems that are not entirely human (Rock and Degeling,

2015). The non-human world includes animals, plants, microbes, environments and technologies (Rock et al., 2009). The term 'One Health' is increasingly being used in veterinary medicine to refer to interdependence between the health of people, animals and entire ecosystems and this term is gaining prominence in human public health as well. The One Health approach has been predominantly applied to pathogens that can be transmitted from animals to people (i.e., zoonotic diseases), but it has implications that extend well beyond the prevention and control of infectious diseases (Green, 2012; Rock et al., 2009; Zinsstag et al. 2011). This shift follows from recognizing that non-human animals along with environments and settings contribute materially to the health and wellbeing of people (Rock and Degeling, 2015).

Indigenous worldviews and knowledge about health and wellbeing preceded the evolving concept of One Health in veterinary and human medicine (Green, 2012). Therefore, the One Health concept provides a useful framework in understanding current structural and systemic forces that have threatened the relationship that Indigenous people have to their land and animals. This is demonstrated in the introduction of Aboriginal farming in Canada under colonial and treaty processes that threatened Indigenous culture and identity pertinent to their health and wellbeing.

28.4 Canadian case example: Aboriginal farming

Aboriginal people in Canada were introduced to crop farming when they were relocated to reserves in order to assimilate them in mainstream culture and to 'civilize' them. Experts were sent by Indian Affairs to teach on-reserve populations how to farm (Miller, 2000). There were specific provisions in the treaties to provide the people with farming implements and seeds.

Bovine spongiform encephalopathy and First Nation cattle producers

On 20 May 2003, a single cow in Wanham, Alberta, tested positive for bovine spongiform encephalopathy (BSE), or what is commonly referred to as 'mad cow disease'. Almost immediately more than 40 countries closed their borders to animals suspected of having the disease (cattle, sheep, goats, bison, elk, deer), meat products and animal by-products originating from Canada. Canada's federal and provincial governments responded swiftly by introducing a number of financial intervention programmes to aid cattle producers who were financially impacted by the crisis. While cattle producers from across the country took advantage of various federal and provincial support programmes, anecdotal reports emerged that First Nation cattle producers had not benefited from government programmes. The Indigenous Land Management Institute at the University of Saskatchewan reports that most First Nation producers in the province failed to even apply for government funding despite potentially qualifying for millions of dollars of government aid.

However, crop farming on the reserves was set up to fail. The Indian Act (1876) was established with the fundamental goal of assimilating the First Nations (Miller, 2000) and Indian Agents micromanaged reserve life. This micromanagement included all facets of reserve agriculture. Many reserves were located in areas not suited to farming crops (e.g., maize, wheat), and many grain seeds and farming implements promised to First Nations never materialized (Miller, 2000). On-reserve farmers were frustrated by government policies of control and emphasis on individualism (e.g., self-reliance) at the expense of traditional collectivism in the Indigenous culture, which acted to undermine their efforts (Tang, 2003). Rudolph and McLachlan (2013) describe that commercial agriculture radically altered the landscape and eradicated the food sovereignty of Indigenous communities. Today, Indigenous farmers in Canada are still disadvantaged, as they cannot leverage reserve lands for operating loans from banks (SWDM, 2010). This also poses impacts related to economic choice and opportunity for Indigenous communities (Richmond et al., 2005). Indigenous farmers may not be part of local or regional associations through which other farmers are reached and

their relationship to the federal government regulatory bodies will not necessarily be the same (see box for an example concerning BSE).

Effective participation of Indigenous peoples in decision-making

Indigenous people have different connections to both national and provincial governments and therefore to agricultural departments than non-Aboriginal peoples. While the health of non-Indigenous people is the responsibility of provinces, for instance, Indigenous peoples' health on reserve in Canada is the responsibility of Health Canada. Treaties are also between First Nations and the government of Canada; therefore, First Nations prefer to negotiate with that level of government. However, in any situation it is best to confirm with a given Indigenous group or First Nations which agency they are accountable to in terms of regulations (see box for an example).

Environment and natural resources

Aboriginal Affairs and Northern Development Canada (AANDC) transfers responsibility and control over lands, resources and the environment to Aboriginal people and northerners through land claim and self-government agreements and devolution to territorial governments. At the same time, AANDC fulfils an important role in developing natural resources and protecting the environment in most First Nations communities and the territories.

The need to consult Indigenous people in the management of natural resources on their land has become a major issue across Canada and internationally. Indigenous people also benefit from a 'duty to consult', which originates from the constitutional protection of their rights and the Crown's fiduciary responsibilities that obliges governments to take measures to avoid infringing on these rights (Newman, 2014). In practice, the meaning of 'consultation' and 'Indigenous participation' is not clear, and often governments or industries may provide information to Indigenous communities or seek their opinions. However, even when information is shared, such consultation processes rarely include Aboriginal peoples in decision-making and do not fully take Indigenous rights into account (Newman, 2014). Limited participation of Indigenous communities in decision-making on the management and use of natural resources poses an infringement on Indigenous rights and autonomy. A number of cases in Canada have been reported where Indigenous communities were not involved in the decision-making about government or industry practices on their land: oil sand production on First Nation reserves (Passelac-Ross and Potes, 2007; Hipwell et al.,

2002), forestry management (Wyatt, 2008) and commercial fishery (Richmond et al., 2005).

Canadian First Nations have been active since the 1970s in negotiating co-management arrangements with the Canadian government that would increase their participation in decisions concerning the land and use of natural resources. These negotiations have transformed and continue to transform the way in which resource management is undertaken in various Canadian provinces (Agrawal, 1995). Environmental decision-making has historically been the domain of government bureaucrats trained in the scientific tradition, who may have little understanding of the cultural context in which Indigenous people live. With the advent of increased self-determination in many regions (e.g., land claims, treaty entitlement settlements), Indigenous people are seeking to increase their role in environmental decision-making, as it directly concerns their traditional lands (Purcell and Onjoro, 2002). By promoting the recognition and use of their traditional knowledge in environmental decision-making, Indigenous people will have a greater capacity to contribute to, and thus exert control over, decisions pertaining to their traditional lands. In co-management of natural resources worldwide, Indigenous peoples not only seek greater control over land and resources, but aim for processes that will lead to management decisions that are closer to their values and worldviews, reflecting to a wider extent the traditional knowledge that they possess about the land (Purcell and Onjoro, 2002).

Scientists, managers and policymakers are now recognizing the value of Indigenous knowledge. By employing traditional knowledge, a greater depth of environmental information can be brought to bear, along with a more holistic understanding of the relationships among living beings and their environments (Huntington, 2000). In Canada, governments, industrial corporations, and other organizations have tried to promote meaningful consideration of Indigenous knowledge in environmental and land-use decision-making, acknowledging that such consideration can foster more culturally appropriate and environmentally sustainable relationships between Indigenous peoples and their environment. Examples of Indigenous participation in environmental decision-making is observed in the forest sector and mining sector.

Efforts to promote the capacity of Indigenous people to bring Indigenous knowledge in environmental decision-making have, however, not lead to any meaningful changes in the engagement of Indigenous people in decision-making. This is especially concerning with regard to the use of their land and resources, primarily because government and industry has failed to overcome certain significant barriers to involving Indigenous people in environmental decision-making. These barriers include government and industry difficulties in understanding the values, practices and context underlying Indigenous knowledge; and political barriers, resulting from an unwillingness to acknowledge Indigenous knowledge that may conflict with the agendas of government or industry. Indigenous knowledge has normally been transferred using an oral tradition. Western scientists value written texts. In addition, the critical ontology of Indigenous peoples (i.e., their worldview) as characterized by Kovach (2009, p. 49) is 'all we can know for sure is our own experience'. This knowledge is 'nested in place and kinship systems' (Kovach, 2009, p. 67). Western scientists may have a difficult time respecting such knowledge and granting it credibility, let alone privileging it in decisions about the land and animals. Agrawal (1995) suggests that the tendency to create a distinction between Indigenous and scientific knowledge poses challenges to integrate both Indigenous and scientific knowledge. Instead, Agrawal (1995) argues that there is a need to move beyond this distinction between the different forms of knowledge and to work towards building bridges across the Indigenous and scientific divide.

28.5 Conclusion

Scholars of Indigenous research methodology discuss creating an ethical space for engagement between Indigenous peoples and western society (Kovach, 2009; Fletcher, 2003; Smith, 2009). Creation of this space requires a level of cultural competency beyond familiarization with the special cultural symbols or practices of a given nation or tribe. Oelke et al., (2013) present a range of competencies from sensitivity, awareness and competency to safety and advocacy. Acquiring these competencies requires an effort on the part of the researcher or practitioner of public health to understand their own cultures (ethnic, academic, sports, etc.) and how these shape their own experiences. They can then move on to learning about and from Indigenous cultures, ontologies and epistemologies and how relationships can be built to improve research and practice. The One Health model is a benefit to opening conversations and building cross-cultural cooperation and dialogue. It is a step in reconciling worldviews. Researchers and practitioners would also be wise to understand the experience of Indigenous peoples with research and interventions in the past so as to begin building a relationship with Indigenous peoples that is founded in a long-term goal of reconciliation.

References

Aboriginal Affairs and Northern Development Canada (1996). *Royal Commission Report on Aboriginal Peoples*, www.aadnc-aandc.gc.ca/eng/1307458586 498/1307458751962.

Adelson, N. (2000). *Being Alive Well: Health and the Politics of Cree Well-Being*. Toronto: University of Toronto Press.

Agrawal, A. (1995). Dismantling the divide between indigenous and scientific knowledge. *Development and Change*, 26(3), 413–439.

Armitage, A. (1995) *Comparing the Policy of Aboriginal Assimilation: Australia, Canada, and New Zealand.* Vancouver: UBC Press.

Asch, M. (2014). *On Being Here to Stay: Treaties and Aboriginal Rights in Canada.* Toronto: University of Toronto Press.

Barrera-Bassols, N. and Zinck, A. (2003). 'Land moves and behaves': Indigenous discourse on sustainable land management in Pichataro, Patzcuaro Basin, Mexico. *Geografiska Annaler*, 85(3–4), 229–245.

Bartlett, J.G. (2003). Involuntary cultural change, stress phenomenon and Aboriginal health status. *Canadian Journal of Public Health*, 94, 165–167.

Bastein, B. (2004). *Blackfoot Ways of Knowing: The Worldview of the Siksikaitsitapi.* Calgary: University of Calgary Press.

Beckford, C.L., Jacobs, C., Williams, N. and Russell, N. (2014). Aboriginal environmental wisdom, stewardship, and sustainability: lessons from the Walpole Island First Nations, Ontario, Canada. *The Journal of Environmental Education*, 41, 239–248.

Boulton-Lewis, G.M., Pillay, H.K., Wilss, L & Lewis, D.C. (2002). Conceptions of health and illness held by Australian Aboriginal, Torres Strait Islander, and Papua New Guinea health science students. *Australian Journal of Primary Health*, 8(2), 9–16.

Brown, R. (2001). Australian Indigenous mental health. *Australian and New Zealand Journal of Mental Health Nursing*, 10(1), 33–41.

Burgess, C., Johnston, F.H., Bowman, D. and Whitehead, P.J. (2005). Healthy country: healthy people? Exploring the health benefits of Indigenous natural resource management. *Australian and New Zealand Journal of Public Health*, 29, 117–122.

Burgess, C.P., Johnston, F., Berry, H.L., McDonnell, J., Yibarbuk, D., Gunabarra, C., Mileran, A. and Bailie, R.S. (2009). Healthy country, healthy people: the relationship between Indigenous health status and 'caring for country'. *Medical Journal of Australia*, 190, 567–572.

Committee on Indigenous Health (1999). *The Geneva Declaration on the Health and Survival of Indigenous Peoples.* Geneva: World Health Organization.

Cornell, S. (2004). *Indigenous Jurisdiction and Daily Life: Evidence from North America*, www.gtcentre. unsw.edu.au/ publications/ papers/ docs/ 2005/ 6_StephenCornell.pdf.

Fletcher, C. (2003). Community-based participatory research relationships with Aboriginal communi-

ties in Canada: an overview of context and process. *Pimatisiwin: A Journal of Aboriginal and Indigenous Community Health*, 1(1), 28–62.

Garnett, S., Sithole, B., Whitehead, P., Burgess, C., Johnston, F. and Lea, T. (2009). Healthy country, healthy people: policy implications of links between Indigenous human health and environmental condition in tropical Australia. *The Australian Journal of Public Administration*, 68(1), 53–66.

Green, J. (2012). One Health, One Medicine, and critical public health. *Critical Public Health*, 22, 377–381.

Hipwell, W., Mamen, K., Weitner, V. and Whiteman, G. (2002). *Aboriginal Peoples and Mining in Canada: Consultation, Participation & Prospects for Change.* Ottawa: The North-South Institute.

Hudson-Rodd, N. (1998). Nineteenth century Canada: Indigenous place of disease. *Health & Place*, 4(1), 55–66.

Huntington, H.P. (2000). Using traditional ecological knowledge in science: methods and applications. *Ecological Applications*, 10(5), 1270–1274.

Institute for Aboriginal Peoples Health (2013). Indigenous or Aboriginal. *Aboriginal Health Research News*, 2, 1–4.

Isenberg, A. (2001). *The Destruction of the Bison: An Environmental History, 1750–1920.* Cambridge: Cambridge University Press.

Kingsley, J., Townsend, M., Phillips, R. and Aldous, D. (2009). 'If the land is healthy . . . it makes the people healthy': the relationships between caring for country and health for the Yorta Yorta Nation, Boonwurrung and Bangerang tribes. *Health & Place*, 15, 291–299.

Kirmayer, L.J., Brass, G.M. and Tait, C.L. (2000). Introduction, the mental health of Aboriginal peoples: transformation of identity and community. In L.J. Kirmayer, M.E. Macdonald and G.M. Brass (eds), *The Mental Health of Indigenous Peoples.* Montreal: McGill University, pp. 5–26.

Kovach, M. (2009). *Indigenous Methodologies: Characteristics, Conversations, and Contexts.* Toronto: University of Toronto Press.

Lutschini, M. (2005). Engaging with holism in Australian Aboriginal health policy – a review. *Australian and New Zealand Health Policy*, 2(15), 1–10.

Miller, J.R. (2000). *Skyscrapers Hide the Heavens: A History of Indian–White Relations in Canada*, 3rd edn. Toronto: University of Toronto Press.

Morrison, D. (2011). Indigenous food sovereignty – a model for social learning. In H. Wittman, A.A. Desmarais and N. Wiebe (eds), *Food Sovereignty in*

Canada: Creating Just and Sustainable Food Systems. Halifax: Fernwood Publishing, pp. 97–113.

Newman, D. (2014). *Revisiting the Duty to Consult Aboriginal Peoples*. Saskatoon: Purich Publishing.

Oelke, N., Thurston, W.E. and Arthur, N. (2013). Intersections between interprofessional collaborative practice, cultural competency and primary healthcare. *Journal of Interprofessional Care*, 27(5), 367–272.

Passelac-Ross, M. and Potes, V. (2007). *Crown Consultation with Aboriginal Peoples in Oil Sands Development: Is it Adequate, is it Legal?* Calgary: Canadian Institute of Resources Law.

Purcell, T. and Onjoro, E.A. (2002). Indigenous knowledge, power and parity: models of knowledge integration. In P. Sillitoe, A. Bicker and J. Pottier (eds.), *Participating in Development: Approaches to Indigenous Knowledge*. New York: Routledge, pp. 162–188.

Richmond, C. and Ross, N. (2009). The determinants of First Nation and Inuit health: a critical population health approach. *Health & Place*, 15, 403–411.

Richmond, C., Elliot, S.J., Matthews, R. and Elliott, B. (2005). The political ecology of health: perceptions of environment, economy, health and well-being among 'Namgis First Nation'. *Health and Place*, 11, 349–365.

Rock, M. and Degeling, C. (2015). Public health ethics and more-than-human solidarity. *Social Science & Medicine*, 129, 61–67.

Rock, M.J., Buntain, B., Hatfield, J. and Hallgrímsson, B. (2009). Animal–human connections, 'One Health', and the syndemic approach to prevention. *Social Science & Medicine*, 68, 991–995.

Rudolph, K.R. and McLachlan, S.M. (2013). Seeking Indigenous food sovereignty: origins of and responses to the food crisis in northern Manitoba, Canada. *Local Environment: The International Journal of Justice and Sustainability*, 19(9), 1079–1098.

Scougall, J. (2002). Away from Wadjelas: the significance of urban place for the Tkalka Boorda Aboriginal community. *Urban Policy and Research*, 20(1), 57–72.

Smith, L.T. (2009). *Decolonizing Methodologies: Research and Indigenous Peoples*. London: Zed Books.

SWDM (2010). *First Nations and Métis Farming*. Saskatchewan Western Development Museum, http://wdm.ca.

Tang, E. (2003). *Agriculture: The Relationship Between Aboriginal and Non-Aboriginal Farmers*. Saskatoon: Western Development Museum/Saskatchewan Indian Cultural Centre Partnership Project.

Wilson, L. and Ellender, I. (2002). Aboriginal versus European perspectives on country. *Philosophy Activism Nature*, 2, 55–62.

WHO (1986). Ottawa Charter for Health Promotion. In *International Conference on Health Promotion: The Move Towards a New Public Health*. Ottawa: World Health Organization, Health and Welfare Canada, Canadian Public Health Association.

Wyatt, S. (2008). First Nations, forest lands, and 'aboriginal forestry' in Canada: from exclusion to comanagement and beyond. *Canadian Journal of Forest Research*, 38, 171–180.

Zinsstag, J., Schelling, E., Waltner-Toews, D. and Tanner, M. (2011). From 'One Medicine' to 'One Health' and systemic approaches to health and well-being. *Preventative Veterinary Medicine*, 101, 148–156.

appendix

Searching for One Health information: guidance for students

Lorraine Toews, Bonnie Buntain and Michelle North

Abstract

The ability to conduct high quality One Health research, or apply the latest One Health approach to practice, is directly related to the ability to access high quality information. There are a number of constraints to literature searches restricting practitioners' access to high-quality information especially in rural areas and in low and middle-income countries with poor internet connectivity and access to library information resources including training. These constraints will need to be addressed before true One Health practice can be implemented on a global scale. This appendix aims to address some of the difficulties associated with finding One Health information by providing guidance on internet search methods and numerous resources to facilitate the search process.

The challenge of One Health literature searches

Using the One Health approach is, by definition, public health practice involving many disciplines and stakeholders. Modern practitioners of veterinary and human preventive medicine are exposed to a growing arsenal of publications touting One Health as a way to solve complex health challenges in human and animal populations impacted by social and ecosystem determinants of health (Min et al., 2013). Practitioners and researchers require access to research-based information for One Health programme research, education and outreach, but face many barriers and challenges in locating and accessing this information (Revere et al., 2007).

The literature supporting a One Health approach is multidisciplinary and dispersed across a wide variety of journals and government resources (Alpi, 2005). This literature is indexed in many different research databases, mainly in accordance with academic disciplinary parameters, so researchers and practitioners must often search multiple databases to locate the literature they require (Alpi, 2005). Each of the One Health disciplines has its own distinctive conceptual frameworks and terminology, so searchers must often use different search terms in each database to ensure complete information retrieval. Whether the purpose of a search is to inform a One Health practice decision, or to produce research on the conceptual framework of One Health, the searcher must account for the varying terminology in his or her search strategies. To complicate matters further, the indexing terms used in many health research databases often do not reflect the full range of concepts present in the human and veterinary medicine public health literature (Alpi, 2005), making precise and complete One Health literature searches very challenging.

In addition to peer-reviewed publications, grey literature is a key source of information for One Health practice. Grey literature is 'that which is produced on all levels of government, academics, business and industry in print and electronic formats, but which is not controlled by commercial publishers' (New York Academy of Medicine, 2014). The types of grey literature that are particularly important for One Health are: conference proceedings, meeting abstracts and reports from government agencies, professional societies, and policy and research institutes. Although much grey literature is posted on the internet, inconsistent organization and indexing, and vulnerability to changes in political priorities and website restructuring, result in it being difficult to retrieve (Alpi, 2005).

Additional barriers to accessing this information are faced by One Health practitioners who are not affiliated with post-secondary or healthcare institutions or government agencies. In most countries, only libraries associated with these institutions are subscribed to peer-reviewed electronic journals and research databases, and access to the resources is limited to students and employees only. Consequently, One Health practitioners who are not affiliated with these institutions do not have access to much of the research-based information they require.

One Health practitioners and researchers in low and middle-income countries (LMICs) face similar barriers in accessing research-based information. While a growing number of peer-reviewed electronic journals are open-access and freely accessible on the internet, a significant number are still available only by subscription. The subscription fees for some journals and research databases put them out of reach for many institutions in these countries. In addition to the lack of access to these critically important information resources, LMIC One Health practitioners and researchers often lack access to the services and expertise of professional librarians, who can provide training in the selection of appropriate databases and effective online search techniques (Alpi, 2005). LMIC One Health practitioners and researchers may also lack access to adequate information technology infrastructure and support, resulting in limited or inconsistent internet access. When submitting articles to peer-reviewed journals, LMIC One Health practitioners and researchers may also encounter bias toward the health issues of developed- rather than developing nations (McMichael et al., 2005). Finally, many journals from developing nations are not indexed in major databases such as PubMed or Agricola, so references from these journals are more difficult to locate. To address some of these issues, the World Health Organization and its regional offices initiated several programmes and partnerships with major publishers to provide developing countries with access to biomedical and health sciences e-journals, e-books and reference resources, as well as training in the use of these resources. Publicly funded non-profit institutions in most LMICs are eligible to register for these programmes (Van Essen et al., 2014).

How to conduct a One Health literature search

The nature and purpose of your research will determine whether your search needs to be brief and focused, comprehensive or something in between. To help decide what kind of search you should do, ask yourself:

- What is my end-product? For example, support for a professional practice decision, a systematic review, scoping review (Grant and Booth, 2009) or policy paper?
- Do I only need key papers, or do I need to retrieve all papers relevant to my topic?
- Do I need to retrieve only published journal literature or also unpublished studies and reports?

Translate your research question(s) into search question(s)

- State your topic as a question or series of concise questions.
- From these question(s), parse out the key concepts that you want to be present in your search results. Usually you will have two to four key concepts per question, which will become the building blocks of your search strategy.
- Define any limits, such as research study design, publication date, language, age group, gender and geographic location that you want to apply to your search results. For comprehensive searches, it is wise to apply limits with caution, because you may inadvertently exclude relevant papers by doing this prematurely.

For some topics, the PICO (Population, Intervention, Comparison, Outcome) framework is helpful in defining the key concepts of a search question:

- What is the *population* group or species of interest? For example, Maasai in East Africa, or poultry in Southeast Asia.
- What is the *problem*, issue, disease or condition of interest? For example, what are the social or gender inequity elements and environmental factors of the problem? What elements identify the problem as complex?
- What is the main *intervention* of interest? For example, government policy, public health intervention, treatment or diagnostic/screening test, an environmental exposure, etc.?
- What is the main *alternative intervention*? For example, what is the current gold standard treatment or intervention for the problem or condition of interest? Is the solution sustainable? Is the intervention transdisciplinary in nature?
- What is the *outcome* of interest? For example, what is the One Health practitioner/researcher/institution trying to accomplish, measure, improve or influence?

Develop search terms

For each key concept in your search question, identify several search terms. You may need to

Table A1 Examples of turning key concepts into search terms using Boolean search operators

Concepts	Search terms
beef cattle	cattle **OR** bovine
antimicrobial resistance	antimicrobial resistance **OR** antibiotic resistance **OR** AMR
metaphylaxis	metaphylactic **OR** metaphylaxis **OR** prophylactic **OR** prophylaxis

modify these terms after you have done some preliminary searching. Factors to consider include:

- synonyms or similar terms;
- initialisms (e.g., BSE for bovine spongiform encephalopathy);
- spelling variants (anaemia or anemia);
- brand and generic drug names;
- cultural variations in terminology (dairy barn versus cowshed).

Select research databases and search engines

Identify and prioritize the research databases needed to locate the types of literature you need. Select databases that index literature in the academic disciplines that address your topic. See later in this Appendix for a list of core databases that index peer-reviewed journal literature and a core list of government agencies and non-governmental institutions that post freely available grey literature reports on their websites. Research librarians at post-secondary or healthcare institutions and government agencies can provide advice on which research databases are most suitable for your topic and your purposes.

Use effective search strategies

The key concepts from your search question(s) form the building blocks of your search strategy. The specific search strategies you use will vary depending on the nature of your project and the database search software. Research librarians can provide in-depth assistance in crafting the optimal search strategies.

Conduct a preliminary scoping search in one or two core databases. Scan titles and abstracts of search results for additional search terms, and for themes and key authors. Then adjust your search question(s), search terms, search strategy and choice of databases accordingly.

Text-word searching

A text-word search looks for any occurrence of your search terms, usually in the title and abstract of the database record. For complete retrieval, be sure to search for all the sub-concepts that are part of your topic. For example, for the topic of disease prevention, also search for immunization, infection control protocols, disease surveillance and so on. Text-word searches can be done in most research databases, as well as in Google and Google Scholar.

Many databases have an advanced search function with several search boxes for each key concept, where you can type the synonyms for each key concept in a separate search box as shown in Table A2.

Table A2

Concept	disease control* **OR** vaccine* **OR** immuniz* **OR** cull*
	AND
Concept	johne* disease **OR** paratuberculosis
	AND
Concept	cattle

Boolean search

The Boolean search terms AND and OR are used in online research databases to connect search terms and tell the search software how to process your search request. AND narrows your search and OR broadens your search. Synonyms or similar terms within each concept should be connected with OR, and the key concepts that you want present in your final search should be connected with AND.

Truncation

Placing the database truncation symbol at the end of word stems retrieves the variant endings of the word. In most databases this symbol is an asterisk. For example, searching for therap* will retrieve therapy, therapies, therapist and therapeutic.

Parentheses

In databases where there is only one search box, the synonyms for each key concept should be placed in parentheses as follows: (disease control OR vaccine* OR immuniz* OR cull*) AND (johne* disease OR paratuberculosis) AND cattle.

Subject heading searching

Some databases assign subject heading index terms to each database record to describe the content of the article. If you are searching for an abstract concept or a multidisciplinary, multifaceted topic, conducting a subject heading search can greatly increase the relevance and completeness of your search because this way of searching takes advantage of the intellectual analysis of article content done by the indexer. Consult the help section within each database for details on subject heading searches.

Modifying your search results

After reviewing your preliminary search results, you may need to modify your search strategy to make it broader or more focused. Below are strategies that can be used in most research databases and also in Google and Google Scholar.

Strategies to broaden your search to get more results.

- Reframe your question to make it broader and more general.

- User broader, more general subject headings and text-words.
- Remove the least important concept from your search.
- Add synonyms for each search concept. Check relevant records for subject headings or text-words, then use these in your search.
- In text-word searches, use the truncation symbol (usually an asterisk) at the end of word stems to retrieve word variations.
- Apply fewer or no limits to your search results.
- Use both subject heading and title/abstract text-words for the broadest search.
- Search in more than one database.

Strategies to focus your search to obtain fewer results

- Reframe your question to make it more specific.
- Use more specific subject headings and text-words.
- Add another concept to your search.
- Use fewer or no synonyms within a search concept.
- Use fewer or no truncation symbols.
- Apply fewer or no limits to your search results.
- In text-word searches, use less or no truncation symbols.
- Use either subject heading or text-words but not both.
- Search only in the core database(s) for your topic.

Conclusions

Conducting literature searches and accessing research-based information either to support One Health practice or research is challenging due to the multidisciplinary and dispersed nature of the relevant literature, variant conceptual frameworks and terminology, and the skills required for effective literature searching.

Additional challenges are faced by One Health practitioners and researchers in LMICs due to the costs of database and e-journal subscriptions, the lack of access to library and information technology support, and the biases of journal literature and research databases toward health issues of developed countries over developing countries. Continued support of international open access and research capacity building programmes is needed to extend access to bio-medical and health sciences literature to all One Health researchers and practitioners in LMICs. One Health researchers and practitioners in developed countries who collaborate with their peers in developing countries need to be aware of the limitations their LMIC colleagues face, both in knowing how to search the literature and in accessing full-text documents.

Core research databases and search engines

Below are some of the core research databases used to locate peer-reviewed journal literature. Some of these databases also index conference proceedings and meeting abstracts. Databases that require a paid subscription to access are denoted by a dollar symbol. All other databases are freely available on the internet.

Table A3 Core research databases

Database	$	Website	Description/fields
Agricola		http://agricola.nal.usda.gov	Animal science, veterinary medicine, agriculture.
Anthropology Plus	$		Anthropology.
Arctic and Antarctic Regions	$		International literature on polar regions.
CAB Abstracts	$	www.cabi.org/publishing-products/online-information-resources/cab-abstracts	Agriculture, environment, veterinary sciences, applied economics, food science and nutrition.
EconLit	$		Economics literature.
Environment Complete	$		Agriculture, ecosystem ecology, marine science, pollution and waste management, environmental technology and law, public policy, social impact and urban planning.
ERIC (Education Resources Information Center)		http://eric.ed.gov	Education.
GEOBASE	$		Human and physical geography, ecology, geology, oceanography and development studies.
Global Health	$	www.cabi.org/publishing-products/online-information-resources/global-health	International public health including literature from developing countries.
Google Scholar		scholar.google.com	Multi-disciplinary search engine to locate scholarly articles, theses, books from academic publishers, professional societies and universities.

Table A3 continued

Database	$	Website	Description/fields
HINARI Databases		http://extranet.who.int/hinari/en/browse_database.php	Databases developed by the World Health Organization that index literature of developing countries in Africa, Southeast Asia and Latin America.
PAIS: Public Affairs Information Service	$		Public and social policy of business, economics, law, international relations, public administration and government.
PsycINFO	$	www.apa.org/pubs/databases/psycinfo	Psychology.
PubMed		http://pubmed.gov	Medicine, nursing, dentistry, veterinary medicine, molecular biology, health care system, preclinical sciences.
Scopus	$	www.elsevier.com/solutions/scopus/content	International, multi-disciplinary abstract and citation database of peer-reviewed journal literature, conference proceedings, trade publications and quality web sources.
Sociological Abstracts	$		Sociology.
Virtual Health Library (Portuguese, Spanish)		www.bireme.br/php/index.php	Free, internet library of healthcare databases and resources developed by the Latin American and Caribbean Center on Health Sciences Information (also known as BIREME), a specialized centre of the Pan-American Health Organization/World Health Organization.
Web of Science	$	http://wokinfo.com	International, multidisciplinary abstract and citation database of peer-reviewed journal literature and conference proceedings.
Wildlife and Ecology Studies	$		International literature on wildlife, wildlife ecology, habitat and wildlife management.

Open access journals

Directory of Open Access Journals (DOAJ), http://doaj.org, full-text of open access journal articles.

Selected websites to locate grey literature

To locate full-text grey literature, either search using Google www.google.com or browse the publications posted on the websites listed in Table A4.

Table A4 Websites to locate grey literature

Database	Website	Description
Canada Food Inspection Agency	www.inspection.gc.ca	Canadian federal government food safety regulations and publications.
Centre for Evidence-Based Conservation	www.cebc.bangor. ac.uk/index.php. en?menu=0&catid=0	Systematic reviews on effectiveness of management and policy interventions on the natural environment.
Centers for Disease Control and Prevention (USA)	www.cdc.gov	US national public health institute publications, statistics.
Cochrane Collaboration Public Health Group	http://ph.cochrane.org/ finding-public-health-reviews	Systematic reviews of the effects of population-level public health interventions from international teams of researchers.
Environmental Evidence Library of Systematic Reviews	www. environmentalevidence. org/completed-reviews/ page/7	Database of systematic reviews and systematic maps from the UK Centre for Environmental Evidence.
Food and Agriculture Organization of the United Nations	www.fao.org	Publications from UN agency dealing with most aspects of food including livestock production and health, food security and aquaculture.
Health Canada	www.hc-sc.gc.ca/index-eng.php	Publications from Canadian federal government health department.
National Collaborating Centres for Public Health (Canada)	www.nccph.ca/en/home. aspx	Centres publish reports on aboriginal health, determinants of health, public policy, infectious diseases, environmental.
Partners in Information Access for the Public Health Workforce (USA)	http://phpartners.org	Extensive lists of resources including veterinary public health and environmental health.
Health Evidence (McMaster University)	www.healthevidence.org	Quality-rated systematic reviews evaluating the effectiveness of public health interventions.
Health Systems Evidence (McMaster University)	www. mcmasterhealthforum. org/hse	Repository of syntheses of research evidence about health systems governance, financial and delivery arrangements, implementation strategies, economic evaluations, descriptions of health system reforms.
OIE – World Organization for Animal Health	www.oie.int	Publications, statistics from international agency dealing with animal disease, veterinary services, animal welfare and related trade issues.
Public Health Agency of Canada	www.phac-aspc.gc.ca/ index-eng.php	Publications from Canadian government national public health agency.
US Animal & Plant Health Inspection Service (APHIS)	www.aphis.usda.gov/wps/ portal/aphis/home	Publications from US Department of Agriculture Department on biotechnology, animal disease, animal welfare and related trade issues.

Table A4 continued

Database	Website	Description
US Foreign Agricultural Service	www.fas.usda.gov	Publications from US agriculture department tasked with enhancing exports and global food security.
World Health Organization	www.who.int/en	International reports, statistics from United Nations public health agency.

Table A5 Programmes that provide developing countries with access to biomedical and health sciences literature

Programme	Website	Description
AGORA	www.aginternetwork.org/en	Agriculture.
BIREME Virtual Health Library (Pan American Health Organization)	www.bireme.br	Latin American and Caribbean Center on Health Sciences Information.
EVIPNet Evidence Informed Policy Network	global.evipnet.org	Policy network sponsored by the World Health Organization that promotes partnerships at the country level in order to facilitate both policy development and policy implementation through the use of the best scientific evidence.
HINARI	www.who.int/hinari/en	Health.
INASP International Network for the Availability of Scientific Publications	www.inasp.info	International development charity working with a global network of partners to improve access, production and use of research information and knowledge.
OARE	www.unep.org/oare/en	Environment.
Research4Life	www.research4life.org	A public-private partnership of the World Health Organization with major publishers that provides developing countries with access to biomedical, agriculture and environmental sciences e-journals, e-books, reference resources and databases. Journals from developing countries are included. Publicly-funded non-profit institutions in most low and middle income countries are eligible to register.
INASP International Network for the Availability of Scientific Publications	www.inasp.info	International development charity working with a global network of partners to improve access, production and use of research information and knowledge.

Programme	Website	Description
WHO Global Health Library	www.globalhealthlibrary.net/php/index.php	International platform and virtual space for collection, organization, dissemination and access to reliable health sciences information sources developed by the World Health Organization and the Pan American Health Organization.

Search tutorials and resources

Centre for Evidence Based Medicine: Finding the Evidence (Oxford), www.cebm.net/category/ebm-resources/tools/finding-the-evidence

Environmental Health & Toxicology (US Department of Health & Human Services) Tutorials, http://sis.nlm.nih.gov/enviro/guides.html

CADTH Finding the Evidence: Literature Searching Tools in Support of Systematic Reviews, www.cadth.ca/en/resources/finding-evidence-is

Canadian Agency for Drugs and Technologies in Health grey literature resource list, search checklist and search filters

O'Connor, A.M., Anderson, K.M., Goodell, C.K. and Sargeant, J.M. (2014). Conducting systematic reviews of intervention questions I: writing the review protocol, formulating the question and searching the literature. *Zoonoses and Public Health*, 61(S1), 28–38.

Public Health Information and Data Tutorial, http://phpartners.org/tutorial/index.html

PubMed Tutorials, www.nlm.nih.gov/bsd/disted/pubmed.html

Research4Life, www.research4life.org/training

Training for HINARI, AGORA, OARE, reference management software and more

Systematic reviews: CRD's guidance for undertaking systematic reviews in healthcare

University of York Centre for Reviews and Dissemination 2009, www.york.ac.uk/inst/crd/index_guidance.htm

One Health terminology

Below are brief descriptions of the conceptual frameworks and terminology published in One Health papers and in the grey literature. Searchers must take this terminology into account when conducting searches about One Health conceptual frameworks and approaches.

- **One Medicine:** 'There is no difference of paradigm between human and veterinary medicine. Both sciences share a common body of knowledge in anatomy, physiology, pathology, on the origines of diseases in all species' (Schwabe, 1984).
- **One Medicine/One Health:** Puts more emphasis on veterinary and human comparative medicine (Zinsstag et al., 2011; Kahn et al., 2007).
- **One Health:** 'The collaborative efforts of multiple disciplines working locally, nationally, and globally, to attain optimal health for people, animals, and our environment' (AVMA, 2014). Because veterinarians recently have brought this concept back to light, the focus of many examples using a One Health approach is often zoonoses.
- **Ecohealth:** A research approach with Canadian roots that responds to both new and longstanding environmental challenges affecting human, animal, and ecosystem health, impeding development of sustainable solutions. Ecohealth researchers work across disciplines, engage communities and decision makers (transdisciplinary), and seek local and

traditional knowledge to inform health and environmental policies to safeguard human health (Charron, 2012).

- **Ecosystem services and human health:** The products of ecosystems that prevent disease and promote human health. Ecosystem services are: fresh water; food, timber, fibre and fuel; biological products (natural medicines); nutrient and waste management, processing and detoxification; regulation of infectious disease; cultural, spiritual and recreational services; and climate regulation (Millennium Ecosystem Assessment, 2005).
- **Health system services:** The laws, policies, programmes, infrastructure, education and related institutions that deliver healthcare in the broadest sense (human, animal, agricultural, and environmental). This definition creates a space in which to study and understand systems and their related impacts on health (WHO, 2010, 2014).
- **Global health:** Promoted by the Institute of Medicine 2008 and being adopted by Canadian global health researchers 'is an area for study, research, and practice that places a priority on improving health and achieving equity in health for all people worldwide. Global health emphasizes transnational health issues, determinants, and solutions; involves many disciplines within and beyond the health sciences and promotes interdisciplinary collaboration; and is a synthesis of population-based prevention with individual-level clinical care' (Koplan et al., 2009).
- **Transdisciplinary approach or framework:** is when scientists from different disciplines involve both individuals and decision-makers from the affected communities as co-researchers thus creating socially robust solutions (Charron, 2012).

References

Alpi, K.M. (2005). Expert searching in public health. *Journal of the Medical Library Association*, 93, 97–103.

AVMA (2014). *One Health: It's All Connected*, www.avma.org/KB/Resources/Reference/Pages/One-Health.aspx.

Charron, D.F. (2012). *Ecohealth Research in Practice: Innovative Applications of an Ecosystem Approach to Health*. New York: Springer.

Grant, M.J. and Booth, A.A. (2009). A typology of reviews: an analysis of 14 review types and associated methodologies. *Health Information and Libraries Journal*, 26, 91–108.

Kahn, L.H., Kaplan, B. and Steele, J.H. (2007). Confronting zoonoses through closer collaboration between medicine and veterinary medicine (as 'One Medicine'). *Veterinaria Italiana*, 43, 5–19.

Koplan, J.P., Bond, T.C., Merson, M.H., Reddy, K.S., Rodriguez, M.H., Sewankambo, N.K., Wasserheit, J.N. and Consortium of Universities for Global Health Executive Board (2009). Towards a common definition of global health. *Lancet*, 373, 1993–1995.

McMichael, C., Waters, E. and Volmink, J. (2005). Evidence-based public health: what does it offer developing countries? *Journal of Public Health*, 27, 215–221.

Millennium Ecosystem Assessment (2005). *Ecosystems and Human Well-Being: Synthesis*, 2nd edn. Washington, DC: Island Press.

Min, B., Allen-Scott, L.K. and Buntain, B. (2013). Transdisciplinary research for complex One Health issues: a scoping review of key concepts. *Preventive Veterinary Medicine*, 112, 222–229.

New York Academy of Medicine (2014). *Grey Literature Report in Public Health*, www.greylit.org.

Revere, D., Turner, A.M., Madhavan, A., Rambo, N., Bugni, P.F., Kimball, A. and Fuller, S.S. (2007). Understanding the information needs of public health practitioners: a literature review to inform design of an interactive digital knowledge management system. *Journal of Biomedical Informatics*, 40, 410–421.

Schwabe, C.W. (1984). *Veterinary medicine and human health*, 3rd edn. Baltimore: Williams & Wilkins.

Van Essen, C., Mizero, P., Kyamanywa, P. and Cartledge, P. (2014). HINARI grows: one step closer to health information for all. *Tropical Medicine and International Health*, 19, 825–827.

WHO (2010). Key Components of a Well Functioning Health System, www.who.int/healthsystems/publications/hss_key/en.

WHO (2014). Health Services, www.who.int/topics/health_services/en.

Zinsstag, J., Schelling, E., Waltner-Toews, D. and Tanner, M. (2011). From 'One Medicine' to 'One Health' and systemic approaches to health and well-being. *Preventive Veterinary Medicine*, 101, 48–56.

Index